LEARNING DSM-5-TR® BY CASE EXAMPLE

BY

Michael B. First, M.D.
Andrew E. Skodol, M.D.

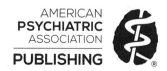

AMERICAN
PSYCHIATRIC
ASSOCIATION
PUBLISHING

If you wish to buy 50 or more copies of the same title, please go to www.appi.org/specialdiscounts for more information.

American Psychiatric Association Publishing
800 Maine Avenue SW, Suite 900
Washington, DC 20024–2812
www.appi.org

Library of Congress Cataloging-in-Publication Data
Names: First, Michael B., 1956– author. | Skodol, Andrew E., author. |
    American Psychiatric Association Publishing, issuing body.
Title: Learning DSM-5-TR by case example / by Michael B. First, Andrew E. Skodol.
Description: Updated first edition. | Washington, D.C. : American Psychiatric
    Association Publishing, [2025] | Includes bibliographical references and index.
Identifiers: LCCN 2024012149 (print) | LCCN 2024012150 (ebook) |
    ISBN 9781615375509 (paperback ; alk. paper) | ISBN 9781615375516 (ebook)
Subjects: MESH: Diagnostic and statistical manual of mental disorders
    (Fifth edition, text revision) | Mental Disorders—diagnosis | Case Reports
Classification: LCC RC473.D54 (print) | LCC RC473.D54 (ebook) | NLM WM 40
    | DDC 616.89/075—dc23/eng/20240814
LC record available at https://lccn.loc.gov/2024012149
LC ebook record available at https://lccn.loc.gov/2024012150

British Library Cataloguing in Publication Data
A CIP record is available from the British Library.

LEARNING DSM-5-TR® BY CASE EXAMPLE

We dedicate this book to our colleagues with whom we have worked with pleasure on its predecessors: the DSM-III, DSM-III-R, DSM-IV, and DSM-IV-TR Casebooks and *Learning DSM-5 by Case Example*.

Robert L. Spitzer, M.D. (1932–2015) led the Biometrics Research Department at the New York State Psychiatric Institute for several important decades. A courageous and brilliant scientist, he is often described as the most influential psychiatrist of the twentieth century. He led the development of the *Diagnostic and Statistical Manual of Mental Disorders*, Third Edition (DSM-III), which for the first time provided diagnostic criteria for all recognized mental disorders and which revolutionized psychiatric assessment and diagnosis. His legacy also includes many important rating scales and instruments, including the *Structured Clinical Interview for DSM* (SCID) and the Patient Health Questionnaire (PHQ). He was the first author of the DSM-III, DSM-III-R, DSM-IV, and DSM-IV-TR Casebooks, all bestsellers in the field of psychiatry and related disciplines.

Janet B.W. Williams, M.S., Ph.D. (1947–) was the stalwart "second-in-command" of the Biometrics Research Department at the New York State Psychiatric Institute for many years. She is the widow of Robert Spitzer and mother of their three children. She is well-known for her work in developing instruments for the assessment of psychopathology in mental health and primary care settings. She was the Text Editor of DSM-III and DSM-III-R, a co-author of the *Structured Clinical Interview for DSM* (SCID), and co-author of *Learning DSM-5 by Case Example*. Her talents in wielding a sharp "editor's pencil" on the DSMs and companion DSM Casebooks have been much appreciated and would make W. Strunk and E.B. White proud.

Miriam (Mimi) Gibbon, M.S.W. (1932–2009) was a treasured colleague and friend. A Research Scientist at the New York State Psychiatric Institute for many years, Mimi was a co-author of the DSM-III, DSM-III-R, DSM-IV, and DSM-IV-TR Casebooks and a co-author of the *Structured Clinical Interview for DSM* (SCID). A superb diagnostician and teacher, she also had a natural talent for coming up with creative and pithy names for cases in the DSM Casebooks.

About the Authors

Michael B. First, M.D., is Professor of Clinical Psychiatry at Columbia University Vagelos College of Physicians and Surgeons, and Research Psychiatrist (retired), Division of Behavioral Health and Policy Research, at New York State Psychiatric Institute in New York, New York.

Andrew E. Skodol, M.D., is Research Professor of Psychiatry at University of Arizona College of Medicine in Tucson, Arizona.

Contents

Introduction

Learning DSM-5-TR by Case Example is designed to help undergraduate, graduate, and postgraduate students in psychology, psychiatry, social work, counseling, and psychiatric nursing learn about DSM-5-TR diagnoses using a case-based approach. It is an updated version of the 2017 book *Learning DSM-5 by Case Example*, co-authored by Michael B. First, Andrew E. Skodol, Janet B.W. Williams, and Robert L. Spitzer. The 2022 publication of DSM-5-TR necessitated that this volume be updated to include information relevant to making DSM-5-TR diagnoses, as well as to incorporate the new information contained in the DSM-5-TR text. The present authors acknowledge that most of the cases first appeared in the previous edition of this book and are grateful to be able to continue to use these cases to teach about psychopathology as the field evolves.

Most experienced clinicians make a DSM-5-TR diagnosis not by systematically applying DSM diagnostic criteria, but instead by matching a patient's symptoms to "prototypes" of the DSM disorders that the clinician has internalized over the years and that are based on their own clinical experience seeing patients with particular diagnoses. We aim in this book to accelerate the process of developing the reader's own internalized prototypes by first describing each DSM-5-TR disorder in prototypical terms and then illustrating how these prototypes present in real-life clinical settings, with the goal of bringing the DSM-5-TR disorders "to life." These real cases have been drawn from our own clinical experience and from the practices of a large number of clinicians who have contributed cases to our DSM-III, DSM-III-R, DSM-IV, and DSM-IV-TR Casebooks over the years (as well as the prior edition of this book, *Learning DSM-5 by Case Example*), among them many well-known experts in particular areas of diagnosis and treatment. The identities of the patients have been disguised by altering such details as age and occupation and, occasionally, locale. We have titled each case to make them easier to remember and reference.

Learning DSM-5-TR by Case Example is organized by chapters corresponding to the 19 disorder classes in the DSM-5-TR Classification. Each chapter begins with a general presentation of the manifestation of the various diagnoses within that diagnostic class. A table succinctly summarizing the characteristic features of each individual disorder in that class is included, with some exceptions noted later in this Introduction. After the introductory content, sections follow for the various diagnoses in the diagnostic class. DSM-5-TR diagnostic criteria for each disorder are cross-referenced to the corresponding DSM-5-TR page on which they begin. Each section begins with a description of the individual disorder; its hallmark features and, when known, its prevalence (i.e., percentage of a population affected with the disorder); sex ratio (i.e., prevalence in men/boys vs. women/girls); age at onset of symptoms; clinical course (e.g., single episode with recovery, recurrent, acute, chronic); associations with suicidal ideation, attempts, or death by suicide; degree of functional impairment; and frequency of other commonly co-occurring disorders. This introduction of each disorder is followed by cases based on disguised real patients, with discussions of each case. Because the presence of multiple co-occurring diagnoses is common, many cases meet criteria for disorders in addition to the one that the case illustrates, and the case discussion includes commentary about these other possible diagnoses.

This book includes at least one case for each mental disorder included in DSM-5-TR, with some exceptions noted below. One of the specific hallmarks of mental disorders is the wide range of presentations of the same disorder that are encountered in real life. Because a major focus of the book is on teaching students to appreciate diagnostic "heterogeneity," we include several different cases for many disorders that vary with respect to symptom presentation, gender, age, clinical course, associated impairment in psychosocial functioning, and developmental factors.

The discussion following each of the cases elaborates on the ways in which the case material fits the prototype presented in the initial disorder description or highlights those features illustrative of the case's diagnostic heterogeneity. For Schizophrenia, for example, because of both its importance as a mental disorder and its considerable symptom diversity, we include five cases (see Section 2.1) that demonstrate heterogeneity in symptom presentation, such as follows: delusions and hallucinations (see "Under Surveillance," p. 49) vs. disordered speech and behavior (see "Eating Wires," p. 51) vs. prominent negative symptoms (see "Low Life Level," p. 52); age at onset, including early onset (see "Star Wars," p. 56) vs. late onset (see "The Witch," p. 53); and developmental life span issues, such as Schizophrenia in an adolescent (see "Star Wars," p. 56).

The heterogeneity in diagnosis in DSM-5-TR can often be noted by the use of so-called diagnostic "specifiers" to further characterize each individual case. For example, Major Depressive Disorder has specifiers for severity (Mild, Moderate, Severe), course (In Partial Remission, In Full Remission), and symptom presentation (e.g., With Melancholic Features, With Atypical Features, With Mood-Congruent vs. Mood-Incongruent Psychotic Features, With Seasonal Pattern, etc.). Therefore, the book includes nine different cases of Major Depressive Disorder (see Section 4.2) in order to illustrate such heterogeneity, including cases of melancholic depression (see "Stonemason," p. 119), atypical depression (see "It's Typical," p. 123), psychotic depression (see "Three Voices," p. 120), postpartum depression (see "New Mom," p. 124), childhood depression (see "A Perfect Checklist," p. 127), seasonal depression (see "Rx Florida," p. 131), and persistent depression (see "A Child Is Crying," p. 125).

This book does not include separate cases for each of the various Mental Disorders Due to Another Medical Condition as they mainly differ from one another by the type of symptom caused by the medical condition. Similarly, the book does not include separate cases for each of the Substance-Related Disorders included in DSM-5-TR as they mainly differ according to the substance class that is involved. Most of the Other Specified disorders are not discussed, and Unspecified disorders are not included, as noted later in this Introduction.

- The DSM-5-TR diagnostic construct "Mental Disorder Due to Another Medical Condition" refers to presentations in which psychiatric symptoms are the direct pathophysiological consequence of another medical condition. DSM-5-TR includes separate diagnoses for the various psychiatric presentations (i.e., psychotic symptoms, catatonia, bipolar symptoms, depressive symptoms, anxiety symptoms, obsessive-compulsive symptoms, delirium, other neurocognitive symptoms, and changes in personality) that may be caused by a nonpsychiatric medical condition. From a learning perspective, each of these presentations are conceptually the same and differ only in regard to the presenting symptoms, so we have included cases for a representative subset of disorders: Catatonic Disorder Due to Another Medical Condition (see "Mute" in Section 2.6), Depressive Disorder Due to Another Medical Condition (see "Toy Designer" in Section 4.5), Anxiety Disorder Due to Another Medical Condition (see "The Outdoorsman" in Section 5.8), Major Neurocognitive Disorder Due to Another Medical Condition (see "The Hiker" and "Certified Public Accountant" in Section 17.2), and Personality Change Due to Another Medical Condition (see "Coma" in Section 18.11).
- Substance-Related Disorders include psychiatric presentations (Substance Use Disorder, Substance Intoxication, Substance Withdrawal, Substance-Induced Mental Disorder) that are related to one (or more) of the DSM-5-TR substance classes (i.e., alcohol; caffeine; cannabis; phencyclidine and other hallucinogens; inhalants; opioids; sedative-, hypnotic-, or anxiolytics; stimulants [cocaine, amphetamine-type, and other stimulants]; tobacco; and other or unknown).

  Reflective of the wide variety of possible psychiatric presentations that can be caused by a variety of types of substance and medications, DSM-5-TR includes at least 88 separately codable substance-related presentations (see Table 1, "Diagnoses associated with substance class," in DSM-5-TR, p. 545). Because each of these presentations are conceptually the same and differ only in regard to the presenting symptoms and the causative substance, we have included cases from only a representative subset of disorders: Methylphenidate-Induced Psychotic Disorder, With Onset During Intoxication (see "Agitated Businessman," Section 2.7) and Alcohol-Induced Psychotic Disorder, With Onset During Withdrawal (see "Threatening Voices" in Section 2.7); Ofloxacin-Induced Bipolar and Related Disorder (see "Sleepless Mother" in Section 3.4); Stimulant-Induced Sleep Disorder (see "Mystery Mastery" Section 12.10); Paroxetine-Induced Sexual Dysfunction (see "Bad Side Effect," Section 13.8); Alcohol Withdrawal Delirium ("Thunderbird," Section 17.1); and Alcohol-Induced Major Neurocognitive Disorder ("Chief Petty Officer," in Section 17.2).
- There are many patients who are diagnostically evaluated for whom no specific DSM-5-TR diagnosis applies because their presentation does not meet the full diagnostic requirements for any of the specific DSM-5-TR disorders. There are two circumstances where this can happen: cases in which the patient's presentation falls below the required diagnostic threshold in terms of severity or duration (e.g., having only three of the required five or more symptoms of Major Depressive Disorder or six symptoms lasting 10 days instead of the required 2 weeks) and cases in which the presentation is not a recognized diagnosis in DSM-5-TR (e.g., olfactory reference disorder, in which the individual is persistently preoccupied with

the belief that they emit a foul or offensive body odor). Such cases would be diagnosed as having one of the various Other Specified Mental Disorders offered in DSM-5-TR, with the clinician having the option to record the reason for not meeting criteria in the name of the diagnosis (e.g., Other Specified Depressive Disorder, depressive episode with insufficient symptoms; Other Specified Obsessive-Compulsive and Related Disorder, olfactory reference disorder). In some circumstances, the clinician is unable to make a specific DSM-5-TR diagnosis because there is insufficient information available to work with, such as in an agitated patient who is hearing voices in the emergency room who is unable to provide a psychiatric history. In such cases, one of the various Other Specified or Unspecified Mental Disorder diagnoses would be given (e.g., Unspecified Schizophrenia Spectrum and Other Psychotic Disorder). Because the aim of this book is to teach the prototypical presentations of the various DSM-5-TR disorders and because by definition the Other Specified and Unspecified presentations do not correspond to any of the prototypical DSM-5-TR presentations, not all Other Specified diagnoses are featured. Therefore, with only a handful of these exceptions, all of the cases in this book meet diagnostic criteria for at least one DSM-5-TR disorder.

This book is designed to teach students about the diagnosis of psychopathology. Thus, case descriptions emphasize information about the manifestations of mental disorders needed to make a diagnosis and may not include information that is nonetheless clinically important, such as childhood history or family history. Also, the cases do not consistently include information about treatment, as the focus of this book is on learning DSM-5-TR diagnoses. However, because many of the specifiers, especially those for the mood disorders, are included in DSM-5-TR to assist with selecting the best treatment, we have included the specifics of treatment in such cases. For example, because the main purpose of the "With Seasonal Pattern" specifier in Major Depressive Disorder is to identify that subgroup of patients most likely to respond to bright light therapy, this treatment is referred to in the case that illustrates seasonal depression (see "Rx Florida" in Section 4.2). In other instances, we have included information about treatment if we felt that it would likely be of particular interest to the reader.

We have mostly selected cases that illustrate single DSM-5-TR disorders because of this book's emphasis on including examples of prototypic presentations of DSM-5-TR disorders. The reader should be aware that in real life clinical settings, comorbidity (i.e., the presence of more than one DSM-5-TR diagnosis at the same time) is actually the rule, rather than the exception. A number of cases in this book do reflect the presence of more than one diagnosis, and in such cases, we do comment on the presence of these additional diagnoses.

The discussions in *Learning DSM-5-TR by Case Example* are framed in terms of how each case either illustrates a diagnostic prototype or demonstrates an aspect(s) of diagnostic heterogeneity, unlike the discussions of cases in our earlier DSM casebooks (for DSM-III, DSM-III-R, DSM-IV, and DSM-IV-TR), which were geared to teaching the application of diagnostic criteria and the process of differential diagnosis. In some instances, however, it is informative to consider alternative diagnoses for a particular case, in order to understand the critical differences among types of psychopathologies that might be easily confused. In these cases, we make an effort to describe the diagnostic alternatives and refer the reader to other cases in this volume that illustrate the alternatives.

Cases in our prior DSM casebooks appeared in no particular order and the diagnosis for each case was revealed only in the discussion section. In contrast, this book is organized according to the order of the diagnostic groupings as they appear in the DSM-5-TR, to facilitate the process of learning about the DSM-5-TR diagnostic classes and categories through the illustrative case examples. We have taken the liberty of altering the DSM-5-TR order in which disorders appear within some of the chapters when a different order seems to make more sense from an educational perspective (e.g., Sexual Dysfunctions are organized according to the phases of the sexual response cycle rather than alphabetically as they are in DSM-5-TR).

In the prior edition of this book (*Learning DSM-5 by Case Example*), we limited the cases to conditions included in DSM-5. For this edition, we have included four new cases in a new Chapter 20, "Cutting-Edge Conditions." These comprise two cases from proposed disorders in DSM-5-TR "Conditions for Further Study": Attenuated Psychosis Syndrome (see "High Risk," Section 20.1) and Internet Gaming Disorder (see "Globally Connected," Section 20.4); and two cases of diagnoses included in the current edition of the World Health Organization's *International Classification of Diseases*, 11th Revision (ICD-11): Olfactory Reference Disorder (see "I Stink," Section 20.2) and Compulsive Sexual Behavior Disorder (see "Don Juan," Section 20.3).

Finally, our book concludes with an alphabetical index of case names to facilitate the reader's retrieval of cases of interest, and a comprehensive alphabetical index of diagnoses and related cases, with the patient's gender, age, and disorder subtype/ specifier information, in addition to a standard textbook index.

Teachers and students of abnormal psychology and psychopathology should find these cases useful as illustrations of various types and presentations of psychopathology. Although this book is designed primarily for students or trainees, it may also be of value to experienced clinicians, facilitating their understanding of the new concepts and terminology in DSM-5-TR. All clinicians, regardless of their level of experience and training, may benefit from reading descriptions of cases that are examples of diagnostic categories rarely seen in their own treatment settings. Similarly, other professionals, such as primary care physicians, internists, and attorneys, may find the cases instructive. Finally, these cases provide an historical point of reference as illustrations of diagnostic concepts in the United States in the early twenty-first century.

Acknowledgments

We would like to thank Paolo Fusar-Poli, M.D.; Bonnie Gorscak, Ph.D.; Jon E. Grant, J.D., M.D., M.P.H.; Meg S. Kaplan, Ph.D.; Richard B. Krueger, M.D.; Katherine A. Phillips, M.D.; and M. Katherine Shear, M.D., who prepared new cases for this book. We would also like to thank those at American Psychiatric Association Publishing who assisted in the production of this book, and most especially Ann M. Eng, for her meticulous editing, which greatly enhanced the clarity of what we've written.

We also gratefully acknowledge the contribution of case material supplied by our colleagues listed below, which originally appeared in the DSM-III, DSM-III-R, DSM-IV, and DSM-IV-TR Casebooks, as well as the prior edition of this book, *Learning DSM-5 by Case Example*.

Gene Abel, M.D.
Henry David Abraham, M.D.
Jacob Abraham, M.D.
Hagop Akiskal, M.D.
Nancy Andreasen, M.D., Ph.D.
Rena Appel, M.D.
Robert L. Arnstein, M.D.
Lorian Baker, Ph.D.
Mark S. Bauer, M.D.
Stephen Bauer, M.D.
Robert Benjamin, M.D.
Fred S. Berlin, M.D., Ph.D.
Angela Bonavoglia, M.S.W.
John M.W. Bradford, M.B.,
    FRCPC, DABPN, FRCPsych
Joan Brennan, Ph.D.
Allan Burstein, M.D.
Justin D. Call, M.D.
Dennis Cantwell, M.D.
Mark Chalem, M.D.
Michelle O. Clark, M.D.
Paula J. Clayton, M.D.
Emil Coccaro, M.D.
David E. Comings, M.D.
Anthony J. Costello, M.D.

George C. Curtis, M.D.
Robert L. Custer, M.D.
Pedro L. Dago, M.D.
Carlo C. DiClemente, Ph.D.
Steven L. Dilts, M.D., Ph.D.
Norman Doidge, M.D.
Steve Dummit, M.D.
Jean Endicott, Ph.D.
Armando R. Favazza, M.D.
Marc D. Feldman, M.D.
Max Fink, M.D.
Leslie M. Forman, M.D.
Allen J. Frances, M.D.
Eve Freidl, M.D.
Andrew J. Freinkel, M.D.
Richard Friedman, M.D.
Abby J. Fyer, M.D.
Paul H. Gebhard, Ph.D.
Miriam Gibbon, M.S.W.
Yonkel Goldstein, Ph.D.
Donald Goodwin, M.D.
Jon E. Grant, J.D., M.D., M.P.H.
Arthur H. Green, M.D.
Richard Green, M.D.
Stanley I. Greenspan, M.D.

Elaine Shapiro, Ph.D.
Lawrence Sharpe, M.D.
Michael Sheehy, M.D.
Meriamne Singer, M.D.
Stephen Sorrell, M.D.
David A. Soskis, M.D.
David Spiegel, M.D.
Laurie Stevens, M.D.
Alan Stone, M.D.
Michael Stone, M.D.
Richard P. Swinson, M.D.
Ludwik S. Szymanski, M.D.
Donn L. Tippett, M.D.
Marcus Tye, Ph.D.
William M. Valverde, M.D.

Susan Vaughan, M.D.
Fred R. Volkmar, M.D.
B. Timothy Walsh, M.D.
Arnold M. Washton, Ph.D.
Betsy P. Weiner, M.D.
Paul A. Wender, M.D.
Katherine Whipple, Ph.D.
Ronald Winchel, M.D.
George Winokur, M.D.
Ken Winters, Ph.D.
Hans-Ulrich Wittchen, Ph.D.
Michael Zaudig, M.D.
Charles H. Zeanah Jr., M.D.
Charlotte Zitrin, M.D.
Kenneth J. Zucker, Ph.D.

Disclosures of Interest

The following authors of this book have indicated a financial interest in or other affiliation with a commercial supporter, a manufacturer of a commercial product, a provider of a commercial service, a nongovernmental organization, and/or a government agency, as listed below:

Michael B. First, M.D., receives publishing royalties from American Psychiatric Association Publishing.

Andrew E. Skodol, M.D., receives royalties from American Psychiatric Association Publishing and UpToDate.

CHAPTER 1

Neurodevelopmental Disorders

Neurodevelopmental Disorders are mental disorders with an onset during the developmental period, usually taken to mean infancy, childhood, and adolescence. Most of these disorders have an onset during childhood, before the person enters school. Most of the disorders involve "deficits" that result in impairment in personal, social, academic, or occupational functioning. Deficits may be relatively circumscribed and involve specific problems in communication or learning, as in Communication Disorders and Specific Learning Disorder, respectively. Other deficits may be more global and involve general problems in social skills or intelligence, as in Autism Spectrum Disorder or Intellectual Developmental Disorder, respectively. Some Neurodevelopmental Disorders involve behavioral "excesses" (i.e., behaviors that are more frequent or intense when compared with normal children of the same age and gender), as well as deficits. Autism Spectrum Disorder involves both deficits in social communication and behavioral excesses, such as repetitive behaviors and insistence on sameness. Prototypical Attention-Deficit/Hyperactivity Disorder involves both deficits in attention and excesses in activity.

Neurodevelopmental Disorders often occur together, such that a child with Autism Spectrum Disorder often has Intellectual Developmental Disorder, and a child with Attention-Deficit/Hyperactivity Disorder often has Specific Learning Disorder. (Table 1–1 lists characteristic features of Neurodevelopmental Disorders.) Neurodevelopmental Disorders may also be accompanied by other mental disorders that are not classified as neurodevelopmental, such as Depressive Disorders (see Chapter 4) or Disruptive, Impulse-Control, and Conduct Disorders (see Chapter 15).

TABLE 1–1.	Characteristic features of Neurodevelopmental Disorders
Disorder	**Key characteristics**
Intellectual Developmental Disorder (Intellectual Disability)	Deficits in intellectual functions
	Deficits in adaptive functioning and failure to meet standards for personal independence and social responsibility
	Onset during the developmental period
Language Disorder	Difficulties in acquisition and use of language
Speech Sound Disorder	Difficulty with speech sound production that interferes with speech intelligibility or prevents verbal communication
Childhood-Onset Fluency Disorder (Stuttering)	Disturbance in normal fluency and time patterning of speech
Social (Pragmatic) Communication Disorder	Difficulties in social use of verbal and nonverbal communication
Autism Spectrum Disorder	Deficits in social communication and social interaction
	Restricted, repetitive patterns of behavior, interests, or activities
Attention-Deficit/ Hyperactivity Disorder	Pattern of inattention and/or hyperactivity-impulsivity
	Some symptoms present prior to age 12 years
	Some symptoms present in two or more settings (e.g., at home, school, or work; with friends or relatives; in other activities)
Specific Learning Disorder	Difficulties learning and using academic skills
Developmental Coordination Disorder	Acquisition and execution of coordinated motor skills substantially below that expected for age
Stereotypic Movement Disorder	Repetitive, driven, and seemingly purposeless motor behavior
Tic Disorders	Sudden, rapid, recurrent, nonrhythmic motor movement or vocalization

INTELLECTUAL DEVELOPMENTAL DISORDERS

1.1

Intellectual Developmental Disorder (Intellectual Disability)

Intellectual Developmental Disorder, also known as Intellectual Disability and formerly known as Mental Retardation, is a disorder characterized by "deficits in general mental abilities, such as reasoning, problem solving, planning, abstract thinking, judgment, academic learning, and learning from experience"

(DSM-5-TR, p. 35). As stated in DSM-5-TR (p. 35), "The deficits result in impairments of adaptive functioning, such that the individual fails to meet standards of personal independence and social responsibility in one or more aspects of daily life, including communication, social participation, academic or occupational functioning, and personal independence at home or in community settings." The diagnosis is made on the basis of clinical assessment and is confirmed by the use of individually administered and psychometrically valid, comprehensive, and culturally appropriate tests of intelligence (i.e., IQ tests). Individuals with Intellectual Developmental Disorder have scores of approximately two standard deviations or more below the population mean, including a margin for measurement error (generally ±5 points). On tests with a standard deviation of 15 and a mean of 100, this would be reflected by a score of between 65 and 75 (70±5 points). Because IQ test scores are approximations of conceptual functioning, they may be insufficient to assess reasoning in real-life situations and mastery of practical tasks. For example, a person with an IQ score above 70 may have such severe problems in social judgment, social understanding, and other areas of adaptive functioning that the person's actual functioning is comparable to that of individuals with a lower IQ score. Thus, clinical judgment is always needed in interpreting the results of IQ tests.

Adaptive functioning involves adaptive reasoning in three domains: conceptual, social, and practical:

- The conceptual (academic) domain involves competence in memory, language, reading, writing, math reasoning, acquiring practical knowledge, problem solving, and judgment in novel situations, among others.
- The social domain involves awareness of others' thoughts, feelings, and experiences; empathy; interpersonal communication skills; friendship abilities; and social judgment, among others.
- The practical domain involves learning and self-management across life settings, including personal care, job responsibilities, money management, recreation, self-management of behavior, and school and work task organization, among others.

Intellectual Developmental Disorder is estimated to affect 10 per 1,000 in the general population. Globally, the prevalence is higher in middle-income countries than in high-income countries. Differences in prevalence may be due to differences in exposures to risk factors, such as perinatal injury or chronic social deprivation, that are associated with lower socioeconomic status and limited access to quality health care. Overall, males are more likely to be affected than females.

Deficits have an onset during the developmental period but may not be present at birth. The age at onset and other characteristic features depend on the underlying etiology. In DSM-5-TR, the diagnosis of Intellectual Developmental Disorder refers to the presence of deficits in intellectual and adaptive functioning—the cause of the intellectual and adaptive deficits, if known, is indicated by giving an additional diagnosis (e.g., Down syndrome). Causes may be genetic, such as in Down syndrome, in which case the child also has characteristic physical features evident from birth. Causes may also include illnesses such as meningitis, encephalitis, or head trauma during the developmental period.

Intellectual Developmental Disorder can be at different levels of severity (i.e., mild, moderate, severe, or profound). Severity is determined by levels of adaptive functioning in the conceptual, social, and practical domains of functioning rather than strictly by IQ, because adaptive functioning determines the amount of support needed. For example, in Severe Intellectual Developmental Disorder, in the conceptual domain, the individual would generally have little understanding of written language or of concepts involving numbers, quantity, time, and money. In the social domain, this individual's speech and communication would be quite limited in vocabulary and grammar, perhaps using single words or phrases, and would be focused on the here and now within everyday events. In the practical domain, the person would require supervision at all times and requires support for all activities of daily living, including meals, dressing, bathing, and elimination. The course of Intellectual Developmental Disorder is usually lifelong, although there may be some fluctuations in severity over time.

Intellectual Developmental Disorder co-occurs with many other mental disorders. Commonly co-occurring neurodevelopmental and other mental disorders include Attention-Deficit/Hyperactivity Disorder, Depressive and Bipolar Disorders, Anxiety Disorders, Autism Spectrum Disorder, Stereotypic Movement Disorder, Impulse-Control Disorders, and Major Neurocognitive Disorder. Individuals with co-occurring mental disorders are at increased risk for suicide. Intellectual Developmental Disorder is also associated with physical disorders, such as cerebral palsy and epilepsy, and with general health problems, such as obesity. Outcomes of co-occurring disorders may be adversely affected by the presence of Intellectual Developmental Disorder.

Global Developmental Delay (DSM-5-TR, p. 46) is a category in DSM-5-TR without diagnostic criteria. It is a diagnosis reserved for individuals under age 5 years who, although failing to meet expected developmental milestones in several areas of intellectual functioning, cannot be diagnosed with Intellectual Developmental Disorder because the clinical severity level cannot be reliably assessed at this young age. This is a "holding" diagnosis indicating the need for reassessment at a later date.

Down Syndrome

Eric, a 15-year-old boy, was brought to the emergency room by his mother who, clutching the on-call psychiatric resident's arm, pleaded, "You've got to admit him; I just can't take it anymore." The patient had been taken home from a special school by his mother 6 months previously. The mother showed the resident papers from the school that indicated that Eric's IQ was 45. He had had several residential placements, beginning at age 8. On visiting days, the boy always pleaded with his mother, "Mommy, take me home?" After a year or so away, Eric would be brought home by his mother, who had always been racked by guilt because of his intellectual impairments and her inability to manage him in the home. The patient was an only child whose parents had been divorced for the past 4 years. The father had moved to another city.

During the last 6 months at home, Eric had increasingly become a behavior problem. He was about 5'9" tall and weighed close to 200 pounds. He had become destructive of property at home—breaking dishes and a chair during angry tantrums—and then, more recently, physically assaultive. He had hit his mother on the arm and shoulder during a recent scuffle that began when she tried to get him to stop banging a broom on the apartment floor. The mother showed her bruises to the resident and threatened to call the mayor's office if the hospital refused to admit her son.

On examination, Eric was observed to have the typical signs of Down syndrome, including thick facial features, slightly protruding tongue, epicanthal fold of the eyelids (skin fold of the upper eyelid), and simian crease (a single line instead of three) on the palms of the hands. With indistinct and somewhat slurred speech, the boy insisted that he "didn't mean to hurt anybody."

Discussion of "Down Syndrome"

The need for placement in special schools since age 8 suggests that Eric has had significant deficits or impairments in adaptive functioning. His IQ of 45 is consistent with deficits in general intellectual functioning. Although detailed information on Eric's conceptual abilities, social functioning, and capacities for self-care are not immediately evident, he needs to be cared for in specialized settings outside the home. Thus, the combination of deficits in intellectual functioning and adaptive functioning, with onset since birth, indicate the diagnosis of Intellectual Developmental Disorder (DSM-5-TR, p. 37) of at least Moderate severity. In Eric's case, Intellectual Developmental Disorder is due to Down syndrome, which would be an additional diagnosis made alongside the diagnosis of Intellectual Developmental Disorder.

The diagnosis of Intellectual Developmental Disorder should be made when the criteria are met, regardless of the presence of another diagnosis. As is often the case for individuals with Intellectual Developmental Disorder, Eric presents for admission because of destructive and aggressive behavior, not because of impairment in intellectual functioning. His aggressive behavior has been present during the past 6 months; nevertheless, the additional diagnosis of Conduct Disorder (see "Shoelaces" in Section 15.3) is probably not justified because Eric has none of the other characteristic features of Conduct Disorder, such as stealing, lying, and running away from home.

The Enigma

A psychiatrist specializing in patients with Intellectual Developmental Disorder received a call from a pediatric colleague referring 17-year-old Libby. Libby was described as "cured from depression" and needing only follow-up medication.

Libby's arrival created a commotion in the waiting room. She was a small, slender person, markedly agitated and restless, who screamed unintelligibly in a high-pitched voice while her anxious parents tried to calm her. She looked far from being "cured."

The parents provided the following history: When Libby was under 1 year old, she was diagnosed with severe mental retardation. Extensive diagnostic evaluations failed to determine the etiology of her intellectual deficits. She has always been physically healthy. Libby is an only child, was reared at home, and attended special classes in public schools. She had been cheerful, friendly, and affectionate. She was nonverbal but managed to communicate through gestures and vocalizations. She learned some household tasks and liked to help her mother around the house.

Libby had never been separated from her parents until 6 months ago, when the parents went to Europe for a week and left Libby with a housekeeper. On their return, they found her agitated, unresponsive to their requests, and uninterested in her usual activities. She cried frequently, slept poorly, ate little, and spent most of the time roaming around the house aimlessly. The parents felt guilty about having gone away and tried to make amends by spending all their time with Libby and trying to do things with her that would make her happy.

Libby's parents wondered if she might be physically ill, but an examination and tests by her pediatrician were negative. The pediatrician gave her an anti-anxiety drug, diazepam, 2 mg three times a day, but it had no effect. The school psychologist thought that Libby's behavior was an attention-getting device, reinforced by her parents' indulgence; he suggested setting firm limits and referred them to a child guidance clinic, where they were informed by the child psychiatrist that Libby was punishing them for abandoning her when they went on their vacation. The child psychiatrist suggested giving Libby unlimited attention and affection.

When this regimen only made matters worse, another psychiatrist was consulted. She thought that Libby might be depressed and prescribed an antidepressant medication. Libby did not improve. In desperation, the parents called every psychiatric hospital in the area, trying to have Libby admitted, but none were willing to take her. As one admitting social worker explained, psychiatric hospitals generally have no experience treating intellectually disabled, nonverbal patients. Libby was finally hospitalized on a pediatric ward, where an extensive medical evaluation failed to disclose the cause of her condition.

Libby's pediatrician decided to treat her in the hospital for a "psychotic depression." He therefore increased the antidepressant medication and added an antipsychotic drug. Libby started to eat better, slept throughout the night, and was somewhat less agitated. She was discharged but soon suffered a relapse. She again became irritable and agitated, slept poorly, and experienced a decrease in appetite.

During the diagnostic interview with the specialist, Libby was extremely agitated. She screamed often, in a high-pitched voice; would not sit in one place; and tugged at her mother's arm, indicating she wanted to go home.

The dosage of the antidepressant medication was gradually decreased and eventually discontinued. For the next 3 months, Libby's mood and behavior varied. For several weeks she was calmer, and then she would again start to scream and become extremely agitated, aggressive, and very distractible.

Detailed family history disclosed that a maternal aunt suffered from "depression" and responded well to maintenance treatment with the mood-stabilizing medication lithium. Therefore, Libby was started on lithium, 300 mg/day, which was increased to 600 mg/day until her serum level was in a therapeutic range, between 0.5 and 0.7 mEq/L. She improved steadily and gradually, and within a few months was her "old self" again. Her improvement continued even after the antipsychotic medication was gradually discontinued over several months.

Discussion of "The Enigma"

This case illustrates the difficulty in diagnosing people with Severe Intellectual Developmental Disorder (DSM-5-TR, p. 37) who are unable to describe their subjective experiences. Libby seems depressed and agitated but cannot tell people about her persistent depressed mood. It seems reasonable to make a provisional diagnosis of Major Depressive Disorder (DSM-5-TR, p. 183) based on her crying, being uninterested, and having decreased appetite, insomnia, and psychomotor agitation, even though she has not consistently responded to antidepressant medication. Libby's pediatrician diagnosed a "psychotic depression," but we see no evidence of psychotic symptoms and assume that the antipsychotic medication was intended primarily to control her psychomotor agitation.

The specialist who treated this patient noted the following, with which we concur:

> Patients like Libby are often dismissed as cases of nonspecific behavior disorders peculiar to intellectually disabled persons, or as exhibitions of "attention-getting behaviors" due to overprotection by parents as compensation for their guilt feelings. In fact, Libby's case was seen by some as an example of the latter mechanism.

Libby's clinical presentation was in marked contrast to her usual condition. It was dominated by irritable mood, agitation, distractibility, and sleep disturbance, all of which are included in the diagnostic criteria for Manic Episode (DSM-5-TR, p. 140). Her screaming could be seen as an equivalent of pressured speech. Symptoms such as grandiosity, flight of ideas, and excessive involvement in pleasurable activity could not, of course, be described by a severely intellectually challenged and nonverbal person. The clinical presentation was cyclic, and the periods of crying, decrease in activities, loss of appetite, and insomnia suggest Major Depressive Disorder. The family history was positive for a lithium-responding "depression." It is possible that Libby was in a Major Depressive Episode when the antidepressant medication was prescribed, and although she improved at first, she then developed manic symptoms apparently triggered by the medication. Therefore, a diagnosis of Bipolar I Disorder (DSM-5-TR, p. 139) seems most appropriate.

COMMUNICATION DISORDERS

1.2
Language Disorder

Language Disorder is characterized by "persistent difficulties in the acquisition and use of language across modalities (i.e., spoken, written, sign language, or other) due to deficits in comprehension or production" (DSM-5-TR, p. 47). The child may exhibit reduced vocabulary, deficits in grammar, limited sentence structure, or impairment in discourse, such as not being able to use words and connect sentences to explain something or to have a conversation. The difficulties place the child at a level substantially below that of their age group and interfere with social and academic functioning. The problems are not due to hearing problems, any motor dysfunctions, other medical or neurological conditions, or Intellectual Developmental Disorder (see Section 1.1). Impairments may be in expressive abilities (i.e., the production of verbal material) or in receptive abilities (i.e., the understanding of language messages) or both.

Due to sex differences in the development of early communication, boys have higher rates than girls of all Communication Disorders. Language Disorder present at age 4 years is likely to be stable over time and persist into adulthood, at which time it can adversely affect the ability of the person to function occupationally. Children with receptive language impairments have a poorer prognosis than those with only expressive problems. Communication Disorders commonly co-occur with other Neurodevelopmental Disorders, other mental disorders (e.g., Anxiety Disorders), and some medical conditions (e.g., seizure disorders).

Broken Home

Don, age 3 years 7 months, has had a complicated early medical history, including having been born 11 weeks premature with hyaline membrane disease (a lung disease in newborn babies that prevents the lungs from proper expansion) and later having bilateral hernia repairs. Early developmental milestones were within normal limits: he began sitting at 6 months, crawling at 10 months, walking at 13 months, and saying words at 12 months. When Don turned 3 years old, his mother noted that his speech seemed far less well developed than that of his playmates, although most of them were younger than he was. He did not attend nursery school and had been subjected to a number of moves because of parental problems and divorce.

During the examination, Don was slow to warm up. He was extremely difficult to understand and had to augment most of his utterances with gestures to make himself understood. Most of his sentences consisted of single words that were mispronounced (e.g., "gun" was "dub," "scissors" was "duh-duh") or demonstrated limited vocabulary (e.g., "fish" was "pet"). Don could follow commands such as "Get the red book and bring it to the table," could point out body parts and objects in the room, and could produce drawings that seemed quite sophisticated for his age.

Discussion of "Broken Home"

Normal developmental milestones rule out Intellectual Developmental Disorder as an explanation for Don's speech difficulties. Significantly, Don's speech difficulties are not in articulating certain speech sounds but rather in finding the proper words to express himself. This rules out Speech Sound Disorder (DSM-5-TR, p. 50) and suggests a Language Disorder (DSM-5-TR, p. 47). The fact that Don apparently has no difficulty understanding language indicates an expressive type of Language Disorder, which has a better prognosis.

Bye-Bye

A 5-year-old boy named Zach was evaluated by a psychologist because of problems in school. He had begun kindergarten 8 months earlier and had had problems getting along with the other children and the teacher from the beginning. The teacher had called numerous parent conferences throughout the school year to report that the boy seemed angry and frustrated, had great trouble handling the natural conflicts that occur among children, seemed at times not to understand her instructions, and was difficult to understand. Very recently, there had been some improvement, however, in that Zach was now playing with the other children, whereas he had started out staying mostly by himself. The parents reported that Zach was taking phenobarbital for a seizure disorder but was otherwise healthy, and that there were no problems at home.

During the examination, Zach was very quiet and shy, and his mother had to remain in the room. He stared at the examiner and seemed to be agreeable but often did not respond to questions or requests. He sometimes produced inappropriate responses, and the examiner was unsure of the boy's grasp of the task. For example, when given a pencil and a toy car and told to "put the pencil on the car," Zach stared at the examiner, put the car on the floor, and began to draw with the pencil. Verbalizations from the boy were very limited: he did tell the examiner his name, but he generally pointed to objects when asked to name them. When asked to define objects (car, pencil, etc.), he only gestured to show their use. When leaving the examination room, Zach said, "me go" and "bye-bye" to the examiner.

Discussion of "Bye-Bye"

Zach has difficulty understanding what people say and making himself understood. Such disturbance in language development can also be seen in Intellectual Developmental Disorder (see Section 1.1), Autism Spectrum Disorder (see Section 1.6), and Specific Learning Disorder (see Section 1.8). The absence of any reference to delayed developmental milestones or deficits in adaptive functioning, such as late walking or inability to dress himself, suggests that Zach has normal intelligence. His ability to grasp the purpose of common objects (e.g., pencils and cars) suggests the presence of inner language and, along with the absence of bizarre behavior, rules out Autism Spectrum Disorder (see "Echo" in Section 1.6). Thus, Zach received the diagnosis of Language Disorder, involving both reception and expression (DSM-5-TR, p. 47). Children with both receptive and expressive language difficulties are more challenging to treat and often do not have as good an outcome as children with only expressive problems.

1.3
Speech Sound Disorder

The characteristic feature of Speech Sound Disorder is "persistent difficulty with speech sound production that interferes with speech intelligibility or prevents verbal communication of messages" (DSM-5-TR, p. 50). The speech production problem is sufficiently severe as to interfere with social activities and academic achievement. The speech difficulties are not caused by any condition that is either 1) congenital (i.e., present at birth), such as a cleft palate or cerebral palsy; or 2) acquired, such as hearing loss or traumatic brain injury.

The DSM-5-TR diagnosis requires that the onset of the speech problem is in the early developmental period. Although normal speech development is a gradual process, most children have intelligible speech by age 3 years and speak most words correctly by age 5. Boys are more likely to have Speech Sound Disorder than girls. Speech problems usually improve with treatment and thus are rarely lifelong. However, when the child also has a Language Disorder, the speech disorder has a poorer prognosis and the child may also have a Specific Learning Disorder (see "Slow Learner" in Section 1.8).

Wabbit

André, a 6-year-old in first grade, came to the clinic with his mother, who reported that her son was humming and making odd noises, was having problems speaking properly, and was reversing letters when writing. André's teacher sent a report stating that André was a "very good" student in reading readiness, phonics, and sports; was average in art; and seemed to have problems only in speech.

On examination, this friendly and handsome boy conversed intelligently on a number of topics. Speech errors noted during conversation included "wab-bit" for *rabbit*, "bwown" for *brown*, "dis" for *this*, and "wewwow" for *yellow*. The Wechsler Preschool and Primary Scale of Intelligence and the Wide Range Achievement Test (WRAT) were administered, and André received the following scores: performance IQ, 135 (significantly above average); verbal IQ, 120 (above average); reading grade level, 1.8; spelling grade level, 1.4; arithmetic grade level, 1.8. The grade-level scores on the WRAT indicated that André was performing academically slightly above grade level. The administrator noted that on the WRAT, when asked to spell "cat," André spelled it "ɔat," with a reversed c.

Discussion of "Wabbit"

André's problem is that he has difficulty articulating various sounds, particularly r, l, and th, which, in addition to s, z, ch, dzh, and zh, are among the later-acquired speech sounds. These most frequently misarticulated sounds are sometimes referred to as the "late eight." André's ability to understand language and to express himself rules out a Language Disorder; his above-average intelligence rules out an Intellectual Developmental Disorder (see "Down Syndrome" in Section 1.1); and his normal social development rules out an Autism Spectrum Disorder (see "Echo" in Section 1.6). Thus, a diagnosis of Speech Sound Disorder (DSM-5-TR, p. 50) is made.

Frequent letter reversals may raise the question of an additional diagnosis of Specific Learning Disorder, With Impairment in Written Expression (see Section 1.8). However, a certain number of letter reversals are normal at age 6, and the Specific Learning Disorder diagnosis is given only if an individually administered test reveals scores significantly below expected levels.

1.4
Childhood-Onset Fluency Disorder (Stuttering)

Persistent "disturbances in the normal fluency and time patterning of speech that are inappropriate for the individual's age and language skills" (DSM-5-TR, p. 51) are the hallmarks of Childhood-Onset Fluency Disorder. The types of disturbances include sound and syllable repetitions, sound prolongations of consonants and vowels, pauses within words, pauses in speech, circumlocutions (i.e., word substitutions to avoid problematic words), word production accompanied by physical tension, and monosyllabic whole-word repetitions (e.g., "I-I-I see him"). The disturbances may be severe enough to cause anxiety that interferes with social or academic functioning and must not be caused by a speech-motor or sensory deficit or a neurological problem, such as a stroke or head trauma. The disorder is commonly referred to as stuttering. Notably, this dysfluency is often absent when the child is reading orally, singing, or talking to pets or inanimate objects.

By definition, the onset of Childhood-Onset Fluency Disorder is in childhood, with the majority of cases developing by age 6 years. The majority of affected children recover. The severity of the problem at age 8 predicts recovery or persistence into adolescence and beyond. Boys and men are more often affected than girls and women. Childhood-Onset Fluency Disorder can occur with other Neurodevelopmental Disorders and with Social Anxiety Disorder.

Don't Worry

A worried psychiatrist and his wife were referred to a speech therapist for a consultation about their 3-year-old son Aaron. The psychiatrist explained that he and his wife had first noticed several months previously that at times Aaron had been "stuttering." When this happened, he would get stuck on words or initial syllables, often repeating them many times until he was finally able to finish the sentence. Sometimes, he was unable to finish the sentence and just gave up. These periods initially were rare but had become much more frequent in the last few weeks, and now Aaron was visibly upset when they occurred. A few days earlier he had become so frustrated that he began striking his head with his fist in an effort to get the words out.

Aaron's parents knew that transient stuttering, particularly among boys, was common. However, they now wondered if something needed to be done to make sure that the problem did not become chronic. They had consulted their pediatrician, who tried to reassure them, but the pediatrician's own slight but noticeable stuttering was disconcerting to them, to say the least.

The speech therapist told the parents that it was important to maintain their own composure during Aaron's episodes of distress and not to complete his sentences for him. She sympathized with their concern but said that most likely the stuttering would go away and would not leave any permanent emotional scars. The speech therapist was correct. Over the next few months, the stuttering gradually resolved, and Aaron, now age 4, is an articulate child without any trace of speech difficulty.

Discussion of "Don't Worry"

Although Aaron's father was a psychiatrist, a layperson would also have had little trouble making this diagnosis. Childhood-Onset Fluency Disorder (Stuttering) (DSM-5-TR, p. 51) is a marked and persistent impairment in the normal fluency and time patterning of speech that is inappropriate for the child's age. In Aaron's case, as in most cases, it was manifested by prolongations and repetitions of sounds and syllables. The severity of the stuttering usually varies from situation to situation and is more severe when there is special pressure to communicate.

1.5
Social (Pragmatic) Communication Disorder

Social (Pragmatic) Communication Disorder, a disorder introduced in DSM-5, is defined as "persistent difficulties in the social use of verbal and nonverbal communication" (DSM-5-TR, p. 54). This category was added to describe individuals who have the social communication component of Autism Spectrum Disorder but who are not considered to be part of the autism spectrum because they do not meet the criterion for restricted, repetitive pattern of behavior, interests, or activities. The word *pragmatic* is added to the diagnostic label to emphasize that social communication is essential for social participation, the development of social relationships, academic achievement, and occupational performance.

The characteristic deficits in using communication for social purposes may be manifested as an inability to share information with others in a manner that is appropriate to the social context; the inability to change style of communication to match the context or the needs of the listener; a difficulty following rules for conversation, such as taking turns in speaking; and difficulty understanding inferences, idioms, humor, and metaphors that depend on context for their meaning. The problems of Social Communication Disorder, like most other Communication Disorders, must interfere with social relationships or academic and occupational functioning. They should not be due to a neurological condition or to other mental disorders that may include problems with social communication as part of the clinical picture, including Intellectual Developmental Disorder (see Section 1.1), Autism Spectrum Disorder (see Section 1.6), or Global Developmental Delay (DSM-5-TR, p. 46).

Children ages 4–5 years should be able to participate in social communication adequately. Milder forms of Social Communication Disorder may not be apparent until early adolescence when social interactions become more complex. The outcome of Social Communication Disorder is quite variable; some children improve substantially over time and others continue to have difficulties persisting into adulthood. Even among those who have significant improvements, the early deficits may cause lasting impairments in social relationships and behavior.

Social Gaffes

Clifford, age 13, is in seventh grade at his local middle school. Although his academic performance has always been on grade level, his teachers and parents describe him as "a little bit immature" and as "a late bloomer." Clifford met all of his motor milestones on time, always showed an interest in his peers, and liked "all the typical little boy stuff—cars, trains, planes, video games, and so on"; however, his mother laments, "Clifford almost always seemed to be running a step behind." Clifford was late to begin talking, and although he had a handful of single words by age 18 months, he did not really begin to string words together until he was approaching his third birthday. He received speech therapy from preschool to third grade, for both his delayed use of language and his difficulties with sibilant "s" or "sh" sounds.

Even as a middle school student, Clifford continues to have some difficulties with verbal communication. He talks loudly, despite frequent reminders to use his "indoor voice," and when in a small group setting, he will talk over the conversations of other kids, sometimes on topics that are largely irrelevant to the group's conversational context. At times he sounds a bit pedantic, especially when talking about his gaming activities, a topic he frequently brings to the fore. When he gets excited about a topic, like his favorite basketball team clinching the division title, he will talk on and on without even seeming to pause for breath and can be quite difficult to follow.

Math is Clifford's favorite subject, and he is fascinated by all computer-related things. He loves video games, especially those of the action and first-person shooter genres. He is a huge basketball fan and follows his favorite professional and college teams religiously. He used to play on his school recreational team but quit last year, complaining, "I spend so much time on the bench, and then the coach and the other kids are always yelling at me, 'Pass the ball!' when it's finally my turn on the court!"

Clifford has had few close friends. Children he spends time with usually share his interest in video games and online activities, and Clifford refers to kids who are merely online contacts as his "friends." He used to spend more time playing outdoors with other children in the neighborhood, but these interactions are now mostly limited to "shooting hoops" in Clifford's driveway, and even these "games" often end in shouting matches and hurt feelings.

Despite his social difficulties, Clifford's mother and teacher both note that Clifford is not a "mean" kid. He wants to have friends and sometimes goes out of his way to try to do nice things for others; unfortunately, his efforts often fall flat. He does not seem to be able to read others' body language or nonverbal cues, and his mother will joke, "*subtle* is not a word in Clifford's vocabulary."

He frequently comes across as insensitive to the feelings of his peers, pointing out their failings, inadequacies, and mistakes, even in public settings, without stopping to think about the impact his words might have. On the one hand, he teases others with comments that he believes to be jokes but that are sometimes hurtful. On the other hand, many of his peers' jokes go over his head, especially puns and double entendres. If an adult calmly points out to him that he has hurt another child's feelings, Clifford typically will, with prompting, apologize and appear to be genuinely sorry, but in the absence of outside intervention, he is not likely to realize when his words or actions have crossed a line, and he repeats the same social gaffes time and time again.

Discussion of "Social Gaffes"

Clifford has a difficult time in social interactions with others. He is unable to communicate with his friends in conversation, often "talking over" them about topics that are not relevant to the context of the conversation. He cannot modulate his conversational tone (he talks loudly despite the teacher's reminders to use his "indoor voice," and he often sounds very formal and pedantic). He will talk on and on without regard to others involved in the conversation and will say things that are hurtful. He is unable to read body language or nonverbal cues in interacting with others, and he is very poor at understanding things like puns or double entendres that depend on context for their interpretation. These severe problems in social communication interfere especially with his peer group interactions and cause impairment in social functioning (he has few close friends and considers some kids he only knows online to be his friends). Clifford's persistent difficulties in the social use of verbal and nonverbal communication all add up to the clinical picture of Social (Pragmatic) Communication Disorder (DSM-5-TR, p. 54).

Social communication deficits are also prominent in Autism Spectrum Disorder (see Section 1.6). However, a person with Autism Spectrum Disorder also has restricted or repetitive patterns of behavior, interests, and activities. One might wonder if Clifford's interest in video games is an example of restricted interests; however, he has demonstrated other interests, such as in toys when he was little and in playing and following basketball as an adolescent. Clifford appears to have had a Speech Sound Disorder (DSM-5-TR, p. 50) during preschool that responded to speech therapy.

Autism Spectrum Disorder

1.6
Autism Spectrum Disorder

Autism Spectrum Disorder was introduced in DSM-5 and is character-ized by 1) "persistent deficits in social communication and social interaction across multiple contexts" and 2) "restricted, repetitive patterns of behavior, interests, or activities" (DSM-5-TR, p. 56). This diagnosis subsumes most cases of DSM-IV Autistic Disorder, Asperger's Disorder, and Pervasive Developmental Disorder Not Other-wise Specified.

The deficits in social communication in Autism Spectrum Disorder are evidenced by 1) deficits in social-emotional reciprocity, such that there is limited back-and-forth conversation or sharing of interests or feelings; 2) deficits in nonverbal communica-tion, such as poor eye contact, lack of facial expression, or understanding or use of gestures; and 3) deficits in developing, maintaining, and understanding relation-ships, such as difficulties adjusting behavior to the social context, poor peer relation-ships, or lack of interest in peers.

Restricted, repetitive patterns of behavior may include stereotyped motor move-ments, use of objects, or speech. For example, a child with Autism Spectrum Disorder may line up toys, flip objects over and over, or "echo" something that someone else has said (echolalia). The child may insist on inflexible adherence to daily routines (e.g., taking the same route to school, eating the same food every day), be pathologi-cally resistant to change (e.g., becoming very distressed at apparently small changes, such as the altered packaging of a favorite food), or have ritualized patterns of behav-ior (e.g., repetitive questioning, pacing of a perimeter). They may have highly re-stricted and fixated interests that tend to be abnormal in intensity or focus (e.g., a toddler strongly attached to a pan, a child preoccupied with vacuum cleaners, an adult spending hours writing out train timetables). Some fascinations and routines may relate to apparent hyperreactivity—or hyporeactivity—to sensory input, which can be manifested through extreme responses to specific sounds or textures, excessive smelling or touching of objects, fascination with lights or spinning objects, and some-times apparent indifference to pain, heat, or cold.

Some individuals with Autism Spectrum Disorder have prodigious capacities or abilities that exceed those of almost all "normal" people; these are called "savant abil-ities" and are usually in one or more of five major areas: art, music, calendar calcula-tion, math, and spatial skills. The most common kind of savant is the "calendrical savant," who can calculate the day of the week for any given date. Although individ-uals with such abilities attract a lot of attention in the media and in literature and movies, only a small minority (fewer than 10%) of individuals with Autism Spectrum Disorder have such abilities.

The signs and symptoms typically become evident in the child's early developmental period (i.e., between ages 12 and 24 months) but may not become fully manifest until social demands exceed the child's capacities. Some children have developmental delays, whereas others may seem to be developing normally and then regress. Social, occupational, or other important areas of functioning are adversely affected. The severity of Autism Spectrum Disorder is based on both the deficits in social communication and the restricted, repetitive behaviors. Severity level is rated based on level of support needed: level 1: "requiring support"; level 2: "requiring substantial support"; or level 3: "requiring very substantial support." Further variability in the diagnosis can be noted with the following specifiers because of the disorder's high frequency of co-occurrence with other disorders and conditions: With or Without Accompanying Intellectual Impairment; With or Without Accompanying Language Impairment; Associated With a Known Genetic or Other Medical Condition or Environmental Factor; Associated With a Neurodevelopmental, Mental, or Behavioral Problem; and With Catatonia.

The prevalence of Autism Spectrum Disorder is estimated at nearly 1% worldwide. Rates have risen in recent years, due to either expanded definitions of the disorder, increased awareness among health care personnel and the public about these conditions, a true increase in the incidence of the disorder, or some combination of factors. In the United States, prevalence of Autism Spectrum Disorder is estimated at between 1% and 2% (children and adults), with lower prevalence among African American and Latinx children compared with White children, even after taking into account differences in socioeconomic resources. Initial diagnosis is often made considerably later in socially oppressed and racialized children than in White children. African American children with Autism Spectrum Disorder are more often misdiagnosed with Adjustment Disorder or Conduct Disorder than are White children.

Autism Spectrum Disorder is diagnosed three to four times more often in boys than in girls and age at diagnosis is usually later in females. Girls are more likely to have co-occurring Intellectual Developmental Disorder (see Section 1.1), and in the absence of Intellectual Developmental Disorder may go unrecognized because they have a milder form of the disorder. The course of the disorder is usually toward improvement over time, although only a minority of individuals live and work independently. Those with superior verbal and intellectual skills may find places to work that match their interests and skills.

Individuals with Autism Spectrum Disorder are at greater risk of death by suicide compared with those without the disorder. Children and adolescents with Autism Spectrum Disorder are also prone to self-harm and increased suicidal thoughts, plans, and attempts.

Autism Spectrum Disorder is frequently associated with other Neurodevelopmental Disorders, such as Intellectual Developmental Disorder, Language Disorder, Specific Learning Disorders, Developmental Coordination Disorder, and Attention-Deficit/Hyperactivity Disorder. Anxiety and Depressive Disorders are common, as is Avoidant/Restrictive Food Intake Disorder.

Echo

Reed, age 3½, a firstborn child, was referred at the request of his parents because of his uneven development and abnormal behavior. His delivery had been difficult, and he had needed oxygen at birth. His physical appearance, motor development, and self-help skills were all age appropriate, but his parents had been uneasy about him from the first few months of life because of his lack of response to social contact and to the usual baby games. Comparison with their second child (who, unlike Reed, enjoyed social communication from early infancy) confirmed their fears.

Reed appeared to be self-absorbed and aloof from others. He did not greet his mother in the morning or his father when he returned from work, and, if left with a babysitter, he tended to scream much of the time. He had no interest in other children and ignored his younger brother. His babbling had no conversational intonation. At age 3 years, he could understand simple practical instructions. His speech consisted of "echoing" some words and phrases he had heard in the past, with the original speaker's accent and intonation; he could use one or two such phrases to indicate his simple needs. For example, if he said, "Do you want a drink?" he meant he was thirsty. He did not communicate by facial expression or use gestures or mime, except for pulling someone along and placing their hand on an object he wanted.

He was fascinated by bright lights and spinning objects, and would stare at them while laughing, flapping his hands, and dancing on tiptoe. He also displayed the same movements while listening to music, which he had liked from infancy. He was intensely attached to a miniature car, which he held in his hand day and night, but he never played imaginatively with this or any other toy. He could assemble jigsaw puzzles rapidly (with one hand because of the car held in the other), whether the picture side was exposed or hidden. From age 2, he had collected kitchen utensils and arranged them in repetitive patterns all over the floors of the house. These pursuits, together with occasional periods of aimless running around, constituted his entire repertoire of spontaneous activities.

The major management problem with Reed was his intense resistance to any attempt to change or extend his interests. If someone removed his toy car, disturbed his puzzles, retrieved a kitchen utensil from his pattern for its legitimate use in cooking, or tried to make him look at a picture book, the action would precipitate a temper tantrum that could last an hour or more, with Reed screaming, kicking, and biting himself or others. These tantrums could be cut short by restoring the status quo. Otherwise, playing his favorite music or taking a long car ride was sometimes effective.

His parents had wondered if Reed might be deaf, but his love of music, his accurate echoing, and his sensitivity to some very soft sounds, such as those made by unwrapping a chocolate in the next room, convinced them that this was not the cause of his abnormal behavior. Psychological testing gave him a mental age of 3 years in non-language-dependent skills (fitting and assembly tasks) but only 18 months in language comprehension.

Discussion of "Echo"

Reed demonstrates marked impairment in reciprocal social interaction and in verbal and nonverbal communication, as well as a markedly restricted repertoire of activities, all beginning early in life. He does not seem interested in other children and never wanted to play "baby games" with his parents. His speech is limited and peculiar (echoing words and phrases of others), and his play is abnormal in that he never engages in imaginative play. His interests are markedly restricted and stereotyped (doing puzzles, though with the uncanny ability to do them with the picture side down, and making patterns with kitchen utensils), and he has stereotyped motor mannerisms (flapping of his hands). These behaviors, beginning in the early developmental period, are the characteristic signs of classic Autism Spectrum Disorder (DSM-5-TR, p. 56).

The Roman

Ronald, a 19-year-old man living in London, was brought by his parents to a social worker who specialized in working with families of developmentally challenged children.

The history revealed that he was the youngest of four children, the older siblings noted to be intelligent and well-adjusted. Unlike the others, he had a difficult birth and had some episodes of cyanosis (bluish discoloration of the skin because of inadequate oxygenation of the blood) in the first 48 hours. He was somewhat delayed in motor and language development, but not enough to cause his parents to ask for advice. He was a quiet, self-contained baby and child, and presented no obvious problems. Ronald was close to his siblings, and he fitted in as the passive member of the group: he never initiated play but did what he was told. In retrospect, his parents remembered that he never seemed to engage in imaginative pretend play, but they did not worry about this at the time. He tended to have poorly coordinated gross motor movements as an infant (e.g., rolling over, sitting up) and was somewhat slower than his siblings in learning to dress himself and perform other motor tasks. He spoke very little and then mostly in response to questioning, but his speech was grammatical, and his vocabulary was adequate. His vocal intonation was always rather odd, with unusually spaced rises and falls in the intonation of his speech; he used few or no gestures when talking and tended to avoid eye contact, but none of these abnormalities elicited enough concern in his parents or teachers to warrant referral for help.

Ronald went to the same schools as his siblings. He had very specific habits and routines with respect to school. He walked the exact same route every day, insisted on sitting in the same seat even in activities or classes where seats were not assigned, and organized his desk and books at home in a precise way that only he could replicate. He coped with schoolwork because of his good rote memory and reading skills, but he was poor at arithmetic and did less well in all subjects in later school years, as understanding of more abstract ideas was demanded. He was naive and immature, which tempted some classmates to tease him, but he was protected from serious bullying by his popular and lively older siblings. He never developed any real friendships with peers outside of his family.

Ronald learned to read before starting school, probably from watching TV commercials. By about age 7 years, he had begun to read books on the ancient Romans and their archaeological remains found in England. He had amassed a prodigious number of facts about the ancient Romans, which he would recite on questioning, but he could not enter into any discussion that required a deeper understanding of the historical context. He spent all his spare time in the pursuit of anything Roman, except when pulled into games with his siblings.

As a teenager Ronald remained a loner, with no interest in girls. He decided that he wanted to be an archaeologist, working on Roman remains. He managed to pass some school examinations at age 16 and stayed on to take the higher exams at age 18. (Students in the United Kingdom take the General Certificate of Secondary Education examinations, usually in about 8–10 subjects that must include English and Mathematics at age 16, and then take Advanced Level examinations, also known as A-level examinations, at age 18.) By this time, all his siblings had left the school, and Ronald missed their protection. He had great difficulty in studying for the higher exams. From being rather silent, he began to talk more and more about Roman remains, regardless of the evident boredom of his unwilling audience. He seemed sure that he was destined to become a world-famous archaeologist. His consuming preoccupation with Roman remains alienated him from many of his peers. His parents became concerned that this goal was unrealistic and worried what would become of him as he grew older.

Discussion of "The Roman"

The long history of oddities in Ronald's social behavior, beginning in early childhood, suggests an Autism Spectrum Disorder. Children with difficulties in communication may have a Language Disorder (see "Broken Home" in Section 1.2), but although Ronald was quiet and spoke little as a child except when answering questions, his speech was grammatical, and his vocabulary was adequate. Children whose difficulties are confined to the social use of communication (either verbal or nonverbal) may have Social (Pragmatic) Communication Disorder (see "Social Gaffes" in Section 1.5).

Certainly, Ronald had significant impairment in his interest in and ability to make friends, and he exhibited some deficits in social communication skills (e.g., he was always the passive member of a group; he never initiated play but did what he was told; his speech intonation was always rather odd; he used few or no gestures when talking and tended to avoid eye contact).

In addition, however, Ronald had an interest in sameness, and he adhered to specific routines surrounding school activities (e.g., walking daily the same route to school, sitting in the same seats, arranging his desk in a certain way). He also had restricted patterns of interests and activities as he grew up, being preoccupied with all things Roman. He "amassed a prodigious number of facts" on this subject, and would talk endlessly about these facts, whether or not he had an interested audience. These ritualized patterns of behavior and restricted interests are not a part of the clinical picture of Social (Pragmatic) Communication Disorder, but instead suggest the diagnosis of Autism Spectrum Disorder (DSM-5-TR, p. 56). Given that the impairments that characterize Autism Spectrum Disorder occur on a continuum ranging from mild to severe, DSM-5-TR recommends that the severity be indicated separately for the social communication domain and for the restricted, repetitive interests domain. In Ronald's case, we would consider his social communication impairment to be at the mildest level (level 1), which DSM-5-TR labels as "requiring support." According to DSM-5-TR (p. 58), individuals at this level of impairment have "difficulty initiating social interactions, and [have] clear examples of atypical or unsuccessful responses to social overtures of others." The severity of restricted interests is also at the mildest level, which according to DSM-5-TR entails "inflexibility of behavior [that] causes significant interference with functioning" (p. 58). In Ronald's case, his consuming interest in Roman remains has greatly contributed to his social isolation.

The British psychiatrist who submitted this case noted that Ronald's disorder has been referred to as Asperger's Syndrome, a higher functioning form of autism characterized by difficulties in social communication and highly restricted and fixated interests, but typically normal language and intelligence. Although Asperger's Syndrome was a separate disorder in DSM-IV (which was in effect from 1994 to 2013), it is now encompassed by the diagnosis of Autism Spectrum Disorder in DSM-5 (introduced in 2013 and continued in DSM-5-TR).

Rocking and Reading

Betsy, age 22 years, was referred for evaluation by the staff of her group home. She had been placed in the group home 3 months earlier, following court-ordered "deinstitutionalization" from a large residential facility for the "mentally retarded." The evaluation was requested because Betsy "didn't fit in" with other clients and had developed some problem behaviors, particularly aggression directed toward herself and, less commonly, toward others. Unlike other clients in the group home, she tended to "stay to herself" and had essentially no peer relations, although she did respond positively to some staff members. Her self-abusive and aggressive behaviors usually were triggered by changes made in her routine. Self-abusive behavior consisted of repeated pounding of her legs and biting of her hand.

Betsy had been placed in residential treatment when she was 4 years old and had remained in some kind of residential setting ever since. Her parents had both died by the time she was 18, and she had no contact with her only sibling. At the time of her transfer to the group home, she was reported to have had several abnormal electroencephalograms, but no seizures or other medical problems had been noted. When last given psychological tests, she achieved a full-scale IQ of 55, with comparable deficits in adaptive behaviors.

During the evaluation, Betsy spent much of her time looking at a children's book she discovered in the waiting room. Her voice was flat and monotonic. She was unable to respond to any questions about the book she was reading and reacted to interruptions of her ongoing activity by pounding her legs with her fist. She rocked back and forth continually during the interview. She made eye contact with the examiner initially but otherwise seemed oblivious of everyone around her. She did not initiate activities, imitate the play of the examiner, or respond to attempts to interest her in alternative activities, such as playing with a doll. From time to time she repeated a single phrase in a monotonic voice, "Blum, blum." Physical examination revealed extensive bruises covering most of her lower extremities.

Betsy was the product of a normal pregnancy, labor, and delivery. She was noted to have been an unusually easy baby. Her parents had first become concerned when she failed to speak by age 2. Motor milestones were also delayed. Her parents initially thought she might be deaf, but this was obviously not the case, because she responded with panic to the sound of a vacuum cleaner. As a young child, Betsy had been noted to "live in her own world," had not formed attachments to her parents, had idiosyncratic responses to some sounds, and always became extremely upset when there were changes in her environment.

By age 4, Betsy was still not speaking, and placement in the state institution was recommended following a diagnosis of "childhood schizophrenia." In the year after her placement, Betsy began speaking. However, she did not typically use speech for communication; instead, she merely repeated phrases over and over. She had an unusual ability to memorize and became fascinated with reading, even though she appeared not to comprehend anything she read. She exhibited a variety of stereotyped repetitive behaviors, including body rocking and head banging, requiring a great deal of attention from the staff.

Discussion of "Rocking and Reading"

Betsy has long-standing problems, including impairment in social interaction (lack of awareness of others and gross impairment in peer relations). Although she has some speech, it is markedly abnormal in its production (monotonic) and in its form and content (she repeats the same phrases over and over). She exhibits repetitive stereotyped behaviors (rocking) and a markedly restricted range of interests. All of these, beginning in early childhood, establish the diagnosis of Autism Spectrum Disorder (DSM-5-TR, p. 56). The presentation in a girl is much less common than in a boy. Because stereotyped movements are part of the definition of Autism Spectrum Disorder—as noted in Criterion B1 (DSM-5-TR, p. 56), "Stereotyped or repetitive motor movements, use of objects, or speech (e.g., simple motor stereotypies, lining up toys or flipping objects, echolalia, idiosyncratic phrases)"—an additional diagnosis of Stereotypic Movement Disorder should be given only when "stereotypies cause self-injury and become a focus of treatment" (DSM-5-TR, p. 67). Given that Betsy's behavior is self-injurious (biting her hand, head banging), she should receive an additional diagnosis of Stereotypic Movement Disorder (DSM-5-TR, p. 89). Of note, DSM-5-TR also includes a symptom code for noting the presence or history of nonsuicidal self-injury to alert clinicians to this problem and to the need to address it in treatment. However, the proposed criteria for Nonsuicidal Self-Injury Disorder (in DSM-5-TR Section III, "Conditions for Further Study") indicate that the behavior should not be "part of a pattern of repetitive stereotypies" (Criterion F) or "better explained by another mental disorder" such as Autism Spectrum Disorder; and thus, the codes for nonsuicidal self-injury should not be used with the diagnosis of Autism Spectrum Disorder.

Although some cases of Autism Spectrum Disorder are associated with normal or, more rarely, high IQ, this case illustrates the frequent coexistence of Intellectual Developmental Disorder (DSM-5-TR, p. 37) and Autism Spectrum Disorder, especially in girls (i.e., "on psychological testing, she had an IQ of 55, with comparable deficits in adaptive functioning"). When this occurs, the diagnosis of Autism Spectrum Disorder can be noted with the specifier With Accompanying Intellectual Impairment to indicate this important limitation in the person's ability to function independently. Moreover, the diagnosis of Intellectual Developmental Disorder should also be given.

At the time of Betsy's placement in the state institution, she received a diagnosis of "childhood schizophrenia." The concept of autism was coined in 1911 by the Swiss psychiatrist Eugen Bleuler to describe a symptom of the most severe cases of schizophrenia. For much of the twentieth century, autism was considered a form of "childhood schizophrenia" as both conditions shared problems with language and social interactions. There is now considerable evidence, however, from family and longitudinal studies that Autism Spectrum Disorder and adult psychosis are not related. Nowadays, the term "childhood schizophrenia" refers to cases of adult schizophrenia with an onset during childhood. Such cases of childhood schizophrenia are very rare, afflicting about 1 in 10,000 children.

ATTENTION-DEFICIT/ HYPERACTIVITY DISORDER

1.7
Attention-Deficit/ Hyperactivity Disorder

Attention-Deficit/Hyperactivity Disorder (ADHD) is defined as "a persistent pattern of inattention and/or hyperactivity-impulsivity that interferes with functioning or development" (DSM-5-TR, p. 68). For the diagnosis to be made, the onset of signs of inattention or hyperactivity-impulsivity should be present before age 12 years; the symptoms should be present for at least 6 months in at least two settings (e.g., at home, school, or work; with friends or relatives; in other activities); and the symptoms should clearly interfere with social, academic, or occupational functioning.

Signs of inattention include not paying attention to details and making careless mistakes, having difficulty sustaining attention in tasks or at play, not listening when spoken to, not following through on instructions and failing to finish tasks, having difficulty organizing tasks and activities, avoiding or disliking tasks that require sustained mental effort, often losing necessary things, being easily distracted, and often forgetting things while engaged in daily activities.

Signs of hyperactivity and impulsivity include fidgeting, leaving one's seat when expected to remain seated, running about or climbing inappropriately, being unable to play or engage in leisure activities quietly, being "on the go" as if "driven by a motor," talking excessively, blurting out answers before questions have been completed, having difficulty waiting one's turn, and interrupting or intruding on others.

Clinical presentation of ADHD varies in terms of the degree to which symptoms of inattention or hyperactivity-impulsivity predominate: the specifier Predominantly Inattentive Presentation can be noted for cases in which there are multiple signs of inattention but few signs of hyperactivity-impulsivity; the specifier Predominantly Hyperactive/Impulsive Presentation can be noted for cases in which there are many signs of hyperactivity or impulsivity but few signs of inattention; and the specifier Combined Presentation can be noted for cases with many signs of both inattention and hyperactivity-impulsivity. The specifier In Partial Remission is used when symptoms have decreased but functional impairment persists. The disorder may also be noted as Mild, Moderate, or Severe, based on both the number of signs that are present and their impact on psychosocial functioning.

Many other mental disorders have signs and symptoms of distractibility, disorganization, and impulsivity and need to be considered before a diagnosis of ADHD is made. These include Schizophrenia (see Chapter 2), which may be characterized by disorganization; Bipolar and Related Disorders and Depressive Disorders (see Chapters 3 and 4, respectively), which may be characterized by psychomotor agitation, restlessness, and impaired impulse control; Anxiety Disorders (see Chapter 5), which may be characterized by agitation; Substance Intoxication or Withdrawal (see Chapter 16), which may be characterized by distractibility and impulsivity; and Personality Disorders (see Chapter 18), such as Antisocial and Borderline Personality Disorders, which may be characterized by impulsivity. ADHD should not be diagnosed if the symptoms are better explained by one of these other conditions.

ADHD is estimated to occur in about 7% of children worldwide and about 3% of adults. The disorder is diagnosed more often in males than in females (2:1 in children, 1.6:1 in adults). Females are more likely than males to present primarily with signs of inattention rather than hyperactivity. ADHD is most often diagnosed during elementary school years, and it tends to persist into early adolescence. In later adolescence, hyperactivity may improve, but problems with inattention and impulsivity often persist. Some individuals with ADHD may develop antisocial behaviors in adolescence or early adulthood (e.g., Conduct Disorder; see Section 15.3) and may go on to have Antisocial Personality Disorder (see Section 18.5). ADHD can seriously affect academic achievement, social relationships, and occupational potential. If associated with antisocial behavior, ADHD may increase the risk of substance use problems and/or incarceration. Traffic accidents and injuries of various types are associated with ADHD. ADHD is a risk factor for suicidal ideation and behavior in children and adults.

Daydreamer

Pavel was 11 years old when first brought for a psychiatric consultation by his parents for problems he has had "since he was born." His parents described him as being socially immature and as always having trouble making friends. His mother said she views Pavel as unhappy, whereas his father described him as being unfocused and lazy. They reported that the then-current school year had been particularly hard. He was being picked on and seemed to always do and say the wrong thing.

Pavel was a "demanding" baby. He never seemed to sleep, and he cried a lot. His developmental milestones were within normal limits. As a toddler, he was "on the quiet side."

Pavel maintained a B average in elementary school, but his grades dropped in seventh grade. His father admits to being very demanding and feels that Pavel constantly wastes time when studying, daydreaming instead of focusing on homework. The father reports that his son's absent-minded behavior was evident when he became a member of the traveling basketball team in sixth grade. Pavel's father, an assistant coach on the team, observed that Pavel "got lost on the court" and was socially less mature than the other players. His mother says that Pavel usually starts the school year on a positive note, but as the work becomes more difficult and complex, he becomes disorganized. At meals Pavel has trouble following the conversation. During the summer he has less trouble, because he is physically coordinated and spends a lot of time in sports activities. However, in day camp he made only one friend, and since starting sleepaway camp at age 8, he has never developed a social network. The camp director reported that Pavel had difficulty following instructions. Pavel's mother, age 40, has a master's degree in audiology. His father, age 41, has a master's degree in business administration from an Ivy League college and is a successful investment banker. The marriage is described as "excellent," and Pavel seems to be the only focus of conflict. His father is disappointed and irritated with Pavel, and his mother is protective and worried. He has two younger brothers, ages 9 and 7, who have no emotional problems.

Pavel had to be coerced by his mother to attend the evaluation. He says he has trouble making friends and he does not do as well in school as he should. His favorite subjects are math and English, even though he does poorly in both. He says that he fights with his parents and his father's criticism can make him cry. He is afraid that coming to see a psychiatrist must mean that he is crazy. He says he has no problem sleeping, his appetite is excellent, and he loves to watch TV for hours, especially sports events. He has no friends and spends his weekends alone. He cannot understand why people do not like him. He admits that in school he has trouble keeping his attention on his work and that his mind wanders while the teacher talks. At camp things are okay when he is playing sports, but he has no close friends. He prefers tennis to team sports because "it's easier to pay attention when you know the ball is always coming to you." He wishes that it would be easier to keep friends, that he and his father would stop fighting, and that he could eventually become a professional basketball player.

School reports consistently state that Pavel has poor organizational skills. He is able to sit for 10–15 minutes but frequently gets drinks of water or makes bathroom trips. He has poor concentration. During one-to-one tutoring, he can accomplish a lot, and Pavel is evaluated as bright by his tutor. No disciplinary problems are reported in school.

Several of Pavel's teachers completed the Conners' Teacher Rating Scale, which assesses hyperactivity, impulsivity, and attention. The teachers indicated that he had a short attention span, was easily distracted, daydreamed often, and consistently failed to finish things he started. The neuropsychological testing data indicated problems with attention and processing speed. Pavel did poorly on a spatial relations test, a timed complex task requiring rapid processing of information. He also did poorly on following oral directions that required attention to both visual and verbal detail. On the Wide Range Assessment of Memory and Learning, he did well on memory tasks that are meaningful but poorly on memory tests of randomly connected information.

Pavel began taking methylphenidate, a stimulant that paradoxically has a calming effect on children with ADHD, 2 months after the evaluation and coinciding with the beginning of the school term. His academic performance during eighth grade improved dramatically. He received all As and Bs, except for a C in social studies. Conners' Teacher Rating Scale scores showed significant improvement on measures of inattention.

Pavel's relationship with his parents improved, and his mother claimed that everyone was getting along better. Pavel reported making two new friends from the basketball program, and his mother reported that classmates have called him to set up playdates. Pavel's blood pressure, pulse, height, and weight were monitored. No adverse side effects to the medication were reported.

Discussion of "Daydreamer"

Pavel's problems seem to fall into two general categories: 1) he has trouble focusing and paying attention, and 2) socially, he is immature and unable to make friends. It is likely that his problems with focusing and paying attention contribute to his social difficulties. In any case, his social problems are not severe enough to consider Autism Spectrum Disorder (see Section 1.6), and there is no evidence of Social Anxiety Disorder (see "No Friends" in Section 5.4).

Pavel's problems with focusing and paying attention have been apparent since he began school. Over the years he has displayed difficulty paying attention to details, sustaining attention to particular tasks, listening to instructions, and finishing what he has begun. In addition, he appears to be easily distracted. These are the symptoms of inattention that are required for the diagnosis of ADHD (DSM-5-TR, p. 68). This disorder usually involves symptoms of hyperactivity and impulsivity (see "Into Everything," below). Because Pavel has few, if any, of these symptoms, the diagnosis would be further specified as Predominantly Inattentive Presentation.

Into Everything

Evan, age 9 years, was referred to a child psychiatrist at the request of his school because of the difficulties he creates in class. Twice during this school year, he has been suspended for a day. His teacher complains that Evan is so restless that his classmates are unable to concentrate. He is hardly ever in his seat, and he roams around the class, talking to other children while they are working. When the teacher is able to get him to stay in his seat, Evan fidgets with his hands and feet and drops things on the floor. He never seems to know what he is going to do next and may suddenly do something quite outrageous. His most recent suspension was for swinging from the fluorescent light fixture over the blackboard. Because he was unable to climb down again, the class was in an uproar.

His mother says that Evan's behavior has been difficult since he was a toddler, and that as a 3-year-old he was unbearably restless and demanding. He has always required little sleep and would awake before anyone else. When he was small, "he got into everything," particularly in the early morning, when he would awaken at 4:30 or 5:00 A.M. and go downstairs by himself. His parents would wake up later to find the living room or kitchen "demolished." When he was 4 years old, Evan managed to unlock the door of the apartment and wander off into a busy main street; fortunately, he was rescued from oncoming traffic by a passerby. He was rejected by a preschool program because of his difficult behavior; eventually, after a very difficult year in kindergarten, he was placed in a special behavioral program for first and second graders. He is now in a regular class for most subjects but spends a lot of time in a resource room with a special teacher. When with his own class, he is unable to participate in games because he cannot wait for his turn.

Psychological testing has shown Evan to be of average ability, and his achievements are only slightly below expected level. His attention span is described by the testing psychologist as "virtually nonexistent." He has no interest in TV and dislikes games or toys that require any concentration or patience on his part. He is not popular with other children. At home, he prefers to be outdoors, playing with his dog or riding his bike. If he does play with toys, his games are messy and destructive, and his mother cannot get him to keep his things in any order.

Evan has been treated with a stimulant that included both amphetamine and dextroamphetamine in small doses (5–10 mg/day). While taking the drug, he was much easier to manage at school in that he was less restless and possibly more attentive.

Discussion of "Into Everything"

Evan's behavior demonstrates the characteristic inattention, impulsivity, and hyperactivity of ADHD (DSM-5-TR, p. 68). He primarily shows symptoms of hyperactivity and impulsivity: he often fidgets, has difficulty remaining seated, runs about or climbs in situations where it is inappropriate, and has difficulty waiting his turn. He also shows some symptoms of inattention: he cannot sustain attention, does not seem to listen to what is being said to him, and strongly dislikes activities that require sustained attention.

The diagnosis of ADHD requires that some of the characteristic symptoms be present in two or more situations, such as at school and at home, to help prevent the diagnosis of ADHD in cases in which the disturbed behavior is apparently situation specific. In Evan's case, it is clear that his disturbed behavior occurs both at home and at school. The diagnosis also requires that the onset of symptoms be before age 12. Evan's symptoms apparently began when he was 3 years old.

Of the three subtypes of ADHD, the appropriate designation for Evan would be Predominantly Hyperactive/Impulsive Presentation because the signs of hyperactivity and impulsivity far outnumber the signs of inattention.

A Wandering Mind

Noreen Hamilton, a 35-year-old clerk and mother of three children, applied for treatment at a mental health clinic with the complaint that "My mind wanders. It's hard for me to keep my attention on one task, and I get distracted so easily." She also described herself as disorganized, restless, irritable, and bad-tempered. She tended to overreact emotionally and was often depressed for days at a time. Her relationship with her longtime lover had begun to unravel. The couple had frequent arguments, exacerbated by Ms. Hamilton's temper. Her lover complained that "problems just never get solved." She also found it difficult to handle her two boys, whom she described as "hyperactive."

The psychiatrist asked the patient's mother to complete a questionnaire in which she was asked to recall Ms. Hamilton's behavior as a child. The results placed Ms. Hamilton in the 95th percentile for childhood "hyperactivity." Although Ms. Hamilton's memories of her own childhood were sketchy, she recalled being a disciplinary problem and often being sent to the principal's office in elementary school. She dropped out of high school. She received no treatment as a child, but at age 20 and again at age 23, she saw a counselor because she had difficulty "coping." Her marriage, which had been very stormy, terminated after the birth of her third child, when Ms. Hamilton was age 25, and she again briefly went to counseling. Finally, 2 years ago she went to the community mental health clinic and was given antidepressant medication, which she took for several months without any noticeable improvement.

The psychiatrist started Ms. Hamilton on atomoxetine, a nonstimulant medication FDA approved for the treatment of ADHD in adults. She experienced a clear-cut and substantial response to this drug, characterized by marked improvement in her concentration, organization, restlessness, temper, handling of stress, affective lability, and "the blues."

Discussion of "A Wandering Mind"

Ms. Hamilton's chief complaints—that her mind wanders, she has trouble keeping her attention on one task, and she is easily distracted—are typical of adults with ADHD. Her problem with attention and focusing is one of the cardinal symptoms of the disorder, and her mother confirms that as a child Ms. Hamilton had hyperactivity, the other characteristic feature.

The long-term problems with mood lability, interpersonal relationships, and difficulty controlling anger suggest a possible diagnosis of Borderline Personality Disorder (see "Disco Di" in Section 18.1). However, she does not have any of the other characteristic features of the disorder, such as identity problems, frantic efforts to avoid abandonment, suicidal behavior, or chronic feelings of emptiness.

When first presenting to the clinic, Ms. Hamilton had the following typical features of attention deficit: difficulty sustaining attention, difficulty organizing tasks, and distractibility. As a child, she probably had other symptoms, such as failing to attend to details and having problems following through on instructions. Because Ms. Hamilton has some symptoms of the disorder but not the full syndrome—a situation that is typical when the disorder persists into adulthood—the diagnosis is ADHD, In Partial Remission (DSM-5-TR, p. 69).

When an adult complains of inattentiveness, distractibility, affective lability, problems controlling temper, and impulsivity, the clinician should be alert to the possibility of the persistence of this childhood disorder. Such patients frequently also have an unusually high energy level, although this was apparently not the case with Ms. Hamilton.

SPECIFIC LEARNING DISORDER

1.8
Specific Learning Disorder

Specific Learning Disorder involves "difficulties learning and using academic skills…despite the provision of interventions that target those difficulties" (DSM-5-TR, p. 76). Difficulties can include slow, inaccurate, or effortful reading of words; trouble understanding the meaning of what is read; problems with spelling words; difficulties with written expression; difficulties mastering numbers and calculation; or problems with mathematical reasoning (e.g., applying mathematical concepts or procedures to solve problems).

- The specifier With Impairment in Reading describes impairment in word reading accuracy, reading rate or fluency, or reading comprehension. *Dyslexia* is a word often used to describe problems with accurate and fluent word recognition, decoding, or spelling; however, additional difficulties, such as problems with reading comprehension, are important to specify separately with use of this term.
- The specifier With Impairment in Written Expression describes problems in spelling accuracy, grammar or punctuation accuracy, or organization of writing.
- The specifier With Impairment in Mathematics describes problems with number sense, memorization of arithmetic facts, accurate or fluent calculation, or accurate mathematical reasoning. *Dyscalculia* is a term that can be used to refer to problems with processing numerical information, learning arithmetic facts, and performing accurate or fluent calculations; however, additional difficulties, such as problems with math reasoning are important to specify separately with use of this term.

Specific Learning Disorder begins during the school-age years. It becomes manifest when academic demands exceed the young person's abilities. Individual testing, as well as clinical observation, are needed to document that the child is performing below expectations for their age, and the difficulties should be severe enough to adversely affect academic or occupational functioning or impact daily life negatively (e.g., the person cannot read signs or instructions on consumer products). Moreover, the learning difficulties are not better explained by the presence of generalized intellectual disabilities, uncorrected visual or auditory acuity, other mental or neurological disorders, psychosocial adversity, lack of proficiency in the language of academic instruction, or inadequate educational instruction.

Worldwide, rates of Specific Learning Disorder in school-age children range from 5% to 15%, making them very common mental disorders. In adults, the prevalence is unknown. Specific Learning Disorder is two to three times more common in males than in females. Impairments in reading, written expression, and mathematics frequently co-occur with each other and with other Neurodevelopmental Disorders (e.g., ADHD, Autism Spectrum Disorder) and other mental disorders (e.g., Anxiety and Depressive Disorders). Specific Learning Disorder may be associated with suicidal thoughts and behaviors in adolescents and adults.

Slow Learner

Janet, age 13 years, has a long history of school problems. She failed first grade—she said because her teacher was "mean"—and was removed from a special classroom after she kept getting into fights with other children. Currently in a normal sixth-grade classroom, she is failing reading; barely passing English, arithmetic, and spelling; but doing satisfactory work in art and gym. Her teacher described Janet as "struggling with learning and memory problems," noting that Janet has difficulties learning in a group setting and requires a great deal of individual attention.

Janet's medical history is unremarkable except for a tonsillectomy at age 5 and an early history of chronic otitis (ear infection). She sat up at 6 months, walked at 12 months, and began talking at 18 months, all within normal limits. Examination revealed an open and friendly girl who was very touchy about her academic problems. She stated that she was "bossed around" at school but had good friends in the neighborhood. On the Wechsler Intelligence Scale for Children, Janet's full-scale IQ score was 97 (average), and her grade-level scores on the Wide Range Achievement Test were 4.8 for reading, 5.3 for spelling, and 6.3 for arithmetic.

Discussion of "Slow Learner"

The differential diagnosis of academic problems includes consideration of poor schooling, Intellectual Developmental Disorder, Attention-Deficit/Hyperactivity Disorder, Oppositional Defiant Disorder, Conduct Disorder, and Specific Learning Disorder. In Janet's case, because her classmates are passing when she is not, it is reasonable to rule out inadequate schooling as an explanation for Janet's academic difficulties. Her average intelligence and reasonable overall functioning rule out a diagnosis of Intellectual Developmental Disorder. Although there is a mention of "fights with other children" and "difficulties learning in a group setting," there is certainly no description of other behaviors that would justify a diagnosis of Attention-Deficit/Hyperactivity Disorder (see "Into Everything" in Section 1.7), Oppositional Defiant Disorder (see "No Brakes" in Section 15.1), or Conduct Disorder (see "Seizure" in Section 15.3).

There is positive evidence suggesting that Janet has a Specific Learning Disorder, With Impairment in Reading (DSM-5-TR, p. 77): she not only seems to have particular difficulty with reading in school, but she also performs significantly below her expected grade level on a reading achievement test. Her reading score of 4.8 is more than 1 year below her expected reading level (and even further below grade level if the clinician considers that Janet should probably be in the seventh or eighth grade). Given her impairment in reading, it is reasonable to regard her fighting and difficulty learning in a group setting as associated features of her Specific Learning Disorder.

Ed Hates School

Ed, age 9½ years, is failing in school, as evidenced by extensive school reports from his teacher and from a school psychologist. The teacher reports that he is failing in arithmetic, spelling, and science, and that he is doing average work in reading, art, history, and gym. She states that he does not work well on his own but that he tries.

The psychologist reports that Ed has been tested frequently over the past several years with the Wechsler Intelligence Scale for Children and has consistently scored in the average to high average range. On the Stanford-Binet Intelligence Scales in third grade, Ed received an intelligence score of 95 (about average), and on the Stanford Achievement Test, he received grade-level scores of 3.0 on reading achievement and 1.0 on math achievement. In fourth grade, Ed was tested with the Wide Range Achievement Test; he received grade-level scores of 4.4 for reading, 3.9 for spelling, and 2.8 for arithmetic. Most recently, 2 months ago, in the fifth grade, the Peabody Individual Achievement Test was administered. He received age-level scores of 10 years 3 months for reading, 8 years 6 months for math, and 9 years 2 months for spelling.

Examination revealed a quiet but personable boy who expressed concern about his schoolwork and "just really hates to go to school."

Discussion of "Ed Hates School"

Why is Ed failing in school? He has a normal intelligence and is motivated, and there is no evidence that schooling is inadequate. The extensive achievement testing consistently reveals that his greatest difficulty is with arithmetic, and it is only in this area that both his school performance and test results indicate a level of achievement significantly below expected levels. These findings suggest a diagnosis of a Specific Learning Disorder, With Impairment in Mathematics (DSM-5-TR, pp. 76–77).

Although the teacher reports that Ed is failing also in spelling and science, a diagnosis of Specific Learning Disorder, With Impairment in Written Expression, is not appropriate because the achievement testing indicates that Ed is not performing significantly below the expected level in spelling.

MOTOR DISORDERS

1.9
Developmental Coordination Disorder

The diagnosis of Developmental Coordination Disorder may apply when the "acquisition and execution of coordinated motor skills is substantially below that expected given the individual's chronological age and opportunity for skill learning and use" (DSM-5-TR, p. 85). Manifestations of these difficulties may include clumsiness, such as dropping things or bumping into objects, or generally slow or inaccurate performance of motor skills. For example, a child may be unable to catch a ball, ride a bike, put together a puzzle or model, use eating utensils, or write. These problems must be severe enough to significantly impact activities of daily living or interfere with academic or occupational functioning. Furthermore, the motor skills deficits are not the result of a visual problem or of a neurological condition that affects motor movement, such as cerebral palsy or muscular dystrophy (both congenital disorders of muscle tone and movement).

The prevalence of Developmental Coordination Disorder is 5%–8% in children ages 5–11 years. Boys are more likely to be affected than girls. The onset of Developmental Coordination Disorder is in early childhood. The course of the coordination problems is relatively stable, with persistence into adolescence in a majority of children. In adults, poor coordination may interfere with the ability to drive a car or use tools and, therefore, the disorder can continue to present challenges for adaptive daily living. Developmental Coordination Disorder frequently occurs with other Neurodevelopmental Disorders, with ADHD being the most commonly associated disorder (about 50% co-occurrence). Co-occurring disorders may contribute to impairment in motor skills and may independently interfere with activities of daily living.

He Breaks His Toys

Juan, age 8 years, was brought to a clinic for evaluation by his mother, who said, "There is something wrong with his brain." When asked to be more specific, she replied with a vague litany of complaints that were frequently self-contradictory.

"He was always slow to learn things, slower than any of my other children. But I know Juan is really very smart. Sometimes he just amazes me with what he remembers or can figure out. He doesn't do much, for example, at school or with activities outside school. Sometimes I think it's because he's lazy, and other times I think he's depressed, and other times I think maybe it's because he is sick a lot. He gets a lot of stomachaches. He's really such a sweet boy. I mean, he's so nice with his three sisters and our pets. But sometimes he's so nasty I get afraid. For example, he gets frustrated with some of his toys and then he gets destructive. He's broken more toys than all of my other three children put together. He seems to like people, but he only has one friend at school. He refuses to try out for soccer or anything like that where he could play with the other boys. Sometimes I think he just doesn't care about anything. He's always dropping dishes and things around the house."

A more detailed history revealed that the pregnancy, birth, and early medical history had been unremarkable, but minor problems had appeared in Juan's first year of life. These included being slow to sit up, crawl, and walk. Because Juan was the fourth child in the family, his mother had not "had time" to record the actual ages when he reached these milestones. She could only pinpoint that "he was much older than any of the other children when he did finally manage to do those things," adding that the pediatrician had nonetheless assured her that Juan was not intellectually disabled. "A good thing he did," she laughed, "because later when Juan had so much trouble learning to use the knife and fork, and to tie his shoelaces, and to button his shirts, I did worry about that."

Asked if there were any remaining concerns along these lines, the mother replied, "none at all." Apparently, Juan excelled in reading and did well in all his other school subjects, except for handwriting and physical education.

His medical history was also unremarkable. During his preschool years, Juan had only "the normal childhood illnesses" (chicken pox, earaches, and flu) and "an awful lot of bruises and scraped knees." The stomachaches had started "sometime around age 7," but again, the pediatrician had assured Juan's mother that they were not cause for concern.

Examination revealed a pleasant but rather quiet boy with appropriate affect, good concentration, and apparently normal cognitive skills. Although quiet and reserved, Juan did not appear apathetic—indeed, he became quite enthusiastic when describing a book he had just read. During the interview, Juan denied any problems in school or with peers. When specifically asked, he did admit to occasional stomachaches and to nonparticipation in group activities, which he attributed to simply "not liking that stuff."

Psychological testing performed in the school setting revealed above-average intelligence and academic performance. However, Juan scored well below the norm on the Bruininks-Oseretsky Test of Motor Proficiency, a test of motor development requiring tasks involving running, balancing, coordination, and motor speed. The psychologist noted, however, that Juan showed good concentration and attention during the testing.

Discussion of "He Breaks His Toys"

Many features of Juan's case are typical of Developmental Coordination Disorder (DSM-5-TR, p. 85). These include late gross motor milestones (standing, sitting, and walking), early history of bruises (from bumping into things and falls), reported "destructiveness" (dropping things or breaking toys when trying to manipulate them), and difficulty with tasks requiring fine motor coordination (buttoning clothes, tying shoelaces, and handwriting) and with sports, such as ball games.

The stomachaches, "laziness," "depression," and "apathy" probably represent Juan's efforts to avoid physical education class, tests in which handwriting is necessary, and the embarrassment of repeated failures in team sport situations. Similarly, Juan's "bad temper" and "frustration" are probably not evidence of disturbance in attention or conduct, but rather a manifestation of his motor difficulties. As often happens, it is these secondary problems that cause the parents to seek professional attention.

Some may wonder why a disorder of physical coordination appears in a classification of mental disorders. It is true that the defining features of the disorder are more "physical" than "behavioral" or "psychological," and therefore it could be argued that the disorder is more properly a physical rather than a mental disorder. However, the disorder seems reasonably classified with the other Neurodevelopmental Disorders of childhood because its behavioral consequences (e.g., irritability and avoidance behavior) are typically treated by mental health professionals.

1.10
Stereotypic Movement Disorder

Stereotypic Movement Disorder is characterized by "repetitive, seemingly driven, and apparently purposeless motor behavior" (DSM-5-TR, p. 89). Typical stereotypic motor movements or behaviors include hand shaking or waving, body rocking, head banging, self-biting, or self-hitting. Such behaviors are clearly maladaptive and interfere with social and academic functioning and may result in self-injury. In cases in which self-injury may be the most serious consequence of this disorder and may constitute a medical emergency, this behavior is noted with the specifier With Self-Injurious Behavior. In other cases, Stereotypic Movement Disorder may be specified as Associated With a Known Genetic or Other Medical Condition, Neurodevelopmental Disorder, or Environmental Factor (e.g., Lesch-Nyhan syndrome [a rare inherited endocrine disorder causing a buildup of uric acid in the body, gout, kidney problems, neurological symptoms, and self-mutilation]; Intellectual Developmental Disorder; fetal alcohol syndrome). When present, these are also noted.

Some simple stereotypic movements, such as rocking back and forth, are common among typically developing young children. Complex stereotypic movements, such as arm waving or flapping or head banging or other potentially self-injurious behaviors, may be seen in about 3%–4%. Among individuals with Intellectual Developmental Disorder living in residential facilities, 10%–15% engage in stereotypy and self-injury. The repetitive behaviors of Stereotypic Movement Disorder ordinarily begin within the first 3 years of life. In most children, these problems will resolve over time or with intervention. Among individuals with Intellectual Developmental Disorder, the behaviors are more persistent. Motor stereotypies are also among the manifestations of Autism Spectrum Disorder (see "Rocking and Reading" in Section 1.6); an additional diagnosis of Stereotypic Movement Disorder is not given in such cases unless the stereotypies cause self-injury and become a focus of treatment.

The Pretzel

Victor, a legally blind 14-year-old boy with Severe Intellectual Developmental Disorder, was evaluated when he transferred to a new residential school for children with multiple disabilities. Observed in his classroom, he was noted to be a small boy who appears younger than his age. He kept his hands in his pockets and spun around in place. Periodically, he approached his teacher, kissed her, positioned himself to receive a return kiss, and clearly enjoyed the contact with her. When offered a toy (which had to be held very close to his eyes), he took it and manipulated it for a while. When Victor was prompted to engage in various tasks that required him to take his hands out of his pockets, he began hitting his head with his hands. If his teacher held his hands, he hit his head with his knees. He was very adept in contorting himself, so he could hit or kick himself in almost any position, even while walking. His face and forehead were covered with black-and-blue marks.

Only a sketchy past history was available. Victor was a premature baby, weighing only 2 pounds at birth. Retinopathy of prematurity (abnormal blood vessels of the retina of the eyes leading to retinal detachment and consequent blindness) and severe mental retardation were diagnosed early in his life. His development was delayed in all spheres, and he never developed language. Comprehensive studies did not disclose the etiology of Victor's developmental disabilities other than prematurity. He lived at home and attended a special education program. His self-injurious behaviors developed early in life, and when his parents tried to stop him, he became aggressive. He gradually became too difficult for them to manage, and at age 3 years he was placed in a special residential school. The self-abusive and self-restraining behavior (i.e., keeping his hands in his pockets) was present throughout his stay there, and virtually all the time he was taking one antipsychotic medication or another. He carried a diagnosis of "cerebral dysfunction." Although the psychiatrist's notes mentioned improvement in Victor's self-injurious behavior, other notes described it as continuing and fluctuating. He was transferred to the new school because of his lack of progress and the difficulties others had in managing him as he became bigger and stronger. His intellectual functioning was within the 34–40 IQ range. His adaptive skills were poor. He required full assistance in self-care, could not provide for his own simplest needs, and required constant supervision for his safety.

In a few months, Victor settled into the routine in his new school. His self-injurious behavior fluctuated. It was reduced or even absent when he restrained himself by holding his hands in his pockets or inside his shirt, or even by manipulating some object with his hands. If left to himself, he could contort himself, while holding his hands inside his shirt, to such a degree that he was nicknamed "Pretzel." Because the stereotypic self-injurious and self-restraining behaviors interfered with his daily activities and education, these became a primary focus of a behavior modification program. For a few months he did well, especially when he developed a good relationship with a new male teacher, who was firm, consistent, and nurturing. With him, Victor could engage in some school tasks. When the teacher left the school, however, Victor regressed. To prevent injuries, the staff started blocking his self-hitting with a pillow. He was offered activities he liked, and he could engage in them without resorting to self-injury. After several months, his antipsychotic medication was slowly discontinued, over a period of 11 months, without any behavioral deterioration.

Discussion of "The Pretzel"

Apparently, Victor suffered brain injury and retinopathy as a result of premature birth. His presentation meets criteria for Severe Intellectual Developmental Disorder (DSM-5-TR, p. 37) because of his significantly low intellectual and adaptive functioning, as well as the onset of the disturbance during the developmental period. For many years he has exhibited repetitive, driven, nonconstructive, inappropriate behaviors, some of which have resulted in damage to his face. Self-restraint, frequently seen in cases involving self-injurious behavior, is present as well. The self-injurious and self-restraining behaviors are the main obstacles to Victor's being able to function even minimally and, therefore, are a major focus of treatment.

Because of Victor's lack of communicative language, it is not possible to ascertain whether the motivation for his behaviors is in response to obsessions, as would be expected in Obsessive-Compulsive Disorder (see "Lady Macbeth" in Section 6.1). However, when self-injurious behavior occurs in Obsessive-Compulsive Disorder (e.g., excessive hand washing), the goal is not the self-injury, as it appears to be in this case. In Victor's case, the lack of language and the presence of self-stimulating behaviors (e.g., body spinning, object manipulation) might at first glance suggest an Autism Spectrum Disorder (see "Echo" in Section 1.6), but unlike individuals with this disorder, Victor has an ability to relate to his caregivers and form basic attachments (within the limits of his Intellectual Developmental Disorder). After ruling out these other disorders, the psychiatrist made the relatively nonspecific diagnosis of Stereotypic Movement Disorder, With Self-Injurious Behavior (DSM-5-TR, p. 89).

Tic Disorders

1.11
Tic Disorders

A *tic* is defined as "a sudden, rapid, recurrent, nonrhythmic motor movement or vocalization" (DSM-5-TR, p. 93). As noted in DSM-5-TR,

> Tics are classically categorized as either simple or complex. *Simple motor tics* are characterized by the limited involvement of specific muscle groups, often are of short duration, and can include eye blinks, facial grimaces, shoulder shrugs, or extension of the extremities. *Simple vocal tics* include throat clearing, sniffs, chirps, barks, or grunting.... *Complex motor tics* are of longer duration and often include a combination of simple tics such as simultaneous head turning and shoulder shrugging. Complex tics can appear purposeful, such as head gestures or torso movements. They can also include imitations of someone else's movements (*echopraxia*) or sexual or taboo gestures (*copropraxia*). Similarly, *complex vocal tics* have linguistic meaning (words or partial words) and can include repeating one's own sounds or words (*palilalia*), repeating the last-heard word or phrase (*echolalia*), or uttering socially unacceptable words, including obscenities, or ethnic, racial, or religious slurs (*coprolalia*). (DSM-5-TR, p. 94)

DSM-5-TR includes three specific Tic Disorders, which differ based on whether both motor and vocal tics are present and whether the tics have persisted for more than 1 year. In Tourette's Disorder, the classic Tic Disorder, both multiple motor and one or more vocal tics have been present but not necessarily at the same time. The tics typically wax and wane but must have persisted for more than 1 year for a diagnosis of Tourette's Disorder to be made. The tics are not caused by substances of abuse (e.g., stimulants) or by other medical conditions (e.g., Huntington's disease—an inherited condition that affects the integrity of nerve cells in the brain). If the individual has had exclusively vocal tics or exclusively motor tics over the course of more than 1 year, the diagnosis is Persistent (Chronic) Motor or Vocal Tic Disorder. The type of tic—motor or vocal—is noted. This diagnosis is not made if the patient has ever had Tourette's Disorder (i.e., the current presence of only motor or vocal tics is not a result of the waxing and waning of tics in a person with a history of both types). The diagnosis of Provisional Tic Disorder is made when single or multiple motor and/or vocal tics have persisted for less than 1 year.

Tics are fairly common in childhood, but most do not persist. In the United States, the prevalence of clinically identified cases is estimated at 3 per 1,000 and is lower among African American and Latinx individuals. The prevalence of Tourette's Disorder in school-age children in Canada is estimated to be 3 to 9 per 1,000, making it a rare disorder. Boys are two to four times more commonly affected with tics than girls. The onset of tics is usually between ages 4 and 6 years. Tics are usually most severe when the child reaches age 10 or 12. Tics commonly improve over the course of adolescence, although tics may persist into adulthood.

Prepubertal children with Tic Disorders are at risk of having comorbid ADHD, Obsessive-Compulsive Disorder, and Separation Anxiety Disorder. Teenagers and adults are more likely to develop Depressive and Anxiety Disorders and Substance Use Disorders. The fact that Tic Disorders are included in DSM-5-TR does not necessarily indicate that Tic Disorders should be considered mental disorders. Although Tic Disorders have been diagnoses in DSM since its first edition (1952), more recently there has been movement toward considering Tic Disorders to be neurological conditions. For example, the National Institute of Neurological Disorders and Stroke and the World Health Organization consider Tic Disorders to be neurological conditions. Nonetheless, for practical reasons, Tic Disorders continue to be included in DSM-5-TR because of their frequent co-occurrence with other neurodevelopmental disorders.

Individuals with Tourette's Disorder or Persistent (Chronic) Motor or Vocal Tic Disorder are at substantially elevated risk of suicide attempts and death by suicide. Persistence of tics beyond young adulthood and prior suicide attempt are the strongest predictors of suicide death.

Embarrassed

Sal Borelli, a 43-year-old married man, was referred to a psychiatrist for evaluation in 1991 because of unremitting tics. At age 13, he had developed a persistent eye blink, soon followed by lip smacking, head shaking, and barking-like noises. Despite these symptoms, he functioned well academically and eventually graduated from high school with honors. He was drafted during the Vietnam War. While he was in the army, his tics subsided significantly but were still troublesome and eventually resulted in a medical discharge. He married, had two children, and worked as a semiskilled laborer and foreman. When he was age 30, his symptoms included tics of the head, neck, and shoulders; hitting his forehead with his hand and with various objects; repeated throat clearing; spitting; and shouting out, "Hey, hey, hey; la, la, la." Six years later, noisy coprolalia (uncontrollable use of obscene language) started: he would emit a string of profanities, such as "Fuck you, you cock-sucking bastard," out of the blue in the middle of a sentence and then resume his conversation.

Over the next 7 years, Mr. Borelli's social life became increasingly constricted because of his symptoms. He was unable to go to church or to the movies because of the cursing and noises. He worked at night to avoid social embarrassment. His family and friends became increasingly intolerant of his symptoms, and his daughters refused to bring friends home. He was depressed because of his enforced isolation and the seeming hopelessness of finding effective treatment. After completing the evaluation, the psychiatrist decided to try pimozide, an antipsychotic medication that is approved for the treatment of tics.

The pimozide had a dramatic effect in that it eliminated 99% of Mr. Borelli's symptoms. He resumed a normal social life and was no longer depressed. When last seen, many years later, he continued to do well on the same maintenance dosage of pimozide.

Discussion of "Embarrassed"

Mr. Borelli has the characteristic features of Tourette's Disorder (DSM-5-TR, p. 93): multiple motor and one or more vocal tics (involuntary cursing or shouting); persisting for more than 1 year; with onset before age 18; and not attributable to the physiological effects of a substance or nonpsychiatric medical condition.

Compulsions

Alan, a 10-year-old boy, is brought for consultation by his mother because of "severe compulsions." The mother reports that the child at various times has to run and clear his throat, touch the doorknob twice before entering through any door, tilt his head from side to side, rapidly blink his eyes, and suddenly touch the ground with his hands by flexing his whole body. These "compulsions" began 2 years ago. The first was the eye blinking, and then the others followed, with a waxing and waning course. The movements occur more frequently when Alan is anxious or under stress. The last symptom to appear was the repetitive touching of doorknobs. The consultation was scheduled after the child began to make the middle finger sign while saying "fuck."

When examined, Alan reported that most of the time he did not know in advance when the movements were going to occur except for the touching of doorknobs. On questioning, he said that before he felt he had to touch a doorknob, he got the thought of doing it and tried to push it out of his head, but he could not because it kept coming back until he touched the doorknob several times; then he felt better. When asked what would happen if someone did not let him touch the doorknob, he said he would just get mad; he reported that he had a temper tantrum once when his father tried to stop him. Alan explained that the touching of the doorknobs did not really bother him—but what did was all the "other stuff" that he could not control.

During the interview the child grunted, cleared his throat, turned his head, and rapidly blinked his eyes several times. At times he tried to make it appear as if he had voluntarily been trying to perform these movements.

Past history and physical and neurological examinations were all normal, except for Alan's abnormal movements and sounds. His mother reported that her youngest uncle had had similar symptoms when he was an adolescent, but she could not elaborate any further. She stated that she and her husband had always been "very compulsive," which she clarified as meaning only that they were quite well organized and stuck to routines.

Discussion of "Compulsions"

Alan's mother describes his difficulties as "compulsions," where Alan's description of what goes on in his mind before he touches doorknobs seems to describe an obsession with an accompanying compulsion. He first gets the intrusive thought of touching the doorknob. He tries to resist the thought but is unable to do so; in response to this obsession, he then touches the doorknob twice. He acknowledges that if he resisted the compulsion to touch doorknobs, he would be extremely uncomfortable. However, because these obsessions and compulsions apparently do not cause marked distress, do not significantly interfere with his functioning, and are not particularly time-consuming, the diagnosis of Obsessive-Compulsive Disorder (see "Lady Macbeth" in Section 6.1) would not be given.

Alan is most disturbed by his motor tics (e.g., tilting his head from side to side, blinking his eyes, flexing his whole body) and verbal tics (e.g., clearing throat, saying "fuck"). Because the motor tics involve a series of coordinated movements, they are considered complex motor tics. The combination of motor and verbal tics with duration of over 1 year establishes the diagnosis of Tourette's Disorder (DSM-5-TR, p. 93).

It is sometimes difficult to distinguish a complex motor tic from a compulsion because the observed behavior can be similar. A tic is an involuntary, sudden, rapid, recurrent, nonrhythmic stereotyped motor movement or vocalization. In contrast, a compulsion is an intentional voluntary act that is either performed in response to an obsession or according to rules that must be applied rigidly. Alan, like many patients with Tourette's Disorder, also has obsessions and compulsions, even if not sufficiently impairing to warrant the additional diagnosis of Obsessive-Compulsive Disorder.

CHAPTER 2

Schizophrenia Spectrum and Other Psychotic Disorders

The Schizophrenia Spectrum and Other Psychotic Disorders diagnostic class in DSM-5-TR includes a number of disorders that differ on the basis of required symptoms and duration. The words *mad, crazy,* or *insane* have often been used by the public and historically to describe people suffering from and exhibiting the various signs of the disorders in this chapter. *Psychosis* is a broadly defined term characterized by thinking, behavior, and emotions that are so impaired that they indicate the person experiencing them has lost contact with reality. In DSM-5-TR, psychotic symptoms involve abnormalities in one or more of the following five domains: hallucinations, delusions, disorganized thinking (speech), grossly disorganized or abnormal motor behavior (including catatonia), and negative symptoms. Each of the disorders in this chapter is defined in terms of symptoms from one or more of these five domains.

- *Hallucinations:* A *hallucination* is a false sensory perception that occurs in the absence of an external stimulus and that has the qualities of a real perception. Hallucinations are distinguished from illusions, which involve distorted or misinterpreted real perceptions (e.g., perceiving a pile of clothes on the floor of a darkened room to be a crouching animal); from dreams, which involve perceptions that occur during sleep; and from imagery (e.g., imagining, daydreaming), which does not mimic real perceptions and is under voluntary control. Hallucinations can occur in any sensory modality: auditory hallucinations involve perceptions of sound (usually voices, but can be noises, music, or other sounds); visual hallucinations involve perceptions of visual stimuli; olfactory hallucinations involve perceptions of smell; gustatory hallucinations involve perceptions of taste; tactile hallucinations involve perceptions of touch, such as being stroked or of bugs crawling on the skin; and somatic hallucinations involve sensations that are perceived as coming from within the body, such as feeling electric shocks.

- *Delusions:* A *delusion* is a fixed false or idiosyncratic belief that is firmly held despite being contradicted by what is generally accepted as reality or by evidence to the contrary. The distinction between a delusion and a strongly held idea or belief that is false and idiosyncratic but not delusional is sometimes difficult to make and depends in part on the degree of conviction with which the belief is held. An individual with a delusion will continue to insist on the veracity of the belief no matter what the contradicting evidence. Religious beliefs can be particularly difficult to differentiate from delusions with a religious theme. Although dictionary definitions of *delusion* typically specify that the person's belief is false, this requirement cannot be applied to religious and other beliefs shared within a particular subculture (e.g., in the supernatural), because there is usually no way to establish whether these kinds of beliefs are true or false. Instead, a shared belief within a religion or subculture is generally not considered to be delusional because the belief is widely shared by members of that group. Only when a person's belief deviates markedly from the tenets of the person's religious or subcultural framework is it considered delusional. For example, when a religious Catholic person believes that they have a guardian angel, this is not considered a delusion because such beliefs are widely shared among many Catholics. Believing, however, that the guardian angel has been controlling the person's actions against their will would be evidence of a delusion, because guardian angels are not considered to have such powers in Catholicism.

- *Disorganized thinking or speech:* Fragmented or disorganized thinking is a feature of many psychotic disorders, particularly Schizophrenia. Disorganized thinking is most evident in the way a person speaks or writes. Individuals with disorganized thinking tend to have trouble maintaining their train of thought. This difficulty is commonly referred to as *loosening of associations*, which is characterized by shifts from one topic to another in ways that are only obliquely related or completely unrelated. The person may respond to a question with an unrelated answer or start sentences with one topic and end somewhere completely different, sometimes referred to as *tangentiality*. When disorganized speech is extreme, the person's speech may become totally incoherent, a phenomenon referred to as *word salad*. Other manifestations of disorganized speech include the use of *neologisms* (made-up words or phrases that have meaning only to the individual), *perseveration* (the persistent repetition of words or ideas even when another person attempts to change the topic), and *clanging* (speech in which ideas are related only by similar or rhyming sounds rather than actual meaning).

- *Grossly disorganized or abnormal motor behavior (including catatonia):* This domain of symptoms involves extremely abnormal behaviors. Disorganized behaviors characteristic of psychotic disorders are not goal directed and may include childlike silliness, bizarre dressing (wearing multiple overcoats on a hot day), and unpredictable and untriggered aggressiveness and agitation. Catatonic behaviors occur in the context of a markedly decreased awareness of the environment and may be exhibited as a dramatic reduction in activity to the point that all voluntary movement stops, or as a dramatic increase in activity that is disconnected from what is going on in the person's surroundings. See Section 2.6 ("Catatonia Associated With

Another Mental Disorder/Catatonic Disorder Due to Another Medical Condition") in this chapter for a more detailed description of the varied behaviors that are considered catatonic.

- *Negative symptoms:* These symptoms are deficits in normal mental functioning that typically account for a substantial portion of the functional impairment associated with Schizophrenia but are less prominent in the other psychotic disorders in this diagnostic class. Among the most important negative symptoms are diminished emotional expression (sometimes referred to as *flattened affect*) and avolition. Individuals with diminished emotional expression appear to lack emotions; they may not make eye contact, may not change facial expressions, may speak without inflection or in a monotone, or may not add hand or head movements that normally provide emotional emphasis in speech. *Avolition* is characterized by a lack of motivation to initiate and perform self-directed, purposeful activities. Individuals with avolition may stay at home for long periods of time rather than seeking out work or peer relations. Other negative symptoms include diminished ability to experience pleasure (known as *anhedonia*) and greatly diminished speech output (known as *alogia*).

The disorders covered in this chapter include Schizophrenia (a persistent psychotic disorder with a mixture of different types of psychotic symptoms that persist for at least 6 months, accompanied by a decline in functioning); Schizophreniform Disorder (a briefer psychotic disorder lasting for at least 1 month but less than 6 months, which often progresses to Schizophrenia); Schizoaffective Disorder (a persistent psychotic disorder with a mixture of psychotic and mood symptoms), Delusional Disorder (persistent delusions for at least 1 month without other psychotic symptoms), Brief Psychotic Disorder (psychotic symptoms that resolve within 1 month), Catatonia (a syndrome of catatonic symptoms), Substance/Medication-Induced Psychotic Disorder (delusions or hallucinations due to substance or medication use), and Other Specified Schizophrenia Spectrum and Other Psychotic Disorder (psychotic presentations that do not meet criteria for one of the specific Schizophrenia Spectrum and Other Psychotic Disorders); see Table 2–1 for characteristic features. DSM-5-TR also includes Psychotic Disorder Due to Another Medical Condition (hallucinations or delusions due to the direct effects of a nonpsychiatric medical condition on the central nervous system) in this diagnostic class as well, but this book does not include a case for this specific condition. (Refer to Section 4.5 for a case of Depressive Disorder Due to Another Medical Condition or Section 5.8 for a case of Anxiety Disorder Due to Another Medical Condition for illustrations of how nonpsychiatric medical conditions can cause psychiatric presentations.) DSM-5-TR also lists Schizotypal Personality Disorder among the Schizophrenia Spectrum and Other Psychotic Disorders, because of evidence that there is a genetic relationship between the two disorders (i.e., relatives of people with Schizophrenia are at increased risk of having Schizotypal Personality Disorder and vice versa) and because some of the symptoms and abnormal patterns in brain chemistry, brain structure, and brain functioning found in people with Schizophrenia can also be found in people with Schizotypal Personality Disorder. However, because Schizotypal Personality Disorder is also conceptualized as a personality disorder in DSM-5-TR, its criteria set and full discussion are included in

TABLE 2–1.   **Characteristic features of Schizophrenia Spectrum and Other Psychotic Disorders**

Disorder	Key characteristics
Schizophrenia	Active-phase symptoms (delusions, hallucinations, disorganized speech, grossly disorganized or catatonic behavior, negative symptoms) lasting at least 1 month
	Duration of symptoms: 6 or more months
	Level of functioning in one or more major life areas is markedly below the level achieved prior to onset
Schizophreniform Disorder	Active-phase symptoms (delusions, hallucinations, disorganized speech, grossly disorganized or catatonic behavior, negative symptoms) lasting at least 1 month
	Symptoms last for less than 6 months
Schizoaffective Disorder	Periods in which Major Depressive or Manic Episodes overlap with active-phase symptoms of Schizophrenia
	Periods in which there are delusions or hallucinations for at least 2 weeks in the absence of Major Depressive or Manic Episodes
Delusional Disorder	Persistent delusions without other psychotic symptoms lasting at least 1 month
Brief Psychotic Disorder	Delusions, hallucinations, or disorganized speech lasting less than 1 month
Catatonia	Psychomotor disturbance characterized by a wide range of symptoms that may involve decreased motor activity, decreased engagement during the interview or physical examination, or excessive and peculiar motor activity
Substance/ Medication-Induced Psychotic Disorder	Delusions or hallucinations due to the direct effects of a substance or medication on the central nervous system
Other Specified Schizophrenia Spectrum and Other Psychotic Disorder	Symptoms characteristic of a Schizophrenia Spectrum and Other Psychotic Disorder that cause clinically significant distress or impairment in functioning that do not meet the full criteria for any of the disorders in the Schizophrenia Spectrum and Other Psychotic Disorders diagnostic class

the DSM-5-TR Personality Disorders chapter; as is done likewise in this book's chapter on Personality Disorders (see Section 18.8).

Several DSM-5-TR disorders that sometimes include psychotic symptoms as part of their presentation are not included in this chapter. These include Mood Disorders with psychotic features (see Chapter 3, "Bipolar and Related Disorders," for psychotic forms of Bipolar I Disorder, and Chapter 4, "Depressive Disorders," for psychotic forms of Major Depressive Disorder); disorders with distorted beliefs, such as Body Dysmorphic Disorder or Obsessive-Compulsive Disorder, in which the person's insight is so impaired that they become completely convinced that the distorted beliefs are true (see Chapter 6, "Obsessive-Compulsive and Related Disorders"); and Neurocognitive Disorders such as Delirium and Major Neurocognitive Disorder, which may involve delusions or hallucinations as associated features (see Chapter 17, "Neurocognitive Disorders").

2.1
Schizophrenia

Schizophrenia is the most severe and debilitating of the Schizophrenia Spectrum and Other Psychotic Disorders included in DSM-5-TR. It is characterized by a range of cognitive, behavioral, and emotional dysfunctions that include impairments in perception, inferential thinking, fluency and productivity of thought and speech, behavioral monitoring, cognition, and the ability to express emotions and be motivated. To meet criteria for a diagnosis of Schizophrenia, the symptoms must persist for at least 6 months, at least 1 month of which is characterized by particularly severe and impairing symptoms known as *active-phase symptoms*. Moreover, the symptoms must be severe enough to have had a significantly negative impact on the person's psychosocial functioning with respect to maintenance and quality of employment, interpersonal relations, or academic achievement. No single symptom by itself is indicative of Schizophrenia (i.e., is pathognomonic); the diagnosis involves the recognition of a constellation of signs and symptoms associated with impaired psychosocial functioning.

The characteristic active-phase symptoms may be thought of as falling into two broad categories: 1) *positive symptoms,* which reflect an excess or distortion of normal mental functions; and 2) *negative symptoms*, which reflect a diminution or loss of normal mental function. DSM-5-TR divides the positive symptoms into four types: delusions (which can be understood as distortions or exaggerations of inferential thinking), hallucinations (distortions in perception), disorganized speech (distortions in language, communication, and thought processes), and grossly disorganized or catatonic behavior (distortions in behavioral monitoring). Negative symptoms in Schizophrenia include avolition (deficits in the initiation of goal-directed behavior) and diminished emotional expression (restrictions in the range and intensity of emotions). At least two different types of symptoms must be present for a significant amount of time during the same 1-month period, and at least one of the symptom types must be a delusion, hallucination, or disorganized speech. If all of the symptoms are of the same type (persecutory delusions and grandiose delusions), the criteria for Schizophrenia are not met. Moreover, if the symptoms are confined to the disorganized/catatonic behavior and negative symptom types (i.e., none of the symptoms are from the delusions type, hallucinations type, and disorganized speech type), the criteria for Schizophrenia are also not met. There is tremendous heterogeneity in the diagnosis—patients with Schizophrenia can have widely different presentations with the only common feature being the persistence of the symptoms and their negative impact on psychosocial functioning.

Many individuals with Schizophrenia go through an early phase (known as the *prodromal phase*), which is a forerunner to the first active phase of the illness (sometimes referred to as the *first psychotic break*), and most individuals with Schizophrenia go through *residual phases* in between active phases. These prodromal and residual phases consist of milder versions of the positive symptoms as well as negative symptoms. For example, some individuals during prodromal or residual phases may have unusual perceptual experiences, such as sensing the presence of an unseen force. Others may express a variety of odd or unusual beliefs that are not so firmly held by the person so as to be considered delusions (e.g., having a strong feeling that other people are conspiring to harm them).

Although some mood symptoms such as depression, irritability, and expansive mood may occur at times in patients with Schizophrenia, such symptoms are present for a minority of time during the whole disturbance. Otherwise, the diagnosis would be Schizoaffective Disorder (see Section 2.3).

Drugs and medical conditions can cause hallucinations and delusions: a diagnosis of Schizophrenia should not be made if the psychotic symptoms are a manifestation of drug use or if they are due to a nonpsychiatric medical condition such as a brain tumor or hyperthyroidism. Given that individuals with Schizophrenia Spectrum and Other Psychotic Disorders often abuse drugs (especially cannabis), it is important to determine whether psychotic symptoms are the result of drug use (i.e., a Substance/Medication-Induced Psychotic Disorder) and thus not indicative of a diagnosis of Schizophrenia (see Section 2.7 for a discussion of how to make this determination).

Similarly, if the psychotic symptoms are a manifestation of an underlying nonpsychiatric medical condition, the diagnosis is Psychotic Disorder Due to Another Medical Condition rather than Schizophrenia. Clues that the psychotic symptoms may be due to a nonpsychiatric medical condition include a close temporal relationship between the onset (and offset) of the psychotic symptoms and the course of the nonpsychiatric medical condition and atypical features such as an unusually late age at onset.

Even though cognitive impairment is not among the defining symptoms of Schizophrenia, it is common in Schizophrenia and is strongly linked to academic (school) and occupational (work) impairment. Individuals with Schizophrenia tend to have problems with attention and memory, especially with regard to planning and organization to achieve a goal. They also often lack insight into the fact that they have a mental illness (known as *anosognosia*). Issues with cognitive impairment, attention, memory, and lack of insight can make the treatment of Schizophrenia quite challenging because these features can lead to nonadherence with a medication regimen, the mainstay of treatment.

Schizophrenia affects between 0.3% and 0.7% of the population and occurs slightly less often in women than in men. Prodromal symptoms of Schizophrenia commonly occur in the teenage years, but the psychotic features of Schizophrenia typically emerge between the late teens and early 30s and tend to be earlier for men (peak onset in early 20s) than women (peak onset in late 20s). Although onset before adolescence is rare, cases do occur in young children. Approximately 5%–6% of individuals with Schizophrenia die by suicide, about 20% attempt suicide on one or more occasions, and many more have significant suicidal ideation. Rates of co-occurrence of Schizophrenia with Substance-Related Disorders are high, and over half of individuals with Schizophrenia have a Tobacco Use Disorder and smoke regularly.

Under Surveillance

Arthur Stanton is a 44-year-old single, unemployed man brought into the emergency room by the police for striking an elderly neighbor in his apartment building. He stated, "That damn bitch—she and the rest of them deserved more than that for what they put me through."

He has been continuously ill since age 22. During his first year of law school, he gradually became more and more convinced that his classmates were making fun of him. He noticed that they would snort and sneeze whenever he entered the classroom. When a girl he was dating broke off her relationship with him, he believed that she had been "replaced" by a look-alike. He called the police and asked for their help to solve the "kidnapping." His academic performance in school declined dramatically, and he was asked to take a leave of absence and seek psychiatric care.

Mr. Stanton got a job as a fulfillment center warehouse associate, which he held for 7 months. While working in that position, he had been getting an increasing number of distracting "signals" from coworkers, and he became more and more suspicious and withdrawn. It was during this time that he first reported hearing voices. He was eventually fired and soon thereafter was hospitalized for the first time, at age 24. He has not worked since.

Mr. Stanton has been hospitalized 12 times, the longest stay being 8 months. However, in the last 5 years he has been hospitalized only once, for 3 weeks. During the hospitalizations, he has received various antipsychotic medications. Medication has been prescribed for him as an outpatient, but he usually stops taking it shortly after leaving the hospital. Aside from twice-yearly lunch meetings with his uncle and his contacts with mental health workers, he is totally isolated socially. He lives on his own, cooking and cleaning for himself, and manages his own financial affairs, including a modest inheritance. He reads the *Wall Street Journal* daily.

Mr. Stanton maintains that his apartment is the center of a large communication system that involves all of the major TV networks, his neighbors, and apparently hundreds of "actors" in his neighborhood. There are secret cameras in his apartment that carefully monitor all of his activities. When he is watching TV, many of his minor actions (e.g., going to the bathroom) are soon directly commented on by the announcer. Whenever he goes outside, the "actors" have all been warned to keep him under surveillance. Everyone on the street watches him. His neighbors operate two different "machines"; one is responsible for all of his voices except the "joker." He is not certain who controls this voice, which "visits" him only occasionally and is very funny. The other voices, which he hears many times each day, are generated by this machine, which he sometimes thinks is directly run by the neighbor whom he attacked. For example, when he is going over his investments, these "harassing" voices constantly tell him which stocks to buy. The other machine, which he calls "the dream machine," puts erotic dreams into his head, usually of "Black women."

Mr. Stanton describes other unusual experiences. For example, he recently went to a shoe store 30 miles from his house in the hope of getting some shoes that would not be "altered." However, he soon found out that like the rest of the shoes he buys, special nails had been put into the bottom of the shoes to annoy him. He was amazed that his decision concerning which shoe store to go to must have been known to his "harassers" before he himself knew it, so that they had time to get the altered shoes made up especially for him. He realizes that great effort and "millions of dollars" are involved in keeping him under surveillance. He sometimes thinks this is all part of a large experiment to discover the secret of his "superior intelligence."

At the interview, Mr. Stanton is well-groomed, and his speech is coherent and goal directed. His affect is only mildly blunted. He was initially very angry at being brought in by the police. After several weeks of treatment with an antipsychotic medication failed to control his psychotic symptoms, he was transferred to a long-stay facility with the plan to arrange a structured living situation for him.

Discussion of "Under Surveillance"

Mr. Stanton's long illness, characterized by multiple hospitalizations for Schizophrenia, apparently began with delusions of reference (the belief that unrelated occurrences in the external world have a special significance or meaning), which in Mr. Stanton's case was his conviction that his classmates were making fun of him by snorting and sneezing when he entered the classroom. Over the years, his delusions have become increasingly complex and bizarre (his neighbors are actually actors; his thoughts are monitored; a machine puts erotic dreams in his head). In addition, he has prominent hallucinations of different voices that harass him. Given that all of the required elements of Schizophrenia are present (i.e., delusions and hallucinations lasting for over 20 years; severe impairment in Mr. Stanton's ability to work or develop interpersonal relationships with others; and absence of a sustained mood disturbance, a nonpsychiatric medical condition, or substance use that can account for the disturbance), the diagnosis of Schizophrenia is made (DSM-5-TR, p. 113).

As noted in the beginning of the case, Mr. Stanton's Schizophrenia resulted in violence. As a consequence of Mr. Stanton's delusion that his elderly neighbor was operating the machine that caused him to hear voices, he assaulted her to get her to turn off the machine. If the neighbor had decided to press charges against Mr. Stanton, it is likely that he would end up being judged to have diminished capacity to make rational decisions or to exert control over his behavior as a result of his delusions and, depending on the legal standard in the state in which he was tried, may not have been held criminally responsible for his behavior. Although individuals with Schizophrenia are significantly more likely to be violent than other members of the general population, the proportion of societal violence attributable to Schizophrenia is actually quite small (less than 5%).

Eating Wires

Emilio Rodriguez is a 40-year-old man who looks 10 years younger. He is brought to the hospital by his mother because she is afraid of him; it is his 12th hospitalization. He is dressed in a ragged overcoat, bedroom slippers, and a baseball cap and wears several medals around his neck. His affect ranges from anger at his mother ("She feeds me shit…what comes out of other people's rectums") to a giggling, obsequious seductiveness toward the interviewer. His speech and manner have a childlike quality, and he walks with a mincing step and exaggerated hip movements. His mother reports that he stopped taking his medication about a month ago and has since begun to hear voices and to look and act more bizarrely. When asked what he has been doing, he says, "eating wires and lighting fires." His spontaneous speech is often incoherent and marked by frequent rhyming and clang associations.

Mr. Rodriguez's first hospitalization occurred after he dropped out of school at age 16, and since that time he has never been able to attend school or hold a job. He has been treated with various antipsychotic medications during his hospitalizations, but he does not continue to take medication when he leaves, so he quickly becomes disorganized again. He lives with his elderly mother; however, he sometimes disappears for several months at a time and is eventually picked up by the police as he wanders in the streets. There is no known history of drug or alcohol abuse.

Discussion of "Eating Wires"

Mr. Rodriguez is suffering from the same severe illness as Mr. Stanton in the previous case (see "Under Surveillance"), in that both men have various persisting psychotic symptoms leading to poor functioning, but Mr. Rodriguez's Schizophrenia presentation (DSM-5-TR, p. 113) is quite different. It is dominated by disorganized behavior, as evidenced by his being dressed in a ragged overcoat, bedroom slippers, and a baseball cap; incoherent speech characterized by frequent clang associations ("eating wires and fighting fires"); and, most recently, auditory hallucinations (hearing voices). As is unfortunately all too common in Schizophrenia, Mr. Rodriguez's multiple hospitalizations are related to his repeatedly discontinuing his antipsychotic medications. It is not clear whether his lack of medication adherence is due to his lack of insight that he has a mental illness and needs to take medication to stay well, his not liking the side effects of the medication, or his chronic disorganization interfering with his ability to be adherent.

Low Life Level

Louise Larkin is a pale, stooped woman of 39 years whose childlike face is surrounded by scraggly blond braids tied with pink ribbons. She was referred for a psychiatric evaluation for possible hospitalization by her family doctor, who was concerned about her low level of functioning. Her only complaint to him was, "I have a decline in self-care and a low life level." Her mother reports that there has indeed been a decline but that it has been over many years. In the last few months, Ms. Larkin has remained in her room, mute and still.

Twelve years ago, Ms. Larkin was a supervisor in the occupational therapy department of a large hospital, living in her own apartment, and was engaged to a young man. He broke the engagement, and she became increasingly disorganized, wandering aimlessly in the street and wearing mismatched clothing. She was fired from her job, and eventually the police were called to hospitalize her. They broke into her apartment, which was in shambles—filled with papers, food, and broken objects. No information is available from this hospitalization, which lasted 3 months and from which she was discharged to her mother's house with a prescription for an unknown medication that she never took to a pharmacy to have filled.

After her discharge, Ms. Larkin's family hoped that she would gather herself together and embark again on a real life, but as the years progressed, she became more withdrawn and less functional. Most of her time was spent watching TV and cooking. Her cooking consisted of mixing bizarre combinations of ingredients, such as broccoli and cake mix, and eating them alone, because no one else in the family would eat her meals. She collected cookbooks and recipes, cluttering her room with stacks of these. Often when her mother entered her room, Ms. Larkin would quickly grab a magazine and pretend to be reading, when in fact she had apparently just been sitting and staring into space. She stopped bathing and brushing her hair or teeth. She ate less and less, although she denied loss of appetite, and over a period of several years lost 20 pounds. She would sleep at odd hours. Eventually she became enuretic, wetting her bed frequently and filling the room with the pungent odor of urine.

On admission to the psychiatric hospital, Ms. Larkin sat with her hands tightly clasped in her lap and avoided looking at the doctor who interviewed her. She answered questions readily and did not appear suspicious or guarded, but her affect was shallow. She denied depressed mood, delusions, or hallucinations. However, her answers became increasingly idiosyncratic and irrelevant as the interview progressed. In response to a question about her strange cooking habits, she replied that she did not wish to discuss recent events in Canada. When discussing her decline in functioning, she said, "There's more of a takeoff mechanism when you're younger." Asked about ideas of reference, she said, "I doubt it's true, but if one knows the writers involved, it could be an element that would be directed in a comical way." Her answers were interspersed with the mantra, "I'm safe. I'm safe."

Ms. Larkin was treated with olanzapine (an antipsychotic medication) in the hospital and was also given clomipramine, an antidepressant medication that is thought to be effective in treating Obsessive-Compulsive Disorder (a disorder that some of the staff thought might account for her strange cooking and eating behaviors). Ms. Larkin improved significantly over a 3-month hospitalization and then returned to her mother's home, enrolled in a day program, and continued in outpatient treatment with her hospital psychiatrist. Her psychiatrist discontinued the clomipramine, believing that Ms. Larkin's "obsessive-compulsive behavior" was actually a symptom of Schizophrenia, but kept her on the olanzapine. Ms. Larkin worked in a cooking group and became so proficient that there were plans to get her a work-study job in a bakery. However, after a few months, she stopped taking her medication because she thought she did not need it anymore and she began to be preoccupied with irrelevant details in the cooking group. Her speech became tangential, and eventually she dropped out of the program and stayed at home ruminating and eating very little. Her personal hygiene deteriorated and, when she lost 30 pounds, she was rehospitalized.

She was treated with a different antipsychotic medication, lurasidone, and was discharged after 6 weeks. Two years after her first admission, she attends a less demanding day program, takes good care of her physical appearance, and demonstrates only very slight tangentiality in her speech.

Discussion of "Low Life Level"

Ms. Larkin's disease course closely follows what the clinician would expect to see in Schizophrenia (DSM-5-TR, p. 113): onset of symptoms in Ms. Larkin's late 20s and an extreme decline in functioning over a period of several years. In contrast to the previous two cases, Ms. Larkin's case is dominated by periods of severe negative symptoms, which are characterized by her inability to take care of herself with respect to eating and basic hygiene and her lack of motivation to do anything other than watch TV and cook. In addition, she has incoherent speech and bizarre disorganized behavior. Unlike the first two cases, there is no evidence that Ms. Larkin has ever experienced either delusions or hallucinations of any kind.

The Witch

Virginia Dubois, a 48-year-old woman, was admitted to the hospital. Her husband reported that she had apparently been well until about 2 months ago when she became anxious, suspicious, and convinced that people in the neighborhood were spying on her and talking about her. She became withdrawn, refused to go outside her home, and on several occasions was observed talking to herself. She neglected her household duties and spent her days wandering through the house, entering one room after the other, opening and closing cupboards and closets, or looking out windows from behind closed curtains.

On admission to the hospital, the patient declared that she could no longer stay at home because "something frightening is going on." She described how, for the previous 2 months, she had been hearing voices without being able to determine where they came from or to whom they belonged. The voices bothered her all the time, except at night when she was asleep. Most of the time she slept well, but whenever she woke up during the night, the voices were there and prevented her from falling asleep again. At times, two or three voices would talk among themselves, telling each other nasty things about her, saying she was a witch who had to be "destroyed." Then again, one or several voices would talk to her directly, telling her obscene things, interrupted by shouts of "Witch, Witch," or insisting that she disappear or else something terrible would happen. At other times, the voices would simply echo her thoughts or keep up a sarcastic running commentary on what she was doing.

On several occasions, Mrs. Dubois declared that she need not give any further details, because the attending clinician, like everybody else, was already aware of what she was thinking. She emphasized the fact that many of those thoughts were not her own but rather were imposed on her by something or somebody she could not identify, perhaps through radiation, waves, or electricity, and that she did, in fact, sometimes feel "electrical discharges" in her body, especially in the genital area. In some way, her neighbors were probably involved in all of this, although she could see no reason why they would be, because she had always been on friendly terms with everybody.

At the beginning of her difficulties, Mrs. Dubois had not felt depressed, but during the last 2 weeks, she had felt low and "down," stating that anyone who was going through what she was experiencing would, naturally, become depressed. She did not feel guilty about anything and was not aware of anything she might have done wrong in the past. She did not wish to die and had never contemplated suicide, but she was afraid that the voices might somehow harm or even kill her.

Mrs. Dubois discussed her problems in a perfectly coherent and understandable way, without ever losing the thread of her thoughts. There was no evidence from the physical examination or laboratory tests of any physical illness or of alcohol or drug use.

Mrs. Dubois was treated with an antipsychotic medication, risperidone 8 mg/day. The voices completely disappeared in about 2 weeks. At discharge, a few weeks later, the dosage of risperidone was reduced to 4 mg/day. She left the hospital in good spirits, looking forward to resuming her household duties and to working in her garden. She was not quite convinced, however, that her voices had been due to some disturbance in her brain; she remained suspicious about her neighbors and hardly ever left her home. In addition, in the subsequent 12 months, she developed an interest in telepathy, clairvoyance, and other similar beliefs that she had previously regarded as "humbug."

During this period, she discontinued her medication on two occasions, and the voices reappeared within 2 weeks. On both occasions the voices disappeared again shortly after she resumed taking antipsychotic medication.

Discussion of "The Witch"

In many ways this vignette is a classic case of Schizophrenia (DSM-5-TR, p. 113). Mrs. Dubois developed a number of persistent psychotic symptoms that significantly interfered with her functioning. These symptoms included hearing voices that kept a running commentary about her actions and that spoke to one another saying that she was a witch who needed to be destroyed; somatic hallucinations involving "electrical discharges" in her genital area; and several delusions, including that people in her neighborhood were spying on her and talking about her and that many of her thoughts were not her own but instead were imposed on her by some kind of outside force. Historically it had been thought that several of the psychotic symptoms she experienced—namely, her belief that her voices conversed with one another and kept up a running commentary, and her belief that the thoughts were not her own but were being inserted into her head (a symptom known as *thought insertion*)—were on their own indicative of the diagnosis of Schizophrenia (i.e., pathognomonic). It is now understood that such symptoms are not necessarily indicative of Schizophrenia but occur in psychotic mania or depression as well. What is unusual about Mrs. Dubois' case is the age at onset. Schizophrenia symptom onset typically occurs between ages 16 and 30; onset after age 45, as in Mrs. Dubois' case, is relatively unusual. Evidence suggests that cases of later-onset Schizophrenia typically have good social functioning before onset, are more likely to have paranoid delusions and hallucinations as opposed to disorganized speech and behavior and negative symptoms, and are more likely to report visual, somatic, and olfactory hallucinations, all of which are true of Mrs. Dubois' case.

Because Mrs. Dubois has been experiencing a variety of psychotic symptoms for 14 months—2 months of hallucinations and delusions before hospitalization and an additional 12 months of residual symptoms with continued paranoia about her neighbors, as well as newly developed beliefs in telepathy and clairvoyance, which affected her functioning (not going out of the house)—the diagnosis of Schizophrenia is appropriate. Although she experienced some depression for a couple of weeks after being admitted to the hospital, it was relatively mild and time limited and, therefore, insufficient to justify a diagnosis of Schizoaffective Disorder (see Section 2.3). At the time of her admission to the hospital, her diagnosis would have been Schizophreniform Disorder (see Section 2.2) rather than Schizophrenia, because at that point her symptoms had lasted only for 2 months and thus would have been too brief to justify a diagnosis of Schizophrenia. (The time frame for the diagnosis of Schizophreniform Disorder is a period of symptoms lasting between 1 month and less than 6 months.)

Star Wars

Jessica, age 15 years, was seen at the request of her school district authorities for advice on placement. She had recently moved into the area with her family and, after a brief period in a regular class, was placed in a class for students with emotional disturbance. She proved very difficult; her understanding of schoolwork was at about the fifth-grade level, although she had an apparently good vocabulary, and she disturbed the class by making animal noises and telling fantastic stories, which made other students laugh at her.

At home Jessica is aggressive, biting or hitting her parents or brother if frustrated. She is often bored, has no friends, and finds it difficult to occupy herself. She spends a lot of time drawing pictures of robots, spaceships, and fantastic or futuristic inventions. Although she has sometimes said she would like to die, she has never made any suicide attempts and apparently has not thought of killing herself. Her mother says that from birth Jessica has been different and that the onset of her current behavior has been so gradual that no definite date can be assigned to it.

Jessica's prenatal and perinatal history is unremarkable. Her developmental milestones were delayed, and she did not use single words until age 4 or 5 years. Ever since she entered school, there has been concern about her intellectual ability. Repeated evaluations have suggested an IQ in the low 70s, with achievement lagging somewhat behind even that expected at this ability level. Although Jessica had relatively few friends growing up, she did have a couple of very close friends with whom she interacted normally.

Her parents report that Jessica has always been difficult and restless and that several doctors have said she not only has low intelligence but also suffers from a serious mental disorder. The results of an evaluation done at age 12, because she was having difficulties in school, showed "evidence of bizarre thought processes and fragmented ego structure." At that time, she was sleeping well at night and was not getting up with nightmares or bizarre requests, although this apparently had been a feature of her earlier behavior. Currently, she is reported to sleep very poorly and tends to disturb the household by getting up and wandering around at night. Her mother emphasizes Jessica's unpredictability, the strange stories that she tells, and the way in which she talks to herself in "funny voices." Her mother regards the stories Jessica tells as childish make-believe and pays little attention to them. She says that since the time Jessica saw her first *Star Wars* movie at age 10, she has been obsessed with ideas about space, spaceships, and the future.

Jessica's parents are in their early 40s. Her father, having retired from military service, now works as an engineer. Jessica's mother has many unusual beliefs about herself. She claims to have grown up in India and to have had a very bizarre early childhood, full of dramatic and violent episodes. Many of these episodes sound highly improbable. Her husband (Jessica's father) refuses to let her talk about her past in his presence and tries to play down both this information from his wife and Jessica's problems. The parents appear to have a rather restricted relationship, in which the father plays the role of a taciturn, masterful head of household and the mother bears the brunt of everyday family duties. The mother, in contrast, is loquacious and very circumstantial in her history giving. She dwells a great deal on her strange childhood experiences. Jessica's brother is now 12 and is an apparently normal child with an average school career. He does not spend much free time in the house or with the family, preferring instead to play with his friends. He is ashamed of Jessica's behavior and tries to avoid going out with her.

In the interview, Jessica presents as a tall, overweight, pasty-looking child, dressed untidily and with a somewhat disheveled appearance. She complains vociferously of her insomnia, although it is very difficult to elicit details of the sleep disturbance. She talks at length about her interests and preoccupations. She says she made a robot in the basement that ran amok and was on the verge of causing a great deal of damage, but she was able to stop it by remote control. She claims to have built the robot from spare computer parts, which she acquired from the local museum.

When pressed for details of how the robot worked, Jessica became increasingly vague. When asked to draw a picture of one of her inventions, she drew a picture of an overhead railway and began stating what appeared to be complex mathematical calculations to substantiate the structural details, but which in fact consisted of meaningless repetitions of arithmetic symbols (e.g., plus, minus, divide, multiply). When the interviewer expressed some gentle incredulity, she blandly replied, "Many people do not believe that I am a supergenius." She also talked about her unusual ability to hear things other people cannot hear, and said she was in communication with some sort of creature. She thought she might be haunted, or perhaps the creature was a being from another planet. She could hear his voice talking to her and asking her questions; he did not attempt to tell her what to do. The voice was outside her own head but was inaudible to others. She did not regard the questions being asked of her as upsetting, and they did not make her angry or frightened.

According to her teacher, Jessica's reading is apparently at the fifth-grade level, but her comprehension is much lower. She tends to read what is not there and sometimes changes the meaning of the paragraph. Her spelling is at about the third-grade level, and her mathematics ability is a little bit below that. She works hard at school but very slowly. If pressure is placed on her, she becomes upset, and her work deteriorates.

Discussion of "Star Wars"

Jessica exhibits several psychotic symptoms. She is delusional in that she believes she has made a complicated invention and that she is in communication with "some sort of creature." She has auditory hallucinations of a voice talking to her and asking her questions. The presence of delusions and hallucinations, in the absence of a full manic or depressive syndrome or a nonpsychiatric medical condition or use of a substance that could account for the disturbance, coupled with the significantly negative impact of these symptoms on her psychosocial functioning, indicate a diagnosis of Schizophrenia (DSM-5-TR, p. 113).

Several aspects of Jessica's history raise questions about whether the diagnosis might be better considered as an Autism Spectrum Disorder (see "Rocking and Reading" in Section 1.6). Autism Spectrum Disorder has its onset in early childhood and is characterized by severe difficulties in social interaction and restricted repetitive patterns of behavior, interests, or activities. Although Jessica is reported to have relatively few friends, there is no evidence that she had impaired social interactions when she was younger—her current lack of friends is most likely related to her being shunned by her peers because of her bizarre behavior. Moreover, although her preoccupation with ideas about space, spaceships, and the future to the exclusion of other interests is typical of Autism Spectrum Disorder, there is no evidence of stereotyped or repetitive motor movements, insistence on sameness, or unusual reactivity (either over-reactivity or underreactivity) to sensory input, which are characteristic features of Autism Spectrum Disorder. Most importantly, delusions and hallucinations are not features of Autism Spectrum Disorder.

Another notable aspect of the case is that Jessica's mother also has a number of unusual beliefs, claiming to have grown up in India and to have had a very bizarre early childhood, full of dramatic and violent episodes, many of which sound "highly improbable." Family members of individuals with Schizophrenia are at increased risk for other disorders in the schizophrenia spectrum, specifically Schizoaffective Disorder (see Section 2.3) and Schizotypal Personality Disorder (see Section 18.8). The odd and unusual beliefs reported by Jessica's mother are most consistent with her mother's having a diagnosis of Schizotypal Personality Disorder.

2.2
Schizophreniform Disorder

Schizophreniform Disorder shares a majority of diagnostic features with Schizophrenia except that the duration is between 1 month and less than 6 months, rather than 6 months or longer as required for Schizophrenia. Moreover, there is no requirement, as in Schizophrenia, that the person's level of functioning be markedly below the level achieved before symptom onset. The diagnosis of Schizophreniform Disorder can be used in two different clinical situations: 1) for individuals who have recovered after an episode of psychotic symptoms that lasted between 1 month and less than 6 months; and 2) for individuals who are in the midst of a psychotic episode that so far has lasted less than 6 months, in which case the Schizophreniform Disorder diagnosis would be considered "provisional," as the diagnosis may ultimately be changed to Schizophrenia if the symptoms continue for 6 months or longer. Individuals with Schizophreniform Disorder have a better long-term prognosis than individuals with Schizophrenia, in that they are less likely to experience a future psychotic episode. Four factors are associated with a good prognosis: onset of full-blown psychotic symptoms within 1 month of the first noticeable change in usual behavior and functioning; confusion or perplexity at the height of the psychotic episode; good functioning before the onset of the psychotic episode; and absence of blunted or flat affect. If at least two such factors are present, the specifier With Good Prognostic Features may be given. If not, the specifier Without Good Prognostic Features applies.

About one-third of individuals with an initial provisional diagnosis of Schizophreniform Disorder recover within the 6-month period, and for them Schizophreniform Disorder is their final diagnosis. The majority of the remaining two-thirds of individuals will eventually receive a diagnosis of Schizophrenia or Schizoaffective Disorder.

Late Bloomer

Gabrielle Fielding is a 35-year-old single, unemployed, college-educated woman who was escorted to the emergency room by the mobile crisis team. Concerned about Ms. Fielding's increasingly erratic behavior, Ms. Fielding's sister had contacted the team after failing to persuade Ms. Fielding to visit an outpatient psychiatrist. Ms. Fielding's only prior psychiatric contact had been brief psychotherapy in college.

Ms. Fielding had not worked since being laid off from her job 3 months previously. According to her boyfriend and her roommate (both of whom live with her), during that time period she had become intensely preoccupied with the upstairs neighbors. A few days earlier she had banged on their front door with an iron for no apparent reason. She told the mobile crisis team that the family upstairs was harassing her by "accessing" her thoughts and then repeating them to her. The crisis team took her to the emergency room for evaluation of "thought broadcasting." Although Ms. Fielding denied having any trouble with her thinking, she conceded that she was feeling "stressed" since losing her job and might benefit from more psychotherapy.

After reading the admission note that described such bizarre symptoms, the emergency room psychiatrists were surprised to encounter a poised, relaxed, and attractive young woman, stylishly dressed and appearing perfectly normal. She greeted them with a courteous but somewhat superficial smile. She related to the doctors with nonchalant respectfulness. When asked why she was there, she ventured a timid shrug, and replied, "I was hoping to find out from you!"

Ms. Fielding had been working as a secretary and attributed her job loss to the sluggish economy. She said she was "stressed out" by her unemployment. She denied having any recent mood disturbance and answered "no" to questions about psychotic symptoms, punctuating each query with a polite but incredulous laugh. Wondering if perhaps the crisis team's assessment was of a different patient, the interviewer asked, somewhat apologetically, if the patient ever wondered whether people could read her mind. She replied, "Oh yes, it happens all the time," and described how, on one occasion, she was standing in her kitchen planning dinner in silence, only to hear, moments later, voices of people on the street below reciting the entire menu. She was convinced of the reality of the experience, having verified it by looking out the window and observing them speaking her thoughts aloud.

Ms. Fielding was distressed not so much by people "accessing" her thoughts as by her inability to exercise control over the process. She believed that most people developed telepathic powers in childhood, whereas she was a "late bloomer" who had just become aware of her abilities and was currently overwhelmed by them. She was troubled most by her upstairs neighbors, who for the past couple of months not only repeated her thoughts but also bombarded her with their own devaluing and critical comments, such as "You're no good" and "You have to leave." Their taunts had begun to intrude on her mercilessly, at all hours of the night and day.

She was convinced that the only solution was for the upstairs neighbors to move away. When asked if she had contemplated other possibilities, she reluctantly admitted that she had spoken to her boyfriend about hiring a hit man to "threaten" or, if need be, "eliminate" the couple. She hoped she would be able to spare their two children, whom she felt were not involved in this invasion of her "mental boundaries." This concern for the children was the only insight she demonstrated into the gravity of her symptoms. She did agree, however, to admit herself voluntarily to the hospital.

Once admitted to the hospital, Ms. Fielding immediately began pressing for discharge and disavowed her previous symptoms. Her behavior, thinking, and affect seemed otherwise normal. After 2 weeks of observation, she was discharged to her treating physician's clinic. Within a couple of weeks, however, she again admitted having frightening experiences of hearing voices and of reading other people's thoughts, as well as being unable to develop a plan for finding work. She agreed to try medication.

She was treated with the antipsychotic risperidone, and her frightening hallucinations and belief that she was clairvoyant remitted within a few days. Within 3 months of her discharge from the hospital, she had obtained work with a temporary employment agency. Soon afterward, feeling completely well, she stopped attending the clinic and did not seek follow-up.

Discussion of "Late Bloomer"

Delusions and hallucinations lasting at least 1 month but less than 6 months, in the absence of a Mood Disorder, Substance Use Disorder, or nonpsychiatric medical condition that could account for the disturbance, justify a diagnosis of Schizophreniform Disorder (DSM-5-TR, p. 111). Ms. Fielding's case illustrates that the stereotypical view that individuals with psychotic symptoms constantly act like raving lunatics is often not true. Ms. Fielding appeared perfectly normal to the emergency room staff on first meeting. It was not until the interviewer asked her the right question ("Do you ever wonder whether people could read your mind?") that her delusional thinking became grossly apparent.

Ms. Fielding's presentation has features associated with a good prognosis. Her functioning before the onset of psychotic symptoms was quite good (she was college-educated and was employed as a secretary before she was laid off 3 months before admission), and she did not have blunted or flat affect (i.e., her ability to express and show emotions was not affected). Therefore, Ms. Fielding would be diagnosed with Schizophreniform Disorder, With Good Prognostic Features.

Postpartum Piety

Zela Akerele is a 30-year-old high school teacher living in Lagos, Nigeria. She is married and has five children. The birth of her last child was complicated by excessive bleeding and infection, and Mrs. Akerele was still hospitalized in the gynecology ward 3 weeks after delivery when her gynecologist requested a psychiatric consultation. Mrs. Akerele was agitated and seemed to be in a daze. She said to the psychiatrist, "I am a sinner. I have to die. My time has passed. I cannot be a good Christian again. I need to be reborn. Jesus Christ should help me. He is not helping me." The psychiatrist diagnosed postpartum psychosis and prescribed the antipsychotic chlorpromazine. Mrs. Akerele was soon well enough to go home.

Three weeks later she was readmitted, this time to the psychiatric ward, claiming that she had had a "vision of the spirits" and was "wrestling with the spirits." Her relatives reported that at home she had been fasting and "keeping vigil" through the nights and that she was not sleeping. She had complained to the neighbors that there was a witch in her house. The "witch" turned out to be her mother.

Mrs. Akerele's husband, Peter, who was studying engineering in Europe, hurriedly returned and took over the running of the household. She improved rapidly on chlorpromazine, the same antipsychotic medication she was given the last time she was in the hospital, and was discharged in 2 weeks. Her improvement, however, was short-lived. She threw away her medication and began to attend Mass whenever one was given, pursuing the priests to ask questions about scriptures. Within a week she was readmitted.

On the ward, she accused the psychiatrist of shining powerful torchlights on her and taking pictures of her, opening her chest, using her as a guinea pig, poisoning her food, and planning to bury her alive. She claimed to receive messages from Mars and Jupiter and announced that there was a riot in town. She clutched her Bible to her breast and accused all the doctors of being "idol worshippers," calling down the wrath of her God on all of them.

After considerable resistance, she was finally convinced to accept electroconvulsive therapy (ECT; a procedure, done under general anesthesia, in which small electric currents are passed through the brain, intentionally triggering a brief seizure), and she became symptom-free after six treatments. At this point, she attributed her illness to a difficult childbirth, the absence of her husband, and her unreasonable mother. She saw no further role for the doctors, called for her priest, and began to speak of her illness as a religious experience, similar to the experiences of religious leaders throughout history. However, her symptoms did not return, and she was discharged after 6 weeks of hospitalization.

Discussion of "Postpartum Piety"

This is a case of so-called *postpartum psychosis*, a term which refers to the sudden onset of psychotic symptoms after childbirth. It affects around 1 to 2 per 1,000 females of child-bearing age,[1] which is significantly lower than the prevalence of postpartum blues (affecting over 50% of women)[2] or postpartum depression (affecting around 1 in 7 woman).[3] Although postpartum psychosis is one of the rarer psychiatric disorders, it is almost always considered a psychiatric emergency because of the rapid onset of severe psychotic symptoms and the potential for a catastrophic outcome, such as infanticide or suicide.

DSM-5-TR does not include postpartum psychosis as a separate diagnosis. Instead, the specifier With Peripartum Onset is available to be applied to various DSM-5-TR diagnoses if the onset of the symptoms is during pregnancy or within 4 weeks of delivery. Moreover, the specifier With Peripartum Onset can apply not only to psychotic symptoms associated with pregnancy and delivery but also to the development of mood symptoms. The specifier can be applied to Manic Episodes and Major Depressive Episodes, each of which may be with or without psychotic features, as well as to Hypomanic Episodes, which must occur without psychosis. The specifier also can apply to Brief Psychotic Disorder. Of note, the term *postpartum psychosis* refers only to psychotic symptoms that develop after childbirth.

Most commonly, postpartum psychotic symptoms emerge in the context of a Manic or Major Depressive Episode that develops after delivery. In Mrs. Akerele's case, she developed recurrent, brief psychotic episodes that included delusions of guilt and visual and auditory hallucinations with a religious content, but she had no manic or depressive symptoms. Given that the combination of her delusions and hallucinations lasted longer than 1 month but less than 6 months, and that no drugs or nonpsychiatric medical conditions caused the symptoms (pregnancy and delivery are not considered to be causative medical conditions in DSM), Mrs. Akerele's diagnosis is Schizophreniform Disorder (DSM-5-TR, p. 111). Because DSM-5-TR does not offer the specifier

[1]Raza SK, Raza S: Postpartum Psychosis. Treasure Island, FL, StatPearls Publishing, Jan 2024 31335024.
[2]Howard LM, Molyneaux E, Dennis CL, et al: Nonpsychotic mental disorders in the perinatal period. *Lancet* 384(9956):1775–1788, 2014 25455248.
[3]Carlson K, Mughal S, Azhar Y, et al: Postpartum Depression. Treasure Island, FL, StatPearls Publishing, Jan 2024 30085612.

With Peripartum Onset for the diagnosis of Schizophreniform Disorder, it cannot be officially applied to this diagnosis. Even though ECT is most commonly used as a treatment for severe depression, it can also be effective in treating postpartum psychosis.

2.3
Schizoaffective Disorder

As its name suggests, Schizoaffective Disorder is a hybrid of Schizophrenia/ Schizophreniform Disorder and an affective disorder (an older term for disorders characterized by a disturbance in mood; i.e., Bipolar Disorders and Depressive Disorders). Individuals with Schizoaffective Disorder have periods with overlapping psychotic and mood symptoms—for example, having both paranoid delusions and auditory hallucinations with a Manic Episode or Major Depressive Episode, as well as other periods in which delusions or hallucinations occur in the absence of any significant mania or depression. There are two types of Schizoaffective Disorder, which differ based on the pattern of mood symptoms: 1) individuals who have Manic Episodes (and who also may have Major Depressive Episodes) as part of the presentation are considered to have the Bipolar Type, and 2) individuals with only Major Depressive Episodes are considered to have the Depressive Type. The Bipolar Type may be more common among young adults, whereas the Depressive Type may be more common among older adults.

Several DSM-5-TR disorders may manifest with a mixture of psychotic and mood symptoms and thus must be differentiated from Schizoaffective Disorder. The best way to understand Schizoaffective Disorder is to contrast it with these other conditions:

- Many individuals with Schizophrenia have occasional periods of depression or mania. The main difference between the diagnoses of Schizoaffective Disorder and Schizophrenia is in the proportion of time in which mood symptoms have been present. In Schizoaffective Disorder, significant mood symptoms occur for at least half time that the person has been ill, whereas in Schizophrenia, mood symptoms occur for a minority of the illness duration, if they occur at all.
- Some individuals with Bipolar Disorder or Major Depressive Disorder have psychotic symptoms when in the throes of a mood episode. For example, an individual with Bipolar I Disorder may have a delusion only during Manic Episodes that he is a prophet chosen by God to convince society to stop using fossil fuels, or an individual with Major Depressive Disorder may be convinced only during depressive episodes that her insides are rotting out (see "Praying Athlete" in Section 3.1 for an example of Bipolar I Disorder, With Psychotic Features; and "Stonemason" in Section 4.2 for an example of Major Depressive Disorder, With Psychotic Features). For such patients, the psychotic symptoms occur entirely within the confines of mood ep-

isodes, whereas individuals with Schizoaffective Disorder experience psychotic symptoms at times when they are not having Major Depressive or Manic Episodes.

Distinguishing between Schizoaffective Disorder and Schizophrenia is potentially important because both the treatment and the prognosis are different. The prominent mood symptoms in Schizoaffective Disorder usually require the use of either mood-stabilizing medications (if the individual has both manic and depressive periods) or antidepressant medications (if the person has only depression), in addition to the antipsychotic medication used to treat the psychotic symptoms. Thus, Schizoaffective Disorder, Bipolar Type, and Bipolar I Disorder, With Psychotic Features, are treated similarly, as are Schizoaffective Disorder, Depressive Type, and Major Depressive Disorder, With Psychotic Features. Moreover, in terms of functional outcomes, the long-term prognosis of Schizoaffective Disorder is considered to be better than the prognosis for Schizophrenia but worse than the prognosis for Bipolar I Disorder, With Psychotic Features, and Major Depressive Disorder, With Psychotic Features. Schizoaffective Disorder appears to be about one-third as common as Schizophrenia.

Foster Mother

Sophie Baumann, a 44-year-old mother of three teenagers, presents for treatment of her persisting depression. She gives the following history: About 1 year ago, after an argument that ended her relationship with her lover, she became acutely psychotic. She was frightened that people were going to kill her and heard voices of friends and strangers talking about killing her, and sometimes talking to each other. She heard her own thoughts broadcast aloud and was afraid that others could also hear what she was thinking. Over a 4-week period she stayed in her apartment, had new locks put on the doors, kept the shades down, and avoided everyone but her immediate family. Mrs. Baumann was unable to sleep at night because the voices kept her awake, and she was unable to eat because of a constant "lump" in her throat. She reported not feeling depressed, elated, or overactive during this period and remembers only that she was terrified of what would happen to her. The family persuaded her to enter a hospital, where she was given the antipsychotic medication ziprasidone to treat her psychotic symptoms. Within a few days of being admitted, she recalls losing her energy and motivation to do anything. She then became increasingly depressed, lost her appetite, and woke at 4:00 or 5:00 A.M. daily and was unable to get back to sleep. She could no longer read a newspaper or watch TV because she could not concentrate. The antidepressant venlafaxine was added to the ziprasidone to treat the depression. The delusions and hallucinations remitted within about 6 weeks, and Mrs. Baumann was discharged 2 weeks later on ziprasidone and venlafaxine, with only modest improvement in her depressive symptoms.

Over the past 9 months, Mrs. Baumann's depression has persisted but without recurrence of the psychotic symptoms. During this time, she has done very little except sit in her apartment, staring at the walls. Her children have managed most of the cooking, shopping, bill paying, and so forth. Mrs. Baumann has continued in outpatient treatment, but her depression has continued even after several trials of different antidepressant medication.

In discussing her past history, Mrs. Baumann is rather guarded. There is, however, no evidence of a diagnosable illness before last year. She apparently is a shy, emotionally constricted person who "has never broken any rules." She has been separated from her husband for 10 years, but since that time has had two enduring relationships with boyfriends. In addition to rearing three apparently healthy and very likable children, she cared for a succession of foster children full-time in the 4 years before her illness. She enjoyed doing this meaningful work and was highly valued by the foster care agency. She has maintained close relationships with a few women friends and with her extended family.

Discussion of "Foster Mother"

During her initial 4-week period of illness, Mrs. Baumann demonstrated the characteristic schizophrenic symptoms of delusions (believing people could hear what she was thinking) and auditory hallucinations (hearing voices of friends and strangers talking about killing her) occurring in the absence of any mood disturbance. Shortly after being admitted to the hospital, she developed the characteristic symptoms of a Major Depressive Episode, with depressed mood, poor appetite, insomnia, lack of energy, loss of interest, and poor concentration. After roughly 6 weeks of treatment with an antipsychotic medication, her delusions and hallucinations remitted, but her depression persisted. The temporal sequence of these symptoms (psychotic symptoms without mood symptoms for about 4 weeks, psychotic symptoms occurring with mood symptoms for about 6 weeks, and then persistent depression for another 9–10 months) conforms to the temporal pattern seen in Schizoaffective Disorder (DSM-5-TR, p. 121). Given that Mrs. Baumann had only depressive symptoms and never any evidence of mania, she would be diagnosed with Schizoaffective Disorder, Depressive Type.

2.4
Delusional Disorder

Delusional Disorder is a persistent psychotic disorder in which the primary symptom is one or more delusions (e.g., the fixed belief that a secret government agency has installed cameras and microphones in the person's apartment and office and is monitoring everything the person does) lasting at least 1 month and occurring in the absence of other psychotic signs or symptoms of Schizophrenia (e.g., hallucinations or disorganized speech or behavior). Moreover, apart from the impact of the delusion on the person's functioning (e.g., a person not willing to leave their house because of the conviction that they are being followed by FBI agents), there may be no obvious evidence of mental illness. For example, a person with the delusion that they are being monitored may appear perfectly normal during a conversation until the subject of the government is brought up, whereupon the person might embark on an irrational rant about their being under constant surveillance. This is in marked contrast to a person with Schizophrenia, whose affect, appearance, and social relatedness are likely to be experienced by an observer as odd, bizarre, or just "off" in some way.

Although all individuals with Delusional Disorder must, by definition, have delusions lasting at least 1 month, each case is unique because of the almost infinite variety of fixed false beliefs that can develop. Therefore, DSM-5-TR provides various subtypes of Delusional Disorder according to the predominant theme of the delusional belief:

- The most common form of Delusional Disorder is the Persecutory Type, in which the person is convinced that they are being followed, spied on, poisoned or drugged, or conspired against.
- In the Jealous Type, the person may be convinced that their spouse or lover is being unfaithful despite the lack of supporting evidence.
- Individuals with the Erotomanic Type are convinced that another person, typically someone famous or of a higher social status, is secretly in love with them, which sometimes results in the person stalking the object of their delusion.
- Those with the Somatic Type have a delusion in which the central theme involves bodily functions or sensations, such as the conviction that the person emits a foul odor or that there is an infestation of insects on or under the skin.
- Those with the Grandiose Type might be convinced that they have made some important discovery (e.g., a cure for cancer).
- Delusional beliefs that do not fit into any of these categories are classified as Unspecified Type.

Delusional Disorder is a rare disorder with an estimated prevalence of 0.2%. The Persecutory Type is the most common. Although the Jealous Type is probably more common in men than in women, there are no major gender differences in the overall frequency of Delusional Disorder. Delusional Disorder can start as early as adolescence, but it more typically begins in middle to late adulthood. In the majority of cases, the onset is sudden. The long-term outcome of Delusional Disorder is variable, with a lasting remission occurring in up to half of patients with the disorder.

Contract on My Life

Robert Polsen, a 45-year-old married postal worker and father of two, is brought to the emergency room by his wife because he has been insisting that "there is a contract out on my life." According to Mr. Polsen, his problems began 4 months ago when his supervisor at work accused him of tampering with a package. Mr. Polsen denied that this was true and, because his job was in jeopardy, filed a protest. He was exonerated at a formal hearing; according to Mr. Polsen, "This made my boss furious. He felt he had been publicly humiliated."

About 2 weeks later, Mr. Polsen noticed that his coworkers were avoiding him. "When I'd walk toward them, they'd just turn away like they didn't want to see me." Shortly thereafter, he began to feel that they were talking about him at work. He never could make out clearly what they were saying, but he gradually became convinced that they were avoiding him because his boss had taken out a contract on his life.

This state of affairs was stable for about 2 months, until Mr. Polsen began noticing several "large white cars," new to his neighborhood, driving up and down the street on which he lived. He became increasingly frightened and was convinced that the "hit men" were in these cars. He refused to leave his apartment without an escort. Several times, when he saw the white cars, he panicked and ran home. After one such incident, his wife finally insisted that he accompany her to the emergency room.

Mr. Polsen was described by his wife and brother as a basically well-adjusted, outgoing man who enjoyed being with his family. He had served with distinction in Afghanistan but saw little combat there.

When interviewed in the emergency room, Mr. Polsen was obviously frightened. Aside from his belief that he was in danger of being killed, his speech, behavior, and demeanor were in no way odd or strange. His predominant mood was anxious. He denied having hallucinations and any other psychotic symptom except those noted above. He claimed not to be depressed, and although he noted that he had recently had some difficulty falling asleep, he said there had been no change in his appetite, sex drive, energy level, or concentration.

During the first week of hospitalization, he received the antipsychotic medication risperidone. He remained delusional, however, and became convinced that several of the patients on the ward with Italian names were part of the "hit team" sent to kill him. Over the ensuing 3 weeks, with continued treatment, these beliefs faded. At discharge, 1 month after admission, he stated, "I guess my boss has called off the contract. He couldn't get away with it now without publicity."

Discussion of "Contract on My Life"

Mr. Polsen's only symptom is the delusion that his boss has put a contract out on his life. Given that he does not have any other psychiatric symptoms, apart from anxiety resulting from his belief that hit men are after him, the most appropriate DSM-5-TR diagnosis for him is Delusional Disorder (DSM-5-TR, p. 104). Also, given that the main theme of the delusion is that the boss has taken a contract out on his life, he would be considered to have the Persecutory Type of Delusional Disorder.

Perhaps the main diagnostic challenge when evaluating someone with a possible Delusional Disorder is to determine that the person's belief is in fact evidence of a *delusion*, which is defined as a fixed false or idiosyncratic belief that is based on an incorrect inference about external reality and held despite evidence to the contrary. For delusions that involve situations or phenomena that cannot possibly be true (e.g., "I was abducted by aliens and returned to Earth with a transmitter in my head that is beaming signals back to the aliens so that they can monitor the human race"), the conclusion that the belief is false and thus delusional is straightforward. In the much more common situation, in which the belief involves something that could possibly occur in real life, determining that the belief is a delusion can be much more challenging. In Mr. Polsen's case, his belief that his boss has put a contract out on his life could be true; however, the possibility that his boss would react to Mr. Polsen's prevailing at a grievance hearing by hiring hit men so stretches the bounds of credibility that it is quite clear that Mr. Polsen's belief is delusional.

The case also illustrates the typical "referential" nature of many delusions in which a person sees events, objects, or other individuals in the immediate environment as having particular and unusual personal significance. The first evidence of the beginnings of Mr. Polsen's delusional illness was his perception that coworkers were avoiding him. Most likely he was misinterpreting innocuous random actions of others (e.g., people turning away when he walked toward them) as his being shunned by them. Similarly, once he developed the conviction that his boss had put out a contract on his life, he viewed random events in his environment (e.g., large white cars being driven down his street) through the lens of his distorted belief that he was being stalked by hit men. Another aspect of this case that is typical of a persecutory delusional process is the incorporation of additional individuals (e.g., patients with Italian names) into the person's paranoid belief system.

Several aspects of this case are somewhat atypical. Most individuals with the Persecutory Type of Delusional Disorder are reluctant to seek help. Mr. Polsen, however, was apparently frightened enough to allow his wife to take him to the emergency room. Also, the effectiveness of an antipsychotic medication in Delusional Disorder is unfortunately more the exception than the rule. Although antipsychotic medication is typically helpful for the psychotic symptoms in Schizophrenia, Bipolar Disorder, and Major Depressive Disorder, such medication is often less effective in individuals with Delusional Disorder. Note that with Delusional Disorder, the goal of treatment is often not to eradicate the delusions but to lessen their intensity so that they no longer interfere with the person's functioning. In this case, although Mr. Polsen's beliefs had "faded" (i.e., he felt his boss had "called off the contract"), he still believed that the contract on his life had been real.

Dear Doctor

Myrna Field, age 55, was a cashier in a hospital coffee shop 3 years ago when she suddenly developed the belief that a physician who dropped in regularly was intensely in love with her. She fell passionately in love with him but said nothing to him and became increasingly distressed each time she saw him. Casual remarks that he made to her when buying coffee were interpreted as cues to his feelings, and she believed he gave her significant glances and made suggestive movements, although he never declared his feelings openly. She was sure he did not admit his feelings because he was married.

After more than 2 years of feeling this way, she became so agitated that she had to give up her job; she remained at home, thinking about the physician incessantly. She had frequent, intense abdominal sensations, which greatly frightened her. (These turned out to be sexual feelings, which she did not recognize because she had never been orgasmic before.) Eventually, she went to her family doctor, who found her so upset that he referred her. She was too embarrassed to confide in the male psychiatrist, and it was only when she was transferred to a female psychiatrist that she poured forth her story.

Mrs. Field was born to a single mom and her upbringing was excessively strict. She learned slowly and was always in trouble at home and at school. She grew up anxious and afraid, and during her adult life consulted many doctors because of hypochondriacal concerns. She was always insecure in company. Mrs. Field was married, but the marriage was asexual, and there were no children. Although her husband appeared long-suffering, she perceived him as overly critical and demanding. She could not confide in her husband about her "love affair."

When she was interviewed by the female psychiatrist, Mrs. Field was very distressed and talked under great pressure. Her intelligence was limited, and many of her ideas appeared simple, but the only clear abnormality that was evident was the unshakable belief that her physician "lover" was passionately devoted to her. She could not be persuaded otherwise.

Mrs. Field readily accepted medication, and the doctor prescribed pimozide, an antipsychotic medication that appears to be more effective in Delusional Disorder than other antipsychotic medications. Over a period of 3–4 weeks, Mrs. Field became much calmer, and the delusion became less insistent.

Three years later, Mrs. Field remains well. She and her husband appear content with their marriage, which remains platonic. She occasionally thinks of the physician with some nostalgia and still believes he loves her but is no longer distressed about this. She continues to take her antipsychotic medication.

Discussion of "Dear Doctor"

Mrs. Field's only symptom is a delusion that she is loved by a doctor whom she barely knows and is thus diagnosed with Delusional Disorder, Erotomanic

Type (DSM-5-TR, p. 104). As is typical with delusional thinking, she interprets casual remarks and gestures made by the physician as evidence of his love for her. This type of delusion, in which the individual is convinced that another person, usually more socially prominent than the individual or sometimes a celebrity, is secretly in love with them, is known as an *erotomanic delusion*. Some individuals who stalk celebrities undoubtedly have the Erotomanic Type of Delusional Disorder. Although erotomanic delusions are more common among women, men can be afflicted by them as well. Some of these men can become aggressive, particularly toward companions of the love object whom they view as trying to come between them.

Unfaithful Wife

Marnie Callahan, a 48-year-old woman, took an overdose of sleeping pills. When she recovered, she confided to her family doctor that during the previous 18 months, Casey, her 50-year-old husband, had become increasingly jealous and accusatory. Recently, his accusations had become totally irrational; he was saying that she had multiple lovers, that she had gotten out of bed at night to go to them, and that she was communicating with them by lights and mirrors. Wrong-number telephone calls were "evidence" that men were contacting her, and he believed that cars passing the house at night flashed their headlights as a signal to her. She reported that Casey put tape on the windows and doors, nailed doors shut, and closely measured the location of every piece of furniture. Any change resulted in a tirade about her unfaithfulness. He refused to accept any food or cigarettes from her. During this time, her husband did not physically assault her, and their sexual activity remained at its usual level, but he appeared increasingly distressed and haggard, and lost 15 pounds.

Mrs. Callahan was so disturbed about her husband's behavior that she considered leaving him but was afraid he might become violent. She admitted that her overdose was a "cry for help."

Mr. Callahan was referred for psychiatric assessment and complied willingly. He gave an account similar to his wife's, but with total conviction about her infidelity. Despite his vehemence and his belief in all the various pieces of "evidence," he seemed to have some awareness that something was wrong with him. An interview with a daughter who lived at home corroborated her mother's innocence and her father's irrationality.

The marriage had been stable until the onset of this problem, although Mr. Callahan had drunk heavily as a young man and sometimes had assaulted his wife. His heavy drinking and violent behavior had ceased in his mid-30s, and he had generally been a good husband and provider since then. He had never used street drugs at any time. Mrs. Callahan described him as always being "pigheaded," but he was not normally unduly argumentative and had never previously evinced jealousy. He had attended school up to grade 7.

Mr. Callahan was unexpectedly agreeable to treatment and started taking the antipsychotic medication pimozide, which he continues to take 3 years later. On two occasions this drug has been withdrawn by his psychiatrist, but after a week or two Mr. Callahan reported, "I'm beginning to get funny ideas about the wife again," and he voluntarily resumed the medication.

Discussion of "Unfaithful Wife"

Even though the case starts out with the focus on Mrs. Callahan as the identified patient because of her overdose of sleeping pills, it is soon apparent that it is her husband, Casey, who has the mental illness. Mr. Callahan has a fixed, unshakable belief that his wife is being unfaithful. Of course, simply believing that a spouse or lover is being unfaithful is not evidence of having a mental disorder, especially if the suspicion turns out to be true. In this case, however, both the grossly improbable nature of Mr. Callahan's beliefs about his wife (that she got out of bed at night to rendezvous with her many lovers, and that she was communicating with them by lights and mirrors) and his extreme behavior stemming from his jealous beliefs (putting tape on the windows and doors, nailing doors shut, and measuring the location of every piece of furniture) are strong indicators of the delusional nature of his beliefs. Therefore, the diagnosis is Delusional Disorder, Jealous Type (DSM-5-TR, p. 104). It also appears that Mr. Callahan may have developed a secondary persecutory delusion that his wife was trying to poison him to get him out of the picture, as indicated by his refusal to accept any food or cigarettes from her. Treatment with the antipsychotic medication pimozide, as in the previous case ("Dear Doctor"), was effective in eliminating his delusion, although it appears that continued treatment with the medication is needed to keep Mr. Callahan's jealous delusions at bay.

Fleas

David Wallace, a fit-looking man of 70, consulted a dermatologist, complaining of being infested with fleas for about a year. The dermatologist found no evidence of infestation and referred him for psychiatric consultation. Although very angry about this recommendation, the patient followed through on the referral and gave the following history.

About a year previously, Mr. Wallace had bought a canary and soon noticed that it had fleas. He applied an insecticide, but the fleas "attacked" him and "invaded" his house. He washed his clothes repeatedly, applied many lotions, and saw a number of physicians, but nothing helped. He insisted he could see the fleas. He was distressed and too ashamed to see his friends, so he had become almost completely isolated.

Mr. Wallace had enjoyed good health until 2 years before, when he experienced a severe myocardial infarction. He had made a good recovery and kept himself active. He had given up heavy pipe smoking at that time. He had always been a moderate drinker. There was no personal or family history of emotional problems. He had married as a young man, but his wife had deserted him, and he had lived alone for many years.

When interviewed, Mr. Wallace looked considerably younger than his stated age and was alert and friendly, although he became angry when talking about the "incompetent" doctors who had failed to cure him, and he bristled when asked if the infestation could possibly be due to his imagination. His level of consciousness and cognitive functions were normal; his mood was essentially normal except for some anxiety and, at times, anger. His basic personality appeared stable. His conviction about the infestation was unshakable, but there was no evidence of other false beliefs.

Mr. Wallace reluctantly agreed to take the antipsychotic medication pimozide, although at one point he accused the psychiatrist of "only wanting to dope me to make me forget the fleas." His condition gradually improved, and he continued taking the medication for 6 months before he insisted on stopping the drug because he saw no reason to continue taking it. One year later, he remained cheerful and symptom-free.

Discussion of "Fleas"

It is unclear whether the insects Mr. Wallace "saw" were the result of delusional misinterpretations of normal visual stimuli (e.g., dust mites perhaps, given that canaries do not get fleas) or visual hallucinations with a delusional explanation. Regardless, his primary symptom was a somatic delusion. (Although a diagnosis of Delusional Disorder [DSM-5-TR, p. 104] generally requires the absence of other psychotic symptoms, an exception is made in DSM-5-TR for visual hallucinations that are related to the delusional content, as would be the situation in this case.) As is typical with somatic delusions, Mr. Wallace initially sought help from a series of nonpsychiatric physicians regarding his flea infestation. At some point, Mr. Wallace was referred to a psychiatrist, a recommendation that he agreed to only reluctantly. Despite his resistance to the idea that the fleas might not be real, he did agree to medication treatment, reflecting either his desperation to get help or the possibility that some part of him was aware that the fleas might be a product of his own mind.

2.5
Brief Psychotic Disorder

One feature that the psychotic disorders previously discussed in this chapter—Schizophrenia, Schizophreniform Disorder, Schizoaffective Disorder, and Delusional Disorder—have in common is that the minimum duration of the symptoms is at least 1 month (although in reality these disorders typically last much longer, sometimes for life). The psychotic symptoms in Brief Psychotic Disorder, on the other hand, are by definition *brief*—they can last anywhere from a few days up to 1 month. These brief episodes can include any of the positive psychotic symptoms—delusions, hallucinations, disorganized speech, or grossly disorganized or catatonic behavior—either alone or in combination. In addition to these psychotic symptoms, people suffering from a brief psychotic episode often experience emotional turmoil or overwhelming confusion and have rapid shifts from one intense mood state to another, going from agitation and irritability to depression.

Brief psychotic episodes typically come on abruptly, often after a major life event that would cause any person significant emotional upset, such as the death of a close family member or a severe accident. Because certain drugs of abuse (e.g., cocaine, phencyclidine [PCP]), certain medications (e.g., steroids), and certain nonpsychiatric medical conditions (e.g., epilepsy) can cause psychotic symptoms, such causes should be considered and ruled out before concluding that the diagnosis is Brief Psychotic Disorder.

Brief Psychotic Disorder has the best prognosis of all the psychotic disorders. Although Brief Psychotic Disorder by definition reaches a full remission within 1 month, more than 50% of the individuals experience a relapse. Despite the possibility of relapse, for most individuals, outcome is favorable in terms of social functioning and symptomatology.

Some individuals with certain personality traits, such as suspiciousness, and a tendency toward odd thinking and unusual perceptual experiences have an underlying vulnerability to developing psychotic symptoms, especially under stress.

The Socialite

Dorothea Cabot, a 42-year-old socialite, has never had any mental problems before. A new performance hall is to be formally opened with the world premiere of a new ballet, and Mrs. Cabot, because of her position on the cultural council, has assumed the responsibility for coordinating that event. However, construction problems, including strikes by the workers, have made it uncertain whether finishing details will be completed by the deadline. The set designer has been volatile, threatening to walk out on the project unless the materials meet his meticulous specifications. Mrs. Cabot has had to calm this angry man while attempting to coax disputing groups to negotiate. She has also had increased responsibilities at home because her housekeeper has had to leave to visit a sick relative.

In the midst of these difficulties, her best friend was decapitated in a tragic auto crash. Mrs. Cabot herself is an only child, and her best friend had been very close to her since grade school. People often commented that the two women were like sisters.

Immediately following the funeral, Mrs. Cabot becomes increasingly tense and jittery, and can sleep only 2–3 hours a night. Two days later she happens to see a woman driving a car just like the one her friend had driven. She is puzzled, and after a few hours she becomes convinced that her friend is alive and that the accident and funeral had been staged as part of a plot. Somehow, the plot is directed toward deceiving her, and she senses that she is in great danger and must solve the mystery to escape alive. She begins to distrust everyone except her husband and to believe that her phone is tapped and the rooms in her house are "bugged." She pleads with her husband to help save her life. She begins to hear a high-pitched, undulating sound, which she fears is an ultrasound beam aimed at her. She is in a state of sheer panic, gripping her husband's arm in terror, as he takes her to the emergency room the next morning. She is admitted to the psychiatric unit, where she is treated with risperidone, an antipsychotic medication, and within days her symptoms resolve, and she returns to her normal self.

Discussion of "The Socialite"

Mrs. Cabot's case is fairly typical of Brief Psychotic Disorder. While already under a great deal of emotional stress in the context of her struggles to get a concert hall ready in time for a world premiere of a ballet, her best friend is killed in a horrible automobile accident. These stressors precipitate the abrupt development of a severe psychotic episode, characterized by an elaborate series of connected paranoid delusions: that her best friend was not really killed in a car accident but that the accident and funeral were staged for the purpose of deceiving her. Moreover, she then concludes that she is at the center of a plot to harm her, and that she is under surveillance (believing that the phone is tapped, and the rooms are "bugged"). She then goes on to develop a related auditory hallucination, hearing a high-pitched undulating sound that she fears is an ultrasound beam being aimed at her.

At the time of Mrs. Cabot's admission to the emergency room, her diagnosis is unclear. The first action in such a case is to conduct a thorough medical evaluation to investigate whether drugs, medications, or an as-yet-undiagnosed nonpsychiatric medical condition might have caused her psychotic symptoms; this evaluation requires checking the patient's blood for the presence of drugs. Once these possible causes have been eliminated from consideration, the clinician must determine which of the DSM-5-TR psychotic disorders best explains this presentation. The presenting pattern of symptoms could be the first sign of the acute phase of Schizophrenia, given the fact that Mrs. Cabot has both delusions and hallucinations. However, because the symptoms resolve within a matter of days and she returns to her normal self, the diagnosis is Brief Psychotic Disorder, With Marked Stressor (DSM-5-TR, p. 108).

2.6
Catatonia Associated With Another Mental Disorder/Catatonic Disorder Due to Another Medical Condition

Catatonia is a marked psychomotor disturbance characterized by a wide range of symptoms that may involve decreased motor activity, decreased engagement during the interview or physical examination, or excessive and peculiar motor activity. These symptoms may manifest in a variety of ways. At its most extreme, the decreased motor activity is manifested by *stupor* (a complete lack of psychomotor activity accompanied by a complete disengagement from the surrounding environment). Some individuals with Catatonia show *catalepsy* (maintaining an unusual body posture for an extended period, often against gravity, such as holding an arm outstretched) or *waxy flexibility* (retention of limbs in any position into which they are manipulated by the examiner). During the interview, the patient may show decreased engagement, which can range from *mutism* (a complete lack of verbal responses to questions) to *negativism* (resisting all attempts to be moved, or all instructions or requests to move, without any apparent motivation). Excessive and peculiar motor activity can entail complex behaviors (e.g., repeatedly running up and down a flight of stairs) or be manifested by simple purposeless motor agitation. It may also include facial grimacing, *echolalia* (mimicking another's speech), or *echopraxia* (mimicking another's movements). In severe cases, the patient may need careful supervision to avoid self-harm or harming others.

DSM-5-TR includes Catatonia in the chapter on Schizophrenia Spectrum and Other Psychotic Disorders because catatonic symptoms are included among the characteristic symptoms of Schizophrenia, Schizophreniform Disorder, and Brief Psychotic Disorder. Its placement in this diagnostic class is a bit misleading, however, because Catatonia occurs most commonly in association with severe depression or severe mania. Less often, catatonic symptoms are due to a nonpsychiatric medical condition or are related to medications (e.g., antipsychotic medications) or use of a substance (e.g., cannabis, PCP). A case of Catatonia Associated With Bipolar I Disorder, Current Episode Manic, is included in Chapter 3, "Bipolar and Related Disorders" (see "Praying Athlete" in Section 3.1).

Mute

Cathy Jarvis, a 25-year-old mother with a 3-year history of systemic lupus ery-thematosus (an autoimmune disease in which the body's immune system at-tacks various parts of the body, including sometimes the central nervous system), was admitted to a university hospital in an acute confusional state, with inability to maintain attention or to carry on a coherent conversation, and with marked disorientation to time and place. Before her hospitalization, she had be-come progressively more confused over a number of days and started to be-lieve that the neighbors were watching her. On the day of admission, she had run out of her house and into the street in a state of uncontrollable agitation.

On admission to the hospital emergency room, Ms. Jarvis was given intra-muscular haloperidol, an antipsychotic medication, but by the next morning her clinical picture had changed dramatically for the worse. She had become rigid, mute, uncommunicative, and unresponsive to all questions. She also ex-hibited facial grimacing. The severity and nature of her symptoms fluctuated over time. At times, she became excited, screaming continuously and seem-ing to be responding to auditory and visual hallucinations. At other times, she would be mute and rigid. She required total nursing care with intravenous feeding, catheterization, and four-point restraint (with both arms and legs re-strained so that she would not hurt herself). She received frequent sedation with intravenous lorazepam, a short-acting benzodiazepine. Because she was thought to have lupus cerebritis (a form of lupus that affects the brain), intravenous methylprednisolone, a steroid, was begun, but there was still no improvement in her clinical condition.

During the next 3 weeks, her condition deteriorated. Ms. Jarvis lost consid-erable weight, was unable to stand, and continued to require total nursing care. On day 28 she was referred for ECT, which is known to be effective in treating catatonia. After seven ECT treatments, she gradually responded, sought to feed herself and to stand, was more alert, and recognized her fam-ily. Rigidity was now only occasionally present. A lumbar puncture (spinal tap) demonstrated the presence of antineuronal antibodies in high titer, consistent with a diagnosis of central nervous system involvement with lupus.

Over the next few weeks, periods of lucidity alternated with rigidity, mut-ism, negativism, and staring. By day 90 of Ms. Jarvis's hospitalization, a sec-ond course of ECT was begun. After 10 treatments, she was verbal, euthymic (had normal mood), and cooperative. When seen a year later, she was without evidence of psychiatric disturbance: she was alert, oriented, cooperative, and fully capable of managing her home and taking care of her children. A repeat lumbar puncture revealed the absence of antineuronal antibodies in the cere-brospinal fluid.

Discussion of "Mute"

Before admission, Ms. Jarvis exhibited a number of features of Delirium (i.e., a neurocognitive disorder characterized by problems with attention, disorientation, agitation, incoherence, and delusional thinking; see Section 17.1). On admission, her condition quickly evolved into the clinical syndrome of Catatonia. She alternated between periods of catatonic negativism and stupor (body rigidity, mutism) and periods of catatonic excitement (agitation and psychotic symptoms).

Given Ms. Jarvis's history of lupus and her initial presentation with Delirium, the most likely etiology for the Catatonia in her case is the lupus, as was supported by the presence of antibodies in the cerebrospinal fluid obtained from the lumbar puncture. Because of the clinical significance of both the Delirium and the catatonic symptoms, the diagnosis would be Delirium Due to Systemic Lupus Erythematosus (DSM-5-TR, p. 672) and Catatonic Disorder Due to Systemic Lupus Erythematosus (DSM-5-TR, p. 136). Although Ms. Jarvis received an antipsychotic medication (haloperidol), which can sometimes cause catatonic symptoms, the persistence of the Catatonia long after the administration of haloperidol makes it unlikely that the medication was responsible for her catatonic symptoms. The initial agitation and delusions also suggest the possibility that a Bipolar Disorder With Catatonia might have accounted for the catatonic symptoms. However, the fluctuating course and the absence of other features suggesting a Manic Episode indicate that the catatonic symptoms are unlikely attributed to Bipolar Disorder.

Many instances of Catatonia resolve spontaneously. The intravenous administration of a short-acting sedative often resolves the symptoms, although usually only transiently. For some patients, the definitive treatment is ECT. In fact, regardless of the etiology, catatonic symptoms generally respond to ECT.

2.7
Substance/Medication-Induced Psychotic Disorder

A particularly important part of the diagnostic evaluation of psychotic symptoms is determining whether the symptoms are caused by the direct effects of a substance (an illicit drug or a medication) on a person's brain. This determination is important because of the impact on how such symptoms are managed. Typically, psychotic symptoms that are due to use of an illicit drug or medication will go away on their own once the substance is metabolized out of the person's system. Psychotic symptoms that are judged not to be exclusively attributed to an illicit drug almost always require treatment with antipsychotic medication.

A wide variety of substances are known to cause psychotic symptoms during either intoxication or withdrawal. Psychotic symptoms can occur during intoxication with alcohol; amphetamines and other stimulants such as cocaine; cannabis; hallucinogens; inhalants (e.g., glue and paint thinner); PCP and related compounds such as ketamine; and sedative, hypnotic, and anxiolytic medications. Symptoms also can develop during withdrawal from alcohol and from sedative, hypnotic, and anxiolytic medications. Note that some of the substances listed above (e.g., amphetamines; cannabis; ketamine; sedative, hypnotic, and anxiolytic medications) are prescribed for therapeutic use and can sometimes cause psychotic symptoms even if used as prescribed. The likelihood that a particular individual will develop psychotic symptoms from a particular substance depends both on the dosage (with higher doses being more likely to lead to psychotic symptoms) and individual susceptibility (certain individuals are more likely than others to develop psychotic symptoms when using certain substances).

In addition, a wide variety of other medications used as prescribed are known to cause psychotic symptoms. These include anesthetics and analgesics, anticholinergic agents, anticonvulsants, antihistamines, antihypertensive and cardiovascular medications, antimicrobial medications, antiparkinsonian medications, chemotherapeutic agents (e.g., cyclosporine, procarbazine), corticosteroids, gastrointestinal medications, muscle relaxants, nonsteroidal anti-inflammatory medications, other over-the-counter medications (e.g., phenylephrine, pseudoephedrine), and disulfiram. Toxins known to cause psychotic symptoms include anticholinesterase, organophosphate insecticides, sarin and other nerve gases, carbon monoxide, carbon dioxide, and volatile substances such as fuel or paint.

Figuring out the cause-and-effect relationship between drug or medication use and psychotic symptoms can be particularly challenging. In some cases, the psychotic symptoms can be explained entirely by the substance use—once the person stops using the substance, the psychotic symptoms remit, and the diagnosis of Substance/Medication-Induced Psychotic Disorder would apply. In other cases, someone with a preexisting psychotic disorder (albeit one that may not have been previously diagnosed) may be taking drugs for recreational purposes or as a way of self-medicating either a psychotic disorder or the side effects of prescribed medications.

Usually, the most telling indicator of whether the psychotic symptoms are due to drug or medication use is whether the person is experiencing psychotic symptoms at times other than when they are using the substance. For example, consider an agitated patient who is experiencing paranoid delusions and hearing voices, and who reports having recently taken a dose of PCP. If it is determined after further questioning that the psychotic symptoms either preceded the PCP use or persisted for a couple of weeks after stopping the PCP (well past the point at which the PCP would have been eliminated from the body), then the diagnosis would be Schizophrenia (e.g., if those criteria are met). However, if the patient had no history of psychotic symptoms occurring at times other than when they had taken PCP in the past and if the psychotic symptoms went away on their own a few days to a week after having taken the PCP, the clinician could conclude that this was a PCP-Induced Psychotic Disorder rather than say, Schizophrenia.

Some individuals who have no history of psychotic symptoms may develop psychotic symptoms during drug use that persist long after the drug has left their body. Such individuals are generally considered to have had a preexisting propensity to develop a psychotic disorder that is uncovered as a result of using the drug. Such cases are not considered to be Substance/Medication-Induced Psychotic Disorders, but instead would be diagnosed as a primary psychotic disorder, such as Schizophrenia.

Agitated Businessman

Jeffrey O'Hara, a 42-year-old married businessman, was admitted to the psychiatric service after a 2½-month period in which he found himself becoming increasingly distrustful of others and suspicious of his business associates. He had become convinced that there was a conspiracy among his coworkers to get him fired by setting up "fake accounts," which they were going to use to accuse him of embezzling money from his clients. He also believed that his colleagues were communicating among themselves about this plan by using hand signals. He was making inappropriately hostile and accusatory comments to his clients; he had, in fact, lost several business deals that had been "virtually sealed." Finally, the patient fired a shotgun into his backyard late one night when he heard noises that convinced him that intruders were about to break into his house and kill him.

One and a half years previously, Mr. O'Hara had been diagnosed as having Narcolepsy because of daily irresistible sleep attacks and episodes of sudden loss of muscle tone when he became emotionally excited, and he had begun taking an amphetamine-like stimulant, methylphenidate, a medication indicated for treatment of both Narcolepsy and Attention-Deficit/Hyperactivity Disorder. He became asymptomatic and was able to work quite effectively as the sales manager of a small ice-machine company and to participate in an active social life with his family and a small circle of friends.

In the 4 months before admission, Mr. O'Hara had been using increasingly larger doses of methylphenidate to maintain alertness late at night because of an increasing amount of work that could not be handled during the day. He reported that during this time, he often could feel his heart race and had trouble sitting still.

Discussion of "Agitated Businessman"

When Mr. O'Hara is admitted to the hospital, his symptomatic presentation of paranoid and referential delusions lasting 2½ months is consistent with a diagnosis of Delusional Disorder. Only when the patient's medication use is evaluated does it become clear that the correct diagnosis is a Methylphenidate-Induced Psychotic Disorder. Mr. O'Hara's symptoms of Narcolepsy had been successfully treated with methylphenidate for over 1½ years. Methylphenidate, a stimulant that is also a mainstay of treatment of Attention-Deficit/Hyperactivity Disorder, almost never causes psychotic symptoms when taken in normal doses. However, taking advantage of the drug's stimulant properties, Mr. O'Hara took increasingly larger doses on his own to help maintain alertness at night so that he could better handle his increasing workload. Although the medication may have had the positive benefit of improving his productivity, this benefit came with a serious catch—the development of paranoid delusions that resembled a diagnosis of Delusional Disorder. Given the lack of evidence that Mr. O'Hara had any preexisting psychotic disorder, the diagnosis is Methylphenidate-Induced Psychotic Disorder, With Onset During Intoxication (DSM-5-TR, p. 126), and the symptoms would be expected to quickly resolve once he stops taking the high doses of methylphenidate.

Threatening Voices

Gary Davis, a 44-year-old unemployed man, lived alone in a single-room occupancy hotel. He was brought to the emergency room by police to whom he had gone for help, complaining that he was frightened by hearing voices of men in the street below his window talking about him and threatening him with harm. When he looked out the window, the men had always "disappeared." The patient had a 20-year history of almost daily alcohol use, was commonly "drunk" each day, and often had experienced the "shakes" on awakening. On the previous day he had reduced his intake to 1 pint of vodka, because of gastrointestinal distress. He was fully alert and oriented (i.e., he knew the current date, where he was, and who he was) on mental status examination.

Discussion of "Threatening Voices"

In contrast to the previous case of paranoid delusions occurring during increased use of a stimulant, this case illustrates that psychotic symptoms (i.e., Mr. Davis's auditory hallucinations that are experienced as real) can occur as a result of a sudden reduction in the amount of substance used. Mr. Davis had been using large amounts of alcohol every day to the point of daily drunkenness. The fact that he develops the "shakes" on awakening is evidence that he has physiological dependence on alcohol. When such daily heavy alcohol use is interrupted—in Mr. Davis's case because of his gastrointestinal distress—some individuals can develop hallucinations. Because hallucinations (especially visual) can occur as part of delirium tremens (DTs), Alcohol Withdrawal Delirium must also be considered as a possible diagnosis (see "Thunderbird" in Section 17.1). Because Mr. Davis is alert and oriented during the examination, a diagnosis of Delirium (the hallmark of which is disorientation and a clouding of consciousness) is unlikely. Thus, the diagnosis would be Alcohol-Induced Psychotic Disorder, With Onset During Withdrawal (DSM-5-TR, p. 126).

2.8
Other Specified
Schizophrenia Spectrum
and Other Psychotic Disorder

Despite the wide variety of psychotic presentations provided in this chapter as examples of the specific DSM-5-TR Schizophrenia Spectrum and Other Psychotic Disorders, some psychotic presentations do not meet the diagnostic criteria for any of the disorders included in DSM-5-TR. Two such presentations are included below.

Bad Voices

Carmen Perez is an attractive 25-year-old divorced mother of two children. Ms. Perez was referred to a psychiatric emergency room by a psychiatrist who was treating her in an anxiety disorders clinic. After telling her doctor that she heard voices telling her to kill herself, and then assuring him that she would not act on the voices, Ms. Perez skipped her next appointment. Her doctor called her to say that if she did not voluntarily come to the emergency room for an evaluation, he would send the police for her.

Interviewed in the emergency room by a senior psychiatrist with a group of emergency room psychiatric residents and medical students, Ms. Perez was at times angry and insistent that she did not like to talk about her problems, and that the doctors would not believe her or help her anyway.

Ms. Perez first saw a psychiatrist 7 years previously, after the birth of her first child. At that time, she began to hear a voice commenting on her behavior and telling her to kill herself. She would not say exactly what the voice told her to do, but she reportedly drank nail polish remover in a suicide attempt. At that time, she remained in an emergency room for 2 days and received an unknown medication that reportedly helped quiet the voices. She did not return for an outpatient appointment after discharge and continued having intermittent auditory hallucinations at various points over the next 7 years. For example, often when she was near a window, a voice would tell her to jump out, and when she walked near traffic, it would tell her to walk in front of a car.

Ms. Perez reports that she continued to function well after that first episode, finishing high school and raising her children. She was divorced a year ago but refused to discuss her marital problems. About 2 months ago, she began to have trouble sleeping and felt "nervous." It was at this time that she responded to an advertisement for the anxiety disorders clinic. She was evaluated and given an antipsychotic medication. She claims that there was no change in the voices at that time, and only the insomnia and anxiety were new. Ms. Perez specifically denied depressed mood, anhedonia, and any change in appetite, but she did report that she was more tearful and lonely, and sometimes ruminated about "bad things," such as her father's attempted rape of her at age 14. Despite these symptoms, she continued working more than full time as a salesperson in a department store.

Ms. Perez says she did not keep her follow-up appointment at the anxiety disorders clinic because the antipsychotic medication was not helping her symptoms and was making her stiff and nauseated. She denied wanting to kill herself and cited how hard she was working to raise her children as evidence that she would not "leave them that way." She did not understand why her behavior had alarmed the psychiatrist.

Ms. Perez denied alcohol or drug use, and a toxicology screen for various drugs was negative. Physical examination and routine laboratory tests were also normal. She had stopped taking the antipsychotic medication on her own 2 days before the interview.

Following the interview, there was disagreement among the staff about whether to let Ms. Perez leave. It was finally decided to keep her overnight, until her mother could be seen the following day. When told she was to stay in the emergency room, she replied angrily: "Go ahead. You'll have to let me out sooner or later, but I don't have to talk to you if I don't want to." During the night, nursing staff noticed that she was tearful, but she said she did not know why she was crying.

When the mother was interviewed the following morning, she said she did not see a recent change in her daughter. She did not feel that Ms. Perez would hurt herself but agreed to stay with her for a few days and make sure she went for follow-up appointments. In the family meeting, Ms. Perez complained that her mother was unresponsive and did not help her enough. However, she again denied depression and said she enjoyed her job and her children. About the voices, she said that over time she had learned how to ignore them and that they did not bother her as much as they had at first. She agreed to outpatient treatment provided the therapist was a female.

Discussion of "Bad Voices"

Ms. Perez applied to the anxiety disorders clinic because of symptoms of increasing anxiety. The clinic doctor, however, was much more concerned about Ms. Perez's auditory hallucinations than she was and insisted Ms. Perez go to the psychiatric emergency department for immediate evaluation and treatment. His concern was understandable—voices telling a person to kill themself (a type of "command hallucination") are usually a serious red flag that the patient might be at risk of harming themself or others and thus may require immediate intervention. In this case, however, Ms. Perez does not consider the voices to be problematic. Although she did act on the voices once (by drinking nail polish remover), she has not acted on them since. Moreover, despite the intermittent voices, Ms. Perez has functioned relatively well: she has been raising her two children while working "more than full-time" as a salesperson in a department store. According to the patient, she has learned over the years to simply ignore the voices. Although chronic and prominent hallucinations certainly suggest a diagnosis of Schizophrenia, the absence of evidence of disorganization of personality, delusions, or deterioration in level of functioning rules out a diagnosis of that disorder. None of the other DSM-5-TR disorders included in this diagnostic class would apply either. Therefore, the most appropriate diagnosis for her symptoms would be Other Specified Schizophrenia Spectrum and Other Psychotic Disorder, Persistent Auditory Hallucinations (DSM-5-TR, p. 138).

There is considerable evidence that symptoms like auditory hallucinations occur on a continuum in the general population, with community surveys indicating that a significant portion of the general population have experienced at least one hallucinatory experience during their lifetime. Some individuals and advocacy groups (e.g., the Hearing Voices Movement) promote the notion that auditory hallucinations are not necessarily evidence of a mental disorder and suggest that hearing voices should be considered instead as a meaningful and understandable, although unusual, human variation. From this perspective, Ms. Perez's current auditory hallucinations would not be considered evidence of any mental disorder, in which case no diagnosis, except perhaps an Anxiety Disorder, would apply to her.

Sex Problem

Janine Birnbaum is a 43-year-old homemaker who seeks outpatient treatment with a chief complaint of being concerned about her "sex problem"; she states that she needs hypnotism to find out what is wrong with her sexual drive. Her husband, Joseph, supplied the history: He complained that she had had many extramarital affairs, with many different men, all through their married life. He insisted that in one 2-week period, she had as many as 100 different sexual experiences with men outside the marriage. The patient herself agreed with this assessment of her behavior but would not speak of the experiences, saying that she "blocks out" the memories. She denied any particular interest in sexuality but said that, apparently, she felt a compulsive drive to go out and seek sexual activity despite her lack of interest.

Mrs. Birnbaum had been married to her husband for over 20 years. He was clearly the dominant partner in the marriage. The patient was fearful of his frequent jealous rages, and apparently it was he who suggested that she see a psychiatrist to receive hypnosis. The patient maintained that she could not explain why she sought out other men and that she really did not want to do this. Her husband stated that on occasion he had tracked her down, and when he had found her, she acted as if she did not know him. She confirmed this and believed it was due to the fact that the episodes of her sexual promiscuity were blotted out by "amnesia." When the psychiatrist indicated that he questioned the reality of the wife's sexual adventures, the husband became furious and accused the psychiatrist of having sexual relations with her.

Neither hypnosis nor psychotherapy with Mrs. Birnbaum was able to clear her "blocked-out" memory of periods of sexual activities. The patient did admit to a memory of having had two extramarital relationships in the past: the first was 20 years before the time of this evaluation, and the other was just a year before she sought treatment. She stated that the last one had actually been planned by her husband and that he was in the same house at the time. She continued to believe that she had actually had countless extramarital sexual experiences, although she remembered only those two.

Discussion of "Sex Problem"

The clinician's first impression of Mrs. Birnbaum might be that Dissociative Amnesia (see Section 8.2), Neurocognitive Disorder Due to Another Medical Condition (see DSM-5-TR, p. 729), or Substance Use Disorder (see Chapter 16) should be considered to explain Mrs. Birnbaum's episodes of memory loss. However, the plot thickens as evidence accumulates that the husband, the chief informant, has delusional jealousy, believing that his wife is repeatedly unfaithful to him. Apparently, under his influence, his wife has accepted this delusional belief, explaining her lack of memory of the events by believing that she has "amnesia." It would seem that Mrs. Birnbaum has adopted her husband's delusional system and does not really have any kind of "amnesia." This rare shared condition, historically referred to as *folie à deux*, is represented in DSM-5-TR as a "delusional syndrome in the context of a relationship with an individual with prominent delusions" and is not a specific psychotic disorder but is listed as an example of Other Specified Schizophrenia Spectrum and Other Psychotic Disorder (DSM-5-TR, p. 138). This syndrome involves the transfer of delusions from one person (in this case, the husband with delusional jealousy) to another (his wife). In the most common form of this syndrome, the individual who first has the delusions is chronically ill and is typically the influential member of the close relationship with another individual, who is more suggestible and develops the delusion too. The second individual is frequently less intelligent, more gullible, more passive, or more lacking in self-esteem than the primary individual. If the person with the shared delusion is separated from the individual with the primary delusion, the second individual may abandon the delusion.

CHAPTER 3

Bipolar and Related Disorders

Bipolar and Related Disorders are all characterized by mood instability, with periods of abnormally high mood and periods of abnormally low mood. Periods of elevated or euphoric mood are what distinguish the disorders discussed in this chapter from the Depressive Disorders (Chapter 4), which involve only periods of depression.

DSM-5-TR includes two types of episodes involving persistently elevated, euphoric, or irritable mood: Manic Episodes and Hypomanic Episodes. The predominant mood in a Manic or Hypomanic Episode is classically euphoric or expansive, which the individual might describe as feeling "high" or "on top of the world." For some people, the mood change is better characterized as a sustained feeling of being irritable, on edge, impatient, and easily angered. In either case, for the mood to be considered characteristic of a Manic or Hypomanic Episode, it must be accompanied by increased activity or energy, in which the person may describe themself as being "hyper" or "wired." The requirement in DSM-5-TR that the elevated or irritable mood be accompanied by increased activity or energy helps to distinguish a Manic or Hypomanic Episode from "normal" periods of euphoria or irritability that might occur, (e.g., the euphoria during the initial phases of falling in love, irritability in someone in a fraught relationship).

Both Manic and Hypomanic Episodes are characterized by the presence of a "syndrome"—that is, a group of symptoms that characteristically co-occur together. From a strictly symptomatic perspective, Manic Episodes and Hypomanic Episodes are defined by the exact same set of symptoms, yet differ in terms of requirements for minimum duration (at least 1 week for a Manic Episode and at least 4 days for a Hypomanic Episode) and requirements for the degree to which the symptoms impair the person's functioning, as noted in Manic Episode Criterion C and Hypomanic Episode Criterion E (both further described in next paragraph). In addition to the elevated, euphoric, or irritable mood along with increased activity or energy, the syndrome includes an additional seven symptoms, at least three of which much be present (or four if the mood is irritable but not euphoric). Particularly common is increased self-esteem, which can range from uncritical self-confidence to marked grandiosity, and in some people may reach delusional proportions, such as when a previously nonreligious person believes they are on a divine mission to warn the world about an impending apocalypse. Also common is a decreased need for sleep, in which the person feels totally rested after getting hardly any sleep. Other characteristic symptoms include being much more talkative than usual to the point where it may be difficult for others to get a word in edgewise, as well as a phenomenon known as *flight of ideas,* in which there is a nearly continuous flow of rapid speech that jumps from topic to topic, usually based on discernible associations or plays on words, but in severe cases is so rapid as to be disorganized and incoherent. Many individuals with Manic or Hypomanic Episodes experience their thoughts racing through their heads. They may become very distracted by extraneous stimuli in the environment so that, for example, their attention is repeatedly drawn away by sounds coming from outside the room. Individuals in a Manic or Hypomanic Episode are usually much more active than is usual for them in multiple areas of life, including in social situations, at work (in which the person's productivity skyrockets), at home (e.g., taking on long-ignored repair projects), or sexually. For some, this increased activity is expressed as extreme motor restlessness in which they are unable to be still. One of the most damaging symptoms is the propensity toward engaging in reckless behavior without regard to potential negative consequences, such as impulsive sexual indiscretions, engaging in lavish spending sprees, abusing alcohol or drugs, or making impulsive, ill-advised business decisions.

Manic Episodes and Hypomanic Episodes differ, however, in terms of the minimum required duration and by their impact on the person's functioning. To meet the requirements for a Manic Episode, the elevated or irritable mood along with the increased energy or activity, must have been present for most of the day, nearly every day, for at least 1 week, whereas in a Hypomanic Episode, the symptoms need only to have been present for 4 consecutive days. Because most Manic or Hypomanic Episodes last longer than a week, the main differentiating factor is the symptomatic impact on the person's ability to function. To meet criteria for a Manic Episode, the symptoms must be sufficiently severe so as to cause marked impairment in social or occupational functioning (e.g., getting fired from a job because of poor business decisions, seriously damaging a relationship because of sexual indiscretions fueled by manic hypersexuality, going seriously into debt because of reckless overspending). Alternatively, the presence of delusions or hallucinations during the episode (e.g., the individual's unassailable conviction that they have discovered a cure for all forms of cancer) or if the person needs to be hospitalized (usually involuntarily) to prevent harm to self or to others would also justify the diagnosis of a Manic Episode. In contrast, symptoms in a Hypomanic Episode by definition cannot be so severe as to cause marked impairment or necessitate hospitalization.

The following disorders are included in the Bipolar and Related Disorders grouping in DSM-5-TR (see Table 3–1 for summary definitions): Bipolar I Disorder, requiring the presence of at least one Manic Episode (which may have been preceded or followed by one or more Major Depressive Episodes or Hypomanic Episodes); Bipolar II Disorder, requiring at least one Hypomanic Episode and one Major Depressive Episode but no Manic Episodes; Cyclothymic Disorder, characterized by numerous

TABLE 3–1.	Characteristic features of Bipolar and Related Disorders
Disorders	**Key characteristics**
Bipolar I Disorder	At least one Manic Episode that may have been preceded by or followed by Hypomanic or Major Depressive Episodes
Bipolar II Disorder	At least one Hypomanic Episode and one Major Depressive Episode
Cyclothymic Disorder	Numerous periods with hypomanic symptoms that do not meet criteria for a Hypomanic Episode
	Numerous periods of depressive symptoms that do not meet criteria for a Major Depressive Episode
	Present more days than not for at least 2 years; criteria have never been met for a Major Depressive, Manic, or Hypomanic Episode
Substance/Medication-Induced Bipolar and Related Disorder	Prominent and persistent elevated, expansive, or irritable mood due to the direct effects of a substance or medication on the central nervous system
Bipolar and Related Disorder Due to Another Medical Condition	Prominent and persistent elevated, expansive, or irritable mood that is the direct physiological consequence of a nonpsychiatric medical condition, such as hyperthyroidism or traumatic brain injury

periods of hypomanic symptoms and depressive symptoms, none of which are severe enough to be considered Manic, Hypomanic, or Major Depressive Episodes; Substance/Medication-Induced Bipolar and Related Disorder; and Bipolar and Related Disorder Due to Another Medical Condition. Cases have been included in this chapter to illustrate each of these conditions, with the exception of Bipolar and Related Disorder Due to Another Medical Condition.

3.1
Bipolar I Disorder

Bipolar I Disorder (in the past referred to as "manic-depressive illness") is a mood disorder that in most people is characterized by multiple Manic, Hypomanic, and Major Depressive Episodes over the person's lifetime. The name of the condition, which implies both pathological highs and pathological lows, is actually a misnomer because all that is required is a single Manic Episode. Most patients, however, have had multiple Manic Episodes as well as one or more Major Depressive Episodes, and all patients at least temporarily experience hypomanic stages before they progress to a full Manic Episode. The Major Depressive Episodes in Bipolar I Disorder are symptomatically identical to those seen in Major Depressive Disorder (DSM-5-TR, p. 183) and are characterized by periods of depressed mood or loss of interest or pleasure for at least 2 weeks, accompanied by changes in appetite or weight (either increased or decreased), sleeping too little or too much, psychomotor agitation or retardation, low energy and activity, feelings of guilt or worthlessness, difficulty concentrating, and thoughts of suicide.

For many individuals with Bipolar I Disorder, the diagnosis is heralded by the onset of a Manic Episode that may be severe enough to require hospitalization. For other individuals, the disorder begins with one or more Major Depressive Episodes without any previous history of Manic or Hypomanic Episodes, making it appear for quite some time (maybe even years) that the correct diagnosis is Major Depressive Disorder rather than Bipolar I Disorder. It is only when the first Manic Episode develops that the diagnosis is changed from Major Depressive Disorder to Bipolar I Disorder, which almost invariably entails a change in both treatment (i.e., use of mood-stabilizing rather than antidepressant medication) and prognosis. For some of these individuals, the Manic Episode may have been triggered by antidepressant medication or another somatic treatment used to treat the depression, such as bright light therapy or electroconvulsive therapy (ECT). In such cases, the manic symptoms persist at a fully syndromal level well beyond the point at which the physiological effects of the treatment should have worn off. Individuals with Manic Episodes that occur only in the context of treatment are nonetheless considered to have Bipolar I Disorder, under the assumption that the depression treatment caused a Manic Episode to emerge in someone who was already predisposed to develop Bipolar I Disorder.

On the other hand, manic-like episodes not necessarily indicative of Bipolar I Disorder can occur in individuals as a result of intoxication with certain substances, such as amphetamines or cocaine, or as a side effect of certain prescribed medications, such as steroids or stimulant drugs, or can be caused by a nonpsychiatric medical condition such as a brain tumor. Such manic-like episodes do not count toward a diagnosis of Bipolar I Disorder and instead should be diagnosed as either Substance/Medication-Induced Bipolar and Related Disorder or Bipolar and Related Disorder Due to Another Medical Condition.

Although the prototypical presentation of Bipolar I Disorder consists of recurrent episodes of mania and depression, there is considerable diagnostic heterogeneity from case to case with respect to the temporal pattern of the episodes and the symptomatic presentation of the type of episode with which the patient is currently presenting. This heterogeneity is indicated in the DSM-5-TR diagnosis by the use of diagnostic specifiers (diagnostic terms that are added after the name of the diagnosis; e.g., "Bipolar I Disorder, Current Episode Manic, Moderate, With Rapid Cycling"), each of which has particular treatment or prognostic implications:

- Among the most clinically important specifiers are those indicating the type of episode that is the focus of current treatment—that is, whether the person is currently presenting for treatment in the context of an active Manic, Hypomanic, or Major Depressive Episode—because current management needs are quite different for someone who is actively manic versus someone who is depressed.
- Other specifiers are used to indicate clinically relevant aspects of the current episode that may also be useful in guiding management decisions. For example, the

presence of delusions or hallucinations during the episode—indicated by the specifier With Psychotic Features—generally suggests the need for antipsychotic medications as part of the current treatment. Less commonly, individuals in a Manic Episode may experience periods of Catatonia (indicated by the specifier With Catatonia), which is a marked psychomotor disturbance characterized by decreased motor activity, decreased engagement during the interview or physical examination, or excessive and peculiar motor activity (see Section 2.6). Symptoms of anxiety commonly co-occur during Manic, Hypomanic, and Major Depressive Episodes and can be indicated using the specifier With Anxious Distress (see "A Perfect Checklist" in Section 4.2). The presence of severe co-occurring anxiety symptoms is particularly noteworthy because they can increase the risk for suicide. Some individuals experience a mixture of both depressive and manic symptoms during the same episode. The specifier With Mixed Features applies to Manic Episodes that have commingling symptoms more characteristic of a depressive episode, such as periods of intense sadness and feelings of worthlessness, or to Major Depressive Episodes that have commingling symptoms of mania, such as inflated self-esteem or grandiosity (see "The Mixed-Up Waiter" in Section 4.2).

- Certain specifiers (i.e., With Melancholic Features and With Atypical Features) apply only if the person is currently experiencing a Major Depressive Episode (see Section 4.2 for descriptions of these specifiers and illustrative cases—"Stonemason" and "It's Typical," respectively).

- Other specifiers are available for indicating the severity of the current episode (Mild, Moderate, or Severe), and whether the person's condition is currently In Partial Remission (i.e., no longer in an episode but still mildly symptomatic) or In Full Remission (i.e., free of symptoms but typically in need of maintenance treatment to prevent future recurrence of episodes).

- Finally, specifiers are available to indicate certain varieties of Bipolar Disorder that have particular treatment implications, such as regular onset of episodes during particular seasons of the year, which suggests the likely efficacy of morning exposure to bright light. The specifier With Rapid Cycling refers to a particularly severe form of Bipolar I and Bipolar II Disorder in which the person has had four or more Manic, Hypomanic, or Major Depressive Episodes within the past year. The specifier With Peripartum Onset applies to episodes with onset during pregnancy or within the 4 weeks following delivery. Finally, the specifier With Seasonal Pattern applies to episodes that regularly occur during the same particular time of the year (e.g., Manic Episodes occurring regularly in the springtime, or Major Depressive Episodes occurring regularly in the wintertime).

Many individuals with Bipolar I Disorder return to a fully functional level between episodes, although approximately 30% of patients continue to show severe impairment in work role functioning. Typically, the mean age at onset of the first Manic, Hypomanic, or Major Depressive Episode is approximately 18 years, but onset can start during childhood, as well as in individuals in their 60s or 70s. The 12-month prevalence of Bipolar I Disorder in the United States is around 1.5%. Bipolar I Disorder is equally common in men and women, which is in contrast to Major Depressive Disorder, for which rates in women are twice as high as in men. The lifetime risk of suicide in individuals with Bipolar I Disorder is estimated to be 20–30 times greater than in the general population. Co-occurring mental disorders are the norm in Bipolar I Disorder with Anxiety Disorders, Alcohol and Other Substance Use Disorders, and Attention-Deficit/Hyperactivity Disorder co-occurring most frequently.

Radar Messages

Alice Braverman, a 24-year-old copy editor who recently moved from Colorado to New York, comes to a psychiatrist for help in continuing her treatment with a mood-stabilizing medication, lithium carbonate. She describes how she was a successful college student in her senior year 3 years previously, doing well academically and enjoying a large circle of friends of both sexes. In the midst of an uneventful period in the first semester, she began to feel depressed; experienced loss of appetite, with a weight loss of about 10 pounds; had difficulty falling asleep; and was waking several hours earlier than she wanted to.

After about 2 months, these problems appeared to go away, but she then began to feel increasingly energetic, requiring only 2–4 hours of sleep at night, and to experience her thoughts as "racing." She started to see symbolic meanings in things, especially sexual meanings, and began to suspect that innocent comments on TV shows were referring to her. Over the next month, she became increasingly euphoric, irritable, and overly talkative. She started to believe that there was a hole in her head through which radar messages were being sent to her. These messages could control her thoughts or produce emotions of anger, sadness, and the like, that were beyond her control. She also believed that her thoughts could be read by people around her and that alien thoughts from other people were intruding themselves via the radar into her own head. She described hearing voices, which sometimes spoke about her in the third person and at other times ordered her to perform various acts, particularly sexual ones.

Her friends, concerned about Ms. Braverman's unusual behavior, took her to a hospital emergency department, where she was evaluated and admitted to a psychiatric inpatient unit. After a day of observation, a clinician prescribed for her an antipsychotic medication, olanzapine, and a mood-stabilizing medication, lithium carbonate. Over the course of about 3 weeks, Ms. Braverman experienced a fairly rapid reduction in all of the symptoms that had brought her to the hospital. The olanzapine was gradually reduced and then discontinued. She was maintained thereafter on lithium carbonate alone, with the goal of preventing future episodes. At the time of her discharge, after 6 weeks of hospitalization, she was exhibiting none of the symptoms reported on admission, but she was noted to be experiencing some mild hypersomnia, sleeping about 10 hours a night, and had loss of appetite and some feeling of being "slowed down," which was worse in the mornings. She was discharged to live with some friends.

Approximately 8 months after her discharge, Ms. Braverman was feeling back to her normal self and stopped taking the lithium carbonate because she did not feel she needed it and did not like the side effects (hand tremor, thirst, and recurrent diarrhea). She continued to do fairly well for the next few months, but then she began to experience a gradual reappearance of symptoms similar to those that had necessitated her hospitalization, such as needing less sleep and being more talkative than usual. The symptoms worsened, and after 2 weeks, she was readmitted to the hospital with almost the identical psychotic symptoms that she had had when first admitted.

Ms. Braverman responded in days to treatment with olanzapine and lithium carbonate, and again the olanzapine was gradually discontinued, leaving her on lithium carbonate alone. As with the first hospitalization, at the time of her discharge, a little more than a year ago, she again displayed some hypersomnia, loss of appetite, and the feeling of being "slowed down." During the past year, she has continued to take lithium, periodically seeing her psychiatrist so that her serum lithium level is monitored to ensure that it stays within the therapeutic range of 0.6 to 1.2 mEq/L. While continuing to take lithium, she has been symptom-free and functioning fairly well, getting a job in publishing and recently moving to New York to advance her career.

Ms. Braverman's father, when in his 40s, had had a severe episode of depression, characterized by sleeping too much, loss of appetite, being profoundly slowed down, and suicidal ideation. Her paternal grandmother had died by suicide during what also appeared to be a depressive episode.

Discussion of "Radar Messages"

Ms. Braverman was functioning at a high level in college when she developed a 2-month period of subthreshold depressive symptoms (subthreshold in the sense that her three symptoms were not enough to meet the minimum five-symptom requirement for a Major Depressive Episode), which was followed shortly by an episode with characteristic manic symptoms: euphoric and irritable mood, increased energy and activity, decreased need for sleep, pressured speech, and the subjective experience that her thoughts were racing. At the height of the episode, Ms. Braverman developed bizarre delusions (her emotions and thoughts were being controlled by radar messages sent through a hole in her head) and auditory hallucinations (both command hallucinations and voices speaking about her in the third person). Even though these kinds of bizarre psychotic symptoms are more typically characteristic of the active phase of Schizophrenia (see "Under Surveillance" in Section 2.1), in Ms. Braverman's case they are considered part of her Bipolar I Disorder because they occur exclusively during the manic mood disturbance. Given that her psychotic symptoms were not consistent with the typical manic themes of grandiosity and invulnerability, her psychotic symptoms would be considered "mood incongruent." At this stage of her history, her diagnosis would be Bipolar I Disorder, Current Episode Manic, Severe, With Mood-Incongruent Psychotic Features, In Full Remission.

In the absence of any evidence of a substance (such as a stimulant) or a non-psychiatric medical condition (such as hyperthyroidism) that could have been directly causing the mood disturbance, Ms. Braverman's symptoms meet criteria for a Manic Episode. The occurrence of Manic Episodes, even without any Major Depressive Episode, is sufficient to meet the DSM-5-TR criteria for Bipolar I Disorder (DSM-5-TR, p. 139). Even during Ms. Braverman's "down" periods after the Manic Episodes, during which she sleeps excessively, loses her appetite, and feels slowed down, there are not enough symptoms to be considered evidence of a Major Depressive Episode.

Her diagnosis after 6 months of being symptom free is Bipolar I Disorder, Most Recent Episode Manic, With Mood-Incongruent Psychotic Features, In Full Remission (DSM-5-TR, p. 143), which reflects the fact that the most recent episode of mood disturbance that necessitated Ms. Braverman's second hospitalization was also a Manic Episode during which mood-incongruent psychotic features were present. Moreover, at the time of her follow-up visits, because Ms. Braverman has been essentially free of symptoms for at least 6 months (while taking lithium carbonate as a preventive measure), she is currently considered to be in full remission.

Triple Divorcée

Sandra Kovacs, a 37-year-old thrice-divorced woman who works as a paralegal in a prestigious law firm, was hospitalized in a psychiatric hospital because of an attempt to end her life by taking an overdose of sleeping pills. She reported that about 3 months ago, after her chronic mild depression had gotten worse, her psychiatrist switched her antidepressant from citalopram, a selective serotonin reuptake inhibitor, to duloxetine, a selective serotonin-norepinephrine reuptake inhibitor. Within a few weeks of starting the new medication, Ms. Kovacs reported feeling more energetic and confident at work, and requested additional assignments from the law partners. Feeling like she no longer needed to be on an antidepressant, she discontinued the duloxetine without telling her psychiatrist. Over the next several weeks, she continued to feel like she was "on Cloud 9," felt that her thoughts were racing, and found that she could get by on only a couple of hours of sleep. She regularly stayed at work until midnight and went into the office on weekends as well.

Ms. Kovacs reported that "everything came to a head" at a retirement party for one of the partners at the law firm, 3 days before her hospital admission. She went to the party feeling wired, hyper, and "super sexual." She was telling racy jokes in a loud boisterous voice and speaking very rapidly. She ended up "coming on" to the husband of her boss; she even wrote her telephone number down on a napkin, gave it to him, and insisted that he call her after the party. When she groggily woke up the next morning, she realized what she had done and felt that she could never go back to the office and face anyone. Despondent over having ruined the best job she ever had, she took the entire bottle of antidepressant pills along with a bottle of sleeping pills. Ms. Kovacs had planned to meet her mother for brunch the next morning, but when she did not show up and failed to respond to repeated telephone calls, her mother went to her apartment, where she found her daughter and called 911.

Ms. Kovacs reported that she has suffered from episodes of depression since her 20s. Her first episode, at age 23, had been triggered by marital separation, but she could suggest no explanation for subsequent episodes—"I just seem to sink into a gloomy despair." Although her depression responds at least partially to treatment, with her mood lifting to the point where she can go back to work and function fairly normally, her mood never completely gets better, and she also feels at least somewhat depressed between episodes. Over the years she has received intermittent individual psychotherapy as well as small doses of all kinds of antidepressant medications. She has not had any prior episodes of elevated or irritable mood but notes that her maternal uncle had been diagnosed with "manic depression" and was in and out of psychiatric hospitals for much of his life.

Discussion of "Triple Divorcée"

From ages 23 to 37, Ms. Kovacs' mood disturbance resembled Persistent Depressive Disorder (DSM-5-TR, p. 193), punctuated by episodes in which her mood got much worse. Recently, after a switch to duloxetine, Ms. Kovacs developed a full-blown Manic Episode with euphoric mood, increased energy and activity, increased self-esteem, decreased need for sleep, rapid speech, racing thoughts, and poor judgment. Even though Ms. Kovacs' episode began shortly after starting the antidepressant duloxetine, the episode is not considered to be a drug-induced mania, as can happen in some people after taking stimulants like cocaine. In drug-induced mania cases, the manic-like symptoms remit once the drug is out of the person's body. In Ms. Kovacs' case, her manic symptoms persisted long beyond the time that the duloxetine was out of her system (typically 4–5 days after stopping) and thus is considered to be indicative of an underlying Bipolar I Disorder, which was "brought out" by the duloxetine; the assumption is that individuals without a propensity to develop Bipolar Disorder would not develop Manic Episodes when exposed to antidepressant treatment. Given that Ms. Kovacs was experiencing six of the seven symptoms of a Manic Episode (everything except distractibility) and that her judgment was clearly impaired, the severity of the Manic Episode would be considered Moderate (DSM-5-TR, p. 139). Thus, the diagnosis for Ms. Kovacs is Bipolar I Disorder, Current Episode Manic, Moderate.

Roller Coaster

When Ernest Eaton's desperate wife finally got him to agree to a comprehensive inpatient evaluation, he was 39 years old and had been unemployed and essentially nonfunctional for several years. After a week during which he was partying all night and shopping all day, his wife said that she would leave him if he did not check into a psychiatric hospital. The admitting psychiatrist found him to be a fast-talking, jovial, seductive man, with no evidence of delusions or hallucinations.

Mr. Eaton's troubles began 7 years earlier, when he was working as an insurance adjuster. He had a few months of mild, intermittent depressive symptoms, anxiety, fatigue, insomnia, and loss of appetite. At the time he attributed these symptoms to stress at work, and within a few months he was back to his usual self.

A few years later, a physician noted an asymptomatic thyroid mass during a routine physical examination. One month after removal of the mass, a papillary cyst, Mr. Eaton noted dramatic mood changes. Twenty-five days of remarkable energy, hyperactivity, and euphoria were followed by 5 days of depression, during which he slept a lot and felt that he could hardly move. This pattern of alternating periods of elation and depression, apparently with few "normal" days, repeated itself almost continuously over the following years.

During his energetic periods, Mr. Eaton was euphoric, optimistic, and self-confident, but also short-tempered and easily irritated. He functioned well on only a couple of hours of sleep per night and sometimes he did not sleep at all for several days at a time. He spoke very rapidly, and people complained that they had trouble getting a word in edgewise during conversations. His judgment at work was erratic. He spent large sums of money on unnecessary and, for him, uncharacteristic purchases that he could not afford, such as a high-priced surround-sound system and several Doberman Pinschers. He also had several impulsive sexual flings. During his depressed periods, he often stayed in bed all day because of fatigue, lack of motivation, and depressed mood. He felt guilty about the irresponsibility and excesses of his prior several weeks. He stopped eating, bathing, and shaving. After several days of this withdrawal, Mr. Eaton would rise from bed one morning feeling better and within 2 days be back at work, often working feverishly, though ineffectively, to catch up on work he had let slide during his depressed periods.

Although both Mr. Eaton and his wife denied that he used any substances other than when he binged on alcohol during his hyperactive periods, he was dismissed from his job 5 years ago because his supervisor was convinced that his overactivity must have been due to drug use. His wife has been supporting him financially ever since then.

When he finally agreed to a psychiatric evaluation 2 years ago, Mr. Eaton was minimally cooperative and noncompliant with several medications that were prescribed, including lithium carbonate, sodium valproate (an anticonvulsant medication that also works as a mood stabilizer), and antidepressant medications. His mood swings continued with few interruptions up to the current hospitalization.

In the hospital, his physical examination, blood chemistry, blood cell counts, MRI of his brain, and cognitive testing were unremarkable. After a week, he switched to his characteristic depressive state.

After 3 weeks in the hospital, Mr. Eaton's mood was stable on sodium valproate. He left the hospital, very quickly found a new job, and did well for the following year. Feeling well, he decided that he did not need the medication and stopped taking the sodium valproate. Within weeks he became extremely manic and had to be hospitalized again.

Discussion of "Roller Coaster"

The diagnosis of Bipolar I Disorder, Current Episode Manic, is not difficult to make in Mr. Eaton's case (DSM-5-TR, p. 139). In his energetic periods, Mr. Eaton had the characteristic symptoms of a Manic Episode: decreased need for sleep, overactivity, overtalkativeness, and excessive involvement in pleasurable activities without thinking of the consequences (overspending, sexual flings). In his depressed periods, his presentation met the symptomatic criteria but not the duration (2-week) criterion for Major Depressive Episodes. Even though his current Manic Episode resulted in his being hospitalized, it does not appear that almost continual supervision was required in order to "prevent harm to self or others" (DSM-5-TR, p. 175), which is required for the Manic Episode to be considered Severe. Thus, the current severity is most appropriately considered Moderate. Because Mr. Eaton had more than four episodes of mania in a 1-year period, separated by brief periods of depression, the specifier With Rapid Cycling applies to his Bipolar I Disorder diagnosis (DSM-5-TR, p. 143).

Not all persons with rapid cycling experience predictable shifts from mania to depression without intervening periods of euthymia (normal mood), as did Mr. Eaton. Rapid cycling usually involves one or more Manic or Hypomanic Episodes, as in this case, but is also diagnosed if all of the episodes are depressed, manic, or hypomanic, as long as they are separated by periods of remission (or switches to the opposite pole).

Mr. Eaton's unusual behavior was attributed to drug use by his employers. It is not uncommon for such an erratic mood pattern to be mistakenly identified as evidence of drug abuse, which should also be part of the differential diagnosis when rapid cycling is being considered. Mr. Eaton's presentation is somewhat atypical in that the rapid cycling form of Bipolar Disorder is much more common in women. Because of high rates of nonresponse to lithium, rapid cycling is often treated with anticonvulsant medications, such as sodium valproate, which was effective for Mr. Eaton.

Wealthy Widow

Anne Kettering, a wealthy 72-year-old widow, is referred for psychiatric evaluation by her children, against her will, because they think she has become "senile" since the death of her husband 6 months previously. After the initial bereavement, which was not particularly severe, Mrs. Kettering had resumed an active social life and become a volunteer at local hospitals. Her family had encouraged this activity, but over the past 3 months, her sons have become concerned about her going to local bars with some of the hospital staff. The referral was precipitated by her announcing her engagement to a 25-year-old male nurse, to whom she planned to turn over her house and a large amount of money. Mrs. Kettering's three sons, by threat and intimidation, have made her accompany them to this psychiatric evaluation. While listening to one of the sons, the psychiatrist also overheard the patient accusing the other two of trying to commit her so they can get their hands on her money.

Initially in the interview, Mrs. Kettering is extremely angry at her sons and the psychiatrist, insisting that they do not understand that for the first time in her life she is doing something for herself, not for her father, her husband, or her children. She then suddenly drapes herself over the couch and asks the psychiatrist if she is attractive enough to capture a 25-year-old man. She proceeds to elaborate on her fiancé's physique and sexual abilities and describes her life as exciting and fulfilling for the first time. She is overtalkative and repeatedly refuses to allow the psychiatrist to interrupt her with questions. She says that she goes out nightly with her fiancé to clubs and bars and that although she does not drink, she thoroughly enjoys the atmosphere. They often go on to an after-hours place and end up breakfasting, going to bed, and making love. After only 3–4 hours of sleep, she gets up, feeling refreshed, and then goes shopping. She spends about $2,000 a week on herself and gives her fiancé about $1,500 a week, all of which she can easily afford.

Mrs. Kettering agrees that her behavior is unusual for someone of her age and social position, but she states she has always been conventional and now is the time to change, before it is too late. She refuses to participate in formal testing of her mental status, saying, "I'm not going to do any stupid tests to see if I am sane." She has no obvious memory impairment and is correctly oriented to time (she knows the current date), to place (she knows she is in a psychiatrist's office), and to person (she is able to state her name). According to the family, she has no previous history of emotional disturbance.

Discussion of "Wealthy Widow"

As the story unfolds, the clinician might wonder whether Mrs. Kettering is suffering only from avaricious children rather than a mental disorder. It does seem, however, that her alternately irritable and expansive mood, pressured speech, decreased need for sleep, and poor judgment (her plan to sign her house over to someone she has met only recently) represent more than a new start in life for someone who has been too "conventional." In fact, all of these symptoms suggest a Manic or Hypomanic Episode, in the absence of a nonpsychiatric medical condition, a substance responsible for the disturbance, or a non-mood Psychotic Disorder (e.g., Delusional Disorder). In a Manic Episode, there is marked impairment in occupational functioning or usual activities or relationships with others. In a Hypomanic Episode, there is an unequivocal change in functioning observable by others, but marked impairment is not present. Even though Mrs. Kettering is wealthy, her plan to sign her house over to her new lover does represent marked impairment in her relationships with others (although she would disagree with this statement). DSM-5-TR offers three levels of severity to choose from based on symptom severity and degree of impairment: Mild (minimum symptom criteria are met for a Manic Episode), Moderate (very significant increase in activity or impairment in judgment), or Severe (almost continual supervision is required in order to prevent physical harm to self or others). In Mrs. Kettering's case, although her symptoms are severe and markedly impair her functioning, they are not putting her or others at risk of physical harm. Thus, the diagnosis is Bipolar I Disorder, Current Episode Manic, Moderate (DSM-5-TR, p. 139). The first appearance of Bipolar I Disorder at age 72 is certainly uncommon. The clinician would want to be careful to rule out the possibility of a nonpsychiatric medical condition, such as a brain tumor or degenerative central nervous system disorder such as Alzheimer's disease, that might be causing a manic-like episode, in which case the diagnosis would be Bipolar and Related Disorder Due to Another Medical Condition. Although Mrs. Kettering appears to be cognitively intact and to have nothing in her history suggesting the presence of a nonpsychiatric medical condition, the onset of such an episode in someone of her age is often indicative of an underlying medical etiology. Because a medical workup to rule out an etiologically related nonpsychiatric medical condition has not yet been done, the diagnosis of Bipolar I Disorder should be considered provisional until the workup is complete.

Praying Athlete

When brought to the emergency room, Dion Robinson, a 24-year-old graduate student, was completely mute and rigid, resisting all attempts to be moved. The friends who had brought him stated that he was playing basketball with them at the student athletic building when he suddenly bent over and put his head down to the floor, made sounds as if he were praying, and became "frozen" in that position for about 15 minutes. Unable to rouse him, his friends called the campus police, who brought him to the emergency room. When interviewed an hour later, Mr. Robinson would only say, "I am communicating directly with Allah."

According to his friends, Mr. Robinson had been getting "hyper" recently, but they emphatically denied that he either used drugs or drank to excess. A call to his girlfriend, whose name and number were provided by his friends, revealed the following: Mr. Robinson had been doing well, with no evidence of unusual behavior, until 1 week before being brought to the emergency department by his friends. He had been living with his girlfriend, going to school, and working at a part-time job. About 1 week ago, he began talking almost nonstop about the "Five Pillars of Islam," which was unusual for him as he previously had no interest in religion. He also stopped sleeping at night and became sexually demanding of his girlfriend. He had begun working out even more than usual at the gym to "burn off excess energy." His girlfriend said that he had had similar symptoms when he was hospitalized 1 year ago; at that time, he left the hospital against medical advice without receiving any follow-up treatment and had become increasingly depressed over the next 3 months. He withdrew from social activities at school and would spend up to 14 hours a day sleeping. At just the point when his girlfriend had decided to break up with him, he spontaneously returned to his normal self. She described him as a friendly, outgoing, energetic young man who was interested in school and athletics, and who performed well both academically and at his part-time job.

In the emergency room, blood and urine toxicology screening for evidence of drug use was negative, as were other medical tests. Physical examination revealed an extremely healthy, athletic young man, who was largely mute and rigidly held his arms against the sides of his body. The hospital chart noted one previous psychiatric admission a year before. The diagnosis for that admission was "Unspecified Psychosis, rule out drug-induced psychosis." Mr. Robinson had been in the hospital only 4 days, during which time he was observed to be hearing voices, and he expressed a delusion that he was communicating directly with Allah.

During the first few days of the current hospitalization, Mr. Robinson was observed to alternate between "rigid posturing," in which he would become frozen into a particular position, resisting attempts by others to move him, and "mild hyperactivity." During one of the times when he was rigid, it was determined by the psychiatrist on the unit that the patient had the symptom of "waxy flexibility," in which his arms could be put into any position, which Mr. Robinson would then hold, as if having been molded as a wax figure. He would then spontaneously become "unstuck" and begin pacing actively around the unit, espousing his newfound faith in Islam to "anyone he could corral."

An antipsychotic medication, risperidone, and a mood-stabilizing medication, lithium carbonate, were prescribed; Mr. Robinson's lithium level was rapidly increased to therapeutic levels over the next 5 days. During this time, his episodes of becoming mute became less frequent, and his hyperactivity between episodes decreased in amplitude. Twelve days after admission, Mr. Robinson's mental status was essentially normal, without hallucinations or active delusions. He was discharged, with follow-up through the university clinic. Mr. Robinson had a mild depression about 1 month after discharge from the hospital; this was managed by increasing his lithium dose. During the year of follow-up, no further psychotic symptoms or Major Depressive or Manic Episodes occurred.

Discussion of "Praying Athlete"

The bizarre behavior (becoming mute and rigid) that is the reason for Mr. Robinson's admission to the hospital is a symptom of Catatonia (see Section 2.6). Traditionally, catatonic symptoms were almost always thought to be evidence of either Schizophrenia or unusual forms of a central nervous system condition. However, it is now understood that the majority of Catatonia cases involve individuals with Depressive or Bipolar Disorders. At least 3 of the 12 symptoms that are part of the syndrome of Catatonia must be present for the diagnosis (DSM-5-TR, p. 135). In Mr. Robinson's case, in addition to the mutism, he has rigid posturing in which he assumes a frozen position, along with waxy flexibility.

In addition to the periods of Catatonia, Mr. Robinson had the classic symptoms of a Manic Episode: his mood was expansive, his friends described him as "hyper," he talked about Islam to "anyone he could corral," he was delusionally grandiose (communicating directly with Allah), he had psychomotor agitation (pacing), he stopped sleeping at night, and he was hypersexual (sexually demanding). Given that the experience of communicating with God is an accepted part of certain religions, it is important to distinguish between a religious delusion (which would be evidence of psychopathology) and a belief that is widely accepted by other members of that person's religious or spiritual community. In Mr. Robinson's case, his belief that he could communicate directly with Allah occurs only in the context of other symptoms of mania; thus, this belief can be considered delusional. In addition, there is a history of what seems to be a Major Depressive Episode: he was extremely depressed, socially withdrawn, and slept 14 hours a day several months ago.

Also characteristic of Bipolar I Disorder is the rapid development of the Manic Episode and the full return to usual functioning between episodes of mood disturbance. Mr. Robinson's grandiose delusion of communicating with God is a typical type of delusion seen in mania, which is referred to as a "mood-congruent" delusion. Therefore, Mr. Robinson is diagnosed with Bipolar I Disorder, Current Episode Manic, With Mood-Congruent Psychotic Features, With Catatonia (DSM-5-TR, p. 139).

You May Keep the Yacht

Jose Lopez was escorted from jail by sheriff's deputies to a locked forensic psychiatry inpatient unit. They brought with them involuntary detention papers citing him as "gravely disabled because of a psychiatric disorder." He was in a jail uniform, chatting cheerfully, incoherently, and rapidly to himself. The accompanying deputy explained to the admitting nurse, "He won't shut up. He's been keeping the other inmates awake for the last 2 nights talking nonsense. The charges are for attempted sexual assault in another state; we don't have any details. He won't talk to us, won't eat any food, refuses to take medicine, and stays naked under the blankets on his cot. He says he's plucking his pubic hair because it increases his virility."

An attending psychiatrist arrived to examine the patient and noted that he was a tall, thin male who appeared his stated age of 35 years. Mr. Lopez had "unruly" hair that was matted and apparently neglected. He was noted to have "intense affect" that was "menacing." His speech was articulate, but rambling, loud, and pressured. His responses were judged to be "guarded" and "questionably reliable." Mr. Lopez gave bizarre responses with loose associations, such as when he was asked to spell the word *world,* and responded, "w-zero-r-l-d. I used the number, but I know it's a letter...it's part of the metric system, world system you know." He denied hallucinations, violent impulses, and any previous psychiatric treatment.

The psychiatrist thought the most likely diagnosis was Schizophrenia, with the need to also rule out drug intoxication. Antipsychotic medication was prescribed, but Mr. Lopez refused it. He also refused the physical examination and laboratory tests, except for urinalysis and a blood test for syphilis. He did later agree to a physical examination and reported to the examining nurse practitioner a history of intravenous heroin use, syphilis infection treated 8 years prior to admission, and a gunshot wound to the heart. The examination revealed no evidence of old scars of gunshot wounds or of track marks. The syphilis serology tests were "nonreactive," indicating no infection with syphilis, and his urine toxicology screen at approximately 72 hours after admission was negative for drugs. On the afternoon of his transfer, Mr. Lopez was released from criminal custody when the sexual assault charges were dropped. He remained involuntarily detained for psychiatric treatment, however, and was transferred to a locked general ward that evening.

On the general ward, Mr. Lopez was cooperative but agitated and unable to sleep. After a few hours he began to complain of homosexual activity by "others" in his room; however, he had no roommates. The staff feared he would lose control over his behavior, and because he continued to refuse medication, they placed him in a seclusion room with the door open. This did not alleviate his agitation, and he began to yell. When the seclusion door was locked, he became calmer, thanked the staff for ensuring his safety, and slept briefly.

The following day, Mr. Lopez was kept in seclusion, where he remained lying on the floor, pacing, or standing in a corner vocalizing to himself. He displayed bizarre, ritualistic movements and was increasingly withdrawn. He refused medication and solid food but did drink fluids. A nurse described him as having a "playful and aloof attitude." He responded to questions by repeating "I refuse, I refuse. I'm in a meeting conducting business." On the fourth day of his hospitalization, the female attending psychiatrist examining him observed "menacing and sexually inappropriate behaviors." On being questioned regarding his refusal of medication, he shouted, "You're not listening" and began making kissing gestures and thrusting his pelvis. Due to persistent symptoms and refusal of medicines, he was presented for court-ordered treatment. At the hearing, Mr. Lopez continued to behave inappropriately, passing flatus and referring to the female court commissioner as "Bette Midler." He lost the hearing due to his lack of ability to rationally refuse the medication. He was offered oral or intramuscular medication and opted to be restrained and receive his first dose of risperidone (an antipsychotic medication) via intramuscular injection. Within 8 hours he agreed to oral medication.

On day 4 of medication, Mr. Lopez was dramatically improved. He was released from seclusion and began to groom himself and attend group therapy. Although he was mostly appropriate, occasional bizarre behaviors were still observed, such as suddenly shaving his head, stating he was "allowing my head to cool down." On mental status examination, he no longer exhibited loose associations, but he continued to be "suspicious," and he declined to provide information regarding his past. He actively lobbied for discharge and requested that the psychiatrist contact his former physician and realtor in a Midwestern state. His only revelations were that his parents were alive, he had four female siblings, and he had been a construction company employee but now received disability due to an industrial accident.

Because the assault charge had been dropped and his psychiatric condition no longer warranted involuntary treatment, the staff attempted to convince him to stay voluntarily. He refused, and the hospital was forced to discharge him. He indicated that he planned to remain in town only long enough to purchase some "superior leather goods," and then he planned to return to the Midwest. Exiting the locked unit door, Mr. Lopez turned to his primary nurse and said, "You've been the best servant I've ever had. You may keep the yacht!"

Discussion of "You May Keep the Yacht"

It is apparent that the admitting psychiatrist in Mr. Lopez's case, having noted a history of violence and perceiving a "menacing," agitated, incoherent large male, was most impressed by these features, which led prematurely to a diagnosis of Schizophrenia. Had it not been for Mr. Lopez's frightening presentation, the psychiatrist might have viewed him as flamboyant rather than as wild and disorganized. He might also have noticed that Mr. Lopez's speech was pressured, he was not sleeping ("He won't shut up. He's been keeping the inmates awake for the last 2 nights talking nonsense"), and he was irritable, physically restless, grandiose, and hypersexual—all symptoms suggesting a possible Manic Episode. The subsequent course, in which Mr. Lopez demonstrated grandiosity and an expansive mood, further supports this diagnosis. In the absence of any information about prior Manic or Major Depressive Episodes, the diagnosis would be Bipolar I Disorder, Current Episode Manic (DSM-5-TR, p. 139). Because of the presence of psychotic symptoms during his episode (e.g., delusions about homosexual activity involving others despite being alone in his cell), the additional specifier With Mood-Incongruent Psychotic Features would also be noted.

3.2
Bipolar II Disorder

Bipolar II Disorder is characterized by a clinical course consisting of one or more Hypomanic Episodes, one or more Major Depressive Episodes, and the absence of any lifetime Manic Episodes. This is in contrast to the requirement for at least one full-blown Manic Episode in Bipolar I Disorder. Individuals with Bipolar II Disorder generally come to clinical attention when they are in a Major Depressive Episode and thus may present as if they have a diagnosis of recurrent Major Depressive Disorder; therefore, it is important to actively inquire about the possible presence of Hypomanic Episodes during nondepressed periods for all patients presenting with a history of recurrent depression, because such individuals typically do not view the Hypomanic Episodes as problematic or even noteworthy. However, for some individuals who experience frequent periods of depressed mood, periods in which their depression lifts may seem like mild euphoria, especially when contrasted to how badly they feel when they are depressed; therefore, it is important to ensure that the person's mood in between depressive episodes is abnormally elevated or irritable and that this mood change is significant enough to be noticeable by others before a diagnosis of a Hypomanic Episode is made, so as to avoid misdiagnosing Bipolar II Disorder in such individuals.

All of the DSM-5-TR diagnostic specifiers discussed in Section 3.1, "Bipolar I Disorder," apply as well to Bipolar II Disorder, except that the specifier With Psychotic Features does not apply to a Hypomanic Episode, which, by definition, cannot have psychotic features (and, if so, would be considered a Manic Episode).

Even though Bipolar II Disorder is thought by some to be a milder form of bipolar disorder than Bipolar I Disorder, this is not necessarily the case. The impairment associated with Bipolar II Disorder results from the Major Depressive Episodes, which can be especially severe, or from the persistent pattern of unpredictable mood changes and fluctuating, unreliable interpersonal or occupational functioning.

Bipolar II Disorder is half as common as Bipolar I Disorder, with a 12-month prevalence rate in the United States of 0.8% (vs. 1.5% for Bipolar I Disorder). Unlike Bipolar I Disorder, in which the gender ratio is equal, Bipolar II Disorder may be more common in women than in men, especially in clinical samples. The average age at onset is in the mid-20s, which is slightly later than for Bipolar I Disorder but earlier than that for Major Depressive Disorder. The illness most often begins with a depressive episode and is not recognized as Bipolar II Disorder until a Hypomanic Episode occurs, which eventually happens in about 12% of individuals initially diagnosed with Major Depressive Disorder. About one-third of individuals with Bipolar II Disorder report attempting suicide at some point in their life. As is the case with Bipolar I Disorder, Bipolar II Disorder is more often than not associated with one or more co-occurring disorders, with Anxiety Disorders being the most common.

Still a Student

Ellen Waters, age 37 years, is a part-time graduate student who lives alone and supports herself by working as a home health aide. She completed course work for a doctorate in sociology 3 years ago but has not yet begun her dissertation. Her psychotherapist referred her for a medication consultation because of Ms. Waters' continuing depressed mood and panic attacks.

Ms. Waters is indeed an unhappy-looking woman and describes being unhappy through much of her life, without any sustained periods of feeling really good. Her father was an alcoholic, and there was always a great deal of strife in her parents' marriage. She denied sexual or physical abuse but felt that her parents were "emotionally abusive" toward her. She was first referred for psychiatric treatment after a suicide attempt at age 14, and there have been many times over the years during which her usual low-level depression became considerably worse, but she did not get treatment.

Two years ago, after she had been seeing her current boyfriend for about 4 years, it finally became clear that he was unwilling to marry her or live with her. She began to get more depressed and to experience acute panic attacks, and it was at that time that she entered psychotherapy.

She says that in the month before the consultation, she was depressed most of the time. She had gained about 10 pounds because she was constantly nibbling on chips or cookies or making herself peanut butter sandwiches. She often awakened in the middle of the night, was unable to go back to sleep for hours, and then overslept the following day, often sleeping up to 18 hours a day. She says that she is always tired and feels like deadweight and that her legs and arms are heavy. She ruminates about her own failures and cannot concentrate on any serious reading.

Ms. Waters' mood is clearly reactive to favorable or unfavorable events. Small attentions from her therapist or her boyfriend can cause her to feel really good for hours at a time. She has an equally extreme reaction to any sort of rejection. If a friend does not return a call, she feels devastated to the point that she cannot work. She then stays at home, overeats, and avoids people.

Ms. Waters' academic and vocational history has been erratic. She has a master's degree in psychology and worked as a counselor for a while but found this work too upsetting. She then began a doctoral program in sociology, but after completing her course work, she interrupted this degree program to train in physical therapy. She has never worked in one job for more than a few years and has spent much of her adult life as a student. Her current romance of 6 years is the longest she has sustained. She lived with a man once previously, but this was a brief and tumultuous relationship. Boyfriends have described her as "needy and clinging," and it appears that her current boyfriend fears her neediness.

Although Ms. Waters reports chronic depression, when asked about "high" periods, she describes many episodes of abnormally elevated mood and increased energy that have lasted for several months at a time. During these times she would function on 3–4 hours of sleep a night, spend hours on the phone catching up with friends whom she never speaks to during those times when she is feeling down, and feel that her thoughts were racing. She was able to get a lot done, but her friends were obviously concerned about the change in her behavior, urging her to "slow down" and "calm down." She has never gotten into any real trouble during these episodes.

Discussion of "Still a Student"

Ms. Waters' long history of mild depressive symptoms suggests the diagnosis of Persistent Depressive Disorder (see "Junior Executive" in Section 4.3) along with recurrent episodes of Major Depressive Disorder (see "Worthless Wife" in Section 4.2). However, her many episodes of elevated mood, decreased sleep, increased activity, and racing thoughts clearly indicate Hypomanic Episodes, which rule out a diagnosis of Persistent Depressive Disorder in favor of a diagnosis of Bipolar II Disorder (DSM-5-TR, p. 150). She currently is experiencing a Major Depressive Episode (weight gain, insomnia, trouble concentrating, self-deprecation, suicidal ideation), so that the Bipolar II Disorder would be further specified as Current Episode Depressed.

In contrast to the so-called typical depressive presentation characterized by trouble sleeping and loss of appetite, Ms. Waters often sleeps 18 hours and has had an increase in appetite. These features are referred to as "reversed vegetative symptoms" and, in the presence of Ms. Waters' rejection sensitivity and depressed mood that brightens in response to positive events, warrant the additional specification of With Atypical Features. Despite its name, "atypical depression" is very common. This clinical picture has been demonstrated to be associated with especially good response to an older type of antidepressant medication called monoamine oxidase inhibitors and poorer response to tricyclic antidepressant medications such as nortriptyline.

3.3
Cyclothymic Disorder

Unlike the other disorders in this chapter, which are episodic—that is, made up of relatively distinct mood episodes (Manic Episodes, Hypomanic Episodes, and Major Depressive Episodes) usually with a period of normal mood in between episodes—Cyclothymic Disorder is a chronic fluctuating mood disturbance with numerous periods of mildly elevated mood that do not meet criteria for a Hypomanic Episode and periods of mildly depressed mood that do not meet criteria for a Major Depressive Episode. For a diagnosis of Cyclothymic Disorder, hypomanic symptoms or depressive symptoms must be present for at least half the time during a period of at least 2 years, and the person cannot have been without mood symptoms for more than 2 months at a time. As a result of the chronic mood changes, individuals with Cyclothymic Disorder are often viewed by others as moody, temperamental, unreliable, or inconsistent. Cyclothymic Disorder can cause significant problems as a result of prolonged periods of cyclical, often unpredictable mood changes, although it is almost always less impairing than Bipolar I or Bipolar II Disorder, in which individuals are often unable to function during Manic or Major Depressive Episodes.

Cyclothymic Disorder usually begins in adolescence or early adult life and usually has an insidious onset and a persistent course. The lifetime prevalence of Cyclothymic Disorder is approximately 0.4%–1%. Prevalence in mood disorders clinics may range from 3% to 5%. In the general population, Cyclothymic Disorder is apparently equally common in men and women.

Car Salesman

Geoffrey Fisher, a 29-year-old car salesman, was referred by his current girlfriend, a psychiatric nurse, who suspected he had a mood disorder, even though Mr. Fisher was reluctant to admit that he might be a "moody" person. According to him, since age 14 he has experienced repeated alternating cycles that he terms "good times and bad times." During a "bad" period, usually lasting 4–7 days, he sleeps 10–14 hours daily and lacks energy, confidence, and motivation—"just vegetating," as he puts it. Often, he abruptly shifts, characteristically on waking in the morning, to a 2- to 3-day stretch of overconfidence, heightened social awareness, promiscuity, and sharpened thinking—"Things would flash in my mind." At such times he indulges in alcohol to enhance the experience, but also to help him sleep. Occasionally, the "good" periods culminate in irritable and hostile outbursts, which often herald the transition back to another period of "bad" days. He admits to frequent use of marijuana, which he claims helps him "adjust" to daily routines.

As a car salesman, his performance has been uneven, with "good days" barely canceling out the "bad days," yet even during his "good days" he is sometimes argumentative with customers and loses sales that appeared sure. Although considered a charming man in many social circles, he alienates friends when he is hostile and irritable. He typically accumulates social obligations during the "bad" days and takes care of them all at once on the first day of a "good" period.

Discussion of "Car Salesman"

Mr. Fisher has had numerous periods in which he has had some symptoms characteristic of both hypomania and depression. Characteristic of the "good days" are overconfidence, increased activity, and poor judgment (promiscuity). These periods come perilously close to meeting the criteria for Hypomanic Episodes, but they do not last sufficiently long (at least 4 days) to meet criteria for a Hypomanic Episode. Similarly, the "bad days," characterized by oversleeping and lack of energy, confidence, and motivation, are of insufficient severity and duration to meet the criteria for a Major Depressive Episode. The chronicity and unpredictable nature of these mood changes have clearly had a negative impact on his life, having negatively affected his performance at work (arguing with customers and losing sales even on good days) and with his friends (alienating friends when he is irritable). Thus, the diagnosis for Mr. Fisher's presentation is Cyclothymic Disorder (DSM-5-TR, p. 159).

3.4
Substance/Medication-Induced Bipolar and Related Disorder

Symptoms that are characteristic of a Manic or Hypomanic Episode (i.e., elevated, expansive, or irritable mood with abnormally increased activity or energy) can be caused by intoxication with certain substances of abuse (i.e., alcohol; phencyclidine; hallucinogens; sedatives, hypnotics, or anxiolytics; amphetamines or cocaine); withdrawal from certain substances of abuse (i.e., alcohol; sedatives, hypnotics, or anxiolytics; amphetamines or cocaine); or as a side effect of certain medications (e.g., corticosteroids, androgens, levodopa). In such cases, a diagnosis of a Substance/Medication-Induced Bipolar and Related Disorder is made. An important exception is the case of a Hypomanic or Manic Episode that occurs after antidepressant medication use and persists beyond the physiological effects of the medication; in this situation, the symptoms are considered an indicator of true Bipolar Disorder rather than Substance/Medication-Induced Bipolar and Related Disorder.

Sleepless Mother

Ingrid Einbach, a 28-year-old woman from the Bavarian countryside of Germany and the mother of two children, had been treated in a dermatology clinic for recurrent skin infections. She is referred to a psychiatric clinic the day she complained to her dermatologist about insomnia, which started after she took her first dose of an oral antibiotic, ofloxacin, that the dermatologist had prescribed.

Following her first sleepless night, Ms. Einbach became unusually cheerful, social, and physically active. She played tennis for hours, saw friends she had not seen in years, and felt "tip-top." She awoke from only 1 hour of sleep feeling rested. After 3 days, she mentioned to her husband that "her thoughts were running away" and that "everything within her was vibrating." Two days later, she consulted the dermatologist who, alarmed by Ms. Einbach's condition, discontinued the ofloxacin and prescribed an antianxiety drug, alprazolam, with instruction to increase the dose over the next 5 days, and made an appointment for her to be seen in the psychiatric clinic that same day.

Ms. Einbach reported no psychiatric history for herself or any family member. Other than the ofloxacin, she had not taken any medications during the 4 weeks preceding her change in mood. Her medical history was unremarkable except for previous hypothyroidism, which had been successfully treated. All laboratory data and medical, gynecological, and neurological findings were within normal limits. Electrocardiogram, electroencephalogram, and a computed tomography scan of her head were all normal.

For the next week, Ms. Einbach complained of "feeling all mixed up." On the one hand, she felt dysphoric and depressed, and complained of loss of energy, indecisiveness, lack of interest, fatigue, and marked loss of appetite. On the other hand, she experienced racing thoughts, felt restless and irritable, and was unable to concentrate. Her affect was labile, alternating between episodes of unprovoked crying and laughing. She also had four panic attacks, one of them witnessed by her private physician, during which she suddenly felt apprehensive, trembled, turned pale, was short of breath, had tachycardia (rapid heartbeat), and almost fainted. On another occasion during a panic attack, she mentioned to her physician that she feared that "something evil had happened" and was worried that he "might be hiding something" from her.

By the 10th day after the beginning of her mood changes, the patient had developed a typical depressive syndrome with a markedly depressed mood, loss of energy, loss of interest in her children, marked loss of appetite, insomnia, and pronounced psychomotor retardation. Two weeks later, her depression seemed to lift shortly after she slept for several consecutive hours for the first time. Within a few days her mood was back to normal.

Discussion of "Sleepless Mother"

Ms. Einbach, who had no prior psychiatric history, developed a variety of psychiatric symptoms during or soon after exposure to a medication that is capable of producing the symptoms (DSM-5-TR, p. 162). The class of antibiotic medication known as the fluoroquinolones are known to have rare psychiatric side effects, including anxiety, depression, insomnia, panic attacks, mania, and psychosis. Ms. Einbach developed insomnia, elevated mood, racing thoughts, and increased activity immediately following taking the medication; soon after stopping the drug, she developed a variety of depressive symptoms (dysphoria, loss of energy, lack of appetite, and loss of interest) that intermingled with the manic symptoms; then she experienced a period with only depressive symptoms. Because of the absence of a history of mood disturbance in the patient or in her family, and because of the close temporal relationship between her having taken the drug and then stopping it and the onset of the mood disturbance, it is reasonable to conclude that the drug was responsible for the manic and depressive disturbances. Therefore, the clinician first makes a diagnosis of Ofloxacin-Induced Bipolar and Related Disorder (DSM-5-TR, p. 162).

A logical assumption is that the panic attacks, which lasted for 5 days, were also triggered by the drug. Therefore, the clinician could give the additional diagnosis of Ofloxacin-Induced Anxiety Disorder, With Panic Attacks (DSM-5-TR, p. 255) or, more parsimoniously, simply list the more prominent Substance/Medication-Induced Bipolar and Related Disorder and think of the panic attacks as an associated feature.

It is reasonable to assume that Ms. Einbach's paranoid ideation (i.e., that the doctor is hiding something from her) is also a reaction to the ofloxacin. However, this feature does not seem marked enough to warrant an additional diagnosis.

CHAPTER 4

Depressive Disorders

Depressive Disorders are among the most common and disabling types of mental disorders worldwide. In earlier editions of DSM, Depressive Disorders were classified along with Bipolar Disorders in a group referred to as Mood Disorders or Affective Disorders, but because Depressive Disorders and Bipolar and Related Disorders have major differences in clinical course, treatment, and presumed etiology, these two groups of disorders were classified separately beginning with DSM-5.

Depressive Disorders are all characterized by "the presence of sad, empty, or irritable mood" (DSM-5-TR, p. 177), along with somatic (physical functions) and cognitive (mental functions) changes that adversely impact an individual's ability to function in major life arenas. Depressive Disorders differ from each other with respect to accompanying clinical features, onset and course, duration, severity, and presumed etiology. Disruptive Mood Dysregulation Disorder, a new disorder in DSM-5, is a disorder of children, characterized by persistent irritability and frequent episodes of extreme behavioral dyscontrol. Major Depressive Disorder is characterized by discrete episodes of changes in mood, cognition, and sleeping and eating patterns that last at least 2 weeks but often much longer. Persistent Depressive Disorder describes a pattern of chronic depression of varying severity that lasts at least 2 years in adults and 1 year in children. Premenstrual Dysphoric Disorder is a specific depressive syndrome in women that begins some time following ovulation in the menstrual cycle and remits within a few days after menses. Finally, depressive syndromes may be caused by a variety of substances of abuse, prescription medications, and other nonpsychiatric medical conditions. Thus, DSM-5-TR includes diagnoses for Substance/Medication-Induced Depressive Disorder and for Depressive Disorder Due to Another Medical Condition. (Table 4–1 lists characteristic features of the Depressive Disorders discussed in this chapter.)

Depressive Disorders, Anxiety Disorders, and Somatic Symptom and Related Disorders are on a continuum of psychopathology known as the "internalizing" spectrum (as opposed to the "externalizing" spectrum; see introduction to Chapter 18, "Personality Disorders") and are particularly associated with the underlying personality trait domain of *negative affectivity* (DSM-5-TR, p. 899). The Depressive Disorders represent disorders characterized mainly by distress, whereas the Anxiety Disorders are characterized mainly by fear or anxiety. Pathological personality traits constitute risk factors for the development of related mental disorders and also help to explain the extensive co-occurrence among related disorders.

TABLE 4–1.   **Characteristic features of Depressive Disorders**

Disorder	Key characteristics
Disruptive Mood Dysregulation Disorder	Severe recurrent temper outbursts manifested verbally or behaviorally occurring three or more times per week
	Persistently irritable or angry mood between outbursts
	Duration at least 12 months
	Outbursts occur in at least two of three settings (i.e., at home, in school, with peers)
	Age of first diagnosis between 6 and 18 years
	Age at onset before 10 years
Major Depressive Disorder	Depressed mood or loss of interest or pleasure for at least 2 weeks
	Other symptoms including appetite and sleep disturbance, psychomotor agitation or retardation, fatigue or loss of energy, feelings of worthlessness or guilt, diminished ability to think or concentrate, recurrent thoughts of death or suicidal thoughts, plans, or attempt
Persistent Depressive Disorder	Depressed mood most of the day, more days than not, for at least 2 years (1 year for children and adolescents)
	Other symptoms including appetite and sleep disturbance, low energy or fatigue, low self-esteem, poor concentration or difficulty making decisions, feelings of hopelessness
	During 2-year period (1 year for children and adolescents), no more than 2 months without symptoms
Premenstrual Dysphoric Disorder	In majority of menstrual cycles over the preceding year, depressive symptoms manifest in final week before onset of menses, start to improve within a few days after menses, and become minimal or absent in the week postmenses
	Confirmed by daily prospective ratings during at least two symptomatic cycles
Depressive Disorder Due to Another Medical Condition	Prominent and persistent period of depressed mood or loss of interest or pleasure
	Disturbance is the direct pathophysiological consequence of a nonpsychiatric medical condition

4.1
Disruptive Mood Dysregulation Disorder

Disruptive Mood Dysregulation Disorder was a new disorder introduced in DSM-5 designed to capture the clinical picture of many children who were formerly (and inappropriately) diagnosed as having childhood Bipolar Disorder. The hallmark symptoms are severe recurrent temper outbursts that a child expresses verbally by yelling and screaming and/or behaviorally by physical aggression toward other people or toward property. The outbursts are "grossly out of proportion in intensity or duration to the situation or provocation" (DSM-5-TR, p. 178). The outbursts occur frequently—on average, three or more times per week—and are far beyond anything seen normally at the child's developmental level. In between the outbursts, the child's mood is persistently irritable or angry most of the time, which is clearly apparent to others, such as the child's parents, teachers, or peers. In fact, the diagnosis is not given unless the temper outbursts and irritable/angry mood are present in at least two of three settings (i.e., at home, in school, with peers) and are "severe" in at least one of these settings. The disturbance should be present for at least 1 year, and the diagnosis is not given if the child has been without symptoms for a period of 3 months or more. Onset must be before age 10 years, and the diagnosis is restricted to children between ages 6 and 18 years. There must be no instances of more than 1 day when the full symptom criteria for a Manic or Hypomanic Episode (DSM-5-TR, pp. 140–141) have been met.

Disruptive Mood Dysregulation Disorder is a very common mental disorder in pediatric mental health settings. Prevalence estimates in general community populations are not clear. It is more common among boys than girls in clinical samples, but consistent sex differences in prevalence have not been found in population samples. The disturbance is persistent, by definition lasting at least 1 year, with perhaps 50% of cases lasting longer. Chronic, severe, nonepisodic irritability rarely turns into Bipolar Disorder (see Chapter 3) over time, which is one reason the diagnosis of childhood Bipolar Disorder was not accurately applicable; instead, this symptom increases the risk of the development of Major Depressive Disorder (see Section 4.2; hence its classification among the Depressive Disorders in DSM-5-TR) or Anxiety Disorders (see Chapter 5) in adulthood. The history of children with Disruptive Mood Dysregulation Disorder often includes other childhood mental disorders, such as Oppositional Defiant Disorder (see "No Brakes" in Section 15.1), Attention-Deficit/Hyperactivity Disorder (see "Into Everything" in Section 1.7), or various Anxiety Disorders (see Chapter 5). Disruptive Mood Dysregulation Disorder is very disruptive to a child's family, school, and peer group functioning. Suicide attempts, dangerous or severely aggressive behavior, and psychiatric hospitalizations are common.

Titanic Tantrums[1]

Dillon, an 8-year-old boy living with his parents and his younger brother, was evaluated because his parents were at their "wits' end" regarding how to handle his explosive outbursts, which were occurring several times a day. Ms. A., Dillon's mother, stated, "It has gotten to the point where I dislike my child."

At the time of the evaluation, Dillon was exhibiting temper outbursts several times a day that lasted approximately 10 minutes, and more intense 30-minute outbursts multiple times a week, during which he became physically aggressive. For example, during a recent tantrum, Dillon kicked and punched holes in his bedroom door, causing such destruction that the door needed to be replaced. Additionally, Ms. A. reported that she always had bruises on her arms from blocking Dillon's strikes. Dillon's parents described him as irritable and cranky for the better part of the day on most days. When irritable, Dillon appeared agitated and restless and often expressed that he wanted to be left alone. Attempts to cheer him up were typically unsuccessful and sometimes worsened his irritability.

Dillon was in the second grade in a restrictive classroom environment, classified under special education as emotionally disturbed. In the past school year, Dillon had been suspended three times—for physical aggression toward school personnel, for throwing a chair in the classroom, and for knocking over a bookcase. Despite his average to superior cognitive abilities, Dillon struggled academically, partly because of the large amount of time he spent out of the classroom due to his disruptive behavior. Teachers noted that Dillon often appeared to be in an irritable, agitated mood and that he rarely smiled or appeared happy. They often felt they were walking on eggshells to avoid his rageful outbursts.

Ms. A. reported that Dillon had always been a difficult child. As a baby, he was colicky and cried incessantly for several hours each day. As a toddler, he threw tantrums multiple times per day, which Ms. A. attributed to the "terrible twos." Unfortunately, Dillon's outbursts escalated as he grew older. By the time Dillon was 5, his temper tantrums included hitting and kicking his parents and throwing breakable objects. His difficulties were also manifest outside the home, as evidenced by his expulsion from prekindergarten because of unmanageable behavior.

Dillon's tantrums and noncompliance at home increased once he entered school, as homework added another source of frustration and negative interactions. He was highly distractible and exhibited strong opposition when asked to do homework. He was constantly restless, fidgeting, and getting out of his seat, and he was difficult to control. He also tried to avoid daily routines,

[1] Adapted from Roy AK, Lopes V, Klein RG: "Disruptive Mood Dysregulation Disorder: A New Diagnostic Approach to Chronic Irritability in Youth." *American Journal of Psychiatry* 171:918–924, 2014. Copyright © 2014 American Psychiatric Association. Used with permission.

such as picking up his clothes and brushing his teeth, and he threw tantrums regularly to avoid them. During this time, Dillon's irritability worsened as well. Around the time he started first grade, he began to appear constantly "on edge" and was easily bothered by little things, such as others sitting too close to him. His mood remained cranky for most of the day, sometimes for several days at a time. When his parents tried to cheer him up by suggesting a fun activity, he would snap, demanding to be left alone. Dillon also started to make hostile attributions regarding his peers' intentions. For example, when playing tag, Dillon would get angry, believing the others had hit him on purpose when they were merely tagging him. He also expressed the negative thoughts that no one liked him, that he did not have any friends, and that his parents did not love him. At times, Dillon had difficulty controlling these thoughts, in episodes that Ms. A. referred to as "mind spirals." Dillon would bring up an angering event out of nowhere, such as being yelled at by his teacher a few days earlier, and remain upset for several hours.

Dillon's outbursts at school led to his classification as emotionally disturbed, and he was moved to a smaller classroom. Despite this more supportive environment, Dillon continued to be disruptive and to have difficulty focusing, following instructions, and completing classwork. He became bored easily and refused to do his work. Over time, Dillon's academic progress declined. Teachers eventually placed fewer academic demands on him to avoid outbursts.

In Dillon's early schooling, he made friends and enjoyed interacting with peers. However, because of his temper tantrums and hostile attributions, his peers began to avoid him. His parents restricted family outings. They stopped attending Mass when Dillon was in second grade because he could not sit still and would throw tantrums in church. They cut back on family gatherings and avoided including Dillon on errands, because of the embarrassment caused by his tantrums.

Dillon's parents and Dillon consulted with a child psychiatrist to discuss medication. The psychiatrist prescribed methylphenidate in the hope that it would improve Dillon's hyperactivity and frustration tolerance and thus reduce his tantrums. Because Dillon's outbursts at home had become a means of avoiding demands, and his parents were unsure about managing them, the parents were referred for parent management training, which offers specific strategies that enhance effective communication and discipline. At the same time, Dillon received individual cognitive-behavioral therapy aimed at teaching him how to better regulate his mood and improve his frustration tolerance. He was taught coping skills to regulate his anger and to identify and relabel distortions that contributed to his hostile reactions. Finally, a school behavior daily report card was developed that functioned like a token economy through which Dillon was rewarded for specific positive behaviors in the classroom.

Discussion of "Titanic Tantrums"

Dillon's behaviors and mood symptoms are consistent with Disruptive Mood Dysregulation Disorder (DSM-5-TR, p. 178). His temper outbursts were frequent (at least three per week), severe, and explosive, causing impairment at home and in school. Between explosive episodes, Dillon's mood was chronically irritable. These symptoms had been present for several years without periods of amelioration. In addition, Dillon's presentation meets criteria for Attention-Deficit/Hyperactivity Disorder, Combined Presentation (see Section 1.7), and Oppositional Defiant Disorder (see Section 15.1). However, according to the note for DSM-5-TR Criterion J (p. 178), when criteria for both Oppositional Defiant Disorder and Disruptive Mood Dysregulation Disorder are met, only the latter diagnosis is assigned. Mania symptoms were not reported in Dillon's case, and his irritable mood was chronic, which ruled out Bipolar Disorder.

The diagnosis of Disruptive Mood Dysregulation Disorder was created to deal with the problem of overdiagnosis of juvenile Bipolar Disorder. Disruptive Mood Dysregulation Disorder is intended to address the mistaken belief that chronic irritability in children is a developmental variant of Bipolar Disorder. The rate of conversion from severe, chronic irritability in children to episodic Bipolar Disorder later in life is very low. Family history studies do not indicate an increase in the number of relatives with Bipolar Disorder in the families of children with chronic irritability. Moreover, various cognitive and emotional processing tests show unique signs of dysfunction in chronically irritable children. Therefore, to discourage clinicians from making a mistaken pediatric bipolar diagnosis, the diagnosis of Disruptive Mood Dysregulation Disorder was added to DSM-5 despite limited empirical data in support of it. Many experts consider Disruptive Mood Dysregulation Disorder to simply be a subtype of Oppositional Defiant Disorder.

Differentiating Disruptive Mood Dysregulation Disorder from actual Bipolar Disorder (see "Radar Messages" in Section 3.1) relies primarily on careful characterization of irritable mood. Disruptive Mood Dysregulation Disorder is characterized by chronic irritability, whereas irritability in Bipolar Disorder is episodic, representing a change from the person's usual state. Thus, the typical mood of Disruptive Mood Dysregulation Disorder is consistently irritable or angry, whereas that of pediatric Bipolar Disorder varies among states of euthymia (i.e., normal mood), depression, and mania.

4.2
Major Depressive Disorder

Major Depressive Disorder is the prototypical Depressive Disorder. It is characterized by periods in which 1) depressed mood and/or 2) markedly diminished interest or pleasure in all or almost all activities occur every day, most of the day, for a continuous period of at least 2 weeks. Additionally, four of the following symptoms occur and together with one or both of the above symptoms constitute a Major Depressive Episode:

- A decrease in appetite leading to significant weight loss or an increase in appetite leading to significant weight gain
- Insomnia or hypersomnia (sleeping too much) nearly every day
- Psychomotor agitation or retardation nearly every day
- Fatigue or loss of energy nearly every day
- Feelings of worthlessness or excessive or inappropriate guilt nearly every day
- Diminished ability to think or concentrate, or indecisiveness, nearly every day
- Preoccupation with thoughts of death, recurrent suicidal ideation with or without a specific plan, or a suicide attempt or plan

The combination of symptoms occurring together are very distressing to the person and cause impairment in social, occupational, or other important areas of functioning. Major Depressive Disorder may be characterized as Mild, Moderate, or Severe, based on the number of symptoms present in excess of those required to make the diagnosis (i.e., a minimum of five of the nine symptoms in Criterion A), the amount of distress caused by the symptoms, and the amount of impairment in psychosocial functioning (DSM-5-TR, p. 183).

Major Depressive Disorder and some other Depressive Disorders also vary by whether or not patients have co-occurring psychotic features (mood-congruent or mood-incongruent), anxious distress, mixed features, melancholic features, atypical features, or Catatonia. These additional features are captured by specifiers in the DSM-5-TR diagnostic system:

- Psychotic symptoms include delusions or hallucinations. *Mood-congruent psychotic features* have content that is consistent with "depressive themes of personal inadequacy, guilt, disease, death, nihilism, or deserved punishment" (DSM-5-TR, p. 213). *Mood-incongruent psychotic features* are those that do not involve these typical depressive themes.
- *Anxious distress* includes such anxiety symptoms as feeling keyed up or tense, feeling unusually restless, having difficulty concentrating because of worry, being fearful that something awful might happen, or the person's feeling that they are losing control of themself.
- *Mixed features* are symptoms of mania or hypomania, such as elevated or expansive mood, inflated self-esteem or grandiosity, excessive talkativeness or pressure of speech, racing thoughts, and increase in energy or goal-directed activity, that occur for the majority of days of a Major Depressive Episode.
- *Melancholic features* include loss of pleasure in all or almost all activities; not reacting positively to usually pleasurable stimuli or when good things happen; having profound despondency, despair, or moroseness (the so-called empty mood); depression that is regularly worse in the morning; waking up very early in the morning; marked psychomotor agitation or retardation; significant anorexia or weight loss; or excessive or inappropriate guilt.

- *Atypical features* are defined as reactivity of mood to positive events, significant weight gain or increase in appetite, hypersomnia, a heavy leaden feeling in the arms or legs ("leaden paralysis"), and a long-standing history of sensitivity to interpersonal rejection.
- *Catatonia*, a syndrome characterized by a marked psychomotor disturbance involving decreased motor activity, decreased engagement with others, or excessive and peculiar motor activity is described in the chapter "Schizophrenia Spectrum and Other Psychotic Disorders" (see Section 2.6) because catatonic symptoms are included among the defining symptoms of Schizophrenia, Schizophreniform Disorder, and Brief Psychotic Disorder.
- Finally, Major Depressive Disorder varies by certain aspects of its clinical course. Major Depressive Disorder can be noted as a Single (one and only one) Episode or as Recurrent Episode. If its onset occurs during pregnancy or within 4 weeks following delivery, it is specified as With Peripartum Onset. If there is a regular pattern of Major Depressive Disorder episode onsets in the fall or winter of the year (not due to any psychosocial reasons, such as winter unemployment), it can be specified as With Seasonal Pattern. Episodes of Major Depressive Disorder can also be noted as In Partial Remission or In Full Remission.

All of these additional features of Major Depressive Disorder are important to note because each has some treatment or prognostic significance (Table 4–2).

The 12-month prevalence of Major Depressive Disorder in the United States is estimated at approximately 7%. Major Depressive Disorder is three times more common in young persons ages 18–29 years than in persons age 60 and older. It is two times more common in women than in men. Women report more atypical symptoms (e.g., increased sleeping and appetite) than men. The prevalence of Major Depressive Disorder has increased in the United States over recent years, especially among young people. The onset of Major Depressive Disorder can be at any age, but there is a large increase in onset around puberty and a peak incidence in the 20s. The course of Major Depressive Disorder is highly variable. A chronic course is associated with underlying depressive personality features; psychotic features; Personality Disorders (see Chapter 18); prominent anxiety and Anxiety Disorders (see Chapter 5); and symptom severity. The course is also adversely affected by poverty, racism, and social marginalization. Major Depressive Disorder occurs in all cultures, although at different rates. In some cultures, and subcultures, somatic symptoms, such as insomnia, pain, and loss of energy, are the most common presenting complaints. Functional impairment in Major Depressive Disorder is also highly variable, but it can be completely incapacitating in some instances. Suicide attempts and completed suicides are possible outcomes: rates of suicide have increased from 10.5 to 14 per 100,000 in the United States since the turn of the 21st century. Women make more suicide attempts, but men's attempts are more likely to be fatal. The presence of co-occurring Borderline Personality Disorder (see "Empty Shell" in Section 18.1), Substance Use Disorder (see Chapter 16), anxiety, nonpsychiatric medical conditions, or functional impairment increase the risk for suicide attempts.

TABLE 4–2. **Clinical utility of specifiers for Major Depressive Disorder**

Specifier	Potential clinical utility
Mild, Moderate, Severe	Treatment selection for Major Depressive Episode (psychotherapy for Mild to Moderate, medication for Moderate to Severe)
With Psychotic Features	Treatment (need for antipsychotic medication)
With Mood-Incongruent Psychotic Features	Possibly shared genetic vulnerability with Schizophrenia
With Anxious Distress	More difficult to treat, higher risk of suicide
With Mixed Features	More difficult to treat, higher risk for developing Bipolar Disorder
With Melancholic Features	Treatment (need for somatic treatment)
With Atypical Features	Treatment (avoid use of tricyclic antidepressant medications)
With Catatonia	Treatment (electroconvulsive therapy)
With Peripartum Onset	Future prognosis
With Seasonal Pattern	Treatment (may benefit from bright light therapy)
In Remission (Partial or Full)	Treatment change vs. maintenance treatment and regular follow-up

Worthless Wife

Connie Russo, a 33-year-old wife and mother of a 4-year-old son, Anthony, is referred by her general practitioner to a psychiatric outpatient program because of her complaint that she has been depressed and unable to concentrate since she separated from her husband 3 months ago after 5 years of marriage. Violent arguments between them, during which Ms. Russo was beaten by her husband, had occurred for the last 4 years of their marriage, beginning when she became pregnant with Anthony. There were daily arguments during which Mr. Russo hit her hard enough to leave bruises on her face and arms. During their final argument, about Ms. Russo's buying an "expensive" tricycle for Anthony, her husband had held a loaded gun to Anthony's head and threatened to shoot him if she did not agree to return the tricycle to the store. Ms. Russo obtained a court order of protection that prevented her husband from having any contact with her or their son. She and Anthony relocated to her parents' apartment, where they are still living.

Ms. Russo, an only child, is a high school and secretarial school graduate. She worked as an executive secretary for 6 years before her marriage and for the first 2 years after, until Anthony's birth. Before her marriage, Ms. Russo had her own apartment. She was close to her parents, visiting them weekly and speaking to them a couple of times a week. Ms. Russo had many friends whom she also saw regularly. She still had several friends from her high school years. In high school, she had been a popular cheerleader and a good student. In the office where she had worked as a secretary, she was in charge of organizing office holiday parties and money collections for employee gifts. She had no past history of depression; there was no family history of violence, mental illness, or substance abuse. Her parents have been happily married for 35 years.

Mr. and Ms. Russo met at work, where he was an accountant. They married after a 3-month courtship, during which time Ms. Russo observed Mr. Russo using cocaine twice at parties. When she expressed concern, he reassured her that he was only "trying it to be sociable" and denied any regular use.

Mr. Russo, a college graduate, is the oldest of three siblings. His father drank a pint of bourbon each night and often beat Mr. Russo's mother. Mr. Russo's two younger brothers both have histories of substance abuse.

During their first year of marriage, Mr. Russo became increasingly irritable and critical of his wife. He began to request that she stop calling and seeing her friends after work, and he refused to allow them or his in-laws to visit their apartment. Ms. Russo convinced her husband to try marital therapy, but he refused to return after the initial two sessions.

Despite her misgivings about her husband's behavior toward her, Ms. Russo decided to become pregnant. During the seventh month of the pregnancy, she developed thrombophlebitis (inflammation of the leg veins) and had to stay home in bed. Her husband began complaining that their apartment was not clean enough and that Ms. Russo was not able to shop for groceries. He never helped her with the housework. He refused to allow his mother-in-law to come to the apartment to help. One morning when he could not find a clean shirt, he became angry and yelled at Ms. Russo. When she suggested that he pick up some clothes from the laundry, he began hitting her with his fists. She left him and went to live with her parents for a week. He expressed remorse for hitting her and agreed to resume marital therapy.

At her parents' and husband's urging, Ms. Russo returned to her apartment. No further violence occurred until after Anthony's birth. At that time, Mr. Russo began using cocaine every weekend and often became violent when he was high.

In the 3 months since she left her husband, Ms. Russo has become increasingly depressed. Her appetite has been poor, and she has lost 10 pounds. She cries a lot and often wakes up at 5:00 A.M., unable to get back to sleep. Since she left her husband, he has been calling her at her parents' home and begging her to return to him. One week before her psychiatric evaluation, Ms. Russo's parents took her to their general practitioner. Her physical examination was normal, and he referred her for psychiatric treatment.

When seen by a psychiatrist in the outpatient clinic, Ms. Russo is pale and thin, dressed in worn-out jeans and a dark blue sweater. Her haircut is unstylish, and she appears older than she is. She speaks slowly, describing her depressed mood and lack of energy. She says that her only pleasure is in being with her son. She is able to take care of him physically but feels guilty because her preoccupation with her own bad feelings prevents her from being able to play with him. She now has no social contacts other than with her parents and her son. She feels worthless and blames herself for her marital problems, saying that if she had been a better wife, maybe her husband would have been able to give up the cocaine. When asked why she stayed with him so long, she explains that her family disapproved of divorce and kept telling her that she should try harder to make her marriage a success. She also thought about what her life would be like trying to take care of her son while working full-time and did not think she could make it.

Ms. Russo received medication and individual psychotherapy for her depression. She also participated in group therapy with other women who had been abused by their spouses.

After 6 months of therapy, Ms. Russo was no longer depressed. She bought new clothes and had her hair cut in a more flattering and youthful style. She found employment as an executive secretary and placed Anthony in a day care center, where she participated in parent programs. She reported that she and Anthony had fun together in the evening and on weekends. She again began seeing her friends. With financial assistance from her parents, she began divorce proceedings against her husband and requested sole custody of Anthony.

Discussion of "Worthless Wife"

When Ms. Russo comes to treatment, she has almost all the characteristic symptoms of Major Depressive Disorder (DSM-5-TR, p. 183). Her mood is persistently depressed; she has lost interest and pleasure in all activities except taking care of her son; she feels worthless, has trouble concentrating, has poor appetite and has lost weight, lacks energy, and has difficulty sleeping. Because she has no history of prior episodes of significant depression, this would be noted as a Single Episode. Ms. Russo's depression has more than enough of the required symptoms of the disorder and significantly affects her role (as a mother) and social functioning, but she has been managing with her parents' help and is not completely dysfunctional. The severity of the episode would therefore be noted as Moderate. Following her excellent response to treatment, her disorder might be considered to be In Full Remission. It would be important to observe her for a period of time to monitor for any recurrence.

Stonemason

Stanley Kozlowski, a previously healthy 55-year-old stonemason, is admitted to a medical service because of loss of appetite and a 50-pound weight loss over the preceding 6 months. His loss of appetite has been accompanied by a burning pain in his chest, back, and abdomen, which he is convinced indicates a fatal abdominal cancer. He is withdrawn and isolated, unable to work, disinterested in friends and family, and unresponsive to their attempts to make him feel better. He awakes at 4:00 A.M. and is unable to fall back asleep. He claims to feel worst in the mornings and to improve slightly as the day wears on. On mental status examination, he is markedly agitated and speaks of feelings of extreme unworthiness. Mr. Kozlowski says that he would be better off dead and that he welcomes his impending demise from cancer. He has no previous history of emotional disturbance or of substance abuse. Physical examination and laboratory tests are within normal limits.

Discussion of "Stonemason"

Mr. Kozlowski does not complain of feeling depressed, but he does complain of a pervasive loss of interest and pleasure. This, plus several of the other symptoms of a depressive syndrome (loss of appetite and weight loss, insomnia, feelings of worthlessness, and recurrent thoughts of death) leading to significant distress and impairment in functioning, suggests the presence of Major Depressive Disorder (DSM-5-TR, p. 183). He is also experiencing various somatic symptoms. The absence of a history of a Manic Episode rules out Bipolar Disorder (see "Radar Messages" in Section 3.1). The normal physical examination and laboratory findings rule out the possibility of a Depressive Disorder Due to Another Medical Condition (see "Toy Designer" in Section 4.5). The absence of a history of medication use or the abuse of substances rules out a Substance/Medication-Induced Depressive Disorder. Because this is Mr. Kozlowski's first episode of depression, it would be specified as Single Episode. Also, because Mr. Kozlowski has a delusion that he has a fatal abdominal cancer, the diagnosis would be further characterized as With Psychotic Features. The somatic delusion that he has a fatal cancer is consistent with the typical depressive themes of a Depressive Disorder (i.e., of disease and death) and therefore would be noted as With Mood-Congruent Psychotic Features.

Mr. Kozlowski also demonstrates melancholic features: loss of pleasure in all, or almost all, activities; lack of reactivity (unresponsive to others' attempts to make him feel better); diurnal mood variation (depression worse in the morning); early morning awakening; significant weight loss; and marked psychomotor agitation. Therefore, the diagnosis would be further specified as With Melancholic Features. According to DSM-5-TR, when psychotic features and melancholic features are both present, both can be noted. Therefore, the final complete diagnosis in Mr. Kozlowski's case would be Major Depressive Disorder, Single Episode, With Mood-Congruent Psychotic Features, With Melancholic Features.

Three Voices

Haruki Takahashi, a 23-year-old man, was admitted to the hospital. He was almost totally mute. His parents reported that he had been apparently well until about 4 years previously when he broke up with his girlfriend. Since then, he had been living at home in Flushing, Queens, New York, spending much time by himself, holding various odd jobs, and unable to pursue any long-term goals. About 4 months before his hospital admission, he decided to go to California to change his environment and find a new job. However, shortly after he arrived there, his parents received a telephone call from him in which he "sounded bad." His father flew to California and found him vigilant, paranoid, and frightened, having seemingly not eaten for several days. The father brought his son home to New York and arranged for him to see a neurologist, who found Haruki to be essentially normal neurologically. Shortly thereafter, Haruki saw a psychologist, who recommended admission to a psychiatric hospital.

On admission, Haruki was sleeping 10–12 hours a night, had little appetite, and had lost perhaps 20 pounds over the last couple of months. He reported a profound loss of energy and did not speak except to give occasional monosyllabic answers to the interviewer's questions. During his first few days in the hospital, the patient showed virtually no interest or pleasure in any activities and spent most of the time sitting on his bed and staring into space. On questioning, he did not complain of any specific feelings of worthlessness, self-reproach, or guilt, and he did not mention thoughts of death or suicide, although it was difficult to be certain about any of these points because of his paucity of speech.

In the hospital, Haruki was seen daily by a medical student who took a great interest in him and gradually gained his trust. Eventually, the patient revealed to the student that he was hearing three distinct voices—the voice of a child, the voice of a woman, and the voice of a man impersonating a woman. The three voices talked among themselves and sometimes talked to him directly. At times, they spoke about him in the third person, and on some occasions, they seemed to echo his thoughts. The voices spoke about many different subjects and did not focus on any specific depressive themes, such as guilt, sin, or death.

On the second day after admission to the hospital, Haruki was started on a regimen of an antipsychotic medication, olanzapine, 5 mg/day, and an antidepressant medication, nortriptyline, at a dosage that was gradually increased to 150 mg/day. For the first 2 weeks, he experienced virtually no improvement. However, by the third week, the patient displayed some increased restlessness. The dosage of olanzapine was reduced to 2.5 mg/day and was eventually stopped entirely by about the end of the third week. On day 23 in the hospital, the patient began to experience a marked improvement in his energy level, and by the end of the fourth week, he was smiling, talkative, sleeping and eating well, and able to reminisce about the hallucinations, which he stated had now completely disappeared. A week later, he was discharged home, on a maintenance regimen of nortriptyline, 150 mg/day, but no other psychotropic medication.

Approximately 8 months after his discharge, Haruki ran out of nortriptyline and did not obtain more from his pharmacy. His symptoms reappeared rapidly over the course of a few days. After a phone call from his parents to his doctor, the nortriptyline treatment was hastily resumed, and the patient again reverted essentially to normal after another week or so.

Haruki's mother had had a postpartum depressive episode of about 1 year's duration that had gradually remitted spontaneously without treatment. In addition, the mother's sister had had a "nervous breakdown" when she was in her 40s that had required her to be hospitalized; she had received a course of 12 electroconvulsive therapy treatments. Since that time, the aunt had had a complete remission and was described as functioning normally.

Discussion of "Three Voices"

Haruki apparently had a 4-year period during which he had some nonspecific difficulties (social withdrawal and inability to pursue long-term goals), followed by an episode of illness with paranoid behavior, bizarre auditory hallucinations, loss of interest and pleasure, anorexia and a 20-pound weight loss, hypersomnia, loss of energy, and psychomotor retardation (paucity of speech and spending most of his time sitting on the bed staring into space). It is interesting that the psychotic symptoms only came to light after the medical student gained the patient's trust; psychotic symptoms can often be hidden by a patient, and it can take some time and the development of rapport (and good powers of observation) to detect psychotic symptoms.

In the past, this clinical presentation might well have been diagnosed as Schizophrenia, the 4-year period being viewed as prodromal to the acute psychotic phase. The patient's loss of interest and pleasure and the other nonpsychotic symptoms would have been considered merely associated features. According to DSM-5-TR, the loss of interest and pleasure and other nonpsychotic symptoms actually constitute a full major depressive syndrome. Because the psychotic symptoms apparently were present only when Haruki had a major depressive syndrome, they are considered a psychotic feature of Major Depressive Disorder. This is true in spite of the fact that the content of the delusions and hallucinations is not consistent with such usual depressive themes as personal inadequacy, guilt, or deserved punishment. Thus, at admission, the patient's diagnosis would be Major Depressive Disorder, Single Episode, Severe, With Mood-Incongruent Psychotic Features (DSM-5-TR, p. 213), a diagnosis that is certainly supported by Haruki's good response to an antidepressant and the family history of depression.

A question raised by this case is the appropriate subclassification of Major Depressive Disorder at the time of the reappearance of the depressive syndrome when Haruki discontinued his medication. Should this be regarded as Major Depressive Disorder, Recurrent, or as the continuation of the Major Depressive Disorder, Single Episode, the symptoms of which had been suppressed by medication? DSM-5-TR considers a 2-month period with no or only one or two mild symptoms of the disturbance to be the minimal amount of time needed to consider a recurrence a different episode. Because this patient's symptoms reappeared after 8 months, we would note it as a recurrent episode, although we recognize that many clinicians might regard the rapid development of symptoms following discontinuation of the medication as indicating that the patient was still experiencing the original Major Depressive Episode.

It's Typical[2]

Settling into a chair in the psychiatrist's office, the young woman sighed and said, "I don't know what's going on, I just don't know." For the past 2 months, Leslie Siegel, a 25-year-old single art student had been struggling with feelings of depression and inadequacy. The depression started when the man she had been seeing, a 42-year-old divorced general contractor, told her that he wanted to "slow down" their relationship, which she had assumed was heading for marriage.

Ms. Siegel found herself crying frequently, not wanting to get out of bed in the mornings, missing classes, fatigued (feeling as though a lead weight had been placed on her shoulders), and constantly eating, "especially chocolate." She had gained 15 pounds, making her noticeably plump compared with her usual thin and lithe figure. She was also experiencing anxiety attacks, which on several occasions had led her to turn around on the subway platform and go home rather than go to school.

Ms. Siegel was convinced that her boyfriend was the only man for her. In the ensuing months, her mood fluctuated with his ambivalence. Whenever she interpreted his behavior or something he said as a sign that they might still work things out, her spirits were buoyed; however, when he was distant or critical, she crashed into despair and self-deprecation. She was unable to separate her mood or her thoughts about her ultimate future from his day-to-day attitude toward her.

Discussion of "It's Typical"

Ms. Siegel clearly has an episode of Major Depressive Disorder (DSM-5-TR, p. 183). She has been persistently depressed for most of the time during the past 2 months, with changes in her interests, eating, sleeping, energy level, and self-concept. The symptoms are causing her significant distress and are interfering with her functioning. Although her depression is in reaction to a stressor—the threatened end of a relationship with the man she hoped to marry—it is more severe than what the clinician would observe in a patient with an Adjustment Disorder, With Depressed Mood (see "Happy Ending" in Section 7.6) or Adjustment Disorder, With Mixed Anxiety and Depressed Mood.

What is somewhat unusual about this case of Major Depressive Disorder is that Ms. Siegel's mood reacts for the better when something positive happens (e.g., she sees something in what her boyfriend does or says that suggests to her that the relationship might still work out). Also, she has gained weight, rather than lost it, and she sleeps too much (missing classes) rather than experiencing

---

[2]Adapted from Skodol AE: *Problems in Differential Diagnosis: From DSM-III to DSM-III-R in Clinical Practice.* Washington, DC, American Psychiatric Press, 1989, pp. 245–246. Copyright © American Psychiatric Press. Used with permission.

insomnia. Finally, she feels like a lead weight is on her shoulders—a sensation referred to as leaden paralysis. These symptoms indicate that her diagnosis would be Major Depressive Disorder, With Atypical Features (DSM-5-TR, p. 212). Although selective serotonin reuptake inhibitor medications are most commonly used to treat most Major Depressive Episodes today, atypical depression has been shown to respond also to monoamine oxidase inhibitor antidepressant medications, such as phenelzine or tranylcypromine.

The anxiety attacks Ms. Siegel has had, which have led her to avoid going to school on several occasions, suggest the additional provisional diagnosis of Panic Disorder (see "Toughing It Out" in Section 5.5), but more information about the nature of the attacks would be necessary to confirm this diagnosis.

New Mom

Maria Jimenez is a 30-year-old married woman who returns to see the psychiatrist who manages her medications. She recently gave birth to her first child, a baby boy, by cesarean section. She is currently on maternity leave from her job as a research analyst at a mutual fund investment company. She had been taking sertraline for about 5 years for social anxiety, but she had discontinued it about 1½ years ago when she decided to try to become pregnant. Although she experienced the return of some of her anxiety symptoms while not taking the medication, she persisted with her plan to be medication-free throughout her pregnancy with the help of her psychotherapist.

Ms. Jimenez's current complaint is of depressed mood with overeating, oversleeping, decreased energy, decreased concentration, and decreased interest in most everything except for the baby and food, all of which began shortly after she was discharged from the hospital 2 months ago and returned home with the baby. She denies suicidal plans or intentions, but she does admit to a "taunting thought" of "what if I somehow ended up hurting myself?" She denies any concerns that she would do anything deliberately harmful to her son. Although her mother lives nearby and has been helping to take care of Ms. Jimenez's son on an almost daily basis, Ms. Jimenez is concerned that she is being neglectful of her husband and baby, and she is feeling guilty and worried that she is being a "bad" mother and might not "bond" with the baby. Her self-esteem has suffered. She is also upset with herself because she has been unable to lose the desired amount of weight after pregnancy and feels "fat and ugly."

Her relationship with her husband has become strained, because the new baby has placed new demands on both of them, and he resents how much time Ms. Jimenez's mother spends in their apartment. Ms. Jimenez's relationship with her mother has always been very close, and her mother has often put pressure on her or criticized her about important aspects of her life, such as where she was working or whom she was dating. Now, her mother is giving advice about baby care, and the patient is all too willing to listen, given that she often feels "not up to the job."

Ms. Jimenez has been in psychotherapy on and off for the past 7 years with a psychologist who specializes in young women's issues. When first seen by the psychiatrist, Ms. Jimenez was diagnosed with Social Anxiety Disorder, because she was experiencing anxiety and fear of embarrassment at business meetings and social gatherings—anywhere that she had to speak or eat in front of other people. She was afraid that other people would see her hands shaking, her face flushing, or her voice wavering. She began to avoid situations such as dinners with friends. The combination of supportive psychotherapy and sertraline had enabled her to manage her anxiety. She was promoted at work and met the man that she eventually married by way of an introduction by her sister.

Discussion of "New Mom"

Ms. Jimenez presents with symptoms of Major Depressive Disorder (DSM-5-TR, p. 183). For much of the time over the past 2 months, she has had depressed mood, loss of interest, increased appetite (with an inability to lose weight), hypersomnia, decreased energy, decreased concentration, guilt about what kind of mother she has been (not merely because she has not felt well), and worries that she might somehow hurt herself. Because these symptoms had their onset within the first 4 weeks following delivery of her baby, the disorder would be noted to be With Peripartum Onset (DSM-5-TR, p. 213).

About 9% of women will experience the onset of a Major Depressive Episode during pregnancy or in the weeks or months following delivery. Ms. Jimenez also has a history of Social Anxiety Disorder (DSM-5-TR, p. 229), which had been under control with medication, but recurred to an extent while she was unmedicated. Mood and anxiety symptoms during pregnancy increase the risk for a postpartum Major Depressive Episode.

A Child Is Crying

Cindy, age 15 years, was brought to a mental health clinic by her father after he received a call from the school counselor, who was concerned that Cindy was depressed and possibly suicidal. Her father had also been concerned about Cindy because she had seemed sad and withdrawn for the past month.

The household consists of Cindy, her father, mother, and two younger siblings. According to Cindy, she has been feeling depressed for most days, with symptoms of low self-esteem and hopelessness ever since she had a fight with her mother 2 years ago. During the fight, her mother threw a pot of hot water and burned Cindy on the shoulder. She was taken to a nearby medical emergency room and treated for the burn. Since then, she has stayed out of her mother's way.

Cindy's mother has a long history of mental problems, with multiple hospitalizations and long-term outpatient treatment. She is reported by the father to be chronically "psychotic" and to have marked mood swings.

There have been many conflicts in the marriage over the years, and the couple is now in the process of getting a divorce and selling their home. For the past 2 years, since the incident with the boiling water, Cindy's mother has occupied the third floor of their house and has had little contact with the family.

Before the incident with her mother, Cindy was very socially involved, taking dance and music lessons, and participating in both church and school activities. She was a straight-A student.

Cindy says that her mood has grown much worse in the last 6 months, from feeling depressed for most days to feeling depressed almost every day, all day long. She worries about her mother and feels that the fight was probably her fault. She has lost interest in school and social activities and has not really paid attention to her schoolwork for the last 6 months. Her grades have dropped from As to Bs and Cs. She is tired all the time and takes a nap when she comes home from school. She has trouble falling asleep at night and often has trouble getting up in the morning.

In the past 3 weeks, Cindy has become anxious and has had two experiences in which she felt "spacey and unreal." She often hears the voice of a young child crying for help, but when she looks to see if there is someone outside the door, there is never anyone there. At times recently, especially when she feels guilty about the fight with her mother, she is convinced that she does not deserve to live, and she has considered killing herself. Three weeks ago, while she was washing dishes, she thought about cutting her wrists with a knife, but the thought of how upset her father would be kept her from doing anything.

The psychiatrist who evaluated Cindy recommended an elective admission to the hospital. However, both she and her father felt that she would be able to follow through with outpatient treatment. She was given the telephone number of the emergency room, and the following day Cindy called to say that the voices were getting worse, and she was afraid she might hurt herself. She was directed to go immediately to the emergency room and was subsequently admitted to the hospital.

Discussion of "A Child Is Crying"

Cindy has been depressed for most days for 2 years. Depressed mood with accompanying symptoms of "low self-esteem" and "hopelessness" for most of the day for more days than not for at least 1 year in a child or adolescent indicates a diagnosis of Persistent Depressive Disorder (DSM-5-TR, p. 193). But in the past 6 months, Cindy has also had the characteristic symptoms of a full Major Depressive Episode (DSM-5-TR, p. 141): unremitting depressed mood, loss of interest in most activities, decreased energy, insomnia, excessive guilt, and thoughts of suicide. More recently, she has had auditory hallucinations of a child crying, which is congruent with her depressed mood, and she has experienced depersonalization (i.e., in her words, she felt "spacey and unreal").

In the absence of a history of either a Manic Episode or Hypomanic Episode or of a substance/medication-induced or a nonpsychiatric medical condition that directly caused the disturbance, the diagnosis of Major Depressive Disorder (DSM-5-TR, p. 183) applies for the most recent 6-month period. It is further noted as Single Episode (because there was no prior episode) and With Mood-Congruent Psychotic Features (DSM-5-TR, p. 213) (because of the hallucinations of a child crying for help). This case illustrates that the characteristic symptoms of Major Depressive Disorder do occur in adolescents. Moreover, in order to indicate that Cindy has had a long-standing depression that has worsened in severity over the past 6 months, DSM-5-TR recommends assigning the additional diagnosis of Persistent Depressive Disorder because it suggests the possibility of a more chronic course for Cindy's depression in the future. DSM-5-TR includes a symptom code for Suicidal Behavior (DSM-5-TR, p. 822) under its Other Conditions That May Be a Focus of Clinical Attention that can be added to any DSM-5-TR diagnosis to alert clinicians to this problem. The symptom code requires that the person has "engaged in potentially self-injurious behavior with at least some intent to die" (DSM-5-TR, p. 822). In Cindy's case, although she has had thoughts of suicide, she has not actually made an attempt and would not warrant the additional code.

A Perfect Checklist

Billy, a 7-year-old child in second grade, was brought to a mental health clinic by his mother because "he is unhappy and always complaining about feeling sick." He lives with his parents, his younger brother, and his grandmother. His mother describes Billy as a child who has never been very happy and never wanted to play with other children. From the time he started nursery school, he has complained about stomachaches, headaches, and various other physical problems, which are most intense in the morning when he is getting ready to go to school. In the last few months, his somatic complaints have escalated, prompting a complete medical examination, including a neurological examination and electroencephalogram (a measurement of electrical activity in different parts of the brain), all of which were normal.

Billy did well in first grade, but now he is having difficulty completing his schoolwork. He takes a lot of time to do his assignments and frequently feels he has to do them over again so that they will be "perfect." Because of Billy's frequent somatic complaints, it is hard to get him off to school in the morning. If he is allowed to stay home, he worries that he is falling behind in his schoolwork. When he does go to school, he often is unable to do the work, which makes him feel hopeless about his situation. To get through the day, he carries a note that he has instructed his mother to write for him: "You are not getting out of school early today. If you feel that you have to do your papers over and over again, please just do the best you can. Do not think about the time of day, and it will go quickly."

His worries have expanded beyond school, and frequently he is clinging and demanding of his parents. When his parents are out later than expected or leave to go shopping or do other routine daily chores without him, he is fearful that "something bad" may happen to them. He sits tensely at the window and watches for their return or walks restlessly around the house before returning again to the window. For the past several weeks, he has insisted that his little brother sleep with him; he is afraid to go to sleep at night alone because "someone might break into the house."

Although Billy's mother acknowledges that he has never been really happy, in the last 6 months, she feels he has become much more depressed. He frequently lies down about the house, saying that he is too tired to do anything. He has no interest or enjoyment in playing. His appetite has diminished. He has trouble falling asleep at night and often wakes up in the middle of the night or early in the morning. Three weeks ago, he talked for the first time about wanting to die and said that maybe he would shoot himself.

Billy's mother became pregnant 2 months after she was married. She did not feel ready for a child. She was hypertensive (had high blood pressure) during the pregnancy and was emotionally upset. Delivery was complicated because of increasing hypertension. At the time of delivery, Billy reportedly went into cardiac arrest. During the first week of his life, he developed projectile vomiting, which persisted for 2 weeks. He had nocturnal Enuresis (bedwetting) until a year ago.

During the assessment, Billy allowed his mother to go to another room to be interviewed; however, after 20 minutes, he became very upset, began crying, and insisted on being taken to her. He then was willing to sit outside the room where his mother was, as long as the door was open, and he could see her.

Billy was unable to finish a symptom checklist (designed for children his age) given at the time of the evaluation. He felt that he had to have a perfect checklist and became very worried about not being able to complete the list. He requested that he be allowed to take the papers home so that he could finish them; although he was told that it was not necessary for him to take the papers home, he insisted on doing so.

Discussion of "A Perfect Checklist"

This case illustrates the occurrence of severe depression in a very young child. Billy is clearly depressed. He has lost interest and enjoyment in playing, and has trouble sleeping, poor appetite, low energy, and suicidal thoughts. Because this is the first episode and the symptoms cause marked impairment in functioning, the diagnosis would be Major Depressive Disorder, Single Episode, Severe (DSM-5-TR, p. 183).

Billy has many other symptoms, including perfectionism, worrying about his performance in school, somatic complaints, and anxiety. He is tense and restless when his parents are away and is afraid to sleep alone. The perfectionism raises the question of whether Billy has Obsessive-Compulsive Personality Disorder (see Section 18.4) or Obsessive-Compulsive Disorder (see Section 6.1); however, he is too young for consideration of a personality disorder diagnosis and there is no evidence of frank obsessions or compulsions. His worrying about his school performance, his sleep disturbance, and his tenseness, restlessness, and fear that something bad might happen to his parents occurring more days than not for at least 6 months suggest the additional diagnosis of Generalized Anxiety Disorder (DSM-5-TR, p. 250).

The diagnosis of Separation Anxiety Disorder (see "Tiny Tina" in Section 5.1) requires at least three of eight symptoms of inappropriate and excessive anxiety concerning separation from those to whom the child is attached. Billy has at least five of these symptoms: distress when anticipating or experiencing separation from major attachment figures, unrealistic worry about possible harm befalling major attachment figures, reluctance to go to school, fear and avoidance of being alone (including clinging), and complaints of physical symptoms on school days. Therefore, a co-occurring diagnosis of Separation Anxiety Disorder (DSM-5-TR, p. 217) can also be made.

Billy's many somatic complaints suggest a Somatic Symptom Disorder (see Section 9.1), but a more parsimonious approach is to regard these symptoms as manifestations of Major Depressive Disorder.

The Mixed-Up Waiter

Andrew Weiglein, age 21 years, is a single man who is currently working at a restaurant as a waiter. He was referred by his family doctor to the walk-in mood and anxiety outpatient clinic for diagnostic clarification and treatment recommendations. His chief complaint is, "I am worried that I might lose my job because my performance has declined a lot over the past month."

Andrew endorses a 4-week history of "feeling and acting differently." He describes that for the past 4 weeks, he has been feeling "really sad" for no apparent reason. He has been unable to identify a trigger that precipitated this sadness and noted that this has never happened to him before. His motivation and enjoyment of working, socializing, and eating have significantly decreased during the past month. He has started to feel somewhat hopeless as well, feeling that he is "stuck working as a waiter" for the rest of his life, which has caused a decline in his self-esteem. He denies any thoughts of self-harm or suicidal ideation. He reports that the quality of his sleep has become quite poor and fragmented, even though he has now increased his time in bed from 8 to 14 hours per night. Notwithstanding the increased time in bed, he reports that he feels "exhausted" and "wired and tired" when he wakes up and has low energy throughout the day.

According to Andrew, his concentration has been significantly affected in many ways. For example, he "never used to need to write down customer food orders—I could remember them all"; however, he has made many mistakes over the past month, and his boss has instructed him to start using a notepad. Customers have also complained that he has been "overly chatty." He has become more easily distracted at work, and customers have complained that he is not listening when they are placing their orders, so they have to repeat themselves numerous times. Andrew also feels that his focus has been affected by "difficulty controlling the speed of my thoughts." He feels that when he is at work, at home, and socializing with friends, his thoughts are constantly racing about "meaningless, unconnected ideas." He denies previously experiencing distractibility, inattention, or racing thoughts earlier in his life. His boss has noticed these changes and has threatened to dismiss Andrew if he does not show improvement in his performance soon.

The possibility of losing his job is particularly concerning to Andrew at the current time because he has accumulated over $10,000 of debt during the past month. He reports daily online purchases of a variety of items (e.g., clothing, gadgets, a laptop, speakers), as well as playing online poker. Before this month, he reports being quite frugal, without any debt and with approximately $5,000 in savings. He would occasionally play online poker, but he had been quite disciplined and maintained a maximum $20 limit per week. This month, he has already lost $1,000 through playing online poker. With this behavior, too, he does not know what the trigger has been, and he feels that all the gambling and online purchases have been fairly impulsive in nature. Andrew denies any impulsive behaviors before this month and denies any current or previous impulsive substance use or sexual encounters. He states he would not have the energy or motivation to go out to "find someone to have sex with or to buy drugs from, so this has not been a problem."

When his family doctor saw him 2 weeks ago, the doctor was apprehensive about prescribing any medication because he was uncertain of the diagnosis. However, the doctor prescribed zopiclone 7.5 mg, a sleep medication to help Andrew sleep at night, and lorazepam 1 mg, an antianxiety medication to use as needed "to take the edge off."

Notably in his family history, Andrew's mother and maternal grandmother have been diagnosed with "depression," and his father has been diagnosed with "manic-depression or schizophrenia…we are not sure." However, because his father was the CEO of a medium-size company, the diagnosis of Bipolar Disorder for his father seems more likely. His father had one hospitalization when he was 25 years old; however, he has been fairly well since then on maintenance lithium therapy.

At the interview, Andrew is well-groomed and appears his stated age. His mood is "very sad," and he appears dysphoric. Although his speech is pressured (rapid, virtually nonstop speech that is usually hard to interrupt), it is of a normal volume. He appears to be quite distracted and difficult to refocus and redirect. His form of thought displays flight of ideas (a rapid shifting of ideas with only superficial associative connections between them). His thought content is significant for ruminating about losing his job. He has no suicidal or homicidal ideation.

Discussion of "The Mixed-Up Waiter"

Andrew has experienced a 4-week period during which he has felt "really sad" and has lost interest in his job and his social life. He has lost his appetite, is not sleeping well (although he spends more hours than usual in bed), feels hopeless about his future, has extreme fatigue and "low energy" throughout the day, and is having trouble concentrating, such that he gets mixed up and forgets customers' orders when he used to be able to remember them without writing them down. In the absence of drug use or a nonpsychiatric medical condition that could cause these symptoms, they are indicative of Major Depressive Disorder (DSM-5-TR, p. 183).

Andrew also reports, however, some additional symptoms not ordinarily associated with depression: he has become more talkative than usual ("overly chatty"), and he feels that he has "difficulty controlling the speed of his thoughts" and has racing thoughts about "meaningless, unconnected ideas." The evaluating psychiatrist observes that Andrew does, indeed, have pressured speech and flight of ideas. In addition, Andrew is impulsively engaging in activities that are causing him harm: buying things that he cannot really afford and playing poker online. His purchases and gambling losses have turned $5,000 in savings into $10,000 in debt in a matter of a month. The presence of three manic-like symptoms during the course of an episode of Major Depressive Disorder are observable by others and are a change from Andrew's usual behavior; however, these symptoms do not meet full criteria for either a Manic or Hypomanic Episode because of the absence of abnormally and persistently elevated, expansive, or irritable mood and the absence of abnormally and persistently increased activity or energy. Instead, these manic-like symptoms justify the addition of the specifier With Mixed Features to the diagnosis of Major Depressive Disorder (DSM-5-TR, p. 211).

Major Depressive Disorder, With Mixed Features, requires close monitoring of the patient's antidepressant medication to guard against precipitation of a full-blown Manic Episode by the antidepressant. If a patient had a history of antidepressant-associated manic symptoms in the past (see "Triple Divorcée" in Section 3.1), which Andrew does not have, then adding a mood-stabilizing medication, such as lithium, carbamazepine, or valproic acid, to the treatment regimen would be considered wise.

Rx Florida

Five winters ago, John Redland, a 42-year-old physician, married with two children, sought treatment for recurrent depression at a university hospital Seasonal Affective Disorder treatment program in Boston. He had stated that over the preceding few weeks, he had felt he was again slipping into a depression.

Dr. Redland said that his first depression occurred at age 21 after he had moved to the Washington, D.C., metropolitan area from Florida, where he had lived until that time. Depressions recurred the next four winters, while he was in college and early in medical school. During the last of those episodes, Dr. Redland was hospitalized and told that because of his recurrent depressions, he was unlikely ever to succeed in becoming a physician, which had been his lifelong goal. He remained depressed and in the hospital for the next year, during which time he was treated with psychotherapy alone. His depression remitted in the spring, and he remained free of depressions for several years, during which time he completed medical school and his internship. However, the winter depressions had returned each year for the 9 years before he applied to the university treatment program.

Dr. Redland came to realize that his depressive episodes seem to follow the same pattern. They start around the first of December (plus or minus 3 weeks) and begin to lift by April. In most years, the onset of depression is gradual, but sometimes it occurs more precipitously, apparently in response to some environmental stress. When depressed, Dr. Redland is lethargic, apathetic, irritable, and pessimistic. His mood is worse in the morning. He cannot sleep through the night. He craves carbohydrates (bread, cake, cookies) and gains weight. He has noticed that his winter clothes are often two sizes larger than his summer ones. He recalls feeling much better during a winter vacation in Bermuda; the mood improvement occurred a few days after he arrived there. However, he relapsed a few days after returning to the northern United States. He also recalls one particularly difficult winter when he worked in Syracuse, New York. These associations between latitude, the weather, and his mood make him wonder whether the climate may actually be influencing his mood changes.

When Dr. Redland first went to the treatment program, he had been treated for several years with psychotherapy and a tricyclic antidepressant, desipramine 175 mg/day, both of which he had found to be "quite helpful." He was maintained on desipramine and placed on "bright light treatment," involving exposure to light from a 10,000-lumen light box (high-intensity light with low emission of ultraviolet light) especially designed for the treatment of seasonal affective disorder. He was treated for 30 minutes each morning, with the light box at a distance of about 18 inches from his face. After 1 week of treatment, he became much less depressed, and his score on the Hamilton Rating Scale for Depression fell from 21 to 8.

After the patient's depression responded, his desipramine dosage was increased to 250 mg/day and he was maintained on light treatment for 15 minutes during the day and again in the evening hours; he remained free of depression when treated with the combination of light and desipramine. Dr. Redland has used lights each winter since then and increases his maintenance dosage of desipramine from 175 mg/day to 250 mg/day during the winter months. He has been virtually free of depression for the last 4 years and is not currently in psychotherapy.

Discussion of "Rx Florida"

There can be little doubt that Dr. Redland suffers from Major Depressive Disorder, Recurrent Episode (DSM-5-TR, p. 183). He has had numerous episodes of persistent depressed mood, disturbed sleep, increased appetite and weight gain, decreased energy, and loss of interest in usual activities. When Dr. Redland first arrived at the depression treatment program, he was once again "slipping into a depression," which was noted as Mild, although in the past his depressions had been Severe.

What is unusual about Dr. Redland's depressions is that they apparently all began in the winter and remitted in the spring. Recurrent Mood Disorders that regularly begin and end during a particular period of the year are commonly called "seasonal affective disorders." Dr. Redland's case illustrates the most common pattern, in which depression begins in fall or winter and ends in spring. Less common patterns involve recurrent depressions or Manic Episodes that begin in the summer and remit in the fall or winter. In DSM-5-TR, the concept of seasonal affective disorder is expressed with the specifier With Seasonal Pattern (DSM-5-TR, p. 214), which requires that the seasonal episodes should have been present during at least each of the past 2 years, with no nonseasonal episodes during the same period. Seasonal episodes should substantially outnumber nonseasonal episodes over the patient's lifetime.

Dr. Redland's weight gain and craving for carbohydrates are typical of cases with seasonal affective disorder. In other ways his case is atypical; most patients with seasonal affective disorder are women, and most complain of increased sleeping (hypersomnia) rather than of disturbed sleep (insomnia).

Like many patients with seasonal affective disorder, during the summer Dr. Redland is able to reduce the dose of antidepressant medication and discontinue the light treatment. In the winter, however, he is unable to stop the light treatment for more than a few days without a return of his depressive symptoms.

4.3
Persistent Depressive Disorder

Persistent Depressive Disorder is characterized by "depressed mood for most of the day, for more days than not," for at least 2 years (1 year for children and adolescents; DSM-5-TR, p. 193). Accompanying the depressed mood, there must be at least two additional symptoms such as poor appetite or overeating, insomnia or hypersomnia, low energy or fatigue, low self-esteem, poor concentration or difficulty making decisions, and feelings of hopelessness. The defining feature of Persistent Depressive Disorder is its chronicity, given that persistence of depression has been demonstrated to be the most important negative prognostic indicator of long-term outcome—more important than the severity of the depression itself. To ensure the chronicity requirement, there should not be a period of 2 months or more during the 2-year period when the individual is without depressive symptoms. To receive a diagnosis of Persistent Depressive Disorder, the individual should never have had a Manic Episode or a Hypomanic Episode (see Chapter 3, "Bipolar and Related Disorders").

Given the precedence of chronicity over severity in the definition of Persistent Depressive Disorder, the severity of the depression during the 2-year period can vary widely from case to case. Some individuals have relatively mild chronic depression, which is below the severity threshold for Major Depressive Disorder. Other individuals with Persistent Depressive Disorder have a background of chronic mild depression punctuated by recurrent episodes of Major Depressive Disorder, a situation that has been referred to as "double depression." Finally, other individuals have severe chronic depression, in which their presentation essentially meets the diagnostic requirements for Major Depressive Disorder every day for the 2-year period. Note that for both of these latter two situations, it is necessary to give the additional diagnosis of Major Depressive Disorder to indicate that the depression has been severe enough to reach the severity threshold of a Major Depressive Episode.

Persistent Depressive Disorder varies by age at onset, which can be specified as Early Onset (before age 21 years) or Late Onset (at age 21 years or older). Persons with Early Onset are more likely to develop Personality Disorders (see Chapter 18) and Substance Use Disorders (see Chapter 16).

The various longitudinal patterns of milder and more severe depressive syndromes described above can be specified for Persistent Depressive Disorder:

- If a person has Persistent Depressive Disorder but has never had an episode of Major Depressive Disorder during a 2-year period, the disorder is further specified as With Pure Dysthymic Syndrome. "Dysthymia" was the term used in DSM editions before DSM-5 to indicate chronic depression below the severity threshold for a Major Depressive Episode.
- If the person has Major Depressive Disorder that has lasted for the entire preceding 2-year period, the disorder is further specified as With Persistent Major Depressive Episode (i.e., chronic Major Depressive Disorder).
- The following two presentations have often been referred to as "double depression":
  - If the person currently has Major Depressive Disorder with periods of 8 weeks or more in the past 2 years when symptoms were below the diagnostic threshold for Major Depressive Disorder, the disorder is further specified as With Intermittent Major Depressive Episodes, With Current Episode.
  - If the person does not currently have Major Depressive Disorder but has had an episode in the preceding 2 years, the disorder is further specified as With Intermittent Major Depressive Episodes, Without Current Episode.

The specifiers In Partial Remission and In Full Remission, the symptomatic specifiers (e.g., With Anxious Distress, With Atypical Features), and the severity specifiers (i.e., Mild, Moderate, Severe) apply to Persistent Depressive Disorder as they do to Major Depressive Disorder (see introduction to Section 4.2).

The course of Persistent Depressive Disorder is by definition chronic. When symptoms rise to the level of a Major Depressive Episode, they will usually subsequently revert to a prior, lower level, but depressive symptoms are much less likely to resolve over a given period of time in the context of Persistent Depressive Disorder than they are in a Major Depressive Episode. The disorder's impact on psychosocial functioning is likely to be as great as or greater than that of Major Depressive Disorder.

Persistent Depressive Disorder is an amalgam of two DSM-IV diagnoses: Dysthymic Disorder (a 2+ year period of depressed mood most of the day, for more days than not but below the threshold for a Major Depressive Episode) and DSM-IV Chronic Major Depressive Disorder (full criteria continuously met for a Major Depressive Episode for at least 2 years). The 12-month prevalence in the United States is approximately 0.5% for DSM-IV Dysthymic Disorder and 1.5% for DSM-IV Chronic Major Depressive Disorder, with prevalence among women approximately 1.5 and 2 times higher than prevalence among men for each of these diagnoses.

Individuals with Persistent Depressive Disorder are at greater risk for Anxiety Disorders, Substance Use Disorders, and Personality Disorders than are people with Major Depressive Disorder. Early Onset Persistent Depressive Disorder is strongly associated with DSM-5-TR Section II Cluster B and C Personality Disorders (see Chapter 18).

Junior Executive

A 28-year-old junior executive, Isabella Garcia, was referred by a senior psychoanalyst for "supportive" treatment. She had obtained a master's degree in business administration and moved to California 1½ years earlier to begin work in a large firm. She complained of being "depressed" and "hopeless" about everything: her job, her husband, and her prospects for the future.

She had had extensive psychotherapy previously. She had seen an "analyst" twice a week for 3 years while in college and a "behaviorist" for 1½ years while in graduate school. Her complaints were of persistent feelings of depressed mood, inferiority, and pessimism, which she claims to have had since she was 16 or 17 years old. Although she did reasonably well in college, she consistently ruminated about those students who were "genuinely intelligent." She dated during college and graduate school but claimed that she would never go after a guy she thought was "special," always feeling inferior and intimidated. Whenever she saw or met such a man, she acted stiff and aloof, or actually walked away as quickly as possible, only to berate herself afterward and then fantasize about him for many months. She claimed that her therapy had helped, although she still could not remember a time when she did not feel somewhat depressed.

Just after graduation, Ms. Garcia married the man she was going out with at the time. She thought of him as reasonably desirable, though not "special," and married him primarily because she felt she "needed a husband" for companionship. Shortly after their marriage, the couple started to bicker. She was very critical of his clothes, his job, and his parents; and he, in turn, found her rejecting, controlling, and moody. She began to feel that she had made a mistake in marrying him.

Recently, Ms. Garcia has also been having difficulties at work. She is assigned the most menial tasks at the firm and is never given an assignment of importance or responsibility. She admits that she frequently does a "slipshod" job of what is given her, never does more than is required, and never demonstrates any assertiveness or initiative to her supervisors. She views her boss as self-centered, unconcerned, and unfair, but nevertheless admires his success. She feels that she will never go very far in her profession because she does not have the right "connections," and neither does her husband; however, she dreams of money, status, and power.

Ms. Garcia's social life with her husband involves several other couples. The men in these couples are usually friends of her husband's. She is sure that the women find her uninteresting and unimpressive, and that the people who seem to like her are probably no better off than she.

Under the burden of her dissatisfaction with her marriage, her job, and her social life, and feeling tired and uninterested in "life," she now enters treatment for the third time.

Discussion of "Junior Executive"

Ms. Garcia's marriage and occupational functioning are severely affected by her chronically depressed mood, low self-esteem, hopelessness, and pessimism. Although she now complains also of loss of interest and energy, it is unlikely that these symptoms represent a significant change from her usual condition. Because her depression and associated symptoms have persisted continuously for more than 2 years, the diagnosis of Persistent Depressive Disorder is considered. Additionally, there is no evidence of a Manic or Hypomanic Episode, the disturbance is not better explained by a persistent psychotic disorder, and Ms. Garcia's symptoms are not attributable to the physiological effects of a substance (e.g., a drug of abuse or a medication) or a nonpsychiatric medical condition (e.g., hypothyroidism); thus, the diagnosis of Persistent Depressive Disorder (DSM-5-TR, p. 193) would be made. In this case, the onset of the mood disturbance in adolescence would be noted as Early Onset. Finally, given that Ms. Garcia has not had any Major Depressive Episodes during her most recent 2-year period of chronic depression, the specifier With Pure Dysthymic Syndrome applies.

Many clinicians would regard Ms. Garcia's depressive symptoms as an expression of a Personality Disorder (see Chapter 18) rather than a Depressive Disorder. They would argue that it is impossible to separate her depressive symptoms from the characteristic and persistent way in which she relates to herself, to others, and to the world, and that treatment should therefore be focused on her characterological style, as well as on the affective symptoms. However, in classifying Persistent Depressive Disorder under the broad rubric of Depressive Disorders, DSM-5-TR makes no assumption that the optimal treatment is necessarily biological or should be directed merely at symptom relief.

Busted Nerves

Norma Jean Luby, a 49-year-old homemaker, was seen in a central Appalachian clinic on referral from her primary care physician for evaluation of depression. She was a pale, neatly and plainly dressed woman, with hair combed straight back and no makeup. Her eyes were filled with tears during most of the interview, although she did not weep openly. She spoke slowly and so softly that at times she was inaudible. She appeared timid, abject, dependent, helpless, and hopeless, claiming she had been ill all of her life, and summed up her situation by stating, "My nerves are busted. I can't do anything."

Mrs. Luby had multiple complaints of pain, including "black ankles," painful "knots" in her neck, "busted discs" in her back, headaches that radiated all over her body, and pelvic and abdominal pain. She described a variety of gastrointestinal and respiratory complaints. It became apparent on conducting a routine review of systems that she would respond positively to every query about the presence of a particular somatic symptom. She said she had been depressed all her life, and it was getting worse. She was sad, helpless, hopeless, and fearful. She had no energy and did little but "sit around the house." She had no interest in anything, and nothing gave her pleasure. She was able to fall asleep but would wake repeatedly during the night and be awake for good before it was light. She had no appetite and had lost 10 pounds over the preceding 2 months. She had had many episodes of weight loss and gain in the past. She said that she "couldn't pay attention to nothing. People are talking to me, and I forget what they are saying right in the middle of things." She also said that she "wasn't interested in nothing, not even TV." From time to time, she thinks she hears voices calling her name; she would look about, but no one was present. Frequent episodes of "smothering" have occurred. At these times, she has felt that she might choke to death. She would become dizzy, her heart would pound, and her hands would tingle.

Mrs. Luby had never had a formal psychiatric evaluation or treatment; however, detailed observations made by her physician in her chart from 25 years ago revealed a picture similar in almost every respect to her current presentation. She has taken multiple "minor tranquilizers" over the years, with no benefit. Aside from mild, self-limited episodes of physical illness, usually infections, her physical examination and laboratory studies were always within normal limits, as they were at the time of this referral.

Mrs. Luby was born and lived all of her life in the central Appalachian Mountains. She attended school through the eighth grade but said she "couldn't learn." She was unable to say how old she was when she stopped going to school and "stayed at home" with her mother and father. All of her siblings left home, but "I stayed home and helped my mother." This was the state of affairs until she met and married her husband, when she was age 23. They have three grown daughters. Her husband, a former coal miner, is drawing disability because of black lung disease.

Mrs. Luby was seen for individual supportive psychotherapy and medication management biweekly for 5 months. The chronicity, fixity, and recalcitrant nature of her symptoms were remarkable. She appeared regularly for sessions and was always on time but displayed little insight into her condition. She had trials on various medications. Finally, while taking trazodone, she reported that her sleep was improved and, consequently, she seemed to feel "a little better" during the day. Based on a review of her medical records for the past 25 years, this is the first time she has reported even a faintly positive response to any psychotropic medication.

Discussion of "Busted Nerves"

Somatic symptoms are a common manifestation of depression in certain cultures and subcultures (see "Cultural Formulation" in DSM-5-TR, p. 860). This case is an example of a syndrome frequently seen in individuals living in rural Appalachia and other rural parts of North America. The syndrome is characterized by a pattern of somatic and emotional complaints that are attributed to "nerves" rather than to specific physical causes or illnesses. Common symptoms include fainting, partial paralysis, forgetfulness and amnesia, inertia and weakness, and inability to do any strenuous physical activity without getting faint, shaky, or "going to pieces." The individuals are often described as fearful and nonassertive, showing surprisingly little resentment over their lot in life. In previous times, similar cases were given the diagnosis of "hysteria."

Because Mrs. Luby responds positively to every query about physical symptoms, Somatic Symptom Disorder (see "Blackout" in Section 9.1) needs to be considered as a diagnosis. However, the patient does not seem to be preoccupied with the seriousness of her symptoms, or to have a persistently high level of anxiety about them, or to have spent excessive time or energy devoted to her symptoms or health concerns—at least one of which is a requirement for the diagnosis of Somatic Symptom Disorder.

Mrs. Luby's chronic mildly depressed mood and associated symptoms of hopelessness, lack of energy, insomnia, poor appetite, and poor concentration indicate a diagnosis of Persistent Depressive Disorder (DSM-5-TR, p. 193). Because she reports that she has been "depressed all her life," it is reasonable to add the specifier Early Onset (i.e., onset before age 21 years). It is unclear whether she also has had superimposed episodes of Major Depressive Disorder (her current state does not appear severe enough to warrant that diagnosis), but if she had one or more episodes in the past 2 years, the specifier With Intermittent Major Depressive Episodes, Without Current Episode, would be added. The episodes of smothering and dizziness suggest a probable additional diagnosis of Panic Disorder (see "Toughing It Out" in Section 5.5).

One question is whether Mrs. Luby should also be diagnosed with a Personality Disorder (see Chapter 18) because of her pattern of timidity, social isolation, and general ineffectiveness, or whether these are symptoms of her underlying Depressive Disorder. Because her personality problems are not aptly described by any specific DSM-5-TR Personality Disorder, there seems to be little advantage to adding a diagnosis of Other Specified or Unspecified Personality Disorder. Furthermore, most patients with long-standing Persistent Depressive Disorder do also show some nonspecific personality disturbances.

Disabled Vet

Roger Albrecht is a 37-year-old man who admits himself to a VA hospital after attempting suicide by taking sleeping pills. He says that nothing in particular prompted this attempt but that he has been very depressed, with only minor fluctuations, since he returned from Iraq 10 years earlier.

He describes a reasonably normal childhood and adolescence. "I never in my life felt like this before I got to Iraq." He had friends throughout high school, always got at least average grades, and never was in trouble with the law or other authorities. He has had many girlfriends but has never married. After high school, he went to technical school, was trained as an electrician, and joined the Army Reserves. He was working in his occupation when he was called up from the Reserves for military service in Iraq. He loathed the violence there, but on one occasion, evidently swept away by the group spirit, he killed a civilian "for the fun of it." This seemed to him totally out of keeping with his character. The memory of this incident continues to haunt him, and he is wracked with guilt. He was honorably discharged from the army after completing an extended tour and has never worked since, except for 3 weeks when an uncle hired him. He has been living on various forms of government assistance.

In the army, Mr. Albrecht began to drink heavily and to use whatever drugs he could get his hands on, abusing most of them, but in the last few years, he has turned to alcohol almost exclusively. He has been drinking very heavily and nearly continually for the past 10 years, with blackouts, frequent arrests for public intoxication, and injuries in barroom brawls. He has acquaintances but no friends. Whenever he "dries out," he feels terribly depressed (as he also does when he drinks); he has made four suicide attempts in the last 7 years. For the month before his latest suicide attempt, Mr. Albrecht had been living in an alcohol-treatment residence, the longest dry period he can remember; all previous attempts at cutting down on his drinking had failed.

Mr. Albrecht presents as a very sad, thoughtful, introspective man with a dignified bearing. In informal conversation, he appears to be of at least normal intelligence. He is not interested in anything and confides that when he sees others enjoying themselves, he is so jealous he wants to hit them; this urge is never evident from his unfailingly courteous behavior. There is no evidence of delusions and no history of hallucinations except during several bouts of Alcohol Withdrawal Delirium in the past. Mr. Albrecht's appetite is normal, as is his sex drive, "but I don't enjoy it." He has trouble falling asleep or staying asleep without medication. He does not have psychomotor slowing. He complains of "absentmindedness."

After 2 weeks at the hospital, Mr. Albrecht still had trouble finding his way around the ward. He seemed very well motivated to cooperate with neuropsychological testing and was extremely distressed by his disabilities. Testing revealed impaired immediate and long-term memory, apraxia (difficulty with complex, coordinated movements), agnosia (inability to interpret sensations and hence to recognize things), peripheral neuropathy (weakness, numbness, and pain from nerve damage in the hands and feet), and constructional difficulties (inability to build, assemble, or draw objects); his IQ measured 66.

Mr. Albrecht has not responded to antidepressant medication. He is sorry that his suicide attempt did not succeed, and he says that if things are not going to get any better, he definitely wants to die.

Discussion of "Disabled Vet"

What occasioned Mr. Albrecht's hospital admission was a suicide attempt, a symptom of his long-standing depression. A 10-year period of depressed mood and anhedonia, with such associated symptoms as sleep difficulties, absentmindedness, and recurrent suicidal acts, suggests chronic Major Depressive Disorder. The episode has lasted for the previous 2 years without a full remission for 2 months or longer, so the diagnosis is Persistent Depressive Disorder (DSM-5-TR, p. 193). Because there is no evidence of a period without significant symptoms of depression, the clinician notes the specifier With Persistent Major Depressive Episode, plus a comorbid diagnosis of Major Depressive Disorder. It does not appear that Mr. Albrecht's depression began when he was an adolescent, so it would be noted as Late Onset. In order to call special attention to his suicide attempt and to track his suicidal behavior over time, and its response (or not) to treatment, a symptom code indicating Current Suicidal Behavior (T14.91XA) should also be added to his Persistent Depressive Disorder diagnosis. Mr. Albrecht is a combat veteran and while serving in Iraq, he witnessed the killing of a civilian (by his own hand), which would qualify as a traumatic event for the purposes of a Posttraumatic Stress Disorder diagnosis. However, although he was haunted by memories of the traumatic event, other symptoms of Posttraumatic Stress Disorder do not appear to be present.

Mr. Albrecht has a long history of heavy drinking; unsuccessful efforts to cut down on alcohol use; reduced involvement in social, occupational, and recreational activities because of alcohol use; and continued drinking despite knowledge of recurrent problems caused by alcohol use (blackouts, frequent arrests, and injuries in barroom brawls). These, together with the history of episodes of withdrawal (Alcohol Withdrawal Delirium), indicate the presence of Severe Alcohol Use Disorder (DSM-5-TR, p. 553).

Furthermore, Mr. Albrecht has severe memory loss and evidence of impairment of higher cortical functioning (apraxia, agnosia, constructional difficulties) and a decrement in intellectual abilities (IQ of 66) that interfere with functioning. Because these symptoms are apparently due to the long history of Alcohol Use Disorder and are not limited to memory loss (as in Alcohol-Induced Major Neurocognitive Disorder, Amnestic-Confabulatory Type), the diagnosis of Alcohol-Induced Major Neurocognitive Disorder (DSM-5-TR, p. 712) is given.

4.4
Premenstrual Dysphoric Disorder

Two groups of signs and symptoms define Premenstrual Dysphoric Disorder in DSM-5-TR:

- The first group consists of classic signs and symptoms of *dysphoria*: affective lability (e.g., sudden changes in mood); marked irritability or anger or increased interpersonal conflicts; marked depressed mood, feelings of hopelessness, or self-deprecating thoughts; and marked anxiety, tension, or feelings of being keyed up or on edge.
- The second group consists of commonly associated symptoms of *depression*: decreased interest in activities, difficulty concentrating, lethargy or lack of energy, marked change in appetite including overeating and craving specific foods, hypersomnia or insomnia, and a sense of being overwhelmed or out of control. Also included in this second group of symptoms are *physical symptoms* such as breast tenderness or swelling, joint or muscle pain, a feeling of bloating, or weight gain.

This diagnosis requires that a woman have a minimum of five total symptoms, with at least one from each of the two groups.

The key to the diagnosis, however, is the relationship of these symptoms to the woman's menstrual cycle. DSM-5-TR states that "in the majority of menstrual cycles, at least five symptoms must be present in the final week before the onset of menses, start to *improve* within a few days after the onset of menses, and become *minimal* or absent in the week postmenses" (DSM-5-TR, Criterion A, p. 197). This pattern should be evident during at least the preceding year. The relationship of the onset and especially the resolution of the symptoms of Premenstrual Dysphoric Disorder to the phases of the menstrual cycle help to distinguish Premenstrual Dysphoric Disorder from an exacerbation of another mental disorder, such as Major Depressive Disorder. Like other mental disorders, Premenstrual Dysphoric Disorder is associated with significant distress and impairment in psychosocial functioning, and it is not merely an exacerbation of another mental disorder or attributable to the physiological effects of a substance or nonpsychiatric medical condition. Because women sometimes misreport the timing of the association of symptoms and the menstrual cycle, the diagnosis is made provisionally until the pattern is confirmed by prospective daily ratings during at least two symptomatic cycles.

Many women experience a variety of cognitive and physical symptoms related to their menstrual cycles, referred to as "premenstrual syndrome." What distinguishes premenstrual syndrome from Premenstrual Dysphoric Disorder is the absence in the former of prominent affective symptoms (e.g., affective lability, irritability or anger, depressed mood, anxiety). Premenstrual syndrome is generally considered a less severe condition.

The 12-month prevalence of Premenstrual Dysphoric Disorder is estimated at 5.8% in menstruating women. In the United States, the prevalence based on prospective ratings of symptoms for two consecutive menstrual cycles is 1.3%. Premenstrual Dysphoric Disorder can begin at any time after menarche. Prevalence may be higher in adolescent girls than in adult women. The disorder may get worse as a woman approaches menopause. Premenstrual Dysphoric Disorder is found in populations worldwide. It may be associated with significant marital conflict and problems with children, other family members, or friends.

Paranoid and Dangerous

Tracy Shaw, age 32, overweight, agitated, and belligerent, was brought to the psychiatric emergency room by the police after she had furiously pushed a chair into a full-length mirror, shattering the mirror, in the principal's office of her child's school. The psychiatrist who examined her described her as "paranoid and dangerous to others" and recommended immediate involuntary hospitalization if she refused to admit herself voluntarily.

Ms. Shaw refused voluntary admission. She stated that her suspicions concerning her child's unfair treatment in school were well-founded and that she would harm no one. She acknowledged that she was particularly tense, irritable, and angry because she was premenstrual. Her husband supported her decision and assumed responsibility for her and for bringing her back to see the psychiatrist the next day. That evening her menses began.

When Ms. Shaw saw the psychiatrist the next day, she appeared to be a "different person." She was relaxed, her anger and irritability had dissipated, and she displayed a sense of humor. However, her conviction that the school principal owed her an explanation of his unfair treatment of her child remained.

Ms. Shaw gave a history of monthly premenstrual symptoms beginning at menarche but worsening since her 20s. The symptoms were not the same every month. Some months she would become depressed, with thoughts of suicide; other months she would crave chocolate and gain 5–10 pounds in 1 week; some months she would break out in hives; and there were months when she had no symptoms. The symptoms were always predictable in their timing, occurring the week before her menses and remitting with onset of menses.

Ms. Shaw was the oldest daughter of a chronically depressed and fearful mother and an alcoholic father. Before marriage, she was the caregiver of her family. Her mother recovered significantly from her depression during Ms. Shaw's adolescence, only to fail rapidly physically and die when her daughter left home and married after high school.

Currently, Ms. Shaw is the mother of four grade-school children and also has primary responsibility for a sibling with alcoholism who is dying of cancer, as well as for her handicapped husband, who has been severely depressed and vocationally incapacitated since surgery 1½ years ago. She lives with her in-laws. Both her husband and his parents have significant alcohol problems.

Ms. Shaw is the family caregiver. "I can't live with myself unless I do it all. I feel guilty if I do something for myself." She can cope with the demands of her life and is not usually depressed, except when she is premenstrual, when "the whole world closes in" and she feels "pulled down."

Discussion of "Paranoid and Dangerous"

The uncontrolled behavior that led to Ms. Shaw's psychiatric evaluation suggested to the psychiatrist that she was psychotic and potentially dangerous to others and therefore in need of involuntary hospitalization. Fortunately, Ms. Shaw was able to convince the psychiatrist that she was not psychotic but that she suffered from episodic difficulties that always occurred in the few days before her menses and remitted when her menses began. Her symptoms vary from cycle to cycle and include depression, anger, irritability, tension, and overeating. Between episodes she is apparently completely free of such symptoms.

This pattern of recurrent dysphoric episodes beginning in the premenstrual phase and remitting with the onset of menses suggests the diagnosis of Premenstrual Dysphoric Disorder (DSM-5-TR, p. 197). To confirm this diagnosis, the psychiatrist needs to ask Ms. Shaw to make daily ratings of her mood and behavior for at least two cycles to validate her impression that the changes are always associated with the menstrual cycle. In addition, it would be necessary to establish that at least five of the dysphoric and other associated symptoms have been present for most of the time during the majority of premenstrual periods over the preceding year and that they impaired her functioning. Selective serotonin reuptake inhibitor medications are effective for many women with Premenstrual Dysphoric Disorder.

4.5
Depressive Disorder Due to Another Medical Condition

When there is evidence that a prominent and persistent period of depressed mood or markedly diminished interest or pleasure in all or almost all activities is the direct pathophysiological consequence of (i.e., caused by) a nonpsychiatric medical condition, then the appropriate diagnosis should be Depressive Disorder Due to Another Medical Condition. The diagnosis can be supported by the clinical history, physical examination, or laboratory tests.

Once the nonpsychiatric medical condition has been diagnosed, then the etiological relationship to depression needs to be established. The development of depression is known to be associated with certain medical conditions, such as stroke, Huntington's disease, Parkinson's disease, traumatic brain injury, Cushing's syndrome, and hypothyroidism. Evidence for an etiological relationship would be a clear temporal association between the onset, exacerbation, or remission of the mood disturbance and the corresponding change in the course of the presumed etiological medical condition. The actual course and outcome, including functional consequences, of a Depressive Disorder Due to Another Medical Condition will depend in large part on the nature of the underlying medical condition and the effectiveness of its treatment.

The characteristics of a Depressive Disorder Due to Another Medical Condition can be noted with certain specifiers. If the full criteria for a Major Depressive Episode are not met, the designation is With Depressive Features. If the full *symptomatic* criteria for a Major Depressive Episode are met, then the specifier is With Major Depressive–Like Episode. If there are also some symptoms of mania or hypomania (see Chapter 3, "Bipolar and Related Disorders") along with the depressive symptoms, then the disorder is noted to be With Mixed Features.

Toy Designer

Two years ago, Ray McKenzie, a 45-year-old toy designer, was admitted to the hospital following a series of suicidal gestures culminating in an attempt to strangle himself with a piece of wire. Four months before admission, his family had observed that he was becoming depressed: when at home he spent long periods sitting in a chair, slept more than usual, and had given up his habits of puttering around the house and watching the evening news on TV. Within a month, Mr. McKenzie was unable to get out of bed in the morning to go to work. He expressed considerable guilt but could not make up his mind to seek help until forced to do so by his family. He had not responded to 2 months of outpatient antidepressant drug therapy and had made several half-hearted attempts to cut his wrists before the serious attempt that precipitated the admission.

Physical examination revealed signs of increased intracranial pressure, and a computed tomography scan showed a large frontal-lobe brain tumor. Mr. McKenzie underwent surgery, and the tumor was removed. Two years following surgery, Mr. McKenzie's wife described to the surgeon how hopeful she initially was following surgery, because Mr. McKenzie's depression seemed to lift. However, he never regained interest in returning to work and has spent all of his time at home. Although Mr. McKenzie makes few complaints, his wife describes him as lacking his former enthusiasm and "spark." In addition, he seems to have trouble concentrating while watching TV.

Discussion of "Toy Designer"

Depressed mood, suicidal gestures, increased sleep, loss of interest, and guilt all suggest a past episode of Major Depressive Disorder. Although Mr. McKenzie's symptoms are identical with those seen in that disorder, it is reasonable to infer that the presurgical disturbance is caused by the frontal-lobe brain tumor; thus, the diagnosis is Depressive Disorder Due to Brain Tumor, With Major Depressive–Like Episode (DSM-5-TR, p. 206). The serious suicide attempt with clear intent to die (strangulation with a piece of wire) that prompted his hospital admission warrants the addition of a symptom code Current Suicidal Behavior (found in "Other Conditions That May Be a Focus of Clinical Attention" in DSM-5-TR, p. 822).

Some clinicians might have preferred to consider this diagnosis provisional, pending the results of surgery in order to better clarify the temporal relationship between the brain tumor and the symptoms of depression. If the depression lifts after removal of the brain tumor, the diagnosis of Depressive Disorder Due to Brain Tumor would be supported. If Mr. McKenzie's depression persists following surgery, the diagnosis would remain equivocal, because there would be no way to definitely rule out Major Depressive Disorder that developed coincidentally.

However, Mr. McKenzie's diagnosis at follow-up is changed from the original diagnosis. The predominant disturbance 2 years after surgery is a marked change in personality, as manifested by Mr. McKenzie's apathy and indifference rather than symptoms of depression. Personality changes are common in Major or Mild Neurocognitive Disorders (see "The Hiker" in Section 17.2); however, in Mr. McKenzie's case, despite some difficulty in concentrating, he demonstrates no evidence of significant cognitive decline. Thus, the follow-up diagnosis is Personality Change Due to Brain Tumor, Apathetic Type (DSM-5-TR, pp. 775–776).

CHAPTER 5

Anxiety Disorders

Anxiety Disorders are characterized by excessive fear or anxiety and resulting avoidance behaviors intended to mitigate the anxiety. The experience of fear and the related emotion of anxiety are normal parts of life. Fear is essential to protect a person from immediate threat and to mobilize the body for quick action to avoid danger. Anxiety, on the other hand, is a future-oriented affective state in which the person anticipates a future threat and experiences a sense of uncontrollability and vulnerability focused on the upcoming event or circumstance. Anxiety leads to a shift in attention toward the source of the danger so that the individual becomes more vigilant for relevant threat cues and, thus, is more likely to experience fear, with the autonomic nervous system arousal necessary for "fight or flight," in the face of a perceived immediate threat. An individual walking home alone at night, for example, may become anxious and begin to scan the environment for noises or shadows that might portend a lurking mugger from whom they would attempt to flee. Fear and anxiety are not always adaptive, however. At times, fear or anxiety can occur in the absence of any realistic threat, or these emotions may be out of proportion to the actual danger posed by the feared object or situation.

Anxiety Disorders differ from one another based on the types of objects or situations that provoke fear or anxiety, the type and pattern of fear or anxiety experienced, and the presence and extent of avoidance behavior. The Anxiety Disorders include Separation Anxiety Disorder, in which a person has fear or anxiety concerning separation from attachment figures (most often parents, but can be offspring or romantic partners for adults); Selective Mutism, in which a person fails to speak in some (usually social) situations; Specific Phobia, in which fear or anxiety is related to a specific object or situation, such as dogs, snakes, heights, or flying; Social Anxiety Disorder, in which the individual has fear or anxiety about social situations involving scrutiny by others; Panic Disorder, in which a person experiences recurrent unexpected "panic" attacks; Agoraphobia, in which the individual has a fear of multiple specific situations from which escape might be difficult; and Generalized Anxiety Disorder, in which the person has ongoing anxiety and excessive worry about a number of events or activities. Anxiety or panic attacks that are the direct pathophysiological consequence of a nonpsychiatric medical condition are diagnosed as Anxiety Disorder Due to Another Medical Condition. (Table 5–1 lists characteristic features of the

TABLE 5–1.   **Characteristic features of Anxiety Disorders**

Disorder	Key characteristics
Separation Anxiety Disorder	Developmentally inappropriate and excessive fear or anxiety concerning separation from those to whom the individual is attached
	Minimum duration of 4 weeks in children, 6 months in adults
Selective Mutism	Consistent failure to speak in social situations in which there is an expectation for speaking
Specific Phobia	Marked fear or anxiety about a specific object or situation
Social Anxiety Disorder	Marked fear or anxiety about one or more social situations in which the individual is exposed to possible scrutiny by others
Panic Disorder	Recurrent unexpected panic attacks (abrupt surges of intense fear or physical discomfort)
Agoraphobia	Marked fear or anxiety about at least two of the following: using public transportation, being in open spaces, being in enclosed places, standing in line or being in a crowd, and being outside of the home alone
	Fear or avoidance of situations because escape might be difficult or help unavailable in the event of incapacitating or embarrassing symptoms
	Situations actively avoided, requiring presence of a companion, or endured with intense fear or anxiety
Generalized Anxiety Disorder	Excessive anxiety and worry about a number of events or activities for at least 6 months
Anxiety Disorder Due to Another Medical Condition	Panic attacks or anxiety due to the direct pathophysiological consequence of a nonpsychiatric medical condition

Anxiety Disorders discussed in this chapter.) Individuals with Anxiety Disorders are often able to reduce their fear and anxiety by avoiding the situations that are the focus of the fear or anxiety. For example, a person with Social Anxiety Disorder who consistently avoids interaction with unfamiliar people may almost never experience fear or anxiety, although at great cost in terms of significantly constricting their life.

5.1
Separation Anxiety Disorder

Separation anxiety—that is, anxiety triggered by being separated from a primary caregiver—is common in infants and small children, typically between ages 6 months and 3 years, and is a natural part of the developmental process. In contrast,

Separation Anxiety Disorder is developmentally inappropriate and involves excessive fear or anxiety about being separated from home or from attachment figures, such as parents or other significant caregivers. The distress may be experienced upon separation or in anticipation of it. The individual often is worried that something untoward will happen to the attachment figure (e.g., the attachment figure will get sick, be injured, or die while separated from the affected person) or that the individual themself will become ill, get lost, be kidnapped, or have an accident leading to a separation from the attachment figure. The fears may be expressed directly or indirectly, such as by refusal to leave home or go to school, refusal to go to sleep, nightmares about separation, or physical symptoms (e.g., headaches, stomachaches, nausea, vomiting) on separation or in anticipation of it. Given that transient separation fears may be common, especially when under stress, DSM-5-TR requires that the separation anxiety persist for at least 4 weeks in children and at least 6 months in adults before the diagnosis is given.

Separation Anxiety Disorder is the most prevalent Anxiety Disorder in children under age 12 years. The 6- to 12-month prevalence of Separation Anxiety Disorder among children is estimated to be about 4%. School-age girls are more likely to have the disorder than boys. The prevalence of the disorder decreases with age, and most children who have it do not experience pathological anxiety as adults. Nonetheless, Separation Anxiety Disorder can be observed in adults. Across 18 countries, the 12-month prevalence has been found to be 1%, with women being more likely to be affected than men. Adults with Separation Anxiety Disorder are typically overconcerned about their offspring and spouses and experience marked discomfort when separated from them. They may also experience significant disruption in work or social experiences because of needing to continuously check on the whereabouts of a significant other.

The onset of the disorder in children can occur at any time during childhood or adolescence and often follows a stressor, such as parental divorce, a natural disaster, a family death, an illness in the patient or a relative, a move, immigration, or the death of a pet. Separation Anxiety Disorder in young adults has an age at onset in late adolescence to the mid-20s and may be precipitated by moving out of the family home, getting involved in a romantic relationship, or becoming a parent. Girls are more likely than boys to engage in school refusal or avoidance because of separation anxiety; boys are more likely to express their anxiety indirectly (e.g., by physical symptoms). Individuals with Separation Anxiety Disorder often severely curtail their independent activities away from home or attachment figures and lead constricted lives.

Tiny Tina

Tina, a small, sweet-faced, freckled 10-year-old, has been referred by a pediatrician, who had been unsuccessful in treating her for refusing to go to school. Her difficulties began on the first day of school 1 year ago when she cried and hid in the basement of her home. She agreed to go to school only when her mother promised to go with her and stay to have lunch with her at school. For the next 3 months, on school days, Tina had a variety of somatic complaints, such as headaches and "tummy aches," and each day would go to school only reluctantly, after much cajoling by her parents. Soon thereafter she attended school only if her parents lifted her out of bed, dressed and fed her, and drove her there. Finally, in the spring, the school social worker consulted Tina's pediatrician, who instituted a behavior modification program with the help of Tina's parents. Because this program was of only limited help, the pediatrician was now, at the beginning of the school year, referring Tina to a psychiatrist.

Tina's mother reported that despite Tina's many absences from school last year, she performed well in school. During this time, she also happily participated in all other activities, including Girl Scout meetings, sleepovers at friends' houses (usually with her sister), and family outings. Her mother wonders if taking a part-time bookkeeping job 2 years ago, plus the sudden death of a maternal grandmother to whom Tina was particularly close, might have been responsible for the child's difficulties.

When Tina was interviewed, she at first minimized any problems about school, insisting that "everything [was] okay" and saying that she got good grades and liked all the teachers. When the psychiatrist pursued the topic of why, then, she often refused to go to school, Tina became angry and gave a lot of "I don't know" responses. She eventually said that kids teased her about her size, calling her "Shrimp" and "Shorty," but she nevertheless gave the impression that she liked school and her teachers. She finally admitted that what bothered her was leaving home. She could not specify why but hinted that she was afraid something would happen, though to whom or to what she did not say. She confessed that she felt uncomfortable when all of her family was out of sight.

Discussion of "Tiny Tina"

All of Tina's problems involve a fear of going to school. The question is whether she is really afraid of school or of separating from her parents. The evidence that she might be afraid of school is her claim that the other children tease her and her willing participation in other activities away from home, such as sleepovers and Girl Scout meetings. However, Tina herself ultimately admits that it is really her fear that something bad will happen when her family is out of her sight that is behind her refusal to go to school. An enforced 6 hours away from her family every day is apparently more troubling to her than an occasional hour at a Girl Scout meeting or, surprisingly, a sleepover, where she is usually accompanied by her sister.

In the absence of a more pervasive disorder, Tina's excessive distress about separation from her family, her unrealistic worry about harm befalling her parents, her reluctance to go to school, and her complaints of physical symptoms on school days—all lasting for longer than 4 weeks—indicate Separation Anxiety Disorder (DSM-5-TR, p. 217).

5.2
Selective Mutism

Selective Mutism is another Anxiety Disorder with a usual age at onset in childhood. The hallmark of Selective Mutism is a "consistent failure to speak in specific social situations in which there is an expectation for speaking" (DSM-5-TR, p. 222), such as at school, although the child continues to speak in other situations (thus, the term "selective"). The failure to speak is not attributable to the child's not knowing the language and is not better explained by a Communication Disorder, such as Childhood-Onset Fluency Disorder (Stuttering), or Autism Spectrum Disorder (see Chapter 1, "Neurodevelopmental Disorders"). The child's refusal to speak interferes with educational achievement and the development of social skills.

Selective Mutism is a relatively rare disorder. Its population prevalence is not known, but studies in clinic and school samples in the United States, Europe, and Israel report point prevalence of from 0.03% to 1.9%. Selective Mutism most commonly appears when the child first enters the school system and is expected to speak in social situations, although some mild signs of the disorder may be apparent earlier. Typically, the child is unable to explain why they will not talk but looks frightened, suggesting the possibility of some kind of Anxiety Disorder. Indeed, Selective Mutism frequently co-occurs with Social Anxiety Disorder; Specific Phobia, such as fear of animals; and Separation Anxiety Disorder. Some children who develop Selective Mutism have mild Communication Disorders or physical disorders that interfere with articulation. Children may "outgrow" the Selective Mutism but continue to have symptoms of Social Anxiety Disorder (see Section 5.4).

Quiet Kevin

Kevin was a playful, attractive 6-year-old who was in first grade in a suburban school when his mother brought him for an evaluation because "he won't speak in school or in any social situations." During the evaluation, he whispered to his mother but would not speak to the interviewer. His mood seemed good, and his affect was very broad—he demonstrated exuberance, some apprehensiveness when he was expected to speak, but no sadness. He agreed with his mother that not speaking was a real problem, and he wanted to overcome it.

Kevin's mother reported that Kevin had been reluctant to speak to people outside of his home since he was about 2 years old. He never answered a greeting, and there were very few people he would talk to if he was away from his home. He did not speak at all in kindergarten. He liked going to parties and playing with others—laughing, running around, and singing—but he would not converse. He did not avoid social situations or strangers. He was taking piano lessons and would play in front of others, but he would not speak. He enjoyed going shopping and would sing out loud in the supermarket, but when people spoke to him, he became mute. At home, he amused himself with games and puzzles, and he played happily with other children.

Kevin had no history of medical problems. His mother described him as a "low-key" child, always easy to get along with, and quite verbal when alone with the family. He had always been very bright and had done well academically.

In kindergarten, he was referred for "play therapy" with a private psychologist, but several months of treatment did not result in any change in Kevin's symptoms.

Kevin was first treated with 4 weeks of behavioral therapy. When this produced no improvement, he was treated with fluoxetine, an antidepressant. After 9 weeks of treatment with fluoxetine, he was talking a little bit in school and talking to his grandparents on the phone. Over the summer, Kevin began to speak to his psychiatrist and to peers in day camp. After 22 weeks, the medication was slowly decreased, and over the next few weeks Kevin's mutism returned with everybody but his immediate family and his psychiatrist. His mood was less exuberant, he was more subdued, and his behavior was more oppositional at home.

At the beginning of the next school term, Kevin initially refused to take medication, but after 10 days—during which he was not speaking to peers and teachers in school—he went back on the medication for 1 month. He returned to his former state of feeling comfortable and exuberant, and he was speaking in school and all social settings. The fluoxetine was gradually discontinued, and by the end of the school year, he was a happy, comfortable, talkative second grader who had been voted president of his class. At this point, he was speaking to everyone, except those teachers who knew him as a mute kindergartner.

Discussion of "Quiet Kevin"

Kevin appeared to be normal in all respects except for his refusal to talk to any people other than his immediate family. This dramatic symptom could hardly be ignored. When, as in Kevin's case, not speaking is not due to lack of familiarity with the language spoken in school or to a Communication Disorder, such as severe Childhood-Onset Fluency Disorder (Stuttering) (see "Don't Worry" in Section 1.4), the symptom is given diagnostic status and is called Selective Mutism (DSM-5-TR, p. 222).

5.3
Specific Phobia

When a person consistently experiences intense fear and anxiety related to an object or situation, a diagnosis of Specific Phobia should be considered. Prototypically, a phobia involves intense fear that is consistently cued by exposure to a particular object or situation, called the *phobic stimulus*. Most individuals will do everything in their power to avoid the phobic stimulus. If the person cannot avoid it, they experience intense fear or anxiety. Irrational fears of objects can occur transiently, and for many people these fears are usually no more than an annoyance because of the ease of avoidance (e.g., having a snake phobia in an urban setting is rarely an issue because exposure to a snake is relatively unlikely). Thus, for an individual to receive a clinical diagnosis of Specific Phobia, the phobia must be persistent (i.e., lasting at least 6 months) and must cause significant distress or impairment in the person's functioning.

Most of the heterogeneity in the diagnosis of Specific Phobia is related to the wide range of stimuli to which people can develop fear. Therefore, DSM-5-TR provides specifiers to indicate the various types of phobic stimuli. These include Animal type for those afraid of certain kinds of animals, such as spiders, insects, or dogs; Natural Environment type for those fearful of certain aspects of the natural environment, such as heights, storms, and water; Blood-Injection-Injury type for individuals afraid of needles, seeing blood, being injured, or seeing someone else injured; Situational type for those afraid of specific situations such as airplanes, elevators, and enclosed places; and Other type for any other phobic stimulus. Because fear or anxiety triggered by social situations or performance in front of others is so common, it has its own diagnosis in DSM-5-TR: Social Anxiety Disorder (see Section 5.4).

Specific Phobia sometimes develops after experiencing a traumatic event (e.g., being bitten by a dog or stuck in an elevator), seeing others experience a traumatic event (e.g., watching someone drown), having an unexpected panic attack in the feared situation (e.g., becoming afraid of going on the subway after developing an unexpected panic attack while on the subway), or seeing extensive media coverage of a frightening event, such as a plane crash. However, many people with Specific Phobia are unable to recall the specific reason for the onset of their phobias.

Typically, individuals with Specific Phobia experience an increase in physiological arousal in anticipation of or during exposure to the feared object or situation, in the form of increased heart rate, increased blood pressure, and sweating. Individuals with the Blood-Injection-Injury type of Specific Phobia typically respond with a vasovagal fainting or near-fainting response that is caused by a drop in heart rate and blood pressure.

Specific Phobia is a common disorder. In the United States, the 12-month community prevalence estimate is approximately 8%–12%. Prevalence in European countries is similar (approximately 6%), but is lower in Asian, African, and Latin American countries (2%–4%). Prevalence rates are approximately 5% in children and approximately 16% in 13- to 17-year-olds. Prevalence rates are lower in older individuals (about 3%–5%), possibly reflecting diminishing severity to subclinical levels. Women are affected twice as often as men, although gender ratios vary across the different phobia types. The Animal, Natural Environment, and Situational types of Specific Phobia are predominantly experienced by women whereas the Blood-Injection-Injury type of Specific Phobia is experienced nearly equally by both sexes.

Thunderstorms

Sheila Antonelli, a 28-year-old stay-at-home mother, sought psychiatric treatment for a fear of thunderstorms that had become progressively more disturbing to her. Although frightened of storms since she was a child, the fear seemed to abate somewhat during adolescence, but had been increasing in severity over the past few years. This gradual exacerbation of her anxiety, plus the fear that she might pass it on to her children, led her to seek treatment.

Ms. Antonelli is most frightened of lightning but is uncertain about the reason for this. She is only vaguely aware of a fear of being struck by lightning and recognizes that this is an unlikely occurrence. When asked to elaborate on her fears, she imagines that lightning could strike a tree in her yard, and then the tree might fall and block her driveway, thus trapping her at home. This possibility frightens her, but she is quite aware that her fear is irrational. She also recognizes the irrational nature of her fear of thunder. She begins to feel anxiety long before a storm arrives. A weather report predicting a storm later in the week can cause her anxiety to increase to the point that she worries for days before the storm. Although she does not express a fear of rain, her anxiety increases even when the weather becomes overcast because of the increased likelihood of a storm.

During a storm, she does several things to reduce her anxiety. Because being with another person reduces her fear, she often tries to make plans to visit friends or relatives or asks her next-door neighbor to come over to her house when a storm is threatening. Sometimes, when her husband is away on business, if a storm is forecast, she and her children stay overnight with a close relative. During a storm, she covers her eyes or moves to a part of the house far from windows, where she cannot see lightning should it occur.

Ms. Antonelli has three young children. She describes her marriage as a happy one and states that her husband has been supportive of her when she is frightened and has encouraged her to seek psychiatric treatment. She is in good physical health, and at the time she entered treatment there were no unusually stressful situations in her life or other emotional difficulties. Her parents separated shortly after she began treatment. Although she found their separation distressing, she felt that her personal supports were adequate and that this occurrence did not necessitate additional attention.

She describes her past history as generally unremarkable in terms of any obvious psychological problems, except her fear of thunderstorms. She feels that she may have "learned" this fear from her grandmother, who also was frightened of storms. She denies panic attacks or any other unusual or incapacitating fears.

Discussion of "Thunderstorms"

Many people feel uncomfortable during thunder and lightning storms, but Ms. Antonelli's persistent fear of this circumscribed stimulus is clearly excessive and causes her considerable distress. Furthermore, her fear and avoidant behavior frequently interfere significantly with her normal routine. These features indicate the presence of a phobia. This case demonstrates a number of important features of Specific Phobia (DSM-5-TR, p. 224). Many people might experience a certain level of fear or anxiety during a severe thunderstorm, especially a particularly violent one. Most of these individuals would not qualify for a diagnosis of Specific Phobia because they are not particularly distressed or functionally impaired by it, and certainly not enough to seek treatment. In Ms. Antonelli's case, her degree of distress and the fact that it exerts such an impact on her life (e.g., needing to stay overnight at the house of a close relative if her husband is out of town when a storm is expected) justify the diagnosis. As is typical with many phobias, Ms. Antonelli's fear goes back to her childhood. This case illustrates one of the many ways phobias can develop—namely, it was "modeled" by another family member. A fear of thunderstorms is an example of the Natural Environment type of Specific Phobia.

Stay Healthy

Jordan Michaels, a 27-year-old computer programmer, seeks treatment because of fears that prevent him from visiting his terminally ill father-in-law in the hospital. He explains that he is afraid of any situation even remotely associated with bodily injury or illness. For example, he cannot bear to have his blood drawn or to see or even hear about sick people. These fears are the reason he avoids consulting a doctor even when he is sick; avoids visiting sick friends or family members; and refuses to even listen to descriptions of medical procedures, physical trauma, or illness. He became a vegetarian 5 years ago to avoid thoughts of animals being killed.

Mr. Michaels dates the onset of these fears to age 9, when his Sunday school teacher gave a detailed account of a leg operation she had undergone. As he listened, he began to feel anxious and dizzy, he sweated profusely, and finally he fainted. He recalls great difficulty receiving immunizations and being subjected to other routine medical procedures through the rest of his school years, as well as numerous fainting and near-fainting episodes throughout his teen and adult years whenever he witnessed the slightest physical trauma, heard of an injury or illness, or saw a sick or disfigured person. When he recently saw someone in a store in a wheelchair, he started wondering if the person was in pain and became so distressed that he fainted and fell to the floor. He was greatly embarrassed, when he regained consciousness, by the crowd of people surrounding him.

Mr. Michaels denies any other emotional problems. He enjoys his work, seems to get along well with his wife, and has many friends.

Discussion of "Stay Healthy"

In this illustration of a Specific Phobia (DSM-5-TR, p. 224), the phobic stimulus is bodily injury or illness. As is common with this type of phobia, a wide variety of situations are avoided: Mr. Michaels avoids having his blood drawn and going to doctors, visiting (or even hearing about) people who are sick, and listening to anything about medical procedures, physical trauma, or illness of any kind. Although his fear of blood and injury has been bothersome and embarrassing because of the fainting spells, his fear has not had a significant impact on his life until recently. Now that his father-in-law is terminally ill in the hospital, Mr. Michaels' inability to visit him is creating enough of a problem to bring Mr. Michaels into treatment.

Mr. Michaels' fear is unrelated to an obsession involving being infected with germs, as might occur in someone with Obsessive-Compulsive Disorder (see "Lady Macbeth" in Section 6.1), and it is not related to a prior traumatic experience such as witnessing mutilation on a battlefield as might occur in someone with Posttraumatic Stress Disorder (see "Flashbacks" in Section 7.3). If it were, an additional diagnosis of Specific Phobia would not be given.

One feature that distinguishes the Blood-Injection-Injury type of Specific Phobia from the other types is the person's physiological response to exposure to the feared stimulus. In other forms of Specific Phobia, individuals respond to exposure with typical sympathetic nervous system symptoms of fear and anxiety, such as racing heart, sweating, and sometimes even a panic attack. In contrast, individuals with the Blood-Injection-Injury type of Specific Phobia experience an initial period of arousal and increased heart rate, followed by a vasovagal (caused by the action of the vagus nerve on blood vessel dilatation and heart rate) drop in heart rate and blood pressure that can lead to fainting.

Notably, DSM-5-TR includes a disorder called Illness Anxiety Disorder (see "The Radiologist" in Section 9.2), which is not in the Anxiety Disorders chapter but instead is classified with the Somatic Symptom and Related Disorders. This condition is characterized by a preoccupation with having or acquiring a serious undiagnosed illness such as cancer and with a high level of general anxiety about health. This disorder is in contrast to Blood-Injection-Injury type of Specific Phobia, in which the primary symptoms are fear, anxiety, and avoidance related to the phobic stimulus of injury or illness. Thus, despite the suggestive name, Illness Anxiety Disorder is quite different from an illness phobia.

5.4
Social Anxiety Disorder

Significant fear or anxiety about being in a social situation in which the person is potentially exposed to the scrutiny of others is indicative of Social Anxiety Disorder. The social situation may involve performance in front of a group (e.g., giving a speech), being observed in public (e.g., eating or drinking), or simply meeting new people or engaging in conversation with others. The person with Social Anxiety Disorder is afraid that they will act in a way that will be embarrassing or humiliating, or will offend others or provoke rejection by others. Similar to Specific Phobias, Social Anxiety Disorder causes the person to either avoid or endure the situation with dread; Social Anxiety Disorder causes fear or anxiety that is out of proportion to any actual threat in the situation, and it leads to anxiety that is very distressing or that interferes with functioning. The anxiety or avoidance is not related to another mental disorder, such as in the case of a person with severe Panic Disorder (see Section 5.5), who avoids social situations because of the fear of having a panic attack, or Body Dysmorphic Disorder (see Section 6.2), in which a person avoids social situations because of embarrassment about their perceived physical defect. Moreover, it is common and often understandable for a person with a medical condition that is characterized by embarrassing symptoms (e.g., severe tremors in a person with Parkinson's disease or severe disfigurement in a person who has been burned) to experience distressing anxiety in social situations. A diagnosis of Social Anxiety Disorder should be given in such circumstances only if the fear and avoidance is out of proportion to the symptom in question (e.g., when a patient with only a slight tremor from Parkinson's disease refuses to leave their house).

Social Anxiety Disorder is one of the more common Anxiety Disorders, with a 12-month prevalence estimate in the United States of approximately 7% in adults. Prevalence in adolescents is roughly half that in adults. The 12-month prevalence in other countries may be lower. It is also somewhat lower in adults over 65. Its onset is usually in early adolescence. The course may wax and wane, but in a substantial number of people, the disorder lasts for several years or more. Women are somewhat more affected than men, although men may be more likely to seek treatment for the disorder presumably because of social expectations to be in public.

Social Anxiety Disorder is associated with school dropout and with decreased well-being, employment, workplace productivity, socioeconomic status, and quality of life. It is also associated with being unmarried or divorced and with less close and supportive friendships. Social Anxiety Disorder often co-occurs with other Anxiety Disorders, Major Depressive Disorder, Substance Use Disorders, Body Dysmorphic Disorder, and Avoidant Personality Disorder.

Mail Sorter

Andy Johnson, a 25-year-old single man, lives with his mother and brother. He works as a mail sorter at the post office, a job he has had since he dropped out of college after 2 years. He came to an anxiety disorders clinic after reading a newspaper advertisement regarding the availability of free treatment for participation in a research study of Anxiety Disorders. His chief complaint is of "nervousness." He says that right now he is "just going through the motions" and wants "to lead a normal life" and go back to college.

During his adolescence and young adulthood, Mr. Johnson had no close friends and usually preferred to be by himself. When he entered college, he formed several close friendships but became "super self-conscious" when speaking to strangers, classmates, and sometimes even friends. He would feel nervous, and his face would become so "stiff" that he had difficulty speaking. He had a "buzzing" in his head, felt as if he were "outside [his] body," had hot flashes, and perspired. These "panic attacks" (his term) came on suddenly, within seconds, and only when he was with people. When a classmate spoke to him, he sometimes "couldn't hear" what the classmate was saying because of his nervousness.

Outside of class, Mr. Johnson began to feel increasingly uncomfortable in social situations: "I think that I was afraid of saying or doing something stupid." He began to turn down invitations to parties and to withdraw from other social activities (e.g., a bowling league). Eventually, he dropped out of college entirely.

Mr. Johnson explains that the reason he chose to work at the post office is that the job does not require him to deal with people. When asked about other things that make him nervous, he says he tries to avoid using public bathrooms, but when he does use them, he feels more comfortable when the lights are dim, when there are few people present, and when he can use a stall rather than a urinal.

Mr. Johnson has two long-standing "best friends" with whom he socializes regularly and feels completely comfortable. However, he has not dated since college, and he totally avoids group settings, such as weddings, parties, or clubs. He has no problem with authority figures and even welcomes constructive criticism from his supervisor at the post office. "My problem is nervousness, not obstinacy."

Discussion of "Mail Sorter"

Mr. Johnson says that he has "panic attacks," and indeed he does get sudden attacks of intense anxiety. However, these always occur in situations that he knows are frightening to him. These expected attacks are quite different from the unexpected panic attacks required for a diagnosis of Panic Disorder (see Section 5.5). Mr. Johnson's anxiety occurs in a variety of different social situations in which he fears that he will do something or act in a way that will be humiliating or embarrassing. This is the hallmark of Social Anxiety Disorder

(DSM-5-TR, p. 229). This diagnosis is given only, as in Mr. Johnson's case, when the distress significantly interferes with the person's normal routine, occupational functioning, or social activities or relationships, or when there is marked distress about having the phobia. The fact that Mr. Johnson has expected panic attacks in the context of Social Anxiety Disorder qualifies for use of the With Panic Attacks specifier, which allows for expected and unexpected panic attacks (DSM-5-TR, pp. 242–243).

Mr. Johnson's chief complaint is "nervousness," and therefore his evaluation focuses on a differential diagnosis of his anxiety symptoms. Were he to seek treatment for the interpersonal problems that have constricted his life, the focus would be on his personality functioning and would have suggested the diagnosis of Avoidant Personality Disorder (see "The Jerk" in Section 18.3). In fact, his symptoms probably also meet the criteria for that disorder in view of his avoidance of activities that involve interpersonal contact, inhibition in interpersonal situations, preoccupation with being criticized or rejected, and general feelings of inadequacy.

On Stage

Doug Phillips is a 33-year-old man who lives in Seattle with his wife. He has been employed as a salesperson for an insurance company since graduating from college. He came to a psychologist, recommended by a friend, complaining of "anxiety at work."

Mr. Phillips describes himself as having been outgoing and popular throughout his adolescence and young adulthood, with no serious problems until his third year of college. At that time, he started becoming extremely tense and nervous when studying for tests and writing papers. His heart would pound, and his hands would sweat and tremble. Consequently, he often did not write the required papers and, when he did, would submit them after the date due. He could not understand why he was suddenly so nervous about doing papers and taking exams when he had always done well in those tasks in the past. As a result of his failure to submit certain papers and his late submission of others, his college grades were seriously affected.

Soon after graduation, Mr. Phillips was employed as a salesperson for an insurance firm. His initial training (attending lectures, completing reading assignments) proceeded smoothly. However, as soon as he began to take on clients, his anxiety returned. He became extremely nervous when anticipating calls from clients. When his business phone rang, he would begin to tremble and sometimes would not even answer it. Eventually, he avoided becoming anxious by not scheduling appointments and by not contacting clients whom he was expected to see.

When asked what it was about these situations that made him nervous, he said that he was concerned about what the client would think of him: "The client might sense that I am nervous and might ask me questions that I don't know the answers to, and I will feel foolish." As a result, he would repeatedly rewrite and reword sales scripts for telephone conversations because he was "so concerned about saying the right thing. I guess I'm just very concerned about being judged."

Although never unemployed, Mr. Phillips estimates that he has been functioning at only 20% of his work capacity, which his employer tolerates because a salesman is paid only on a commission basis. For the last several years, he has had to borrow large sums of money to make ends meet.

Although financial constraints have been a burden, Mr. Phillips and his wife entertain guests at their home regularly and enjoy socializing with friends at picnics, parties, and formal affairs. Mr. Phillips lamented, "It's just when I'm expected to do something for work. Then it's like I'm on stage, all alone, with everyone watching me."

Discussion of "On Stage"

Mr. Phillips' problem is crippling anxiety whenever he feels that he is performing. In college this happened when he had to write papers or take exams. At work it happens whenever he has to talk to clients, either on the phone or face to face. What he fears is that people will observe his anxiety and make him "feel foolish." Significantly, he has no anxiety in social situations that he does not define as being "on stage," and he has never experienced sudden attacks of panic in situations that he did not expect to cause him anxiety (as in Panic Disorder, see "I Could Be Dying" in Section 5.5).

A marked and persistent fear of one or more social or performance situations in which the person is exposed to unfamiliar people or to possible scrutiny by others and fears of acting in a way that will be humiliating or embarrassing are the essential features of Social Anxiety Disorder (DSM-5-TR, p. 229). Social Anxiety Disorder may be limited to a specific phobic stimulus (as in Mr. Phillips' case) or may be generalized to almost all social situations. The most common specific expression of Social Anxiety Disorder is fear of public speaking. Fear of public speaking is usually limited to formal presentations and does not include, as in this case, fear of talking on the telephone. Less common forms of Social Anxiety Disorder are fear of eating in public, fear of writing in public, and fear of using public lavatories. Because Mr. Phillips is able to enjoy social activities in which he feels he is not being judged, and his fear is limited to speaking or performing in public, he has the Performance Only type (DSM-5-TR, p. 230) of Social Anxiety Disorder.

No Friends

Emily is a 7-year-old girl whose mother has brought her to an outpatient mental health clinic for children because of difficulties with peer relationships. A recent telephone call from Emily's second-grade teacher convinced her mother that it was necessary to seek professional help for Emily. The teacher had become increasingly concerned about Emily's reluctance to interact with the other children in the class. During recess, Emily stands off to the side of the playground with her head down, looking extremely uncomfortable. In the classroom, she never initiates conversation with the other children and has great difficulty responding even when approached by another child. It is now 6 months into the school year, and Emily's extreme discomfort around her peers has not improved at all. Indeed, she does not have a single friend in the classroom.

Emily's discomfort in interacting with peers dates back to kindergarten. Her teachers in kindergarten and first grade had commented on her report card that she was very withdrawn and nervous with the other children. However, her second-grade teacher was the first to take an active role in trying to get Emily the help she needed.

Emily's mother had tried repeatedly to get Emily involved with other children in the neighborhood. In fact, she would take Emily by the hand and lead her to neighbors' homes where there were children of the same age to try to make friends for her child. Unfortunately, when she did this, Emily would start to shake or cry and would not be able to say a word to the neighbor's child. Emily has never been invited to a birthday party for another child.

Her behavior at home is quite different. Emily is warm and outgoing with her family, in marked contrast to the withdrawn and anxious child observed by her teachers and peers.

Discussion of "No Friends"

Many children are socially reticent—that is, slow to warm up in an unfamiliar social situation. However, such children generally overcome their initial shyness and do not demonstrate the extreme and persistent social isolation that Emily does. In an adult, Emily's behavior would suggest a possible diagnosis of Avoidant Personality Disorder (see "The Jerk" in Section 18.3). However, because Emily is so young, the diagnosis of a Personality Disorder is not appropriate. Emily is clearly afraid of situations in which she is exposed to unfamiliar people, and the psychiatrist suspects that Emily is afraid of acting in a way that will be humiliating or embarrassing. These features, plus her capacity for social relationships with familiar people (her family), warrant the diagnosis of Social Anxiety Disorder (DSM-5-TR, p. 229). Although somewhat unusual in such a young child, Social Anxiety Disorder can occur in children.

5.5
Panic Disorder

Sudden unexpected attacks of extreme fear or anxiety are the hallmark of Panic Disorder. *Panic attacks* are abrupt surges of intense fear or discomfort that reach a peak of intensity in a matter of minutes. Any number of uncomfortable physical symptoms may occur involving the cardiovascular, respiratory, gastrointestinal, neurological, and other body systems. Symptoms may include palpitations, accelerated heart rate, sweating, trembling or shaking, shortness of breath, choking, chest pain, nausea, dizziness, chills or hot flashes, and numbness and tingling in the extremities. The person may also experience disturbing perceptions or cognitions during the panic attack, including feelings of unreality (i.e., derealization) or being detached from themself (i.e., depersonalization), fear of losing control or going crazy, and fear of dying. Moreover, the person may become so rattled by the panic attack that following an attack, they develop "persistent concern or worry about additional panic attacks or their consequences (e.g., losing control, having a heart attack, 'going crazy')" (DSM-5-TR, Criterion B1, p. 236) or make a significant change in their behavior to try to ward off additional attacks (e.g., avoiding exercise). Behavioral changes often include avoiding places or situations that the person believes are triggering the attacks, such as traveling on public transportation, being in crowds, or even going outside the house. When Panic Disorder causes a person to avoid a number of different places or situations, an additional diagnosis of Agoraphobia (see Section 5.6) may apply.

Panic Disorder is relatively common, with a 12-month prevalence in the general population in the United States and several European countries estimated to be about 2%–3% in adults and adolescents. Significantly lower rates have been found in Asian, African, and Latin American countries. The onset of Panic Disorder is usually in the early 20s. The course is chronic without treatment, but there may be some waxing and waning of symptoms. Women are nearly twice as likely as men to be affected. Panic Disorder can be very impairing. People with the disorder may miss significant amounts of work or school while seeking medical attention from doctors or in emergency rooms. Panic attacks are associated with high medical care utilization, poor quality of life, and increased rates of suicidal thoughts and behaviors. In the general population, 80% of individuals with Panic Disorder had another mental disorder in their lifetimes.

Toughing It Out

Mindy Markowitz is an attractive, stylishly dressed, 25-year-old art director for a trade magazine who comes to an anxiety disorders clinic after reading about the clinic program in the newspaper. She is seeking treatment for "panic attacks" that have occurred with increasing frequency over the past year, often two or three times a day. These attacks begin with a sudden intense wave of "horrible fear" that seems to come out of nowhere, sometimes during the day, sometimes waking her from sleep. She begins to tremble, is nauseated, sweats profusely, feels as though she is choking, and fears that she will lose control and do something crazy, like run screaming into the street.

Ms. Markowitz remembers first having attacks like this when she was in high school. She was dating a boy her parents disapproved of and had to do a lot of "sneaking around" to avoid confrontations with them. At the same time, she was under a lot of pressure as the principal designer of her high school yearbook and was applying to Ivy League colleges. She remembers that her first panic attack occurred just after the yearbook went to press and she was accepted by Harvard, Yale, and Brown. The attacks lasted only a few minutes, and she would just "sit through them." She was worried enough to mention them to her mother, but because she was otherwise perfectly healthy, she did not seek treatment.

Ms. Markowitz has had panic attacks intermittently over the 8 years since her first attack, sometimes not for many months, but sometimes, as now, several times a day. There have also been extreme variations in the intensity of the attacks, with some being so severe and debilitating that she had to take a day off from work.

Ms. Markowitz has always functioned extremely well in school, at work, and in her social life, apart from her panic attacks and a brief period of depression at age 19 when she broke up with a boyfriend. She is a lively, friendly person who is respected by her friends and colleagues for her intelligence and creativity, and for her ability to mediate disputes.

Ms. Markowitz never limited her activities, even during the times that she was having frequent, severe attacks, although she has occasionally stayed home from work for a day because she was exhausted from multiple attacks. She never associated the attacks with particular places. She says, for example, that she is as likely to have an attack at home in her own bed as on the subway, so there is no point in avoiding the subway. Whether she has an attack on the subway, in a supermarket, or at home by herself, she says, "I just tough it out."

Discussion of "Toughing It Out"

Ms. Markowitz describes classic unexpected panic attacks. They hit her unpredictably with a sudden burst of fear and the characteristic symptoms of autonomic arousal: sweating, trembling, nausea, and choking, all severe enough to make her fear she will lose control. Unlike most patients who have such severe panic attacks (see "I Could Be Dying," below), she has never associated particular situations, such as crowded places or public transportation, with having the attacks. Therefore, she does not show any symptoms of agoraphobic avoidance. Thus, the diagnosis is simply Panic Disorder (DSM-5-TR, p. 235). Ms. Markowitz's Panic Disorder is fairly typical in that it is intermittent but has persisted for quite a number of years.

I Could Be Dying

Niyol Begay is a 52-year-old wholesale distributor of automobile parts who awoke in the middle of the night, gasping for breath, sweating, shaking, and having palpitations. He felt his pulse; it was 120. He had the thought, "I could be dying." It was his third attack of the week and at least his tenth that month that had awakened him from sleep. The problem, which had begun 2 years previously, was getting much worse: not only was he having trouble staying asleep because of similar attacks, but after such nights he felt tired all day. He decided to take a friend's advice and seek help from a psychiatrist who specializes in sleep problems.

The psychiatrist elicited this additional history from Mr. Begay: Attacks of panic occurring during the day had begun at age 12 and had recurred every few months since that time. They did not begin to occur during sleep until the patient turned 50, about 2 years earlier. A few months ago, the attacks had become much rarer, after Mr. Begay had discontinued drinking the 8–10 beers he had drunk periodically every weekend for most of his adult life. His weight had fallen from 227 pounds to a mildly overweight 181 pounds, and the mild hypertension he had had for several years had disappeared.

In addition to having the recurrent attacks, for most of his life Mr. Begay had also felt anxious in anticipation of particular situations, including being shut inside airplanes or elevators or traveling in the middle lane of a road. On a limited-access road, he counted the exits until he could leave, fearing that he would have a panic attack.

Mr. Begay described a fear of falling apart if he ever got too far from his "support system," his term for a beer cooler, which he carried with him always, although he rarely drank the beer. In anticipation of an airplane flight, however, he would drink 6–8 beers. He almost always had a company employee, his son, or a friend accompany him, and he particularly disliked plane flights when he was not with a familiar person. The night after he drank, the anxiety attacks occurred, awakening him from sleep.

Mr. Begay ran a successful business and consulted for several others. Recently, however, anxiety had prevented his accepting a huge government contract to set up an international distribution system for retail stores on military bases. He felt he would be too exposed to scrutiny and would therefore fail. He also worried that some long plane flights would be unavoidable.

During the interview, Mr. Begay was highly verbal, informative, cheerful, friendly, and engaging. He talked about uncomfortable subjects frankly and productively. He had two sisters and two daughters with Agoraphobia; one of the daughters was housebound.

Initially, Mr. Begay was thought to have Obstructive Sleep Apnea (recurrent periods of not breathing during sleep; see "Food for Thought" in Section 12.4), on the basis of the loud snoring that he reported, his awakening provoked by drinking alcohol (relieved by weight loss), and the presence of mild hypertension. These symptoms are common in patients with sleep apnea and are presumably related to pulmonary hypertension that develops from insufficient breathing and oxygen desaturation. No evidence for this condition emerged from results of sleep laboratory recording, upper airway examination, or laboratory tests for daytime vigilance.

Discussion of "I Could Be Dying"

Although Mr. Begay's chief complaint is of difficulty staying asleep, it is clear that what keeps waking him up are recurrent panic attacks. He wakes up with typical symptoms of panic attacks: the abrupt onset of difficulty breathing, sweating, shaking, rapid heartbeat, and palpitations. The diagnosis of Panic Disorder (DSM-5-TR, p. 235) is made because Mr. Begay has recurrent unexpected panic attacks with at least four of the characteristic symptoms, as well as concern about the consequences of the attacks (i.e., fear of dying from the attacks).

People with Panic Disorder frequently attempt to avoid places or situations from which escape might be difficult or embarrassing or in which help might not be available in the event of having a panic attack (Agoraphobia). Mr. Begay's history is unusual in that he apparently avoided situations in which he anticipated feeling anxious even before he identified the onset of panic attacks. In any case, he currently avoids airplanes, elevators, and driving in the middle lane of roads because of fears of having a panic attack. Therefore, the additional diagnosis of Agoraphobia (see "No Fluids" in Section 5.6) applies.

This case is unusual from two perspectives. First, it is unusual for patients with Panic Disorder to have panic attacks at night. Second, insomnia is rarely caused by panic attacks that awaken the patient. When, as in this case, persistent insomnia is the predominant symptom requiring independent clinical attention and causes daytime fatigue and distress or impairment in functioning, the additional diagnosis of a Sleep-Wake Disorder is made. Mr. Begay, therefore, would also be diagnosed with Insomnia Disorder, With Mental Disorder (DSM-5-TR, p. 409).

5.6
Agoraphobia

Agoraphobia is defined as marked fear or anxiety triggered by real or anticipated exposure to a variety of situations. DSM-5-TR specifically requires that there be fear or avoidance of at least two of the following situations: 1) using public transportation (e.g., automobiles, buses, trains, ships, or planes); 2) being in open spaces (e.g., parking lots, markets, bridges); 3) being in enclosed spaces (e.g., shops, theaters); 4) standing in line or being in a crowd; or 5) being outside of the home alone. The person fears these situations or avoids them "because of thoughts that escape might be difficult or help might not be available in the event of developing panic-like symptoms or other incapacitating or embarrassing symptoms" (e.g., fear of falling, fear of incontinence) (DSM-5-TR, p. 246). These situations consistently provoke fear or anxiety in the individual, who actively avoids the situations, or endures them with intense fear or anxiety, or requires the presence of an accompanying companion. The fear or anxiety must be persistent, lasting for at least 6 months, and must cause significant distress or impairment in functioning to justify a diagnosis. The diagnosis should not be given if attempts to avoid a situation would be considered reasonable because of its inherent danger, such as not venturing outside at night in a very high-crime neighborhood.

Agoraphobia has an estimated 12-month prevalence in the general population of adults and adolescents of approximately 1.0%–1.7% worldwide. The typical onset of Agoraphobia is in late adolescence or early adulthood. Women are twice as likely to be affected as men. The course of Agoraphobia is typically chronic without treatment, and very few persons have remissions that are spontaneous (i.e., not related to treatment). Other Anxiety Disorders, Depressive Disorders (see Chapter 4), and Substance Use Disorders (see Chapter 16) commonly co-occur with Agoraphobia. People with Agoraphobia may become completely homebound and unable to go to school or work.

No Fluids

Anna O'Reilly, a 32-year-old medical secretary in Dublin, Ireland, is referred to a clinic for treatment of depression. She confides that the reason she is depressed is that for the last 5 months she has been afraid that she will urinate in public. She has never actually done this, and in the safety of her own home she considers the idea that she will actually do this to be nonsensical.

When Ms. O'Reilly is away from home, the fear dominates her thinking, and she takes precautions to prevent its happening. She always wears sanitary napkins, never travels far from home, limits her intake of fluids, has stopped drinking alcohol, and has had her desk at work relocated near a toilet. For the 2 weeks before the consultation, she was unable to go to work because the fear had become so intense.

She vaguely recalls that her deceased father also had a fear of urinating in public. Before leaving for work each day, he urinated several times and avoided drinking any fluids. Her younger sister has been successfully treated for a cleansing ritual in which she had to wash first her left hand and then her right hand exactly 10 times without touching the sides of the sink (probably Obsessive-Compulsive Disorder).

Ms. O'Reilly had psychiatric treatment 10 years earlier, when she began to fear that she had contracted syphilis, even though there was no clinical or laboratory evidence of infection. Prior to 5 months ago, she never feared that she would urinate in public. In addition to this specific fear, she has always been an anxious, insecure person, considered by her family to be overly cautious and perfectionistic. For the past year, she has been upset about her boy-friend's impending return to Pakistan, after completing his medical studies in Ireland. She was divorced 5 years ago and is now living with her 7-year-old son and mother. Her mother disapproves of her boyfriend, and Ms. O'Reilly has felt increasing pressure to end the relationship. She believes that the on-set of her current difficulties coincided with the stress of her relationship with her mother and the threat of her boyfriend's departure from the country.

When interviewed, Ms. O'Reilly is visibly anxious. She remarks that she has been feeling despondent about her problems. She has trouble sleeping and has no energy during the day. Although her appetite is poor, she has not lost any weight.

Ms. O'Reilly was treated with clomipramine, an antidepressant medication that is indicated for the treatment of Obsessive-Compulsive Disorder, initially at a dosage of 10 mg/day, increasing over 2 weeks to 125 mg/day. Her fear that she might urinate in public lessened after 10 days of treatment. Then, to correct her repertoire of avoidance behaviors, a behavioral program was in-stituted in which she was encouraged to leave her home for increasingly lon-ger periods of time until she was able to tolerate the anxiety. Before her boyfriend left the country, Ms. O'Reilly and her son moved away from her mother, and she was able to lead a more independent life. Her medication was phased out after 2 months, and the fear that she would urinate in public did not return. The psychiatrist attributed Ms. O'Reilly's initial improvement to the medication, and her continued improvement to the behavioral program and the changes that she made in her life circumstances, particularly moving away from her mother.

Discussion of "No Fluids"

Ms. O'Reilly has markedly restricted her usual activities because of a fear that she will involuntarily urinate in public. The fear of being in situations from which escape might be difficult in the event of developing an embarrassing or incapacitating symptom is called Agoraphobia. Often, Agoraphobia is a com-plication of Panic Disorder (see Section 5.5), in that a person avoids certain sit-uations that they associate with having had a panic attack. Less common in Agoraphobia is no history of Panic Disorder and the fear of developing some specific symptom, such as loss of bladder control (as in Ms. O'Reilly's case), vomiting, fainting, or having a heart attack. In such cases, the diagnosis is sim-ply Agoraphobia (DSM-5-TR, p. 246).

A reader may wonder why Ms. O'Reilly's condition is not diagnosed as So-cial Anxiety Disorder (see "On Stage" in Section 5.4)—that is, a persistent fear of a situation in which she is exposed to possible scrutiny by others and fears that she may do something (e.g., urinate) that will be humiliating or embar-rassing. In Social Anxiety Disorder, the person is attempting to accomplish a voluntary activity (e.g., speaking, eating, writing, urinating) and fears that the normal activity will be impaired by signs of anxiety (e.g., be unable to speak, choke while eating, tremble while writing, be unable to urinate). In contrast, in

Agoraphobia, the person is afraid of suddenly developing a symptom that is out of their control and unrelated to the activity that they are trying to accomplish (e.g., cardiac distress while shopping, involuntary urination when away from home, dizziness while crossing the street).

5.7
Generalized Anxiety Disorder

When a person has excessive anxiety, worry, and apprehension about a number of events or activities more days than not for a period of at least 6 months, a diagnosis of Generalized Anxiety Disorder may be appropriate. Colloquially, such an individual may be referred to as a "worrywart." Adults with Generalized Anxiety Disorder often worry about routine life circumstances, such as possible job responsibilities, health and finances, the health of family members, misfortune to their children, or minor matters (e.g., doing household chores or being late for appointments). Children with Generalized Anxiety Disorder tend to worry excessively about their competence or the quality of their performance. An individual with this disorder will be unable to control the worry and will experience symptoms such as restlessness or feeling keyed up or on edge, being easily fatigued, having difficulty concentrating or mind going blank, irritability, muscle tension, and sleep disturbance (DSM-5-TR, p. 250). As in other Anxiety Disorders, the fear or anxiety must be significantly distressing or cause impairment in functioning to justify a diagnosis.

Generalized Anxiety Disorder is relatively common, with the 12-month prevalence in the general population in the United States estimated to be approximately 0.9% among adolescents and 2.9% among adults. The mean 12-month prevalence around the world is 1.3%. The 12-month prevalence in older adults, including individuals ages 75 and older, ranges from 2.8% to 3.1% in the United States, Israel, and several European countries. The onset of the disorder usually occurs around age 35, making it a later-onset disorder compared with others in this diagnostic class. Women and adolescent girls are twice as likely as men or adolescent boys to have the disorder. As with other Anxiety Disorders, the course tends to be chronic, with waxing and waning of symptoms across the lifespan, but a low percentage of full remissions. Generalized Anxiety Disorder can cause considerable impairment, particularly in the ability to work effectively. Individuals with Generalized Anxiety Disorder are likely to have a current or past history of other Anxiety and Depressive Disorders, linked by the underlying personality trait of negative affectivity (neuroticism).

Edgy Electrician

Max Schmidt is a 27-year-old married electrician who has experienced anxiety and worry over the past 2 years. He has felt periods of extreme muscle tension and has been easily fatigued, although he also has had difficulty falling and staying asleep. In addition, he reports irritability and a constant "edgy" and watchful feeling that has often interfered with his ability to concentrate. These feelings have been present more days than not, and they have not been limited to discrete periods. Although these symptoms sometimes make him feel "discouraged," he denies feeling depressed and continues to enjoy time spent with his family. He does not take medications regularly, use recreational drugs, or drink alcohol.

Because of these symptoms, Mr. Schmidt had previously seen a family practitioner, a neurologist, an orthopedist, a chiropractor, and an ear-nose-throat specialist. He had been placed on a hypoglycemic (low-sugar) diet, received physiotherapy, and been told he might have "an endocrine problem," although all blood tests were, in fact, normal.

Mr. Schmidt has many worries. He constantly worries about the health of his parents. His father, in fact, had a myocardial infarction (heart attack) 2 years previously but is now feeling well. Mr. Schmidt also worries about whether he is "a good father," whether his wife will ever leave him (there is no indication that she is dissatisfied with the marriage), and whether he is liked by coworkers. Although he recognizes that his worries are often unfounded, he cannot stop himself from worrying.

For the past 2 years, Mr. Schmidt has had few social contacts because of his nervous symptoms. Although he has sometimes had to leave work on days when the symptoms became intolerable, he continues to work for the same company he joined for his apprenticeship following high school graduation. He tends to hide his symptoms from his wife and children, to whom he wants to appear "perfect," and he reports few problems with them as a result of his nervousness.

Discussion of "Edgy Electrician"

Mr. Schmidt's predominant symptoms are excessive and uncontrollable anxiety and worry for most of the time over the past 2 years. This suggests a diagnosis of Generalized Anxiety Disorder. He also has the characteristic associated symptoms of feeling on edge, being easily fatigued, difficulty concentrating, irritability, muscle tension, and sleep disturbance. His worries cause him significant distress and impair his social functioning. The diagnosis of Generalized Anxiety Disorder (DSM-5-TR, p. 250) is made in this case because the symptoms, which have lasted for longer than 6 months, are not attributable to the physiological effects of a substance (e.g., a drug of abuse or a medication) or a nonpsychiatric medical condition (e.g., hyperthyroidism), and are not better explained by another mental disorder (e.g., worrying about having a panic attack, as in Panic Disorder, or being embarrassed in public, as in Social Anxiety Disorder).

Although Mr. Schmidt recognizes that his worries are often excessive and repetitive, they would not be considered to be evidence of obsessions, as occur in Obsessive-Compulsive Disorder (see "Lady Macbeth" in Section 6.1), because they do not have an intrusive and inappropriate quality.

5.8
Anxiety Disorder Due to Another Medical Condition

Anxiety or panic attacks that are the direct pathophysiological consequence of a nonpsychiatric medical condition, such as a pheochromocytoma—that is, a benign tumor of the adrenal gland that secretes norepinephrine (a hormone that causes anxiety)—are diagnosed as Anxiety Disorder Due to Another Medical Condition. This anxiety is in contrast to anxiety that might develop as a psychological response to being diagnosed with a nonpsychiatric medical condition, which might be diagnosed instead as an Adjustment Disorder (see Section 7.6). A diagnosis of Anxiety Disorder Due to Another Medical Condition requires evidence from the history, physical examination, or laboratory testing of a nonpsychiatric medical condition that is known to cause anxiety, as well as other evidence to link the anxiety to the medical condition. Aspects of the clinical presentation that can assist in making the causal connection include 1) the presence of a clear temporal association between the onset, exacerbation, or remission of the medical condition and the anxiety symptoms; 2) the presence of features that are atypical of Anxiety Disorders, such as an unusual age at onset; and 3) evidence in the medical literature that a known physiological mechanism causes anxiety. This disorder is to be distinguished from Illness Anxiety Disorder (see Section 9.2), in which the individual worries about illness but may or may not have another nonpsychiatric medical condition and, if present, the nonpsychiatric medical condition is not physiologically related to the anxiety.

The Outdoorsman

Arne Olsen, a 78-year-old retired lumber company president, sought help for the onset of a series of episodic attacks in which he experienced marked apprehension, restlessness, and the need to be outdoors to relieve his sense of discomfort. He described the most recent event as having occurred at 3:00 A.M. a week earlier: he awoke from sleep and felt "the walls were caving in" on him. He denied that this was related to dreaming and said that he was fully awake at the time. He arose, dressed, and went outside in subzero weather; once outside, he noted gradual improvement (but not full resolution) of his symptoms. Complete resolution took a full day.

In response to pointed questioning, Mr. Olsen denied shortness of breath, palpitations, choking sensations, numbness and tingling, and nausea. He reported trembling and some sweating, together with intermittent dizziness. He imagined that he would die (or lose consciousness) if he could not "escape" from his house. He spoke of a need "to be active."

Mr. Olsen denied recent sleep dysfunction, change in appetite or weight, crying spells, or decreased energy. He had been taking clonazepam, an antianxiety medication, for approximately 2 months for feelings of increased nervousness and tension. He had noted mild memory problems of late.

Further inquiry established a problem with balance and intermittent pain in his right arm, and a complaint of indigestion and intermittent diarrhea. Mr. Olsen had stopped gardening the past summer because of his balance problem. On examination he was found to have a "beefy" red tongue (which he said was painful), difficulty with tandem gait (walking with one foot directly in front of the other) and rapid alternating hand motions, and a mild intention (on movement) hand tremor. He denied urinary incontinence.

Laboratory studies revealed a macrocytic anemia (blood with an insufficient concentration of hemoglobin characterized by red blood cells that are larger than their normal volume) and vitamin B_{12} deficiency. Mr. Olsen was given vitamin B_{12} replacement, and his attacks did not recur.

Discussion of "The Outdoorsman"

Mr. Olsen describes unexpected panic attacks (with trembling, sweating, dizziness, and fear of dying, but without such typical symptoms as palpitations or shortness of breath), suggesting a diagnosis of Panic Disorder (see "I Could be Dying" in Section 5.5). However, careful physical examination and laboratory findings indicate the characteristic features of vitamin B_{12} deficiency due to pernicious anemia, an acquired vitamin B_{12} malabsorption syndrome. Pernicious anemia is characterized by a macrocytic anemia, as well as other symptoms, such as a beefy red tongue, diarrhea, loss of balance, and pain. Because the panic attacks disappeared with treatment of the vitamin deficiency, it is reasonable to assume that the correct diagnosis is Anxiety Disorder Due to Pernicious Anemia, With Panic Attacks (DSM-5-TR, p. 258).

CHAPTER 6

Obsessive-Compulsive and Related Disorders

Obsessive-Compulsive and Related Disorders are characterized by an individual's difficulties in controlling their cognitive processes (e.g., thinking, perceiving) and behaviors, such that these processes and behaviors become overwhelmingly preoccupying (thoughts, urges, or images) and endlessly repetitive (behaviors or mental acts in response to preoccupations). The hallmark disorder in this group, Obsessive-Compulsive Disorder (OCD), is characterized by 1) *obsessions*—recurrent and persistent thoughts, urges, or images that are experienced as intrusive and unwanted by a person and cause the individual marked anxiety or distress; and/or 2) *compulsions*—repetitive behaviors or mental acts that a person feels driven to perform in response to an obsession or according to rigid rules. Other disorders in this group are characterized by preoccupations with perceived physical flaws or defects (Body Dysmorphic Disorder) or with the perceived need to keep essentially useless possessions (Hoarding Disorder). This chapter also includes a case of Olfactory Reference Disorder (characterized by a preoccupation with the belief that one is emitting a foul or offensive body odor or breath), which is a recognized disorder in the International Classification of Diseases, 11th Revision (ICD-11) and is given as an example of an Other Specified Obsessive-Compulsive and Related Disorder in DSM-5-TR (DSM-5-TR, p. 294). Two other disorders are characterized by recurrent body-focused repetitive behaviors that are self-injurious or self-destructive: Trichotillomania (Hair-Pulling Disorder) and Excoriation (Skin-Picking) Disorder. (Table 6–1 lists characteristic features of the Obsessive-Compulsive and Related Disorders discussed in this chapter.)

Obsessive-Compulsive and Related Disorders have a significant anxiety component in that the cognitions cause anxiety in most cases and the behaviors involved often appear to serve an anxiety-reducing function. Obsessive-Compulsive and Related Disorders are all characterized by an individual's extreme difficulty in controlling or inability to control preoccupying thoughts or repetitive behaviors.

In addition to having variations in the types of preoccupations and repetitive behaviors involved, Obsessive-Compulsive and Related Disorders vary by the amount of insight that an affected person has into the unrealistic aspects of their thoughts or

TABLE 6–1.   **Characteristic features of Obsessive-Compulsive and Related Disorders**

Disorder	Key characteristics
Obsessive-Compulsive Disorder	*Obsessions:* Recurrent, persistent, and intrusive thoughts, urges, or images, which the individual attempts to actively ignore, suppress, or neutralize with another thought or action (e.g., performing a compulsion)
	Compulsions: Repetitive, driven behaviors or mental acts performed in response to obsessions applied according to rigid rules; unrealistic or excessive behaviors or mental acts aimed at preventing or reducing anxiety or preventing some dreaded event or situation
Body Dysmorphic Disorder	Preoccupation with perceived defects or flaws in physical appearance
	Repetitive behaviors or mental acts in response to appearance concerns
Hoarding Disorder	Persistent difficulty discarding or parting with possessions
	Accumulation of possessions congests and clutters living areas, compromising their intended use
Trichotillomania (Hair-Pulling Disorder)	Recurrent pulling out of hair resulting in hair loss
Excoriation (Skin-Picking) Disorder	Recurrent skin picking resulting in skin lesions

behaviors. *Insight* refers to the individual's understanding of the origin and nature of their maladaptive attitudes and behavior. For Obsessive-Compulsive and Related Disorders that have a cognitive component (i.e., OCD, Body Dysmorphic Disorder, and Hoarding Disorder), DSM-5-TR includes three insight-related specifiers:

- With Good or Fair Insight indicates that people recognize that their beliefs are definitely or probably not true or that they may or may not be true or that their behavior is problematic.
- With Poor Insight indicates that people think that their beliefs are probably true and are mostly convinced that their behavior is not problematic despite evidence to the contrary.
- With Absent Insight/Delusional Beliefs applies to people who have no insight or are delusional (see introduction to Chapter 2, "Schizophrenia Spectrum and Other Psychotic Disorders") and are completely convinced that their beliefs are true and their behaviors are not problematic (e.g., that there is nothing problematic or abnormal about having every inch of their home filled with old newspapers).

6.1
Obsessive-Compulsive Disorder

The content of the obsessions and compulsions of OCD vary among people with the condition, but certain themes are common. These include themes of *cleaning*, with repetitive thoughts about possible contamination by dirt, germs, or disease and compensatory cleaning behaviors such as excessive hand washing; *symmetry*, with repetitive thoughts about order and behaviors involving repeating, ordering, and counting; *forbidden thoughts*, with aggressive, sexual, or religious thoughts and behaviors such as praying; and *harm*, with fears of harm to self or others and compensatory behaviors such as checking things (e.g., doors, gas ranges and ovens) to see if they are safe or secure. Obsessions cause individuals a great deal of anxiety or distress, and people with them struggle to ignore or suppress them or to "neutralize" them with other thoughts or actions (i.e., compulsions). Compulsions are repetitive behaviors or mental acts that individuals feel "driven" to perform in response to an obsession or according to rigid rules. For example, a person who is worried about becoming contaminated by germs after touching something may feel an irresistible need to scrub and rinse their right hand exactly seven times and then to scrub and rinse their left hand exactly seven times (and perhaps to then start over). Although the compulsive actions in OCD are aimed at preventing or reducing anxiety or preventing some calamity, they are not connected in any realistic way to what they are intended to neutralize or prevent, or they are clearly excessive.

Obsessive thoughts need to be distinguished from "worries," which are usually about real-life concerns. The obsessive thoughts of OCD often are not about real-life concerns and can include content that is odd or irrational and may have a "magical" component. Depressed patients may have recurrent negative thoughts about themselves or their lives (i.e., "ruminations"), but these are not usually experienced as "intrusive" or out of their control. Superstitious behaviors, such as blowing on dice before a roll, avoiding stepping on a sidewalk crack or walking under a ladder, or tossing spilled salt over one's shoulder, have some characteristics of compulsions. Usually, however, these behaviors are performed without a time-consuming ritual, as compared with compulsive rituals, which can go on for hours and severely interfere with a person's social or occupational functioning.

OCD usually begins in late adolescence but may begin earlier or even in childhood. The 12-month prevalence of OCD in the United States is 1.2%, with similar prevalence in countries around the world. Women are slightly more likely than men to have the disorder in adulthood, but boys are more likely than girls to have the disorder in childhood. OCD can be a very impairing disorder. People with OCD can spend inordinate amounts of time engaged in obsessive thinking or with compulsive rituals to the exclusion of other activities, and they may be completely unable to complete schoolwork or job tasks on time. In addition, people with OCD may avoid people or situations that might trigger symptoms (e.g., not going outside for fear of being contaminated by dirt).

They may also cause themselves physical harm (e.g., raw and broken skin from excessive washing). Up to 15% of people with OCD attempt suicide at some point (DSM-5-TR, p. 269). If OCD is untreated, the course can be chronic, and only about 20% of individuals will recover. Other mental disorders, such as Anxiety, Depressive, Tic, Substance Use, Impulse-Control, Personality (e.g., Obsessive-Compulsive Personality Disorder), and other Obsessive-Compulsive and Related Disorders often occur in people with OCD.

Lady Macbeth

Interviewer: Cindy, tell me about when things were the hardest for you. When was that?

Patient: It was around Christmastime last year.

Interviewer: And you were how old then?

Patient: I was 13.

Interviewer: You're 14 now, right?

Patient: Yes.

Interviewer: When things were really at their worst, can you tell me what it was that was disturbing to you at that time?

Patient: Well, the major part about it was that, like all these things that I did, they were really stupid, and they didn't make any sense, but I'm still gonna have to do it, and it was sort of like being scared of what would happen if I didn't do it.

Interviewer: What were the things that you were doing?

Patient: In the morning when I got dressed, I was real afraid that there'd be germs all over my clothes and things, so I'd stand there and I'd shake them for half an hour. I'd wash before I did anything—like if I was gonna wash my face, I'd wash my hands first; and if I was gonna get dressed, I'd wash my hands first; and then it got even beyond that point. Washing my hands wasn't enough, and I started to use rubbing alcohol. It was wintertime and cold weather, and this really made my hands bleed. Even if I just held them under water, they'd bleed all over the place, and they looked terrible, and everyone thought I had a disease or something.

Interviewer: And when you were doing that much washing, how much time every day did that take, if you added up all the different parts of it?

Patient: It took about 6 hours a day. In the morning I didn't have a whole lot of choice, because I had to get up at 6:00 and get ready for school. All I'd do was to get dressed as best I could. I didn't even have time to brush my hair. At the time I never ate breakfast, so all these things—it was just so complex that I didn't have time to do anything.

Interviewer: You also told me about other things in addition to the washing and worrying about dirt—that you would have plans about how you would do other things.

Patient: Okay, well, they were like set plans in my mind that if I heard the word, like, something that had to do with germs or disease, it would be considered something bad and so I had things that would go through my mind that were sort of like "cross that out and it'll make it okay" to hear that word.

Interviewer: What sort of things?

Patient: Like numbers or words that seemed to be sort of like a protector.

Interviewer: What numbers and what words were they?

Patient: It started out to be the number 3 and multiples of 3 and then words like "soap and water," something like that; and then the multiples of 3 got really high, they'd end up to be 123 or something like that. It got real bad then....

Interviewer: At any time did you really believe that something bad would happen if you didn't do these things? Was it just a feeling, or were you really scared?

Patient: No! I was petrified that something would really happen. It was weird, because everyone would always say how sensible I was and intelligent. But it was weird because I tried to explain it in order to really make them understand what I was trying to say and they'd go, you know, like, "Well, that's stupid," and I knew it; but when I was alone, things would be a lot worse than when I was with this group, because if I was around friends, that would make me forget about most of this. But when I was alone, it...like, my mind would wander to all sorts of things and I'd get new plans and new rituals and new ideas, and I'd start worrying more and more about people that could get hurt that I cared about and things that could really go bad if I didn't.

Interviewer: Who were the people you'd worry most would get hurt?

Patient: My family, basically my family.

Interviewer: Any particular people in your family?

Patient: Well, like my grandmother—she's 83 and, you know, I was just worried that...I know that she's old and she's not gonna be around much longer, but I was worried that maybe something I did could cause her to get really, really sick or something.

Interviewer: Had anything like this ever been on your mind before you were 13, when this started?

Patient: Well, let's see...my mother, her family has always been mostly real neat people and extremely clean and so that could have affected it, because I was growing up in that sort of background. But I always like to be clean and neat, and I was never really allowed to walk around the house with muddy shoes or anything like that, so...

Interviewer: But your concerns about clean, about how many times you did things—have they ever gotten in the way of your doing things that you wanted to do?

Patient: Uh-huh. Many times. Like, I was supposed to go somewhere with a friend, and we were gonna leave at 11:00 and I wanted to take a shower before I left. So I had to get up about 6:00 in the morning, and sometimes I just won't even make it with 5 hours to do it....

Interviewer: And that was since you were 13. But what about any time in your life before that—had anything like this ever happened? Or, as far as you know, was this the first?

Patient: It was the first time.

Interviewer: Have you at any time felt that you had some other special idea about forces beyond you...about your being able to control things magically or be in control?

Patient: I'm really scared of supernatural things. I don't like to say that I believe in superstitions and things, but I guess I really do 'cause they frighten me. When I was little, they weren't really bothering me or anything, but now I avoid it as much as I can. Like, the number 13 now, if it came up, you know, it wouldn't bother me, but I'd rather have the number 7 instead.

Interviewer: So you are superstitious, but you've never heard any special voice talking to you or...

Patient: Yeah, I have. It's like…if I tried to describe it, people would think that I saw little people dancing around or something, and that was wrong because all it was, it wasn't like a voice, it was just like a thought.

Interviewer: More like being able to hear yourself think?

Patient: Right.

Interviewer: Have you ever seen things that other people couldn't see?

Patient: No.

Interviewer: I know you are doing very well here in school and on the ward here at the hospital. Do you have any signs left of the problems that you used to have with your rituals and compulsions?

Patient: Well, everyone is compulsive to a point. I can see little things that I'll do. Like, I will go over something twice, or three times, because that's a special number. Like, if I read something and I really don't understand it, maybe I would go over it one more time and then, say, one more time will make it three. But nothing really big. It's been really good, because I have gotten out and taken a shower, and gotten dressed, and washed my face and brushed my teeth, and all that stuff in like half an hour! That's really good for me because I wasn't able to do that before.

Interviewer: So, in general, it's fair to say that there are things that just you would notice now, and probably someone sharing the room with you wouldn't be able to tell the other things you are doing even though you know these little things are there. Good…. Well, thank you very much.

Discussion of "Lady Macbeth"

This adolescent girl articulately and vividly describes what it is like to have a severe form of OCD (DSM-5-TR, p. 265). She has both obsessions and compulsions, and both are significant sources of distress to her, interfere with her functioning, and cause her physical harm. The onset of her problems in adolescence is typical of the disorder.

Cindy's obsessions, with a mixture of themes of contamination and harm, consist of ideas that intrude into her consciousness and are experienced as unwanted. For example, she gets the idea that she may have done something that could cause her grandmother to get sick. Another example is the thought that there are germs on her clothes. The need to neutralize such distressing thoughts has led to various compulsions that are repetitive and that she feels driven to perform according to rules that must be rigidly applied. For example, if she heard a word that suggested germs or disease, she had to undo it ("cross that out") by saying the number 3 and multiples of 3, or words like "soap and water." Although these behaviors were designed to prevent her discomfort or a dreaded event (her grandmother becoming "really, really sick"), the activity was not connected in a realistic way to what it was designed to prevent (i.e., her saying "soap and water" could not, in fact, prevent her grandmother from becoming sick) and was clearly excessive. In addition, she washed her hands for hours to prevent becoming infected by germs, to the extreme that her hands would actually bleed. Although emotionally Cindy reacted as if the dangers were real ("I was petrified that something would really happen"), intellectually she always knew that her fears were irrational and were not about real-life problems (her friends would say that her behavior was stupid, and she knew that it was). Because of Cindy's level of awareness, the specifier With Good or Fair Insight (DSM-5-TR, p. 266) would be noted with her diagnosis. In a few cases (i.e., 4% or less), during a severe episode of the illness, the person may no longer recognize that the obsessions or compulsions are excessive or unreasonable; in such instances the diagnosis would be further designated with the specifier With Absent Insight/Delusional Beliefs.

Obsessive thoughts may be confused with auditory hallucinations (see Chapter 2, "Schizophrenia Spectrum and Other Psychotic Disorders"). This patient recognized that if she described some of her obsessive thoughts to people, they might think that she was hallucinating ("if I tried to describe it, people would think that I saw little people dancing around or something"). However, she is quite clear that it was just her own thoughts that she was experiencing and that she was not hearing a real, other voice external to herself.

OCD is sometimes associated with Obsessive-Compulsive Personality Disorder (see "The Workaholic" in Section 18.4). Whereas OCD involves true obsessions and compulsions (as defined in the introduction to this chapter), Obsessive-Compulsive Personality Disorder involves personality traits such as perfectionism, interpersonal control, and excessive devotion to work or productivity. There is no evidence of Obsessive-Compulsive Personality Disorder in this case.

6.2
Body Dysmorphic Disorder

Body Dysmorphic Disorder involves a preoccupation with "perceived defects or flaws in physical appearance that are not observable or appear slight to others" (DSM-5-TR, p. 271). Like individuals with OCD (see Section 6.1), people with Body Dysmorphic Disorder engage in repetitive behaviors in response to their concerns—but their concerns are centered exclusively on their appearance and on others' responses (as they perceive others' responses) to their appearance. Their behaviors may include, for example, frequently checking how they look in mirrors, repetitively grooming, seeking reassurance about their appearance from others, or comparing how they look to how other people look. People with the disorder may feel ugly, unattractive, abnormal, or deformed. The most common parts of the body that are of concern are the skin, the hair, or the nose, but other body areas, such as eyes, teeth, face, chin, stomach, breasts, legs, and genitals, also can be the focus.

Many individuals with Eating Disorders, particularly those with Anorexia Nervosa (see Section 10.4) or Bulimia Nervosa (see Section 10.5), have body image issues and may be preoccupied with the idea that they are overweight or that some part of their body (e.g., thighs, stomach) is flabby. For such individuals an additional diagnosis of Body Dysmorphic Disorder would be redundant, because those kinds of body image distortions are a feature of their Eating Disorder. Individuals without an Eating Disorder who have such preoccupations could be given a diagnosis of Body Dysmorphic Disorder if such preoccupations are sufficiently impairing. Moreover, some individuals with an Eating Disorder may qualify for an additional diagnosis of Body Dysmorphic Disorder if the focus of preoccupation with appearance is not that they are fat or overweight but rather, for example, that their nose is horribly crooked.

Body Dysmorphic Disorder commonly begins in adolescence. The point prevalence of Body Dysmorphic Disorder in the United States is estimated at 2.4%. It is slightly more common in women than in men. A type that occurs almost exclusively in men is *muscle dysmorphia,* which is a preoccupation with the body as being too small or insufficiently muscular, leading to excessive dieting, exercise, weight lifting, or ingestion of anabolic steroids to increase muscle mass. Body Dysmorphic Disorder is quite commonly seen in dermatology, cosmetic surgery, orthodontia, and oral and maxillofacial surgery practices. It is often a chronic disorder, and people with it can subject themselves to unnecessary and potentially harmful dermatological treatments or surgery. When patients with Body Dysmorphic Disorder undergo treatments, such as dermabrasion (a scraping of the skin to remove damaged layers) or surgery, they are almost invariably unsatisfied with the results (see "Elephant Man," below). For this reason, medical treatments are not likely to be helpful. Some individuals may actually attempt surgery on themselves or attempt suicide. Body Dysmorphic Disorder is very impairing, because affected people will avoid social situations, drop out of school, not work, or even become completely housebound because of their concerns about their appearance. Major Depressive Disorder, Social Anxiety Disorder, Obsessive-Compulsive Disorder, and Substance Use Disorders, commonly co-occur with Body Dysmorphic Disorder.

Elephant Man

Marco Caruso is a shy, anxious-looking, 31-year-old carpenter who has been hospitalized after making a suicide attempt by putting his head in a plastic bag after looking at himself in the mirror. He asks to meet with the psychiatrist in a darkened room. He is wearing a baseball cap pulled down over his forehead and partially covering his eyes. Looking down at the floor, Mr. Caruso says he has no friends, has just been fired from his job, and was recently left by his girlfriend. When the psychiatrist asks him to elaborate, he replies, "It's really hard to talk about this, Doctor. I don't know if I can. It's too embarrassing. Well, I guess I should tell you…after all, I'm in the hospital because of it. It's my nose." "Your nose?" the psychiatrist asks. "Yes, these huge pockmarks on my nose. They're grotesque! I look like a monster. I'm as ugly as the Elephant Man! These marks on my nose are all I can think about. I've thought about them every day for the past 15 years. I even have nightmares about them. And I think that everyone can see them and that they laugh at me because of them.

That's why I wear this hat all the time. And that's why I couldn't talk to you in a bright room…you'd see how ugly I am."

The psychiatrist could not see the huge pockmarks that Mr. Caruso was referring to, even when she later met him in a brightly lit room. Mr. Caruso is, in fact, a handsome man with normal-appearing facial pores. The psychiatrist says, "I don't see any ugly pockmarks. Is it possible that your view of your appearance is distorted, that maybe they're just normal-looking facial pores?"

"That's a hard question to answer," he replies. "I've pretty much kept this preoccupation a secret because it's so embarrassing. I'm afraid people will think I'm vain. But I've told a few people about it, and they've tried to convince me that the pores really aren't visible. Sometimes I sort of believe them. I think that I probably am distorting and that they're not so bad. Then I look in the mirror and see that they're huge and ugly, and I'm convinced that people laugh at them. Then no one can talk me out of it. When people try to, I think they just feel sorry for me and that they're trying to make me feel better. This has affected me in a lot of ways, Doctor," he adds. "It may be hard for you to believe, but this problem has ruined my life. All I can think about is my face. I spend hours a day looking at the marks in the mirror. But I just can't resist. I started missing more and more work, and I stopped going out with my friends and my girlfriend. I got so anxious when people looked at me that I was staying in the house most of the time. Sometimes when I did go out, I went through red lights so I wouldn't have to sit at the light where people might be staring at me. The hat helped a little, but it didn't cover all the marks. I tried covering them with makeup for a while, but I thought people could see the makeup so that didn't really help. The only time I really felt comfortable was when I wore my nephew's Batman mask on Halloween. Then no one could see the marks. I missed so much work that I was fired. My girlfriend stuck it out with me for a long time, but she finally couldn't take it anymore. One thing that was really hard for her was that I started asking her about 50 times a day whether I looked okay and whether she could see the marks. I think that was the last straw. If I had a choice, I'd rather have cancer. It must be less painful. This is like an arrow through my heart."

Mr. Caruso went on to discuss the fact that he had seen a dermatologist to request dermabrasion but was refused the procedure because the doctor "said there was nothing there." He finally convinced another dermatologist to do the procedure, but Mr. Caruso thought it did not help. Eventually, he felt so desperate over the supposed marks that he made two suicide attempts. His most recent attempt occurred after he looked in the mirror and was horrified by what he saw. He told the psychiatrist, "I saw how awful I looked, and I thought: I'm not sure it's worth it to go on living if I have to look like this and think about this all the time." His first suicide attempt had also led to hospitalization, but, because the patient was so ashamed of his appearance concern and thought it would not be taken seriously, he kept it a secret and told the staff only that he was depressed.

Discussion of "Elephant Man"

Mr. Caruso looks normal, but he is preoccupied with a perceived defect in his appearance. This preoccupation has clearly caused him significant distress and has significantly interfered with his functioning (he was fired from his job because of absenteeism, and his girlfriend broke off their relationship). Although this is a fairly severe case of Body Dysmorphic Disorder (DSM-5-TR, p. 271), it is not atypical: occupational, social, and other important areas of functioning may be severely impaired, and suicide attempts are not uncommon. However, the degree of distress and dysfunction associated with this disorder spans a spectrum of severity; some individuals with this disorder—although distressed and perhaps not functioning up to their capacity—are relatively high functioning.

The focus of a person's concern in Body Dysmorphic Disorder commonly involves a facial flaw, as in Mr. Caruso's case—often a perceived defect of the hair, nose, or skin. In some cases, again like Mr. Caruso's, no physical anomaly is actually present. In other cases, a slight physical anomaly is present, but the person's concern is markedly excessive.

Certain repetitive behaviors are present in relation or response to the perceived defect. In Mr. Caruso's case, these include excessive mirror checking, camouflaging grooming activities involving the use of makeup to try to hide his "pores," wearing hats or masks to cover up, and repetitively questioning his girlfriend and other friends about the "defect." Because people with Body Dysmorphic Disorder are often ashamed of their concern, they may keep it a secret, as Mr. Caruso did most of the time and during his first hospitalization, and may not reveal it unless specifically asked about it.

People with Body Dysmorphic Disorder often have poor insight into the fact that the "defect" is imagined or distorted. In addition, it appears that degree of insight may be more accurately conceptualized as spanning a spectrum that ranges from good insight to delusional thinking (see introduction to Chapter 2, "Schizophrenia Spectrum and Other Psychotic Disorders"), along which the person's belief may vary over time. Indeed, at the time of the evaluation described above, Mr. Caruso's insight was fair, which would warrant a diagnosis of Body Dysmorphic Disorder, With Good or Fair Insight (DSM-5-TR, p. 272), but at other times he has appeared to be delusional, which would be noted as "With Absent Insight/Delusional Beliefs."

6.3
Hoarding Disorder

The hallmark of Hoarding Disorder is a "persistent difficulty discarding or parting with possessions, regardless of their actual value" (DSM-5-TR, p. 277). The individual has a perceived need to save the things that are kept, and the thought of getting rid of them causes substantial distress. Individuals with this disorder intentionally hold on to possessions because they believe that the objects may have future utility or are of some aesthetic or sentimental value. The most commonly saved items are newspapers, magazines, old clothing, bags, books, mail, and paperwork, but almost anything can be kept, including animals. The problem of difficulty with discarding possessions leads to an accumulation of them, and the resulting congestion and clutter compromise the use of active living space. Thus, because of the extent of accumulation, a kitchen may not be suitable for cooking, a bed not available for sleeping, or a whole house or apartment completely inaccessible. In some cases, items may also be accumulated outside the home in cars, yards, offices or other places of work, or the homes of friends or family members. Living areas may become unsafe due to risk of fire, falling, or respiratory or other diseases.

Symptoms of hoarding commonly begin in adolescence but, due to their chronic course, increase in prevalence with age. It has been found to be more common in older adults (over 65 years) than in younger adults (30–40 years). Estimates of the prevalence of Hoarding Disorder in the United States and Europe range from 1.5% to 6%. Hoarding Disorder may be equally common in men as in women, but women are more likely to seek treatment for it. Approximately three-quarters of individuals with Hoarding Disorder have another mental disorder: Major Depressive Disorder, Social Anxiety Disorder, and Generalized Anxiety Disorder are the most common.

Something of Value

Eli Wolfe, a 50-year-old man, came to the emergency room of a New York hospital complaining of malaise, fever, and a cough. An upper respiratory infection was diagnosed, but as the doctor was writing out the prescription, Mr. Wolfe tearfully revealed that he had no home to go to, was depressed, and felt that life was not worth living. The psychiatric resident who was called to see the patient obtained the following additional information.

For the past month, Mr. Wolfe had been living in the basement of his apartment building, eating in restaurants, and using a Young Men's Hebrew Association for showers. He was eating and sleeping poorly. His own apartment was so full of newspapers, magazines, and books that he could no longer get in the door, but he could not bring himself to get rid of any of his "stuff."

When he was age 12, Mr. Wolfe began collecting baseball cards, and then books and magazines. His parents were poor immigrants from Eastern Europe, and the idea of holding on to things that might someday be valuable was not strange to them. Eventually, however, the apartment became so cluttered that they threw out much of his collection. He retrieved it from the garbage, and from that point on his "collecting" has been a focus of conflict with both family and employers. He does not go out of his way to obtain things, but once he has a newspaper, book, or magazine, he cannot throw it away because "there might be something of value written in it." The thought of throwing things out makes him extremely anxious, and in the end, he simply cannot do it.

For many years Mr. Wolfe worked as a doorman in elegant apartment buildings, but invariably he was fired because he brought his "stuff" to store in his workplace, and he sometimes got into fistfights with the building maintenance people who tried to throw it out. He was married for 16 years and has a 25-year-old son. His wife finally left him, unable to tolerate his behavior. He rarely sees his son.

Mr. Wolfe first entered treatment not because of his collecting but because, at age 20, "my mood took a turn for the worse. I had a breakdown." He stopped doing virtually everything—working, eating, and sleeping. "It was an effort even to lift my leg." He began seeing a psychiatrist as an outpatient, and over the years has been in therapy much of the time and has been treated with amitriptyline, desipramine, and fluoxetine (all of which are antidepressant medications); quetiapine (an antipsychotic medication); and other medications that he does not remember.

After his divorce 10 years ago, Mr. Wolfe moved some of his collection into his own apartment and rented storage space for the rest. Gradually, his new apartment filled up with newspapers, magazines, and books, and it became a struggle just to get in the front door and make his way to his bed. Finally, last month, after injuring his shoulder trying to push things aside, he abandoned the apartment for a cot in the basement of the building. He understands that his inability to throw out things is irrational, but the thought of starting to do it makes him intolerably anxious.

Mr. Wolfe was admitted to the psychiatric hospital, diagnosed as having Major Depressive Disorder, and started on fluoxetine, an antidepressant that had helped him with his depressed mood in the past. The dosage was gradually raised to 80 mg/day, and after 4 weeks, with considerable pressure from his psychotherapist, Mr. Wolfe was able to clear the foyer of his apartment, so he could at least get in the door. His mood improved, and he began eating and sleeping better. In the succeeding 6 months, he has slowly and methodically discarded bundles of articles. Although he is now able to live in his apartment, it remains cluttered with his things.

Discussion of "Something of Value"

Mr. Wolfe presents with symptoms suggesting depression: depressed mood, difficulty eating and sleeping, and thoughts that life is not worth living. More information about the severity and persistence of these symptoms eventually is collected to determine a diagnosis of Major Depressive Disorder (see "Stonemason" in Section 4.2). However, what is most striking is that there is a long-standing problem with his inability to throw things out—hoarding—that has totally disrupted his life.

Mr. Wolfe's case seems to be a prototypical case of Hoarding Disorder (DSM-5-TR, p. 277), because he has a persistent difficulty parting with possessions—along with a perceived need to save them, distress on the prospect of discarding them, an accumulation of possessions that has made his apartment uninhabitable, and both job (e.g., being fired) and personal (e.g., a divorce from his wife) losses that have resulted from his behavior. His collection of information-containing items, such as newspapers, books, and magazines, is classic.

Hoarding may be part of the picture of Obsessive-Compulsive Personality Disorder (see "The Workaholic" in Section 18.4), because hoarding behavior is actually one of the criteria for that disorder ("Is unable to discard worn-out or worthless objects even when they have no sentimental value"; DSM-5-TR, p. 772) and approximately 50% of those with Hoarding Disorder also have Obsessive-Compulsive Personality Disorder. However, none of the other features of Obsessive-Compulsive Personality Disorder, such as perfectionism or excessive devotion to work, seem to be present in Mr. Wolfe's case.

Hoarding is sometimes seen as part of the disorganized or bizarre behavior of individuals with Schizophrenia (see "Eating Wires" in Section 2.1), but in this case none of the characteristic features of Schizophrenia (e.g., delusions or hallucinations) are present. Mr. Wolfe's anxiety associated with the thought of throwing things away suggests an obsession. However, in true obsessions, such thoughts are experienced as intrusive and unwanted, whereas in Mr. Wolfe's case, they are not. Is the hoarding behavior a compulsion? Compulsions are repetitive behaviors or thoughts in which the individual engages and that are done in a stereotypic manner or in response to an obsession. In contrast, Mr. Wolfe's hoarding is actually the failure to engage in an appropriate behavior (throwing out old and unused newspapers, books, and magazines). Furthermore, he does not follow any stereotyped rules in collecting his books and papers, and his hoarding is not in response to an obsession.

6.4
Trichotillomania
(Hair-Pulling Disorder)

The essential features of Trichotillomania are "recurrent pulling out of one's hair, resulting in hair loss," and "repeated attempts to decrease or stop hair pulling" (DSM-5-TR, p. 281). The hair that is pulled can come from any part of the body, but the most common sites are the scalp, eyebrows, and eyelids. Less commonly, hair may be pulled from axillary, facial, pubic, or perirectal areas. Episodes of hair pulling may be brief and sporadic or may be prolonged and enduring. Hair-pulling behavior causes great distress, including embarrassment, shame, and feelings of being out of control. It may be triggered by negative emotions, such as boredom or anxiety; is often accompanied by an increasing sense of tension before pulling out hairs; and may lead to a sense of pleasure or relief once the behavior has occurred. Individuals who engage in pulling hair from visible places (e.g., from the scalp) may attempt to hide their hair loss with hats, scarves, or wigs.

The 12-month prevalence of Trichotillomania in adults and adolescents is estimated to be 1%–2%. In clinical samples, women are 10 times more likely than men to have Trichotillomania, but in community samples, the gender ratio may be closer to 2:1. The onset is most common at puberty. Even though the course is chronic, symptoms frequently come and go, even without treatment. Hair pulling often interferes with social and occupational functioning and occasionally may be associated with some physical problems, such as skin infections. Commonly co-occurring other mental disorders include Major Depressive Disorder (see Section 4.2) and Excoriation Disorder (see Section 6.5).

Hair

Celeste Nguyen, now age 25, had always thought she was the only person who pulled out her hair. When she was a teenager, her parents made her feel like no other people ever pulled out their eyebrows until none were left. This behavior had been going on since she was 12 years old. In addition to pulling out her eyebrows, she pulled out hair on her head; at times, there have been quarter-size bald patches on her head. In fact, there was a 1-year period (about 5 years ago, when she was a sophomore at college) when she was practically bald.

It always amazed Ms. Nguyen how "together" everyone thought her to be. She earned good grades and got into law school. "If they only knew," she often said to herself. However, through her careful brushing of whatever hair she still had, artful use of scarves, and occasional use of a hairpiece, as well as by avoiding all gym classes, she hid the behavior and its results, and not a soul ever found out. The eyebrows were easy: she just drew in new ones.

She found her hair picking to be a merciless daily habit. Usually, she would be sitting in front of the TV, distractedly watching reruns, when she would notice that her fingers were in her hair, rummaging about, looking for a hair with a nice thick shaft. Then she would rapidly tug with an expertise gained from long experience. Out would come the hair, root and all. Ms. Nguyen would then notice the little pile of hairs accumulating on the arm of the sofa and realize she must have been doing this for many minutes already. She would try to stop, but her nervousness would escalate, and the hair pulling would recommence and go on until the urge just wore itself out. On good days, this activity might end after 10 minutes. On bad days, it could last for an hour.

Ms. Nguyen might never have known that other people had this habit except that a month ago a sudden rainstorm messed up her strategically coiffed hair, exposing the large ratty patch just above her left ear. Horrified that she was now revealed to her coworker Sylvia, Ms. Nguyen was surprised when she heard, "You're a hair puller too?" Three days later, Sylvia took Ms. Nguyen to a self-help group, where she met seven other "pullers," five women and two men. Ms. Nguyen thought she was hearing her own life in other people's words:

I felt like I must be an awful person, with no self-control. That's what my parents said.

High school gym terrified me. I was constantly afraid of my wig coming off.
I figured, who could ever want to marry me. First of all, I'm scared to have
any real sex. I know my hair will come undone. And what if someone does fall
in love with me? How would he react when he realized I did this thing? I had
one boyfriend whom I told that I got messed up by a chemical reaction to a
bad permanent. But I wouldn't be able to say that forever.

I thought I was the only one in the world.

In the self-help group, Ms. Nguyen learned the name of a doctor who specializes in the treatment of Trichotillomania. The doctor prescribed an antidepressant, fluoxetine, which seemed to help substantially for about 3 months. Then the symptoms worsened again, and Ms. Nguyen was switched to clomipramine (another antidepressant that is often used for the treatment of difficult-to-manage OCD). It took a while for her to quit feeling sleepy when she took the medication, but her hair-pulling symptoms improved significantly and stayed that way. Six months later she went to see a hypnotist, which further helped reduce the hair-pulling urge. She now has days, and even weeks, when she does not pull her hair at all, and the symptom is never as bad as it used to be. Surprisingly, the use of the two medications had an unexpected benefit. Even though she felt herself demoralized by her hair pulling, she had never thought of herself as "depressed," but while taking the medication, her mood became much more chipper. She was more enthusiastic about work and felt better about herself when she went out on dates—even before the hair pulling got better. She continues to attend the self-help group and credits it for some of her improvement, particularly in her self-esteem.

Discussion of "Hair"

Ms. Nguyen cannot resist the impulse to pull out her hair. Her hair-pulling behavior is far in excess of the common practice of plucking eyebrows that many women engage in solely for cosmetic reasons (i.e., to improve their physical appearance). In fact, her hair pulling has resulted in extensive hair loss, both on her head and from her eyebrows. When she tries to resist the behavior, she becomes increasingly anxious and inevitably gives in. She apparently derives some relief of tension from the activity. These are the characteristic features of Trichotillomania (DSM-5-TR, p. 281). This case is typical in that the patient is a woman and the onset was during adolescence.

The absence of pleasure associated with the activity and the intrusive quality of the impulse-driven hair-pulling behavior might suggest OCD (see Section 6.1). However, in OCD, the compulsions are in response to an obsession or are performed in a stereotyped way and are often aimed at preventing some dreaded event. It is fairly clear that Ms. Nguyen's hair pulling is not in response to any obsessive thoughts; it happens almost without her awareness. Although her hair pulling is repetitive, it is not performed in a ritualized or rigid fashion, and it does not seem to be intended to ward off any future calamity. Furthermore, in OCD, compulsions usually are not limited to a single behavior, as is the case in Trichotillomania.

6.5
Excoriation (Skin-Picking) Disorder

The hallmark behavior of Excoriation Disorder is "recurrent skin picking resulting in skin lesions" (DSM-5-TR, p. 284). The person with this disorder repeatedly attempts to decrease or stop skin picking. The most commonly picked sites are the face, arms, and hands. Individuals may pick at normal skin or at skin with lesions, such as pimples, calluses, or scabs from prior picking. The most common method involves picking with the individual's fingers, but some individuals use tweezers, pins, or other objects. Picking of the skin can consume hours of the day and may persist for months or years. Skin picking causes significant distress, including embarrassment, shame, and a feeling of being out of control. It may be triggered by negative emotions, such as boredom or anxiety; is often accompanied by an increasing sense of tension before picking the skin; and may lead to a sense of pleasure or relief once the behavior has occurred. Individuals who engage in picking skin from visible places (e.g., from the face or arms) may attempt to hide skin lesions with makeup or clothing.

The lifetime prevalence of Excoriation Disorder is estimated at 3.1% and the current prevalence at 2.1%. Women with Excoriation Disorder outnumber men with the disorder by about 3 to 1. The onset is most commonly at puberty and may begin with acne. Without treatment, the disorder is usually chronic, with some waxing and waning of symptoms. Skin picking often interferes with social and school or work functioning, because some people with Excoriation Disorder will not go out in public. Physical problems, including tissue damage, scarring, and infections, may occur. Treatment with antibiotics or surgery may be required. Obsessive-Compulsive Disorder, Trichotillomania, and Major Depressive Disorder frequently accompany Excoriation Disorder.

Picking

Shelley Kellerman is a 28-year-old single woman who picks at her skin. She began picking at her acne when she was approximately 13 years old. She reports that while in college, she picked more frequently and usually when under stress from examinations. She admits that she often felt or looked for things to pick at even if a skin blemish, bump, or inconsistency was fairly insignificant. For the past 4 years, Ms. Kellerman reports picking on a daily basis. After showering in the morning, she often picks at her face, legs, back, or arms. She also picks at night before going to bed as a way to calm herself from the stress of the day. She picks with her fingernails. When she totals the time per day, Ms. Kellerman realizes that she usually spends approximately 3 hours each day picking at her skin. She refrains from picking while at work or around other people. She usually stops picking when she feels that she has gotten rid of the blemish, she starts bleeding, or the picking begins to cause her pain.

Ms. Kellerman reports an urge or a need to pick and she feels unable to resist this drive. She is embarrassed by the fact that the picking is actually rewarding to her in the sense that when she gets rid of a bump or expresses some pus from a pimple, she feels a sense of accomplishment. In fact, she has even wanted to pick her boyfriend's pimples, and when she is with him, she sometimes cannot stop thinking about or focusing on one of his blemishes. Each episode of picking ends with her feeling ashamed and embarrassed by her behavior. She then tells herself that she will never do it again. This resolve lasts only a day at most, and then she picks again.

Due to the time spent picking in the morning, Ms. Kellerman is often late for work or misses social appointments on the weekends. She worries that her boss may fire her due to her frequent tardiness, but she does not want to explain her situation due to embarrassment. Because the picking has resulted in scarring all over her body, Ms. Kellerman avoids doing things that she would like, such as swimming with friends or wearing shorts and short-sleeved tops. She considers herself an attractive young woman, but the picking has made her feel self-conscious in public. She denies any drug use. Overall, she reports being a fairly happy person who enjoys her life, her friends, and her job. She wishes, however, that she could stop picking, because the behavior has taken a toll on her self-esteem. Ms. Kellerman went to a dermatologist for the problem and was told that there was no point in using topical creams for the blemishes until she got the picking under control. She has had difficulty, however, in finding a psychologist or psychiatrist who understands the problem.

Discussion of "Picking"

Ms. Kellerman feels recurrent, irresistible urges to pick at her skin. She cannot control the urges, no matter how hard she tries. The behavior causes her considerable distress, sometimes makes her late to work (she is afraid she might actually be fired because of lateness), and prevents her from some activities that she would otherwise enjoy, such as swimming. In light of the fact that she considers herself to be attractive and does not pick to improve a flaw in her appearance, as might be the case in Body Dysmorphic Disorder (see "Elephant Man" in Section 6.2), and that she has no evidence of psychosis or history of drug abuse, this would seem to be a classic case of Excoriation (Skin-Picking) Disorder (DSM-5-TR, p. 284). The onset of her disorder coinciding with onset of puberty, when an individual often begins the behavior by picking at acne, is common. Her chronic course is also typical. Excoriation Disorder was added as a new diagnosis in DSM-5 to focus clinical attention on what can be a serious and disabling problem behavior.

CHAPTER 7

Trauma- and Stressor-Related Disorders

Many if not most psychiatric disorders can be triggered or exacerbated by exposure to a traumatic or stressful event. For example, it is not uncommon for individuals who are susceptible to developing a Depressive Disorder to develop a Major Depressive Episode in the aftermath of a stressful life experience. This chapter, however, is limited to those DSM-5-TR disorders in which exposure to a traumatic or stressful event is explicitly a diagnostic criterion. Although transient, acute responses to trauma are common for a few days or weeks, some responses to trauma can develop into disorders when the symptoms and their duration adversely affect the person's life and ability to function. All of the DSM-5-TR Trauma- and Stressor-Related Disorders involve maladaptive psychological distress or behavior following exposure to a traumatic or stressful life event or circumstance. The disorders in this group vary primarily in their requirement for the type of stressor: Acute Stress Disorder and Posttraumatic Stress Disorder (PTSD) require that the stressor involve exposure to actual or threatened death, serious injury, or sexual violence; Reactive Attachment Disorder and Disinhibited Social Engagement Disorder require early childhood exposure to extremes of insufficient care; Prolonged Grief Disorder specifically requires the death of a loved one; and the residual category of Adjustment Disorders requires simply the development of emotional or behavioral symptoms in response to an identifiable stressor. (Table 7–1 lists characteristic features of these Trauma- and Stressor-Related Disorders.)

The type of psychological distress following exposure to a traumatic or stressful event is quite variable. Although such symptoms can often be well understood within an anxiety- or fear-based context, many individuals who have been exposed to a traumatic or stressful event exhibit anhedonic and dysphoric symptoms, externalizing angry and aggressive symptoms, or dissociative symptoms.

TABLE 7–1. **Characteristic features of Trauma- and Stressor-Related Disorders**

Disorder	Key characteristics
Reactive Attachment Disorder	Pattern of inhibited, emotionally withdrawn behavior toward adult caregivers
	Extremes of insufficient care responsible for disturbed behavior
Disinhibited Social Engagement Disorder	Pattern of behavior in which child actively approaches and interacts with unfamiliar adults
	Extremes of insufficient care responsible for disturbed behavior
Posttraumatic Stress Disorder	Exposure to actual or threatened death, serious injury, or sexual violence
	Intrusion symptoms associated with the traumatic event
	Persistent avoidance of stimuli associated with the traumatic event
	Negative alterations in cognitions and mood associated with the traumatic event
	Marked alterations in arousal and reactivity associated with the traumatic event
	Duration of disturbance more than 1 month
Acute Stress Disorder	Exposure to actual or threatened death, serious injury, or sexual violence
	Presence of symptoms of intrusion, negative mood, dissociation, avoidance, and arousal after the traumatic event
	Duration of disturbance 3 days to 1 month
Prolonged Grief Disorder	The death, at least 12 months ago, of a person who was close to the bereaved
	Persistent grief response characterized by yearning/longing for the deceased and/or preoccupation with thoughts or memories of the deceased nearly every day
	Identity disruption, sense of disbelief, avoidance of reminders, intense emotional pain, difficulty reintegrating into life, emotional numbness, loss of meaning in life, and intense loneliness nearly every day—all related to the death
Adjustment Disorders	Emotional or behavioral symptoms in response to identifiable stressor occurring within 3 months of stressor onset
	Stress-related disturbance does not meet criteria for another mental disorder or represent exacerbation of a preexisting mental disorder

7.1
Reactive Attachment Disorder

Reactive Attachment Disorder is a relatively rare disorder of young children—that is, those between ages 9 months and 5 years. A pattern of inhibited, emotionally withdrawn behavior toward adult caregivers is apparent from the child's rarely seeking or responding to comfort when distressed. Persistent social and emotional distress is apparent from the child's minimal social and emotional responsiveness to others, limited positive emotions (e.g., expressions of affection, joy), and episodes of irritability, sadness, and fearfulness even when not threatened. The stressful life circumstances leading to the disorder involve insufficient care of the child as manifested by social neglect such that basic emotional needs for comfort, stimulation, and affection from adult caregivers has been absent; caregivers have been changed so frequently that the opportunities for the child to form attachments have been limited; or the child has been raised in a setting that limits the possibility of selective attachments (e.g., an institutional setting with high child-to-caregiver ratio).

Even among the most severely neglected children, the development of Reactive Attachment Disorder is uncommon. The course of the disorder is usually chronic, lasting at least for several years, in the absence of some remedial exposure to a normal caregiving environment. Reactive Attachment Disorder severely impairs the child's interpersonal relationships with adults and peers and is commonly associated with developmental delays in cognition and language. Malnutrition may be present.

This disorder needs to be distinguished from Autism Spectrum Disorder (see Section 1.6), in which a child also exhibits abnormal social behavior. Children with Reactive Attachment Disorder have a history of severe social neglect, which is rare in Autism Spectrum Disorder. Children with Autism Spectrum Disorder have a restricted range of interests and exhibit repetitive, ritualized behaviors, neither of which is usually seen in Reactive Attachment Disorder. Children with Autism Spectrum Disorder regularly show developmentally appropriate attachment behavior, which is rare in children with Reactive Attachment Disorder.

Grandma's Child

Tanya, age 4 years, was seen for assessment in a child psychiatry clinic at the request of her grandparents. Tanya was the only child of parents who were long-time heroin users. Several months earlier, after not having seen Tanya or her parents for several years, the grandparents were called by a child protection agency in another state and informed that Tanya's parents had been arrested, and Tanya had been placed in foster care. The grandparents applied for and received temporary guardianship.

Soon after Tanya came to live with them, the grandparents noticed that she did not have the verbal skills of a normal 4-year-old and she had problems interacting with them. She rarely sought out either of her grandparents for comfort or protection. She often seemed oblivious and unresponsive to ordinary invitations to hug or play with her grandparents and other relatives. The grandparents later learned from a caseworker that apparently since Tanya was an infant, she had often been left with various friends of her parents, many of whom were also heavy drug users and were often only minimally attentive to her.

On examination, Tanya had mild language delays and marked problems in social interaction. She tended to avoid interaction with either the examiner or her grandparents. When interaction could not be avoided, she became very fearful. After Tanya received several months of consistent care in her grandparents' home, her use of language became much more appropriate for a 4-year-old, but she still had some difficulties responding to her grandparents' attempts to comfort her or play with her.

Discussion of "Grandma's Child"

Tanya displays the characteristic features of Reactive Attachment Disorder (DSM-5-TR, p. 295)—inhibited and emotionally withdrawn behavior, minimal social and emotional responsiveness to her grandparents, and fearfulness—as a result of extremely neglectful care from her parents and her parents' friends with whom she was often left. Also contributing to the development of the disorder in this case are the repeated changes in Tanya's primary caregiver, which prevented the formation of stable attachments. This child also exhibits typical delays in the development of age-appropriate language skills.

The reversal, at least in part, of the syndrome with the provision of an appropriate, caring environment is consistent with the diagnosis. The major differential diagnosis is with Autism Spectrum Disorder (see "Echo" in Section 1.6), which is ruled out in this case because there are no signs of a restricted range of interests or repetitive, ritualized behaviors.

7.2
Disinhibited Social
Engagement Disorder

In addition to Reactive Attachment Disorder, the other DSM-5-TR Trauma- and Stressor-Related Disorder related to social neglect early in life is Disinhibited Social Engagement Disorder. Instead of exhibiting inhibited, emotionally withdrawn behavior toward caregivers, children with Disinhibited Social Engagement Disorder tend to indiscriminately approach and interact with unfamiliar adults. These children show little social inhibition toward strangers, can be overly familiar with them even physically, seem unattached to their adult caregiver, and may readily go off with complete strangers. This pattern of behavior also arises from grossly inadequate caregiving in which basic needs for comfort, stimulation, and affection are not met by caregivers; frequent changes in caregivers preclude formation of stable attachments to others; or opportunities for forming attachments are limited by institutionalization.

The diagnosis is not made before age 9 months, the age at which most children are developmentally able to form attachments to other specific people. In contrast to Reactive Attachment Disorder (see Section 7.1), which is not ordinarily seen in children older than age 5, the course of Disinhibited Social Engagement Disorder is more persistent and may continue into adolescence, especially if neglectful conditions of child rearing persist. Preschool children with this condition are very attention seeking. In middle childhood, there is both verbal and physical overfamiliarity and inauthentic emotional expression (e.g., of love or affection), especially with adults. Adolescents with Disinhibited Social Engagement Disorder have superficial and conflicted peer relationships. The disorder may co-occur with Autism Spectrum Disorder. Co-occurrence with Attention-Deficit/Hyperactivity Disorder (ADHD) and other externalizing disorders is presumably due to common impairments in cognitive inhibitory control.

Going Off With Strangers

Harlow, age 37 months, and her three siblings were referred to an intervention program for maltreated young children. According to Child Protective Services (CPS), Harlow and her siblings were wandering in the family's front yard with no adults in sight, and the agency was contacted. CPS found the home in disarray, with trash and several bottles of alcohol scattered about. The children all had severe diaper rashes and scattered bruises on their bodies. The children had poor hygiene and grooming, as well. Two children were placed in one foster home, and Harlow and her 18-month-old brother went to another.

In the initial home visit by a social worker, 1 week after her placement, Harlow immediately ran up to her and began to hug her, despite never having met the social worker before that home visit. During the visit, Harlow's foster mother reported that when the children were first placed into her home, Harlow and her brother tended to "shovel" food into their mouths at mealtimes, and both drank copious amounts of water. The foster mother also reported that the children were afraid of bath time and protested when it was time to get into the water. The foster mother recalled that a few days after Harlow was placed with her, Harlow ran into the street. This was quite concerning to the foster mother, who had to be vigilant about setting limits and had begun to teach Harlow the boundaries of remaining safe.

When in unfamiliar places with her foster mother, Harlow did not stay close; instead, "she [ran] around all over the place" and did not check back with her foster mother. If separated from her foster mother, Harlow did not seem especially bothered by the separation. The foster mother said that it seemed that

Harlow did not have any "connections" with anyone. She also noted that Harlow seemed to constantly seek attention and that she craved this attention "any way she [could] get it." Harlow often smiled coyly at strangers on the bus, for example.

When Harlow was first placed in foster care, she did not have a preference for any particular adult and was reported to "run up to anybody" without hesitation. When hurt or frightened, Harlow grabbed onto anyone who was around her, whether or not she knew the person. However, she did tend to respond to others' attempts to comfort her. Harlow was always friendly and affectionate with strangers—for example, hugging strangers as if she had "known them for years." When a family friend came to the home to visit, Harlow ran over to the friend, whom she had never met, and hugged her and wanted to be picked up by her. The foster mother said that Harlow would most certainly "go off" with an unfamiliar adult, as demonstrated by Harlow's responses in numerous encounters she had had with strangers since entering foster care. When Harlow encountered strangers, Harlow told them, "I'm going with you."

Discussion of "Going Off With Strangers"

Harlow exhibits behavior that should worry any caregiver. She indiscriminately approaches strangers as if she already knows them, demonstrating no age-appropriate hesitation or reticence. She hugs people she has never met. She has little attachment to her own caregivers and appears as if she would go off with a complete stranger, if not prevented from doing so. She has experienced significant social and physical neglect and physical abuse in her early rearing by her own parents, who are apparently quite troubled people themselves. It is assumed that such neglect and abuse is the cause of the child's social impairments because extremes of inadequate care prevented Harlow from being able to form selective and stable attachments to adult caregivers. In the absence of any signs to suggest the inattention or hyperactivity of ADHD, which might include some degree of social impulsivity (see "Into Everything" in Section 1.7), the diagnosis in this case would certainly be Disinhibited Social Engagement Disorder (DSM-5-TR, p. 298).

7.3
Posttraumatic Stress Disorder

The hallmark feature of PTSD is the development of certain characteristic symptoms in response to an extremely traumatic experience that involves "exposure to actual or threatened death, serious injury, or sexual violence" (DSM-5-TR, p. 301). The person may directly experience threat to life or imminent safety (e.g., by having their life threatened or undergoing actual or threatened serious injury or rape); may witness such an event occurring to another person; may learn about an event occurring to a close family member or close friend (in cases of actual or threatened death of a family member or friend, the event must have been violent or accidental); or may be repeatedly exposed to the gruesome details of the traumatic event(s) through their job (as may occur for first responders to accidents involving many victims or to natural or man-made disasters).

The characteristic pattern of symptoms includes 1) intrusion symptoms, in which the traumatic event is persistently reexperienced; 2) persistent avoidance of stimuli associated with the traumatic event(s); 3) negative changes in cognitions and mood associated with the event(s); and 4) alterations in arousal and reactivity associated with the event(s). The problems must have lasted for more than 1 month and cause clinically significant impairment in functioning. Briefer but similarly intense reactions (lasting 3 days to 1 month) to trauma exposure are diagnosed as Acute Stress Disorder (see Section 7.4).

Intrusion symptoms may take many forms. Common symptoms include recurrent, involuntary, and intrusive distressing memories of the event and recurrent dreams in which the content or the emotion associated with the dream is related to the event. Dissociative reactions (e.g., flashbacks) may occur, in which the person feels or acts as if the traumatic event is happening again. Individuals may experience intense or prolonged psychological distress (e.g., intense fear) or physiological reactions (e.g., sweating, palpitations) from exposure to reminders or to things that symbolize some aspect of the traumatic event (e.g., anniversaries of the traumatic event, experiencing hot humid weather for combat veterans of the South Pacific, seeing someone who physically resembles the perpetrator of a personal attack).

Avoidance of stimuli associated with the event involves deliberately avoiding thoughts, memories, and feelings about the traumatic event, or avoiding activities, objects, situations, or people who are likely to arouse uncomfortable recollections of the traumatic event. For example, a person might distract themself to keep from thinking about a trauma by playing computer or video games, by watching TV, or by using drugs or alcohol to numb themself. Or a person who was seriously injured in an automobile accident on an interstate highway might restrict their driving to only local streets.

Negative changes in cognitions and mood associated with the event include the inability to remember important aspects of what happened during the event; persistent and exaggerated negative beliefs about self, others, or the world (e.g., "I am a bad person," "No one can be trusted," "The world is a completely dangerous place"); persistent distorted thoughts about the cause or consequences of the event that lead a person to blame themself or others; persistent feelings of fear, horror, anger, guilt, or shame; greatly diminished interest or participation in previously enjoyed activities; feelings of detachment or estrangement from others; or persistent inability to experience positive emotions, such as happiness, satisfaction, or love.

Alterations in arousal and reactivity may involve irritability and angry outbursts with little or no provocation, recklessness or self-destructive behavior (e.g., dangerous driving, excessive alcohol or drug use), hypervigilance (i.e., feeling constantly on guard against some perceived future threat), exaggerated startle response, problems concentrating, or sleep disturbance (e.g., trouble falling asleep or staying asleep, or restless sleep).

Some individuals with PTSD also experience persistent or recurrent dissociative symptoms involving either *depersonalization* (i.e., feeling detached from their bodies or as if they are an outside observer of their mental processes or body) or *derealization* (i.e., feeling that their surroundings are unreal, dreamlike, distant, or distorted). These symptoms can be noted with the specifier With Dissociative Symptoms. Individuals with this form of PTSD are more likely to have had repeated traumatization and adverse experiences earlier in life, before onset of PTSD, and are more likely to have increased functional impairment and increased suicidal thoughts and attempts.

PTSD symptoms often begin immediately after the traumatic event, and usually within the first 3 months following exposure, although there may be a delay of months or even years before the full criteria for the diagnosis are met. If more than 6 months elapse between trauma exposure and the full expression of the PTSD syndrome, the specifier With Delayed Expression is used.

PTSD can occur at any age after the first year of life. DSM-5-TR includes age-appropriate modifications to indicators of PTSD for children in general and specifically for those age 6 years and younger. For children in general, repetitive play with traumatic themes related to the event and trauma-specific reenactments in play may replace adult symptoms of distressing memories and flashback-type experiences. For children under age 6, if the traumatic event involves others, it is usually the parent or primary caregiver. In children, psychological distress may not be as apparent, and dreams may not be as obviously related to the traumatic event. Play continues to be an important arena for expressing a young child's emotions, and a child's constriction of play and their social withdrawal are the equivalents of an adult's loss of interest in activities and detachment or estrangement from others, respectively. Finally, some sophisticated conceptual interpretations of the person in relation to the trauma (e.g., self-blame) that a young child would not be expected to have or express are omitted from the criteria for PTSD for a child under age 6 years.

PTSD is more common in the United States than in most Asian, African, or Latin American countries. Lifetime DSM-5-TR PTSD prevalence estimates in the United States range from 6.1% to 8.3% and the 12-month prevalence estimate is 4.7%. It is more common among war veterans and among people whose work puts them at risk for exposure to traumatic events, such as police, firefighters, or emergency personnel. The highest rates are found among survivors of rape, military combat, captivity, and ethnically and politically motivated internment and genocide. Women have higher rates of PTSD than men (8.0% to 11% vs. 4.1% to 5.4% for lifetime prevalence according to DSM-5-TR criteria).

The course of PTSD varies. Some people recover within a few months, whereas others have symptoms for longer than a year or even for many decades. PTSD is associated with increased risk of suicidal thoughts, suicide attempts, and death from suicide. Individuals with PTSD are likely to have at least one other mental disorder, such as a Depressive, Bipolar, Anxiety, Substance Use, or Major Neurocognitive Disorder. Young children with PTSD are likely to have other disorders that occur predominantly in childhood, such as Oppositional Defiant Disorder or Separation Anxiety Disorder.

The Singer

Natasha Blackman is a 27-year-old nightclub singer who was referred to a psychologist by a friend for evaluation. Four months earlier, her boyfriend had been stabbed to death during a mugging one night on a dark street near her house as they were walking home from her work—an attack from which she escaped unharmed. After a period of mourning, she appeared to return to her usual self. She helped the police in their investigation and was generally considered an ideal witness.

Nevertheless, shortly after the recent arrest of a man accused of the murder, Ms. Blackman began to have recurrent nightmares and vivid memories of the night of the crime. In these dreams, she frequently saw blood and imagined herself being pursued by ominous cloaked figures. During the day, especially when walking somewhere alone, she often drifted into daydreams and forgot where she was going. Her friends noted that she began to startle easily and seemed to be preoccupied. Ms. Blackman left her change or groceries at the store or could not remember what she had come to buy. She began to sleep restlessly, and her work suffered because of an inability to focus on the songs. She gradually withdrew from her friends and began to turn down singing jobs. She stopped going out after dark because she was reminded of the night of the murder. She felt considerable guilt about her boyfriend's murder, although she was no able to say exactly why. After experiencing these distressing symptoms for a number of weeks and realizing that they were interfering with her social and occupational functioning, Ms. Blackman asked her friend if she knew someone who might be able to help.

Discussion of "The Singer"

Most people who have experienced a severely traumatic event, such as witnessing a murder, repeatedly think about the event for some time. In this case, however, after a period of grief and then apparent acceptance of what had happened, Ms. Blackman developed a specific syndrome characterized by intrusive recollections of the trauma (vivid memories of the murder and recurrent nightmares), avoidance of places and situations that reminded her of the event (going out after dark, working as a singer), negative changes in her cognitions and mood (withdrawal from friends, feelings of guilt and self-blame), and alterations in arousal (exaggerated startle response, trouble concentrating, sleep disturbance). In addition, her daydreaming and being unable to remember what she intended to buy at a store may be examples of mild dissociative experiences. Thus, assuming that these symptoms have persisted for more than 1 month, Ms. Blackman has a fairly typical case of PTSD (DSM-5-TR, p. 301). The symptoms of the disorder began after a short (4-month) latency period, but because the full syndrome was present within 6 months of the trauma, the specifier With Delayed Expression does not apply.

If Ms. Blackman had experienced only mild and nonspecific anxiety symptoms, her diagnosis would be Adjustment Disorder, With Anxiety (see "Abducted" in Section 7.6).

The Wreck

Enrique Casales is a 40-year-old married carpenter who was involved in a motor vehicle accident that "totaled" his car approximately 2 years ago. He sustained no head trauma or loss of consciousness. He was hospitalized for 1 day with a diagnosis of neck strain and inflammation of the spinal nerve to the trapezius muscle in his back. A course of physical therapy and anti-inflammatory medication was prescribed.

In the months that followed the accident, Mr. Casales experienced occasional involuntary thoughts of it. He had trouble falling asleep, irritability, anxious mood, impaired concentration, and increased appetite, with a 30-pound weight gain. These symptoms tended to wax and wane over the subsequent months. The patient suffered no avoidance behavior and no loss of interest in his usual activities, including sexual interest, and he continued to socialize with his friends. He drove an automobile and was comfortable as a passenger in a car; however, there was some transient anxiety when he drove past the accident site.

Mr. Casales' orthopedic injuries prevented him from returning to work as a carpenter, but he continued to work actively at various "side" businesses. His marital life began to deteriorate as he became increasingly irritable at home. Despite these difficulties, he was able to enjoy himself on a 3-day camping trip with some friends.

After approximately 2 years of physical therapy, Mr. Casales decided to undergo recommended surgery. Mr. Casales tolerated the surgery well, but the procedure left him with a temporary disability (a restriction in range of motion and loss of strength) in his right shoulder and arm. As soon as he returned home, his emotional status changed dramatically. In addition to having concerns about the ultimate outcome of the surgery, he began thinking about the accident continually, despite efforts to avoid such thoughts by distracting himself. He was unable to sleep, in large part because of terrifying dreams that would awaken him and leave him sweating and unable to return to sleep for 2 or more hours. He lost interest in sex and reported that he now "did not care about anybody or anything." He developed an exaggerated startle response to loud noises, such as the honking of a horn or the slamming of a door.

Mr. Casales' postsurgery disability prevented him from driving. When he was a passenger in a car, Mr. Casales became acutely anxious, broke out in a sweat, felt nauseated, and often gave vent to abusive verbal outbursts at other drivers on the road. He had a similar response when passing an accident. He was unable to concentrate on his side businesses. His marital situation deteriorated, because of an increasing sense of emotional isolation from his wife, to the point of a planned divorce. After 6 weeks of symptoms, the patient sought assistance from his orthopedic surgeon, who made a psychiatric referral.

"I am a wreck," Mr. Casales reported to the psychiatric consultant. The psychiatrist treated the patient with an antidepressant, sertraline, and supportive psychotherapy, which resulted in prompt control of his symptoms. During the next 2 months, his postsurgical disability resolved, so that he had full range of motion and nearly full strength. After 6 months, attempts were made to reduce the dosage of sertraline, but the dreams, sleep disturbances, and high level of anxiety promptly returned.

Discussion of "The Wreck"

In considering the diagnosis in this case, it is necessary to distinguish the symptoms Mr. Casales experienced in the months following the trauma of the accident from the more dramatic symptoms that developed immediately following surgery 2 years after the accident. In the months following the accident, Mr. Casales exhibited many nonspecific anxiety symptoms, such as occasional thoughts of the accident, trouble sleeping, and impaired concentration. A Depressive Disorder is ruled out by the absence of depressed mood or loss of interest or pleasure. Had he sought treatment at the time, he may have been diagnosed as having Adjustment Disorder, With Anxiety (see "Abducted" in Section 7.6).

Apparently, Mr. Casales' experience of the accident was reawakened following the surgery. He developed intrusive symptoms associated with the trauma of the accident from which he had narrowly escaped serious injury (thinking about the accident continually, having terrifying dreams of the accident, and distress at being a passenger in a moving car), avoidance of stimuli associated with the accident (trying not to think about it by distracting himself), negative alterations in thinking and mood (loss of interest in everything, feeling estranged from his wife), and symptoms of increased arousal (difficulty staying asleep, exaggerated startle response, difficulty concentrating, outbursts of anger). This clinical picture following a traumatic event that exposes a person to actual or threatened death, serious injury, or sexual violence is characteristic of PTSD (DSM-5-TR, p. 301). What is unusual in this case is that the full clinical picture did not develop immediately or soon after the trauma, but about 2 years later, when the patient underwent surgery for injuries related to the accident. For that reason, Mr. Casales' diagnosis is noted with the specifier With Delayed Expression.

Flashbacks

Michael Bennett, a 23-year-old Vietnam veteran, was admitted to the hospital in 1975 (2 years after the United States ended its direct participation in the Vietnam War), at the request of his wife, after he began to experience depression, insomnia, and flashbacks of his wartime experiences. He had been honorably discharged 2 years previously, having spent nearly a year in combat. He had only minimal difficulties in returning to civilian life, resuming his college studies, and then marrying within 6 months after his return. His wife had noticed that he was reluctant to talk about his military experience, but she wrote it off as a natural reaction to unpleasant memories.

Michael began experiencing symptoms, however, at about the time of the fall of Saigon in April 1975. He became preoccupied with watching TV news stories about this event. He then began to have difficulty sleeping, and at times would awaken at night in the midst of a nightmare in which he was reliving his past war experiences. His wife became particularly concerned one day when he had a flashback while out in the backyard: as a plane flew overhead, flying somewhat lower than usual, the patient threw himself to the ground, seeking cover, thinking it was an attacking helicopter. The more he watched the news on TV, the more agitated and morose he became. Stories began to spill out of him about horrifying atrocities like those he had seen and experienced, and he began to feel guilty that he had survived while many of his friends had not. At times he also seemed angry and bitter, feeling that the sacrifices he and others had made were all wasted.

Finally, he avoided watching TV or reading a newspaper because reports on the war made him so distressed.

The veteran's wife expressed concern that his preoccupation with Vietnam had become so intense that he seemed uninterested in anything else and was emotionally distant from her.

Discussion of "Flashbacks"

This veteran had become totally preoccupied with his painful year in Vietnam. Michael's combat experience obviously involved traumatic events in which he and others were threatened with death. He had intrusion symptoms associated with this trauma (recurrent distressing dreams, dissociative flashbacks). He had persistent negative emotions (feelings of fear and horror) and diminished interest in anything beyond his preoccupation with his time in Vietnam. He had become emotionally distant from his wife. In addition, he had symptoms of increased arousal (disturbed sleep, outbursts of anger, and exaggerated startle response). He eventually began to avoid all sources of war news because of the distress it caused him. This is the full picture of PTSD (DSM-5-TR, p. 301). Michael's disorder is further noted with the specifier With Delayed Expression to indicate that the onset of the symptoms occurred at least 6 months after the trauma.

This patient displayed a common symptom seen in people who experience a life-threatening trauma shared with others: a sense of guilt that they have survived when others have not (survivor guilt).

If Michael were alive today (2024), he would be 72 years old. Male Vietnam War veterans with war zone PTSD have been found to be twice as likely to die over a 25-year period as those without PTSD. Surviving veterans may continue to report PTSD symptoms and have a host of other chronic health issues, including cardiovascular diseases, nervous system disorders, and musculoskeletal disorders, for which they may continue to seek treatment. More recent wars in Iraq and Afghanistan have produced approximately 270,000 veterans who have been evaluated for PTSD, more than half of whom receive some disability benefits for it. These wars have been characterized by multiple and prolonged deployments of service members, which may contribute to these problems.

Memories

Zelda Podlevner, a 49-year-old married Orthodox Jewish woman, was referred to a psychiatrist in 1975 for an evaluation in preparation for an appeal to the board that had previously denied her claim for workers' compensation. Mrs. Podlevner's problems began 6 months earlier, following a fire in the dress factory where she had been employed as a seamstress for 15 years. The fire was minor and easily contained, but the synthetic fabrics that burned had produced an extremely acrid smell. After the fire, Mrs. Podlevner developed abdominal pains, nausea, and heart palpitations. She was hospitalized in an intensive care unit for a week because her doctor suspected asthma or a heart condition. A thorough medical evaluation revealed no evidence of physical illness.

After the patient went home, she felt depressed and so frightened about leaving her apartment that she was unable to go to work. Her symptoms persisted and intensified when her compensation claim was rejected 2 months before the psychiatric evaluation. She had been staying at home, cooking and cleaning, but had no interest in doing anything else.

In the psychiatric interview, she appeared mildly depressed, and said that whatever the decision of the appeals board, she could not bring herself to return to work. She felt comfortable and safe at home, but whenever she had to go out, she became apprehensive, although she could not say exactly what she was afraid of. She felt more comfortable when her husband accompanied her to stores in the neighborhood, but when she had to travel to a different neighborhood (e.g., to go to a doctor's office), she felt uncomfortable despite his presence, afraid that his long sideburns and ethnic garments would attract hostile attention from non-Jews. She had trouble sleeping because of recurrent nightmares of her experiences in a concentration camp over 30 years earlier and found herself dwelling on these memories during the day and unable to concentrate on reading.

Mrs. Podlevner had always been an active and competent person, and she did not understand why she had developed all of these problems since the fire and why she now felt that she was "a dead person." Although she would not describe herself as having been a particularly "happy" person before the fire, she believed that she had been "content." She had always thought about how she would have been a very different person were it not for the war, but she claimed that she was not preoccupied with this thought.

The psychiatrist asked Mrs. Podlevner to talk about her experiences in the concentration camp and learned that she was in Auschwitz in 1943, at age 17. Having been young and healthy, she was selected by Dr. Josef Mengele, the sadistic camp doctor, to be part of the workforce. After the selection, she and hundreds of other women were told to undress and wait for instructions. Because the camp was extremely overcrowded, they were shoved into a strange-looking empty hall without windows. The place had a peculiar odor. When they were transferred a few hours later, she found out that she and the other women had been temporarily kept in a gas chamber. She began to cry as she realized that the smell in the factory fire had brought back the memory of the gas chamber.

The psychiatrist sent his report to the Workmers' Compensation Board. At the hearing, the presiding officer said that he did not want to hear the story again and agreed to full compensation. After being in treatment for 6 months, Mrs. Podlevner was still afraid to go to work but was less depressed. Her therapist said that Mrs. Podlevner was dealing with the feeling that her life stopped when she was age 17.

Discussion of "Memories"

Mrs. Podlevner's case is an example of PTSD, With Delayed Expression (DSM-5-TR, p. 301). The fire in the factory in which Mrs. Podlevner worked had triggered a reliving of her experience in Auschwitz, even though she was not aware of the connection until she spoke with the psychiatrist. A relatively minor event as a small fire uncovered a deeply buried memory of a horrendous experience after many years.

The characteristic symptoms of PTSD are apparent: the traumatic experience of being in a concentration camp is certainly one that involves actual or threatened death of self or others. In Mrs. Podlevner's case, intrusion symptoms associated with the trauma are in the form of nightmares and distressing recollections. She avoids situations that remind her of the trauma (going back to work). She has lost interest in her usual activities, has negative thoughts about herself (feels "dead"), and has symptoms of increased arousal, including difficulty sleeping and concentrating.

The concentration camp at Auschwitz-Birkenau in Poland was liberated on January 27, 1945, by Soviet troops. In 2023, an estimated 240,000 Holocaust survivors were still alive, living in Europe, Israel, the United States, and elsewhere. They are in old age. If Mrs. Podlevner were alive today (2024), she would be 98 years old. Although survivors of the Holocaust are dwindling in number, many of those that are still alive live in poverty and suffer from a host of physical and emotional problems related to their traumatic experiences, in addition to those associated with normal aging.

Sniper

Leah, age 6 years, was referred by her teacher to a child psychologist for evaluation because of her tearfulness, irritability, and difficulty concentrating in class. Two and a half months earlier, Leah had been among a group of children pinned down by sniper fire on her school playground. Over a period of 15 minutes, the sniper killed one child and injured several others. After the gunfire ceased, no one moved until the police stormed the sniper's apartment and found that he had killed himself. Leah did not personally know the child who was killed or the sniper.

Before the shooting, according to her teacher, Leah was a shy but vivacious, well-behaved, and good student. Within a few days after the incident, there was a noticeable change in Leah's behavior. She withdrew from her friends. She began to bicker with other children when they spoke to her. She seemed uninterested in her schoolwork and had to be prodded to persist in required tasks. The teacher noticed that Leah jumped whenever there was static noise in the public address system and when the class shouted answers to flash cards.

Leah's parents were relieved when the school made the referral because they were uncertain about how to help her. Leah had been uncharacteristically quiet when her parents asked her about the shooting incident. At home she had become moody, irritable, argumentative, fearful, and clinging. She was apprehensive about new situations and fearful of being alone, and insisted that someone accompany her to the bathroom. Leah regularly asked to sleep with her parents. She slept restlessly and occasionally cried out in her sleep. She appeared always to be tired, complained of minor physical problems, and seemed more susceptible to minor infections. Her parents were especially worried after Leah nearly walked in front of a moving car without being aware of it. Although she seemed less interested in many of her usual games, her parents noticed that she frequently engaged her siblings in "nurse games," in which she was often bandaged.

When asked about the incident during the interview, Leah said that she had tried very hard to hide behind a trash can when she heard the repeated gunfire. She had been terrified of being killed and was "shaking all over," her heart pounding and her head hurting. She vividly told of watching an older child fall to the ground, bleeding and motionless.

Leah described a recurring image of the injured girl lying in blood on the playground. She said that thoughts of the incident sometimes disrupted her attention, although she would try to think about something else. Lately, she could not always remember what was being said in class. She no longer played in the area where the shooting had occurred during recess or after school. She avoided crossing the playground on her way home from school each day and avoided the sniper's street. She was particularly afraid at school on Fridays, the day the shooting had occurred. Although her mother and father comforted her, she did not know how to tell them what she was feeling.

Leah continued to be afraid that someone would shoot at her again. She had nightmares about the shooting and dreams in which she or a family member was being shot at or pursued. She ran away from any "popping noises" at home or in the neighborhood. Although she said that she had less desire to play, when asked about new games, she reported frequently playing a game in which a nurse helped an injured person. She began to watch TV news about violence and recounted news stories that demonstrated that the world was full of danger.

Discussion of "Sniper"

Leah experienced a traumatic event that involved actual or threatened death or serious injury to herself and to her classmates. Within a few days of the trauma, she began to exhibit the characteristic symptoms of severe PTSD (DSM-5-TR, p. 303). PTSD can occur in children as young as age 1 year. Age-specific indicators of PTSD are to be considered in children age 6 years and younger.

Although adults sometimes have flashbacks in which they actually experience the situation as if it were currently happening, children infrequently reexperience trauma in this way. As is typical for young children, Leah experienced intrusion symptoms that were associated with the trauma in the form of recurrent, intrusive images and recollections of the event, and recurrent, distressing dreams about it. She also incorporated themes from the event into repetitive games and play.

Leah attempted to avoid thoughts and feelings associated with the trauma and places that reminded her of the event. This formerly vivacious little girl now exhibited negative alterations in cognition: she had become apathetic and uninterested in her schoolwork, as well as detached and withdrawn from her former friends. She displayed persistent symptoms of increased arousal, including exaggerated startle reaction (to loud noises), irritability, difficulty concentrating, and sleep disturbance.

Nighttime Visitor

Christina was 8 years old when her guidance counselor at school referred her to a family treatment center because of disruptive, aggressive behavior. Her 11-year-old brother, Don, and her 9-year-old sister, Sara, were also evaluated, together with their mother.

Several months earlier, Christina had been admitted to the hospital with vaginal bleeding and a discharge. A diagnosis of vaginal warts (condyloma acuminatum) was made, and the vaginal culture proved to be positive for gonorrhea. When questioned by a social worker, who was asked by the pediatrician to see the children, Christina revealed that she and Sara had been sexually molested by their father for the past 2 years. According to her, he would come into their bedroom regularly at night and have vaginal intercourse with her and, more rarely, with Sara. The girls noticed that if they were awake, their father often would not bother them. Nevertheless, Christina was so frightened that she would close her eyes and feign sleep during the molestation. Their father threatened them with beatings if they were to divulge the secret, so they had never told anyone.

Their brother, Don, after witnessing one of the molestations, told their mother. She did not believe him and told her husband, who then proceeded to beat Don. In fact, Don had often been beaten by his father. After Don's disclosure, Christina and Sara told their mother what had been happening, but she scolded them for "making up stories."

When the social worker talked with the mother about these events, she admitted that she had suspected that her children were telling the truth, but she was afraid of confronting her husband about his sexual abuse because she feared his murderous rage. During their 12-year marriage, he had frequently beaten her, but she never thought of leaving him because her religion forbade divorce.

After the medical confirmation of the sexual abuse, the children were temporarily placed in foster care, the father was jailed, and the family court cited the mother for neglect because she had failed to intervene to protect the children from their father's sexual abuse. The children were subsequently placed with their maternal grandmother, and later were returned to their mother after she agreed to a psychiatric evaluation and treatment for herself and her children.

During the interview at the family treatment center, Christina presents as a sad, unusually quiet child who rarely smiles. She describes that since the abuse started 2 years ago, she spends most of her time in her room alone doing little more than watching TV. During the day, she tries not to think about what has been happening to her, but at night, she often has difficulty falling asleep and reports nightmares about her father coming into her room. At school, she has stayed away from her friends for fear that they would suspect something was the matter with her and might reject her. When she testified in court, she was certain that she would be sent to jail because she had done something wrong. She also fears that her father will return and attack her. At home, she is generally irritable and often fights with Sara and Don, and she feels "picked on" by her mother, whom she feels has always favored her siblings.

After the evaluation of the family, individual psychotherapy was recommended for Christina, Sara, and their mother. In addition, family treatment was instituted to improve the relationship between the children and their mother and to help establish structure and discipline in the home. Christina's mother was encouraged to allow the children to express their feelings of having been betrayed by her. At home Christina began to overeat and steal money from her mother's purse, as a way of expressing anger toward her mother and of getting more attention.

In the treatment setting, Christina acted frightened and needy, and she clung to her female therapist. She expressed her yearnings for nurturance and safety by caring for doll babies and stuffed animals. She was frequently involved in "traumatic play," in which she acted out various elements of the

trauma. These dramas often involved a witch who poisoned children and dev-
ils and monsters that attacked the children when they tried to run away.

Discussion of "Nighttime Visitor"

Christina's difficulties are almost certainly related to the trauma of having
been repeatedly sexually abused by her father. The stressor criterion for PTSD
(DSM-5-TR, p. 301) requires that the person has experienced or witnessed an
event that involves actual or threatened death, serious injury, or sexual violence. In this case, there has been ongoing repeated sexual abuse; therefore, the
stressor requirement has been met.

Although Christina is a young child, she is older than 6 years, so the adult
definition of PTSD applies. Her intrusion symptoms associated with the
trauma are the nightmares of her father coming into her room. This diagnosis
also requires symptoms indicating persistent avoidance of stimuli associated
with the trauma. Christina tries not to think about what has been happening
to her and distracts herself with TV. She feels estrangement from others (her
classmates), has negative affect and limited positive emotions (she is unusually quiet, feels guilty, rarely smiles), and has diminished interest and participation in significant activities (doing little else than watching TV). In addition,
she has persistent symptoms of increased arousal (difficulty falling asleep,
general irritability and aggression at home).

Christina's reaction to having been sexually abused by her father and not
protected (or even believed) by her mother has included depressed mood,
nightmares about the trauma, anger, inappropriate self-reproach and guilt,
and the feeling that schoolmates might dislike her. These symptoms suggest
the possible additional diagnosis of a Depressive Disorder, but there is no evidence that the depressed mood is accompanied by the characteristic symptoms of a Major Depressive Episode, other than self-reproach and guilt.
Although the sexual abuse went on for 2 years, there is no description of a persistent depressed mood that would justify a diagnosis of Persistent Depressive
Disorder (see Section 4.3). In fact, during this time Christina seems to have
been more frightened than depressed.

7.4
Acute Stress Disorder

The manifestations of Acute Stress Disorder (DSM-5-TR, p. 313) are very
similar to those of PTSD, but the duration of the disturbance lasts from 3 days to 1 month
after exposure to the trauma. The requirements for the characteristics of the stressor

in Acute Stress Disorder are nearly identical to those for PTSD—that is, "exposure to actual or threatened death, serious injury, or sexual violence" (DSM-5-TR, p. 313).

In comparison to PTSD, however, which requires a minimum (at least 1 or 2 symptoms) from each of four categories (i.e., intrusion symptoms, avoidance symptoms, alterations in cognition and mood, and alterations in arousal and reactivity), the symptom requirement for Acute Stress Disorder is for any 9 or more of 14 symptoms regardless of category. There are also fewer symptoms in the list for Acute Stress Disorder (14) than for PTSD (20), with 13 of the 14 coming from the list of 20 PTSD symptoms (see DSM-5-TR, pp. 301–302 and 314). The only symptom unique to Acute Stress Disorder is Criterion B6, "an altered sense of the reality of one's surroundings or oneself (e.g., seeing oneself from another's perspective, being in a daze, time slowing)" (DSM-5-TR, p. 314). The symptoms of Acute Stress Disorder usually begin immediately following the stressful event, but a diagnosis is not given unless they persist for at least 3 days (and up to 1 month).

Fewer than 20% of people who are exposed to traumatic events not involving interpersonal assault develop Acute Stress Disorder. For traumatic events such as assault, rape, and witnessing a mass shooting, rates can be as high as 50%. Like PTSD, Acute Stress Disorder is more common among women, which may be due both to neurobiological differences in stress responses between women and men and to a greater likelihood of exposure to the kinds of events that are associated with the development of Acute Stress Disorder, such as rape and other types of interpersonal violence. Acute Stress Disorder may be a transitory reaction to a severe stressor and may resolve within 1 month, or it may progress to PTSD. Approximately half of the people who develop PTSD had Acute Stress Disorder immediately after the stressor.

Burned

A liaison psychiatrist was called to see Vicky Lawson, a 28-year-old woman, 1 week after she had been admitted to the burn unit of a large municipal hospital. She had incurred a 28% burn injury to her skin in a house fire in which her children, ages 3 and 5, had also been injured and her husband killed. The circumstances of the injury had been quite traumatic in that she was trapped, found it difficult to escape, and risked her own life to save her children.

On examination, Ms. Lawson was alert and oriented, but quite fearful and anxious when asked to describe what had happened. Almost since the patient's admission, nurses noted that she awoke repeatedly during the night, and she reported recurrent nightmares in which she relived the experience of escaping from her home from which she awoke in a sweat. During the day, she sometimes appeared to be in a daze and unaware of her surroundings, whereas at other times she seemed to be hyperalert, was easily startled, and responded fearfully to slight noises, such as the horns of cars passing on the street outside her window. She expressed little joy for the news that her children's injuries were less serious than her own and that they would be fine. The consultation was requested because the nursing staff had become concerned that she did not want to talk about what had happened, seemed unable to remember that her husband had died, and was not working through her grief appropriately.

Discussion of "Burned"

In response to an overwhelming stress, Ms. Lawson is having distressing memories and recurrent distressing dreams (nightmares) of the trauma, negative mood changes (no joy about her children's optimistic prognoses), dissociative symptoms (appearing in a daze, being unable to remember that her husband had died), avoidance behavior (refusal to talk about what had happened), and symptoms of increased arousal (sleep disturbance, hypervigilance, and exaggerated startle response). Because this clinical picture developed in relation to a trauma in which Ms. Lawson and family members were all threatened with death and serious injury and has persisted for nearly a week, the diagnosis would be Acute Stress Disorder (DSM-5-TR, p. 313). This diagnosis takes precedence over Adjustment Disorder (see Section 7.6), which is a residual category for stress-related emotional or behavioral disturbances that are not severe enough to meet the criteria for a more serious disorder.

Eyewitness

Karen Davidoff is a 39-year-old TV reporter who saw a psychologist at her network employee assistance program a few weeks after being an eyewitness at the execution of a murderer. For several years she had been following the story of the inmate as he approached execution. The execution itself was remarkably protracted and gruesome: along with colleagues, she maintained a deathwatch for several hours while various last-minute reprieves were granted and then set aside by judicial bodies. At one point the inmate was actually strapped onto the gurney when a phone call from a federal judge, literally at the last minute, reprieved him, and the inmate was removed from the death chamber alive. When execution finally occurred, Ms. Davidoff and her colleagues watched from a distance of about 10 feet through the windows between the witness room and the death chamber. The inmate's eyes rolled back in his head, and he began gasping for air and drooling as he writhed on the table and struggled at the straps of the gurney. After approximately 5 minutes, his body was still, and he was declared dead by prison authorities.

Ms. Davidoff told the psychologist, "Once you see someone die, you don't forget what it looks like." She felt that her professional role as an objective reporter was helpful to her initially in that it separated her from her emotional response. She recalled, for example, the sensation of her mouth going dry just at the moment of execution, but the sensation was detached from any emotional response. This detached feeling, which she described as "surreal and macabre," persisted for some days after the event. For a week after the execution, she continued to be detached from her feelings and was "in a daze and not like my usual self."

For the last few weeks, since the execution, she has been unable to concentrate on her work, has felt uninterested in it, and has been dissatisfied with it. She was surprised, for example, at her unwillingness to cover a riot that occurred shortly after the execution, a story that she would normally have been very enthusiastic about. Ms. Davidoff has had trouble staying asleep, and often has nightmares of the execution. Additionally, she says that although she tries not to, she thinks of the event at least daily, sometimes having vivid "snapshot" images of the moment of execution.

Discussion of "Eyewitness"

Ms. Davidoff is suffering from the aftereffects of watching a gruesome execution. She reexperiences the trauma in intrusive recollections, nightmares, and flashbacks ("vivid 'snapshot' images"); has a negative mood state manifested by disinterest and lack of excitement and satisfaction in her work; experiences dissociative symptoms of derealization ("surreal and macabre" feelings of detachment) and a reduction in awareness of her surroundings ("in a daze"); attempts to not think about the execution and to avoid work in general; and has difficulty sleeping and trouble concentrating. All of these symptoms suggest the diagnosis of PTSD (see Section 7.3). However, the PTSD diagnosis requires that symptoms persist beyond 1 month, because transient, acute PTSD-like symptoms are quite common following traumatic events, and most people with such symptoms recover in a few days or weeks. In DSM-5-TR, the diagnosis of Acute Stress Disorder (DSM-5-TR, p. 313) is used when PTSD-like symptoms are sufficiently severe to interfere with social or occupational functioning and persist for at least 3 days but less than 1 month.

7.5
Prolonged Grief Disorder

What constitutes an abnormal emotional response to the abrupt loss of a loved one has confounded mental health clinicians and researchers for many years. Grief itself is a normal response to loss and the characteristics and duration of adaptive grief can vary widely from person to person and across cultures. According to DSM-5-TR, prolonged grief in reaction to the death of someone who was close to the bereaved individual must be evident for at least 12 months (6 months for children and adolescents) following the death. The persistent grief is characterized by either "intense yearning/longing for the deceased person" or "preoccupation with thoughts or memories of the deceased person" that has occurred on most days to a clinically significant degree since the death and must be present nearly every day for at least the past month in order to qualify for the diagnosis (DSM-5-TR, p. 322). In addition, clinically significant symptoms, such as feeling as if a part of oneself has died, disbelief that the death really happened, avoidance of reminders that the person is dead, intense emotional pain, difficulty resuming relationships and activities, emotional numbness, feeling that life is meaningless, and intense loneliness have been present to a clinically significant degree on most days since the death and must have occurred nearly every day for at least the past month.

It is estimated that 7%–10% of bereaved adults will experience the persistent symptoms of Prolonged Grief Disorder.[1] Symptoms usually begin within the first few months after the death, although they may be delayed. The course may be particularly prolonged among parents of deceased children. Older age may be associated with an increased risk of prolonged grief after the death of a loved one, such as a spouse or a sibling. Individuals with Prolonged Grief Disorder are at increased risk of thinking about suicide across the life span, especially among those who experience the death of a child. It is not clear, however, that the incidence of actual suicidal behavior is increased. Impairment in psychosocial functioning is ubiquitous, and harmful health behaviors (e.g., smoking and alcohol consumption) may be increased. Prolonged Grief Disorder is also associated with marked increases in risks for serious medical conditions, including cardiac disease, hypertension, cancer, and immunological deficiencies. Prolonged Grief Disorder commonly co-occurs with PTSD, particularly if the death was violent or accidental, and with Substance Use Disorders.

A Good Man Died

Evelyn Smith, a 52-year-old widow, was referred for evaluation after her daughter, Jen, contacted Mrs. Smith's primary care physician out of concern for her mother. Mrs. Smith's husband, Jim, had died in an automobile accident 2 years earlier. Jen and her husband, expecting their first child, had recently moved from the West Coast back to the Northeast to be nearer to her mother, in anticipation of the coming baby.

Jen's child was born 2 weeks earlier, and Mrs. Smith hadn't yet seen the baby. She had planned a visit to see him, but ended up canceling, saying she could not go without her husband, Jim. Jen found this very sad and frustrating, and it worried her. Jen told the doctor that because she had been living at a distance, she had not appreciated how much her mother's life had become very restricted. Her mother avoided most activities that she and her late husband used to do together, places where she might see loving couples, or things that were reminders of Jim—the grocery store, restaurants, church—and no longer would eat at the dining table where she and her husband

---

[1]Szuhany KL, Malgaroli M, Miron CD, et al: Prolonged grief disorder: course, diagnosis, assessment, and treatment. *Focus* 19:161-172, 2021 34690579.

shared meals. Fighting back tears, Jen added, "All she seems to care about is my father and their life together. She only seems happy living in the past, reminiscing. It feels like I lost my mother when my father died." Jen said she had been worried about her mother ever since her father died in the car accident 2 years ago. She kept telling herself that everyone grieves in their own way. Her mother was an emotional person so Jen just thought that it might take her longer to get over this. But now she was concerned that something must be very wrong.

For the first weeks after moving back East, Jen and her husband were preoccupied with settling in their new house and preparing for the new baby. When she saw her mother, it was to have breakfast at a local diner or a quick cup of coffee at her mother's home. During a recent visit, however, when walking by her mother's open bedroom door, Jen noticed that some of her father's belongings appeared to remain just as he may have left them on the day he died—his empty coffee mug untouched on the nightstand, sneakers near the closet—and so she decided to say something. When she suggested that her mother should do something with these things, Mrs. Smith bristled, uncharacteristically snapping that it was not Jen's business to tell her what to do. She later apologized and agreed to see a therapist.

Mrs. Smith told the therapist that, as far as she was concerned, her life ended when her husband died, and that she has felt like an empty shell of a person ever since. She had not previously shared this with Jen because she did not want to hurt or scare her. She even felt torn about meeting her new grandson, because Jim could not wait to become a grandfather. She sometimes thought it would be a good idea to take all of her husband's sleeping pills or to just stop eating and waste away, but she didn't think she would do this because, as she said, "I would never do that to Jen." Still, she often thought that there was little point in living without Jim.

Mrs. Smith was the only daughter and the youngest of four in her family of origin. Her parents drank to excess and frequently fought over money. She was not close to any of her brothers. School was a refuge for her, and she was a good student. At her teacher's urging, she applied to college, where she earned her associate's degree. After graduation she got a job at an accounting firm, where she met Jim.

They both felt it was love at first sight. She told the therapist, "We were soulmates." This was the first important relationship in Mrs. Smith's life, and it felt like a miracle. Jen was born a year after they married. Mrs. Smith felt she was the luckiest woman alive. Her life had turned out so much better than she'd hoped. Jim was generous, friendly, and outgoing. She felt she had married the kindest, most loving man in the world.

On the night he died, Mr. Smith had been at a dinner with his coworkers. Mrs. Smith was invited, but his colleagues liked their alcohol and she felt uncomfortable around them when they were drinking. Jim said he understood and that he'd only stay for a short time. When the phone rang, and she saw the police number on her caller ID, she assumed that one of her brothers was in trouble again. But when the officer asked for Mrs. Jim Smith, she felt anxious and confused. She heard the officer saying that there was an accident, Jim had been taken to the ER, and she should get there immediately. When she arrived, a doctor escorted her into a small room, where he said Jim had not survived. Mrs. Smith remembered thinking the doctor must be mistaken and asking to see him. After barely glancing at her husband's body, she collapsed. She had little memory of the funeral or the days that followed.

In the 2 years since her husband died, Mrs. Smith has not felt like herself. She alternates between feeling numb and feeling overwhelmed with intense loneliness and yearning, sobbing uncontrollably. She keeps wishing she could wake up from this nightmare. When she wakes and is aware of his absence, she feels a wave of intense grief and starts ruminating about how he did not deserve this. She frequently replays scenarios of what could have happened differently—what if she'd gone to dinner that night and they'd left earlier, or later? What if they were both killed?—thinking that would have been better. She feels angry at herself, thinking Jim's death was her fault, blaming herself for not wanting to go to the dinner and causing him to leave the dinner early. When she sees other married couples, she feels envious and bitter, feeling it was unfair that he died when she needed him so much. She often questions why God would take such a good man. She has resumed doing part-time accounting work, which provides some distraction, but her leisure time is occupied cataloging photos and daydreaming about their wonderful life together—until something shakes her from her reverie, and she's flooded with intense longing to hold him in her arms.

Although Mrs. Smith feels empty most days since the death of her husband, is unable to enjoy things that she used to do with him, and expresses some guilt and suicidal thoughts, when questioned by her therapist, she denied other symptoms characteristic of clinical depression: she has not had a significant change in appetite or weight, a significant change in her sleeping patterns, agitation, fatigue, or difficulty concentrating.

Discussion of "A Good Man Died"

Mrs. Smith unexpectedly lost the most important person in her life. That she would experience intense feelings of grief afterward comes as no surprise. In Mrs. Smith's case, however, the grief has been unrelenting for 2 years. She appears to be totally preoccupied with thoughts and memories of her deceased husband, to the point of excluding her daughter and newborn grandson from her daily life. She longs "to hold [her husband] in her arms." She feels "like an empty shell of a person"; she avoids places, people, and activities that remind her of her husband; and she acts as if he had never died (keeping his empty coffee mug on his nightstand, his sneakers where they always were). She alternates between feeling numb and feeling intense loneliness and emotional pain. She feels that there is "little point" in living without her husband. As is typical, Mrs. Smith has contemplated suicide, but believes that she could not act on these thoughts because of the effect it would have on her daughter and her grandson. That these symptoms are present in the current month, have been present for the past 2 years, are distressing and impairing of her functioning, and exceed norms for her sociocultural group indicate a diagnosis of Prolonged Grief Disorder (DSM-5-TR, p. 322).

Being suddenly confronted by the police telephone call with news of the accidental, violent death of a close loved one qualifies for the type of stressor known to be associated with PTSD (see Section 7.3). PTSD and Prolonged Grief Disorder may, in fact, co-occur. There is no indication, however, that Mrs. Smith has experienced intrusive, distressing memories of the phone call; no distressing dreams of having received the call; no flashbacks of receiving the call; and no psychological or physiological distress on hearing a telephone ring. The absence of these symptoms rules out an additional diagnosis of PTSD. Although Major Depressive Disorder and Prolonged Grief Disorder may also co-occur, at no time did Mrs. Smith's presentation meet the diagnostic requirements of a Major Depressive Episode. She has none of the vegetative symptoms of depression (e.g., changes in appetite or sleep), and although she is less interested in doing the things she used to enjoy, it is because they remind her of her life with Jim as opposed to a more general loss of pleasure. She is not agitated, and she is able to concentrate sufficiently to do some accounting work. As is characteristic of Prolonged Grief Disorder, Mrs. Smith's "distress is focused on feelings of loss and separation from a loved one rather than reflecting generalized low mood" (DSM-5-TR, p. 327).

7.6
Adjustment Disorders

Any kind of a stressful life event can result in a distressing emotional or behavioral reaction that causes significant distress or interferes with social or occupational functioning. A stressor may be a single event, such as the breakup of a romantic relationship; a series of events, such as the loss of a job and needing to move; or an ongoing situation, such as having an illness or living in poverty. The stressor might cause or precipitate the recurrence of another mental disorder, such as an Anxiety Disorder or a Depressive Disorder. If the stressor is one that involves exposure to threatened death, serious injury, or sexual violence, and specific other symptoms are present, a diagnosis of Acute Stress Disorder (see Section 7.4) or PTSD (see Section 7.3) may apply. Experiencing the death of a close relative normally causes a grief reaction, which by itself is not considered a mental disorder.

For all other stress-related problems that do not qualify for the diagnosis of another mental disorder and are not considered indicative of normal bereavement, but either cause significant distress that is out of proportion to the severity or intensity of the stressor or cause significant impairment in functioning, the diagnosis is Adjustment Disorder. Adjustment Disorders may manifest in several ways, each of which can be noted as part of the diagnosis with the following subtypes: With Depressed Mood, With Anxiety, With Mixed Anxiety and Depressed Mood, With Disturbance of Conduct, or With Mixed Disturbance of Emotions and Conduct.

By definition, the disturbance in an Adjustment Disorder begins within 3 months of onset of a stressor and lasts no longer than 6 months after the stressor or its consequences have ceased (DSM-5-TR, p. 319). Usually, if the stressor is an acute event, the onset of an Adjustment Disorder is immediate and the problems last no more than a few months. The specifier Acute can be used to indicate the persistence of symptoms for less than 6 months. In the case of an ongoing set of stressful circumstances, such as domestic abuse, the disturbance may persist indefinitely. The specifier Persistent (chronic) can be used to indicate persistence of symptoms for 6 months or longer. Rates of Adjustment Disorder may be higher in women than in men. Adjustment Disorders are associated with an increased risk of suicide attempts and death by suicide.

Happy Ending

Esther Kim, a 24-year-old single nursery school teacher, terminated brief psychotherapy with a psychologist after 10 sessions. She had entered treatment 2 weeks after discovering that the man she had been involved with for 4 months was married and wanted to stop seeing her. She reacted with bouts of sadness and crying, felt that she was falling apart, took a week's sick leave from her job, and had vague thoughts that the future was so bleak that life might not be worth the effort. She felt that she must be "flawed" in some essential way; otherwise, she would not have become so involved with someone who had no intentions of maintaining a long-term relationship. She also felt that others "would have seen it" and that only she was "so stupid" as to have been deceived. There were no other signs of a depressive syndrome, such as trouble concentrating or loss of interest or appetite. She responded to mixed supportive-insight psychotherapy and, toward the end of treatment, began dating a law student whom she met at a local cafe.

Discussion of "Happy Ending"

Ms. Kim's depressive symptoms (sadness and crying, thoughts that the future was bleak) raise the possibility of a Major Depressive Episode. However, because she had no other signs of the depressive syndrome, a diagnosis of Major Depressive Disorder (see "Worthless Wife" in Section 4.2) is ruled out.

The diagnosis of Adjustment Disorder requires that the symptoms that develop in response to the psychosocial stressor be severe enough to be considered "clinically significant" (Criterion B). With few exceptions, the criteria sets for virtually every DSM-5-TR disorder include a "clinically significant" criterion, which requires that the symptoms cause either "clinically significant distress or impairment in social, occupational, or other important areas of functioning." Determining whether this criterion is met can be challenging, given that DSM-5-TR does not offer any concrete guidance for a presentation to be considered "clinically significant," other than it is inherently a clinical judgment—which is one of the reasons why clinical experience is often necessary to making an accurate DSM-5-TR diagnosis. The distress component of the clinical significance criterion for Adjustment Disorder, however, is unique among the DSM-5-TR diagnoses in that the distress must be "marked" as well as "out of proportion to the severity or intensity of the stressor, taking into account the external context and the cultural factors that might influence symptom severity and presentation" (Criterion B1).

In Ms. Kim's case, it seems reasonable to make the judgment that the severity of her distress (her feeling that she was "falling apart," that life might not be worth the effort, and that she was in some way "flawed") was out of proportion to the severity of the stressor (discovering that the man she had been involved with for 4 months was married and wanted to stop seeing her). Thus her diagnosis is Adjustment Disorder, With Depressed Mood (DSM-5-TR, p. 319).

This is a fairly straightforward and typical case of an Adjustment Disorder, which resolved with a brief course of psychotherapy, and is an example of a case with a happy ending.

Abducted

Kaitlyn, a 3-year-old girl, was referred to the mental health clinic by the pediatric clinic at a large Midwestern hospital because her mother reported that her daughter has had a variety of problems for the last 5 months, ever since she had been abducted for 1 month by her father, who lives out of state. According to her mother, although Kaitlyn had been successfully toilet-trained, she wet her bed constantly during the period of abduction. Since that time, she "chews the skin off her fingers below the nails and twists her hands. She is scared of the dark and wakes up seeing things or thinks someone is after her or coming into her room." Kaitlyn describes scary dreams of "monsters" and has trouble sleeping.

Her parents were unhappy and quarreled frequently during their 2 years together. Her father came from a financially poor family and did not complete high school. He always talked as if he had lots of money; however, after they had separated, the mother discovered that he had a long police record, involving rape and assault and battery. He was involved in using illegal credit cards, doing contract work without a license, and not paying state and federal income taxes. There was a warrant out for his arrest in their state.

When interviewed, Kaitlyn had her hair attractively styled with pigtails and wore small red earrings and colorful play clothes. She was cooperative and left her mother with only slight hesitation. She quickly showed the intake social worker that she could tie her own shoelaces with ease. She easily became engaged in play, but her play involved many frightening themes: a father puppet repeatedly scared a baby puppet, a tiger choked a mouse, and a cow was eaten up by a frog.

Discussion of "Abducted"

Kaitlyn's difficulties apparently began 5 months previously when she was abducted by her father. Since that time, she had demonstrated various symptoms of anxiety (e.g., chewing the skin off her fingers, fears of the dark, and nightmares). The persistence of the symptoms for 5 months is most likely in excess of a normal and expected reaction and something that most clinicians would want to treat.

The absence of the multiplicity of symptoms that would suggest a generalized and persistent anxiety state eliminates the diagnosis of Generalized Anxiety Disorder (see "Edgy Electrician" in Section 5.7). There is no evidence that Kaitlyn has any of the other Anxiety Disorders, such as Separation Anxiety Disorder (see "Tiny Tina" in Section 5.1) or Specific Phobia (see "Thunderstorms" in Section 5.3).

Because Kaitlyn's anxiety symptoms were precipitated by a psychosocial stressor (the abduction), do not meet the criteria for another mental disorder, and are causing ongoing distress months after her abduction, her diagnosis is Adjustment Disorder, With Anxiety (DSM-5-TR, p. 319). As this case illustrates, an Adjustment Disorder can occur even in very young children, although some of the distress may be expressed indirectly, as in play (e.g., Kaitlyn's play involved many threatening themes).

Kaitlyn was incontinent during the 1-month abduction by her father, but because her incontinence did not persist, it would not be significant enough to warrant a separate diagnosis of Enuresis (see "Never Dry" in Section 11.1).

No One Hits the Baby

Four-year-old Carol was referred for an evaluation when her teacher made a complaint to the state Central Registry for Child Abuse Reports. A family evaluation by a social worker revealed the following information.

Carol is the older of two children, both of whom live with their parents in a two-bedroom apartment. Her problems began with the birth of her sister 3 months ago. Her teacher noticed a change in her behavior at school. She began pushing other children and hit a classmate with a wooden block, causing a laceration of the classmate's lip. When Carol's teacher took her aside to talk about her behavior, she noticed what seemed to be belt marks on Carol's abdomen and forehead.

Carol's sister was "colicky" and slept for only short periods throughout the day and night. She stopped crying only when her mother held her. Her mother therefore had little time for Carol, and Carol's father took over her care on evenings and weekends. He began to drink more than usual, half a bottle to a bottle of wine each evening, and became increasingly irritable. He and his wife argued over her attention to the infant and the requirement that he take care of Carol. Carol, who was a bright, curious, talkative 4-year-old, asked constant questions and often wanted to hold the baby. When refused, she would lie on the floor and have a tantrum. Since her sister's birth, she had begun to have difficulty falling asleep and awoke repeatedly during the night.

Carol's father was unable to cope with her demands for attention and often told her to shut up and slapped her when she did not obey. On many occasions he responded to her tantrums or repeated questions by hitting her with his belt.

Carol is a small, lively, and attractive girl, dressed in jeans, T-shirt, and sneakers. She relates appropriately and warmly to the evaluating social worker and easily separates from her parents in the waiting room. Her intelligence appears above average, as indicated by her fund of knowledge, vocabulary, and drawings of a person and of geometric forms. About her sister, Carol says, "She's a bad girl. She cries all the time. I get hit when I cry, but no one hits the baby." When asked about fights at school, she replies, "I hit Robert [her classmate] because he pulls my hair." She says she is afraid to go to sleep because she has bad dreams of an old man killing her.

Carol, along with her mother and father, began a family therapy program that included parenting training and behavioral therapy for Carol, coordinated with the school. Her father was persuaded to join Alcoholics Anonymous, has stopped drinking, and has been able to control his anger at his daughter. Six months later, Carol's aggressive behavior had ceased. She was doing well with peers and in her academic work, was sleeping throughout the night, and had stopped having temper tantrums.

Discussion of "No One Hits the Baby"

Although the focus is on the diagnosis of Carol's difficulties because she is the "identified patient," her problems are actually the consequence of her father's psychopathology. Carol's reaction to having a baby sister would likely not have been remarkable were it not for her father's physical abuse of her.

Children who are physically or sexually abused are at risk for developing several disorders. Major Depressive Disorder (Section 4.2), Separation Anxiety Disorder (Section 5.1), Oppositional Defiant Disorder (Section 15.1), and Conduct Disorder (Section 15.3) are frequent initial reactions to sexual or physical abuse. Among adolescents, suicidal behavior and psychoactive substance use are also frequent. It is unclear how often either Acute Stress Disorder or PTSD develops following abuse, although these disorders should be considered. Long-term consequences of abuse that are seen in adults include Major Depressive Disorder, various personality disturbances (e.g., Borderline Personality Disorder; see Section 18.1), and (more rarely) Dissociative Identity Disorder (Section 8.1). Children who themselves have been physically or sexually abused are likely to abuse their own children. The cases in which this kind of multigenerational abuse have been identified have generally involved more serious and long-term abuse than Carol has experienced.

Carol's changed behavior includes temper tantrums at home, fighting with other children at school, having trouble falling asleep, and bad dreams. These few symptoms are not indicative of a syndrome that would justify the diagnosis of any of the disorders in the paragraph above. Therefore, the diagnosis is Adjustment Disorder, With Mixed Disturbance of Emotions and Conduct (DSM-5-TR, p. 319).

CHAPTER 8

Dissociative Disorders

Dissociation is a mental process that causes a lack of connection between a person's conscious awareness and some aspect of themselves, such as memory, sense of identity, self-perception, or subjective experience of reality. Dissociation falls on a continuum of severity. Mild and nonpathological dissociation is common and occurs, for example, when a person daydreams while driving a car and is unable to remember the last few miles driven, or when a person gets completely "lost" in a book. The temporary altered state of consciousness that can occur while a person is intoxicated with certain drugs (e.g., cannabis, hallucinogens, phencyclidine) is also a form of substance-induced dissociation.

When dissociative experiences become problematic and interfere with the person's functioning, one of the three specific Dissociative Disorders included in DSM-5-TR may be present. Dissociative Disorders are characterized by a disruption of the normal integration of consciousness, memory, identity, emotion, and perception. At the most severe end of the continuum of dissociation, a person's sense of identity or self can become so fragmented that two or more separate and distinct personality states alternately control that person's behavior, a condition known as Dissociative Identity Disorder, which was formerly called Multiple Personality Disorder. In Dissociative Amnesia, there is an inability to recall important autobiographical information, usually of a traumatic or stressful nature, which is inconsistent with ordinary forgetting. In Depersonalization/Derealization Disorder, the core features are perceptual abnormalities in which the person experiences either their thoughts and feelings as being unreal (known as *depersonalization*) or their surroundings as unreal (known as *derealization*). (Table 8–1 lists characteristic features of the DSM-5-TR Dissociative Disorders discussed in this chapter.)

Dissociative symptoms, especially depersonalization and derealization, are not necessarily indicative of a Dissociative Disorder and can occur as part of other DSM-5-TR disorders, such as during a Panic Attack (DSM-5-TR, p. 242) or as a response to a traumatic event (e.g., as part of Posttraumatic Stress Disorder; DSM-5-TR, p. 301). Moreover, they may not be indicative of any disorder at all—about one-third of people say they occasionally feel that they are watching themselves in a movie and feel disconnected from their feelings and actions, yet have none of the distress or impairments in functioning experienced with Dissociative Disorders.

TABLE 8–1.   **Characteristic features of Dissociative Disorders**

Disorder	Key characteristics
Dissociative Identity Disorder	Disruption of identity characterized by two or more distinct personality states
	Recurrent gaps in the recall of everyday events
Dissociative Amnesia	Inability to recall important autobiographical information, usually of a traumatic or stressful nature
Depersonalization/ Derealization Disorder	Persistent or recurrent experiences of depersonalization (unreality or detachment with respect to oneself) or derealization (unreality or detachment with respect to surroundings)

8.1
Dissociative Identity Disorder

Dissociative Identity Disorder (formerly known as Multiple Personality Disorder) is the most severe of the Dissociative Disorders. A person with Dissociative Identity Disorder has two or more different personality states, sometimes referred to as "alters" (short for "alternate personality states"). Each alter might have distinct traits, personal history, and ways of thinking about and relating to their surroundings. An alter might even be of a different gender, have their own name, and have distinct mannerisms or preferences. Stress or a reminder of a trauma can act as a trigger to bring about a switch from one alter to another. The person with Dissociative Identity Disorder may or may not be aware of the other personality states and might not have memories of those times when another alter is dominant. Instead, the person's primary symptoms might be episodes of amnesia or time loss. Individuals with this disorder may repeatedly encounter unfamiliar people who claim to know them, find themselves somewhere without knowing how they got there, or find items that they do not remember purchasing among their possessions.

Dissociative Identity Disorder is thought to be a consequence of severe trauma (usually extreme, repetitive physical, sexual, or emotional abuse) during early childhood. The dissociative aspect is thought to be a coping mechanism—the person literally dissociates themselves from a situation or experience that is too violent, traumatic, or painful to assimilate with their conscious self, leading to a fragmentation in sense of identity.

Dissociative Identity Disorder is one of the more controversial disorders included in DSM-5-TR. On the one hand, those clinicians who specialize in its treatment claim that the condition is much more common than generally recognized. They point out that the diagnosis is almost always first made several years after the patient has had the symptoms and therefore after having accumulated many different diagnoses because of the shifting nature of the symptomatology. On the other hand, critics of the disorder question its very existence and claim that most if not all cases are the result either of therapists suggesting the symptoms or of the patient taking on the characteristics of a famous case of the disorder, such as after watching or reading *The Three Faces of Eve* or *Sybil*.

The 12-month prevalence of Dissociative Identity Disorder among adults in a small U.S. community study was 1.5%. Lifetime prevalence of Dissociative Identity Disorder was 1.1% in a representative sample of community-based women in Middle Eastern Turkey. Among those individuals with Dissociative Identity Disorder, women predominate in clinical studies of adult populations but not in clinical studies of child/adolescent populations or in general population studies. More than 70% of outpatients with Dissociative Identity Disorder report having attempted suicide, and multiple attempts and other self-injurious and high-risk behaviors are also commonly reported.

Mary Quite Contrary

Mary Kendall is a 35-year-old social worker who was referred to a psychiatrist for treatment of reflex sympathetic dystrophy (a chronic pain disorder of uncertain etiology) in her right forearm and hand. She has a complex medical history that includes asthma, migraine headaches, diabetes mellitus, and obesity. She was found to be highly hypnotizable and quickly learned to control her pain with self-hypnosis.

Mary was quite competent in her work but had a rather arid personal life. She had been married briefly and divorced 10 years earlier, and she had little interest in remarrying. She spent most of her free time volunteering in a hospice.

As the thorough psychiatric evaluation continued, she reported the strange observation that on many occasions, the gas tank of her car was nearly full when she returned home from work, yet when she got into her car to go to work the next day, the tank was half empty. She began to keep track of the odometer readings and discovered that on many nights, 50–100 miles would be put on the car overnight, although she had no memory of driving it anywhere. Further questioning revealed that she had gaps in her memory for large parts of her childhood.

Because of the gaps in her memory, the psychiatrist suspected a Dissociative Disorder, but it was only after several months of hypnotic treatment for pain control that the explanation for the lost time emerged. During a hypnotic induction, the psychiatrist again asked about the lost time. A different voice suddenly responded, "It's about time you knew about me." The personality (alter) with a slightly different name, Marian, now spoke and described the drives that she took at night as retreats to the nearby hills and seashore to "work out problems." As the psychiatrist got to know Marian over time, it was apparent that she was as abrupt and hostile as Mary was compliant and concerned about others. Marian considered Mary to be rather pathetic and far too interested in pleasing others, and said that "worrying about anyone but yourself is a waste of time."

In the course of therapy, six other personalities emerged, roughly organized along the lines of a dependent-aggressive continuum. Considerable tension and disagreement emerged among these alters, each of which was rather two-dimensional, lacking any depth. Competition for control of Mary was frequent, and Marian would provoke situations that frightened the others, including one who identified herself as a 6-year-old child. The subjective experience of distinctness between some of the personality states was underscored when one rather hostile alter made a suicide threat. The psychiatrist insisted on discussing this with the other alters, and the alter objected that to do so would be a "violation of doctor-patient confidentiality."

The memories that emerged with these dissociated personality states included recollections of physical and sexual abuse at the hands of her father and others, as well as considerable guilt about not having protected the other children in the family from such abuse. She recalled her mother as being less frequently abusive but quite dependent, and forcing Mary to cook and clean from a very early age.

After 4 years of psychotherapy, Mary gradually integrated portions of these personality states. Two similar personalities merged, although she remained partially dissociated. The personality states were aware of one another but continued to "fight" with each other periodically.

Discussion of "Mary Quite Contrary"

Mary's case illustrates several of the typical features of Dissociative Identity Disorder (DSM-5-TR, p. 330). As was discovered during the course of her treatment for chronic pain, Mary was highly hypnotizable. The first clue that she might have Dissociative Identity Disorder was not the emergence of an alternative personality state during an interview but the presence of symptoms indicative of gaps in her memory, such as the unexplained drops in the amount of fuel in her gas tank and the odometer evidence that she had driven 50–100 miles at night without having any memory of having done so. Moreover, Mary reported having gaps in her memory for large parts of her childhood. Only during sessions under hypnosis did it become clear that the reason Mary had memory gaps for those nighttime drives was because another personality state, named Marian, was in control of her behavior during those times. Then, in the course of her therapy, six additional distinct personality states emerged. Ultimately, Mary was able to recall a history of childhood physical and sexual abuse, which is generally believed to be a causal factor in the development of Dissociative Identity Disorder.

8.2
Dissociative Amnesia

Dissociative Amnesia occurs when a person unconsciously blocks out certain information, usually associated with a stressful or traumatic event such as child abuse or intense combat, leaving them unable to remember important personal information. The memory loss may be situation specific (i.e., for a particular incident) or more global, involving a complete gap in memory lasting from months to years. *Localized amnesia*, the failure to recall events during a circumscribed period of time, is the most common form of this disorder. Sometimes the amnesia for an event may be *selective*, so that the person can remember part of a traumatic event but not other parts. Much more rarely, there can be *generalized amnesia*, in which a person has a complete loss of memory for their life history, and in some cases the person may even forget their own personal identity.

Unlike memory loss associated with head trauma or excessive alcohol use ("blackouts"), in which the memories are permanently lost, in Dissociative Amnesia the memories still exist but are deeply buried within the person's mind and cannot be recalled. However, the memories might resurface on their own or after being triggered by something in the person's surroundings. Some episodes of Dissociative Amnesia resolve rapidly (e.g., when the person is removed from combat or some other stressful situation), whereas other episodes persist for long periods of time. Some individuals may gradually recall the dissociated memories years later. Suicidal and other self-destructive behaviors are common among individuals with Dissociative Amnesia and may be a particular risk when the amnesia remits suddenly and overwhelms the individual with intolerable memories.

The 12-month prevalence among adults in the U.S. general population is estimated to be 1.8%. Dissociative Amnesia is more than twice as common in women as in men and can occur in all age groups.

The Sailor

Psychiatric consultation is requested by an emergency department physician for an 18-year-old youth who has been brought into the hospital by the police. Joshua appears exhausted and shows evidence of prolonged exposure to the sun. He identifies the current date incorrectly, giving it as September 27 instead of October 1. He has difficulty focusing on specific questions, but with encouragement he supplies a number of facts. He recalls going sailing with friends on a weekend cruise off the Florida coast, apparently around September 25, when they encountered bad weather. He is unable to recall any subsequent events and does not know what became of his companions. He has to be reminded several times that he is in a hospital, because he expresses uncertainty as to his whereabouts. Each time he is told, he seems surprised.

There is no evidence of head injury or dehydration. Because of Joshua's apparent exhaustion, he is permitted to sleep for 6 hours. On awakening, he is much more attentive but is still unable to recall events after September 25, including how he came to the hospital. There is no longer any doubt in his mind that he is in the hospital, however, and he is able to recall the contents of the previous interview and the fact that he had fallen asleep. He is also able to remember that he is a student at a southern college, maintains a B average, has a small group of close friends, and has a good relationship with his family. He denies any previous psychiatric history and says he has never abused drugs or alcohol.

An interview is then conducted under the influence of amobarbital (colloquially known as "truth serum"), a medication that causes full relaxation with only minimal sedation and is known to facilitate an individual's willingness to relate information that they would otherwise block. During this interview, Joshua relates that neither he nor his companions were particularly experienced sailors capable of coping with the ferocity of the storm they encountered. Although Joshua had taken the precaution of securing himself to the boat with a life jacket and tie line, his companions had failed to do this and had been washed overboard in the heavy seas. He completely lost control of the boat and felt he was saved only by virtue of good luck and his lifeline. Over a 3-day period, he had been able to consume a small supply of food that was stowed away in the cabin. He never saw either of his sailing companions again. Joshua was picked up on October 1 by a Coast Guard cutter and brought to shore, and subsequently the police brought him to the hospital.

Discussion of "The Sailor"

This case illustrates the classic features of the most common form of Dissociative Amnesia (DSM-5-TR, p. 337)—namely, the inability to remember anything about a specific period of time in the past, which in this case involved an extremely traumatic and life-threatening situation. When a patient such as Joshua presents with acute memory loss, however, other specific external causes of memory loss must first be ruled out before a diagnosis of Dissociative Amnesia can be made. A number of medical conditions, such as head trauma or stroke, can lead to the development of a Major Neurocognitive Disorder (see Section 17.2), which may involve acute memory loss along with other cognitive problems. Other medical problems, such as electrolyte imbalances or brain infections, can lead to Delirium (see Section 17.1), a Neurocognitive Disorder characterized by acute confusion and decreased awareness of the individual's environment, as well as memory loss. Intoxication with sedatives or sleeping pills and intoxication resulting from heavy alcohol consumption can result in a blackout in which the person is unable to remember what was happening to them during the period of intoxication. In all of these cases, the memory loss reflects a physical disturbance in brain functioning in which either the memories were never permanently encoded or the ability to access them is permanently gone.

Joshua's initial disorientation and confusion did suggest the possibility that there might have been a physical cause of his memory problem. However, the absence of any evidence of a nonpsychiatric medical problem or history of drug or alcohol use and the fact that his confusion resolved after a night of sleep, leaving him with only the inability to remember what happened during the time period in question, indicated that there was likely nothing physically wrong with his memory. Moreover, his ability to remember the content of his first interview in the hospital indicated that his brain was able to form (and recall) new memories since the accident.

The fact that Joshua's memory loss was caused by psychological stress was finally confirmed by the results of the amobarbital interview. Under the influence of the intravenous sedative, he was sufficiently relaxed to be able to finally have access to the previously blocked memories of what happened to him and his sailing companions on the boat.

Burt Tate

The patient is a 42-year-old man who was brought to the emergency room by the police. He was involved in an argument and fight at the diner where he is employed. When the police arrived and began to question the patient, he gave his name as "Burt Tate" but had no identification. "Mr. Tate" had drifted into town several weeks earlier and begun working as a short-order cook at the diner. He could not recall where he had worked or lived before his arrival in this town. There were no charges against him, but the police convinced him to come to the emergency room for an examination.

When questioned in the emergency room, "Mr. Tate" knew what town he was in and the current date. He admitted that it was somewhat unusual that he could not recall the details of his past life, but he did not appear very upset about this. There was no evidence of alcohol or drug abuse, and a physical examination revealed no head trauma or any other physical abnormalities. He was kept overnight for observation.

When the police ran a background check on the patient, they found that he fit the description of a missing person, Gene Saunders, who had disappeared a month before from a city 200 miles away. A visit by Mrs. Saunders confirmed the identity of the patient as Gene Saunders. Mrs. Saunders explained that for 18 months before his disappearance, her husband, who was a middle-level manager at a large manufacturing company, had been having considerable difficulty at work. He had been passed over for a promotion, and his supervisor had been very critical of his work. Several of his staff had left the company for other jobs, and the patient found it impossible to meet production goals. Work stress made him very difficult to live with at home. Previously an easygoing, gregarious person, he had become withdrawn and critical of his wife and children. Immediately preceding his disappearance, he had had a violent argument with his 18-year-old son. The son had called him a "failure" and stormed out of the house to live with some friends who had an apartment. Two days after this argument, the patient disappeared.

When brought into the room where his wife was waiting, the patient stated that he did not recognize her. He appeared noticeably anxious.

Discussion of "Burt Tate"

Like the patient in the previous case, this patient is also experiencing an inability to recall important personal information that is not explained by drug or alcohol use or a nonpsychiatric medical condition. This case differs in that instead of experiencing localized amnesia for a specific period of his life, the patient has generalized amnesia in which he cannot recall any details about his past life, including his past identity. What also distinguishes this case is that in addition to the memory loss, the patient has assumed a new identity, as a short-order cook named "Burt Tate." This presentation has historically been called a *Dissociative Fugue* (*fugue* from the Latin word for "flight"), a condition that involves the individual's sudden, unexpected travel away from home or customary place of work, which is accompanied by either confusion about personal identity or the assumption of a new identity. Thus, the DSM-5-TR diagnosis for this case is Dissociative Amnesia, With Dissociative Fugue (DSM-5-TR, p. 337).

Dissociative Fugue was a separate disorder from Dissociative Amnesia in DSM-IV but was folded into Dissociative Amnesia in DSM-5 (and DSM-5-TR) because of its rarity and the fact that both disorders involve the individual's inability to recall some or all of their past. The onset of Dissociative Fugue or Dissociative Amnesia is typically linked to one or more severe stressors. In this patient's case, the fugue developed after a sequence of stressful life events, starting with being passed over for a promotion at work, followed by work stress related to an inability to meet production goals, and finally culminating in an argument with his 18-year-old son that ended with the son abruptly moving out of the house. Although considered to be quite rare in real life (with a prevalence of less than 0.2%), the phenomenon of Dissociative Amnesia and Dissociative Fugue is commonly used as a plot device in books, TV shows, and movies (e.g., *The Bourne Identity*).

8.3
Depersonalization/ Derealization Disorder

Depersonalization/Derealization Disorder involves the lack of integration of one or more components of perception and consists of persistent or recurrent episodes of depersonalization, derealization, or both. *Depersonalization*, in which the focus is on the self, involves feeling that the individual's thoughts, feelings, sensations, body, or actions are unreal or that these are somehow detached or estranged from the individual. Typically, individuals with this disorder feel as though they are outside observers of their own mental processes or that they are a robot or an automaton, lacking control of their speech or movements. In some cases, individuals may be unable to accept their reflection (e.g., in a mirror) as their own or may have out-of-body experiences. *Derealization*, on the other hand, involves the feeling that the individual's surroundings are unreal, so that other individuals or objects in the environment are experienced as dreamlike, foggy, lifeless, or visually distorted. Although this disorder involves an alteration in the subjective experience of reality, it is not a form of psychosis, because these individuals maintain the ability to distinguish between their own internal experiences and the objective reality of the outside world. An episode of depersonalization or derealization can last anywhere from a few minutes to many years.

Approximately 50% of the general population has had an episode of depersonalization or derealization, frequently occurring in connection with life-threatening danger, acute drug intoxication (cannabis, hallucinogens, ketamine, ecstasy), sensory deprivation, or sleep deprivation. Depersonalization can also occur as a symptom in many other mental disorders, including Panic Disorder (see Section 5.5), Posttraumatic Stress Disorder (see Section 7.3), and Borderline Personality Disorder (see Section 18.1), as well as in nonpsychiatric medical conditions, such as seizure disorders. When depersonalization occurs independently of other mental or nonpsychiatric medical disorders and is persistent or recurrent and causes clinically significant distress or impairment in functioning, the diagnosis is Depersonalization/Derealization Disorder. This disorder is estimated to occur in about 2% of the general population, with women and men equally affected.

Foggy Student

Edward Martinez, a 20-year-old college student, sought psychiatric consultation at student health because he was worried that he might be going insane. For the past 2 years, he had experienced increasingly frequent episodes of feeling "outside" himself. These episodes were accompanied by a sense of deadness in his body. In addition, during these periods he was uncertain of his balance and frequently stumbled into furniture; this unsteadiness was more apt to occur in public, especially if he was somewhat anxious. During these episodes he felt a lack of easy, natural control of his body, and his thoughts seemed "foggy" as well, in a way that reminded him of having received intravenous anesthetic agents for an appendectomy some 5 years previously.

Edward's subjective sense of lack of control was especially troublesome, and he would fight it by shaking his head and saying "Stop" to himself. This interruptive strategy would momentarily clear his mind and restore his sense of autonomy, but only temporarily, because the feelings of deadness and of being outside himself would return. Gradually, over a period of several hours, the unpleasant experiences would fade. Edward was anxious, however, about their return, and he found them increasing in both frequency and duration.

At the time Edward came for treatment, he was experiencing these symptoms about twice a week, and each incident lasted from 3 to 4 hours. On several occasions, the episodes had occurred while he was driving his car and was alone. Worried that he might have an accident, he had stopped driving unless someone accompanied him. Increasingly, he had begun to discuss this problem with his girlfriend, and eventually she had become less affectionate toward him, complaining that he had lost his sense of humor and was totally self-preoccupied. She threatened to break off with him unless he changed, and she began to date other men.

Edward's college grades remained unimpaired—they had, in fact, improved over the past 6 months, because the patient was spending more time studying than had previously been the case. Although discouraged by his symptoms, the patient slept well at night, had noted no change in appetite, and had experienced no impairment in concentration. He was neither fatigued nor physically "edgy" because of his worry.

Because a cousin had been hospitalized for many years with severe mental illness, Edward had begun to wonder if a similar fate might befall him, and therefore he sought direct reassurance on the matter.

Discussion of "Foggy Student"

Edward is experiencing recurrent episodes, lasting for hours at a time, of feeling "outside himself," which are accompanied by a sense of deadness in his body, a feeling that his thoughts are "foggy," and a sense that he lacks an easy, natural control of his body. Given that his perceptual abnormalities are focused on various aspects of himself (i.e., his body, his thoughts, his ability to control his body) rather than his environment, they are indicative of depersonalization. The distress that Edward experiences, as well as the absence of other mental disorders, substance use, or nonpsychiatric medical conditions that could account for the symptoms, indicates that the DSM-5-TR diagnosis of Depersonalization/Derealization Disorder (DSM-5-TR, p. 343) is most appropriate. Even though patients often have both depersonalization and derealization, in Edward's case there is no evidence of symptoms of derealization, which in any event are not required for the diagnosis of Depersonalization/Derealization Disorder. Although Edward expresses concern that he might be going insane and that he might end up in a mental institution like his cousin, his symptoms are not indicative of a Psychotic Disorder, because he remains aware at all times that the symptoms are a product of his own mind.

CHAPTER 9

Somatic Symptom and Related Disorders

The common feature shared by the DSM-5-TR Somatic Symptom and Related Disorders is a significant focus on somatic (physical) symptoms or physical illness that is associated with significant distress and impairment. Because individuals with these disorders are strongly focused on their physical symptoms, they are most often encountered in medical settings rather than in mental health care settings, and they often resist recommendations that they obtain mental health care treatment for their symptoms. DSM-5-TR disorders in this diagnostic class are as follows:

- Somatic Symptom Disorder, which is characterized by the presence of one or more distressing or impairing somatic symptoms
- Illness Anxiety Disorder, which involves an unjustified preoccupation with having or acquiring a serious illness in the absence of prominent somatic symptoms, accompanied by high levels of anxiety about health
- Functional Neurological Symptom Disorder (formerly known as Conversion Disorder), which involves symptoms of altered motor or sensory function that are not compatible with the symptom pattern of any known neurological condition
- Psychological Factors Affecting Other Medical Conditions, which is diagnosed when psychological or behavioral factors are present that negatively influence the course of a nonpsychiatric medical condition
- Factitious Disorder, in which a person feigns symptoms of a nonpsychiatric medical illness or a mental disorder in the absence of obvious external incentives to do so, such as avoiding work, evading criminal responsibility, or winning a lawsuit. A person's falsification of physical or psychological signs or symptoms can relate either to the person themself (Factitious Disorder Imposed on Self) or to another person, most typically a child under the person's care (Factitious Disorder Imposed on Another).

In prior editions of DSM, these conditions were known as Somatoform Disorders (i.e., psychological symptoms that took the form of somatic symptoms) and were typically diagnosed in individuals with physical symptoms for which no medical explanation could be determined. In such cases, the symptoms were thought to represent a physical manifestation of psychological symptoms (referred to as "somaticizing") and were erroneously viewed as somehow "not real" or "all in the person's head" and best treated by a mental health care professional rather than by a nonpsychiatric medical clinician. For several reasons, DSM-5-TR has moved away from basing these diagnoses on the absence of a medical explanation and instead to basing the diagnosis on the presence of somatic symptoms and the degree of distress about or impairment from them. Most patients who received a DSM-IV somatoform diagnosis rejected the notion that the physical symptoms they experienced as real were declared to be of psychological origin; and thus, they often refused treatment with a mental health care professional, preferring to seek out the help of another medical doctor who would finally get to the bottom of their physical complaints. Moreover, the ability of a mental health care clinician to determine whether a physical symptom is medically unexplained is quite limited. For example, rather than there being no medical basis for a particular physical symptom, the lack of explanation may instead reflect an inadequate medical workup. Given that most medical conditions are also characterized by the presence of distressing or impairing physical symptoms, the disorders in this section include additional requirements that are indicative of the presence of a mental disorder rather than (or in addition to) a nonpsychiatric medical condition. For example, for a diagnosis of Somatic Symptom Disorder, the somatic symptoms must be accompanied by excessive thoughts, feelings, or behaviors related to the symptoms (e.g., appraisal of one's symptoms as being unduly serious). Table 9–1 lists characteristic features of the Somatic Symptom and Related Disorders discussed in this chapter.

9.1
Somatic Symptom Disorder

Somatic Symptom Disorder is characterized by distress or life disruption arising from concerns about physical symptoms. Patients with Somatic Symptom Disorder typically present with multiple current somatic symptoms, although sometimes there is only one severe symptom, most commonly pain. Symptoms may be specific to a particular part of the body (e.g., localized pain) or relatively nonspecific (e.g., generalized fatigue). In some cases, the symptoms represent normal bodily sensations or discomfort that does not generally signify serious disease. Given that it is normal to experience transient somatic symptoms at times, the diagnosis requires that the symptoms be persistent, typically lasting 6 months or longer.

For cases in which Somatic Symptom Disorder is accompanied by a nonpsychiatric medical condition, the disorder is often manifested by the person's excessive level of worry about the implications of the medical condition. For example, a person who has had a complete recovery from an uncomplicated myocardial infarction may behave as an invalid or constantly worry about having another heart attack. Regardless

TABLE 9–1. **Characteristic features of Somatic Symptom and Related Disorders**

Disorder	Key characteristics
Somatic Symptom Disorder	Somatic symptoms that are distressing or result in significant disruption of daily life
	Excessive thoughts, feelings, or behaviors related to the somatic symptoms or associated health concerns
Illness Anxiety Disorder	Preoccupation with having or acquiring a serious illness
	Somatic symptoms are not present or are mild in intensity
	A high level of anxiety about health
	Excessive health-related behaviors or maladaptive avoidance
Functional Neurological Symptom Disorder (Conversion Disorder)	Symptom(s) of altered voluntary motor or sensory function that are incompatible with recognized neurological or medical conditions
Psychological Factors Affecting Other Medical Conditions	Psychological or behavioral factors that adversely affect the course or treatment of a medical condition, that constitute additional health risks for the individual, or that influence the underlying pathophysiology
Factitious Disorder (includes Factitious Disorder Imposed on Self and Factitious Disorder Imposed on Another)	Falsification of physical or psychological signs or symptoms, or induction of injury or disease, either in oneself or in another, in the absence of external incentives

of whether the symptoms are related to an already established nonpsychiatric medical condition, a diagnosis of Somatic Symptom Disorder requires that the somatic symptoms be accompanied by excessive thoughts, feelings, or behaviors related to the somatic symptoms or associated health concerns. Individuals may worry excessively about the symptoms and their possible catastrophic consequences and are very difficult to reassure. Attempts at reassurance are often interpreted as the physician not taking the symptoms seriously. Health concerns often assume a central and sometimes all-consuming role in the individual's life, with the person devoting excessive time and energy to dealing with health concerns. These individuals tend to be very anxious about their health and frequently seem unusually sensitive to adverse drug effects.

Patients with Somatic Symptom Disorder are commonly unaware of any underlying mental illness–related factor in their distress and truly believe that they have physical ailments, so they typically continue to pressure physicians for additional or repeated tests and treatments even after the results of a thorough evaluation have been negative. As noted in DSM-5-TR (p. 351), "The individual's suffering is authentic, whether or not it is medically explained." For some individuals with Somatic Symptom Disorder, the predominant complaint is of chronic pain. DSM-5-TR includes the specifier With Predominant Pain to allow this relatively common presentation to be noted. Other individuals have a particularly chronic and severe presentation in which their entire lives tend to revolve around their somatic complaints. DSM-5-TR includes a Persistent specifier to note such presentations.

Somatic Symptom Disorder is relatively common and is estimated to affect approximately 5%–7% of the adult population. It more often affects women than men. Somatic Symptom Disorder can occur at any time of life but most often begins in early adulthood. The disorder is associated with high rates of comorbidity with Anxiety and Depressive Disorders, each of which co-occurs in up to 50% of cases of Somatic Symptom Disorder.

Blackout

A perplexed internist asked for a psychiatric consultation for Gloria Jackson, a 50-year-old divorced and unemployed secretary, who was hospitalized for a workup of her unusual physical complaints. When first encountered by the psychiatrist, Ms. Jackson was lying in bed in a contorted position, with occasional jerking movements of her arms, once every few seconds. Within 10 minutes, she was sitting up and explaining that she had been having "a seizure" that was "still there, in my spine. At any minute it can break out and overwhelm me again." Her present difficulties began about 8 months previously with nausea, abdominal cramps, and pain in her arms, legs, and back that have kept her bedridden for days at a time, and she has been experiencing "seizures" like the one witnessed by the psychiatrist "several times a week." Ms. Jackson noted that since the seizures started, they are all that she can think or talk about. She reports having gone to a large number of various types of doctors for her current constellation of symptoms ("too many to count"), but none has yet been able to figure out what to do for her. She is very worried that the symptoms are indicative of a "terrible disease" but has no idea what that disease might be.

Ms. Jackson reports having had abdominal pain since age 17, necessitating exploratory surgery that yielded no specific diagnosis. She had several pregnancies, each with severe nausea, vomiting, and abdominal pain; she ultimately had a hysterectomy for a "tipped uterus." Since age 40, she has experienced dizziness and "blackouts," which she eventually was told might be multiple sclerosis or a brain tumor. She continues to be bedridden for extended periods of time, with weakness, blurred vision, and difficulty urinating. At age 43, she was evaluated for a hiatal hernia because of complaints of bloating and intolerance of a variety of foods. She also had additional hospitalizations for neurological, hypertensive, and renal workups, all of which failed to reveal a definitive diagnosis.

Discussion of "Blackout"

Ms. Jackson's chief complaint is her constellation of distressing and disabling physical symptoms, which include nausea, abdominal cramps, pain in her back and extremities, and "seizures." Her physical complaints are accompanied by numerous examples of "excessive thoughts, feelings, or behaviors" related to her symptoms (DSM-5-TR, p. 351), so that her health concerns dominate her thoughts and conversations; she repeatedly seeks out medical evaluations from various doctors; and she fears that her symptoms are indicative of a serious disease, despite the lack of evidence supporting such a worry. Given that Ms. Jackson's current symptoms have persisted for the past 8 months and that the course of her Somatic Symptom Disorder has been characterized by severe symptoms, marked impairment (being bedridden for extended periods of time), and long duration (symptoms starting at age 17), the diagnosis would be Severe Somatic Symptom Disorder, Persistent (DSM-5-TR, p. 351).

Presentations of recurrent unexplained physical complaints having an onset by age 30 and involving multiple organ systems, as in Ms. Jackson's case, were diagnosed as Somatization Disorder in DSM editions prior to DSM-5 and were originally called Briquet's syndrome, first identified by Paul Briquet in 1859. This chronic and pervasive form of Somatic Symptom Disorder is 10 times more common in women than in men.

No Parking

Vanessa Abernathy, a 36-year-old traffic enforcement agent, was referred for psychiatric examination by her lawyer. About 10 months previously, moments after she had written a ticket and placed it on the windshield of an illegally parked car, a man dashed out of a barbershop; ran up to her, swearing and shaking his fist; and hit her in the jaw with enough force to knock her down. A fellow worker came to her aid and summoned the police, who caught the man a few blocks away and arrested him.

Ms. Abernathy was taken to the hospital, where a hairline fracture of the jaw was diagnosed by X-ray. The fracture did not require that her jaw be wired, but she was placed on a soft diet for 4 weeks. Several different physicians, including her own, found her physically fit to return to work after 1 month. The patient, however, complained of severe pain and muscle tension in her neck and back that virtually immobilized her. She spent most of her days sitting in a chair or lying on a bed board on her bed. She talked about her pain incessantly with her family and friends, to the point that her friends stopped calling her because they were sick of hearing her complain. She also enlisted the services of a lawyer because the Workers' Compensation Board was cutting off her payments and her employer was threatening her with suspension if she did not return to work.

Ms. Abernathy shuffled slowly and laboriously into the psychiatrist's office and lowered herself with great care into a chair. She was attractively dressed, was well made up, and wore a neck brace. She related her story with vivid detail and with considerable anger directed at her assailant, her employer, and the compensation board. It was as if the incident had occurred yesterday. Regarding her ability to work, she said that she wanted to return to the job and would soon be severely strapped financially but was physically not up to even the lightest office work.

Ms. Abernathy denied any previous psychological problems and initially described her childhood and family life as "storybook perfect." In subsequent interviews, however, she admitted that as a child, she had frequently been beaten by her alcoholic father, and had once suffered a broken arm as a result, and that she had often been locked in a closet for hours at a time as punishment for misbehavior.

Discussion of "No Parking"

In contrast to the previous case ("Blackout"), in which the patient had a years-long history of multiple somatic complaints affecting various organ systems, in this case, the patient's focus is entirely on her pain symptoms. Chronic pain is quite common; studies indicate that 10%–50% of people around the world have chronic pain. Ms. Abernathy's focus on her pain, combined with the way her life now completely revolves around her pain complaints, justifies the diagnosis of Somatic Symptom Disorder, With Predominant Pain (DSM-5-TR, p. 351).

Given that Ms. Abernathy has retained a lawyer to challenge the Workers' Compensation Board's decision to discontinue payments to her, the question is raised of whether her pain symptoms are being made up or exaggerated so that she will no longer have to earn a living, which would be an instance of Malingering rather than Somatic Symptom Disorder. Malingering is defined as "the intentional production of false or grossly exaggerated physical or psychological symptoms, motivated by external incentives such as…avoiding work [or] obtaining financial compensation" (DSM-5-TR, p. 835). It is not considered to be mental disorder in DSM-5-TR and is included in the DSM-5-TR chapter "Other Conditions That May Be a Focus of Clinical Attention." The apparent genuineness of the patient's suffering and her stated desire to return to work make an interpretation of Malingering less likely.

9.2
Illness Anxiety Disorder

Individuals with Illness Anxiety Disorder overly focus on and think about their physical health and have an unrealistic and uncontrollable fear of having or developing a serious disease. They are so preoccupied with the idea that they are or might become ill that their illness anxiety impairs their social and occupational functioning or causes significant distress. In those cases in which a physical sign or symptom is present, it is often a normal physiological sensation (e.g., feeling lightheaded on standing up too quickly), a benign and self-limited dysfunction (e.g., a brief period of ringing in the ears), or a bodily discomfort not generally considered to be indicative of disease (e.g., belching). If the person has a medical condition or is at high risk for a medical condition (e.g., a strong family history of heart disease), the individual's anxiety and preoccupations about the medical condition or risk factor must be clearly excessive and disproportionate to the severity of the condition.

Individuals with Illness Anxiety Disorder address this preoccupation in a variety of ways. They typically seek out reassurance from family, friends, or health care providers on a regular basis. After doing so, they feel better for a short time, but then they begin to worry about the same symptoms or new symptoms. Some individuals examine themselves repeatedly (e.g., look at their throat in a mirror, check their skin for signs of skin cancer). In some cases, the anxiety leads to maladaptive avoidance of situations (e.g., visiting hospitalized family members) or activities (e.g., exercise) that these individuals fear might jeopardize their health. Individuals with Illness Anxiety Disorder are easily alarmed by news about illness, such as hearing about a friend or even a public figure falling ill or encountering a health-related news story in a newspaper, on TV, or on the internet.

The course of Illness Anxiety Disorder is often chronic, fluctuating in some individuals but steady in others. The disorder most commonly begins during early or middle adulthood and appears to occur equally among men and women. The 1- to 2-year prevalence of health anxiety and/or disease conviction in community surveys and population-based samples ranges from 1.3% to 10%. In medical outpatients, the 6-month to 1-year prevalence rates are between 2.2% and 8%.

In DSM editions prior to DSM-5, this condition was referred to as Hypochondriasis; however, this term was abandoned because of its pejorative connotation.

The Radiologist

Malcolm Davies, a 38-year-old radiologist, is evaluated after returning from a 10-day stay at a famous out-of-state diagnostic center to which he had been referred by a local gastroenterologist after "he reached the end of the line with me." Dr. Davies reports that he underwent extensive physical and laboratory examinations, X-ray examinations of the entire gastrointestinal tract, and endoscopic evaluations of his esophagus, stomach, and colon. Although he was told that the results of the examinations were negative for significant physical disease, he appears resentful and disappointed rather than relieved at the findings. He was seen briefly for a "routine" evaluation by a psychiatrist at the diagnostic center but had difficulty relating to her on more than a superficial level.

On further inquiry about his physical symptoms, Dr. Davies describes occasional twinges of mild abdominal pain, sensations of "fullness," "bowel rumblings," and a "firm abdominal mass" that he can sometimes feel in the left lower quadrant of his abdomen. Over the past 6 months, he has gradually become more aware of these sensations and is convinced that they may be due to a carcinoma of the colon. He tests his stool for occult (i.e., not visible) blood weekly and spends 15–20 minutes every 2–3 days carefully palpating his abdomen as he lies in bed at home. He has secretly performed several X-ray studies on himself in his own office after hours.

Although he is successful in his work, has an excellent attendance record, and is active in community life, Dr. Davies spends much of his leisure time at home on the internet, looking up information about illnesses he worries that he might have. His wife, an instructor at a local school of nursing, is angry and bitter about this behavior, which she describes as "robbing us of what we've worked so hard and postponed so much for." Although she and her husband share many values and genuinely love each other, his behavior is causing a real strain on their marriage.

When the patient was 13 years old, a heart murmur was detected on a school physical examination. Because a younger brother had died in early childhood of congenital heart disease, Dr. Davies was removed from gym class until the murmur could be evaluated. The evaluation found the murmur to be benign (i.e., not harmful), but he began to worry that the evaluation might have "missed something" and considered the occasional sensations of "skipping a beat" as evidence that this was the case. He kept his fears to himself, and they subsided over the next 2 years but never entirely left him.

As a second-year medical student, Dr. Davies was relieved to share some of his health concerns with his classmates, who also worried about having the diseases they were learning about in pathology. He realized, however, that he was much more preoccupied with and worried about his health than they were. Since graduating from medical school, he has repeatedly become immersed in a series of health concerns, each following the same pattern: noticing a symptom, becoming increasingly preoccupied with what it might mean, and having a negative physical evaluation. At times he returns to an "old" concern but is too embarrassed to pursue it with physicians he knows, such as when he discovered a new "suspicious" mole only 1 week after he had persuaded a dermatologist to biopsy one that proved to be entirely benign.

Dr. Davies tells his story with a sincere, discouraged tone, brightened only by a note of real pleasure and enthusiasm as he provides a detailed account of his discovery of a genuine, but clinically insignificant, anomaly in his urethra as the result of an intravenous pyelogram (X-ray of the kidneys and urinary tract made after an intravenous injection of dye) he had ordered himself. Near the end of the interview, the patient explains that his coming in for evaluation now was largely self-motivated, precipitated by an encounter with his 9-year-old son. The boy had accidentally walked in while he was palpating his own abdomen for "masses" and had asked, "What do you think it is this time, Dad?" As he describes his shame and anger (mostly at himself) about this incident, Dr. Davies' eyes fill with tears.

Discussion of "The Radiologist"

Dr. Davies is preoccupied with the idea that he has a serious illness, namely colon cancer. Although his concerns are triggered by somatic symptoms, such as occasional twinges of mild abdominal pain, sensations of "fullness," "bowel rumblings," and a "firm abdominal mass" that he can sometimes feel in his left lower quadrant, he is bothered not so much by the symptoms themselves but rather by the implication that they represent evidence of colon cancer. Although his preoccupation has clearly had a negative impact on his relationship with his wife, it took an encounter with his 9-year-old son to finally motivate him to accept that he had a psychological problem that might benefit from the help of a mental health care professional. The persistent nature of Dr. Davies' preoccupation, his overall high level of anxiety about his health, and his excessive enactment of health-focused behaviors related to his preoccupation, such as repeatedly examining himself for masses and repeatedly testing his stool for signs of blood (a possible indicator of colon cancer), point to a diagnosis of Illness Anxiety Disorder (DSM-5-TR, p. 357). Were his focus on the disabling nature of the symptoms themselves, the diagnosis would be Somatic Symptom Disorder rather than Illness Anxiety Disorder.

9.3
Functional Neurological Symptom Disorder (Conversion Disorder)

Individuals with Functional Neurological Symptom Disorder present with altered voluntary motor or sensory function—such as paralysis of a limb or convulsions—that suggests a possible neurological or nonpsychiatric medical condition. However, following a thorough evaluation, including a detailed neurological examination and appropriate laboratory and radiographic diagnostic tests, it is clearly determined that the person's symptoms are not compatible with any recognized neurological or nonpsychiatric medical conditions. This condition is also known as Conversion Disorder (a name that has its origins in Sigmund Freud's doctrine that unconscious anxiety can be "converted" into physical symptoms such as blindness)—and represents perhaps the last vestige of psychoanalytic theory that appears in DSM.

Motor symptoms in patients with Functional Neurological Symptom Disorder can include weakness or paralysis; abnormal movements, such as tremor; gait abnormalities; and abnormal limb posturing. Sensory symptoms can include altered, reduced, or absent skin sensation, vision, or hearing. Episodes of abnormal generalized limb shaking with apparent impairment or loss of consciousness may resemble epileptic seizures. There may be episodes of unresponsiveness resembling a fainting episode or coma. Other symptoms may include reduced or absent speech volume, inability to speak clearly, and double vision. To qualify for a diagnosis of Functional Neurological Symptom Disorder, the symptoms must be severe enough to cause the person significant distress or to interfere with important areas of functioning.

Although the diagnosis of Functional Neurological Symptom Disorder requires that the symptoms not be better explained by a recognized neurological condition, the diagnosis should not be given simply because results from investigations are normal or because the symptoms seem to be bizarre. The diagnosis requires that clinical findings show clear evidence of incompatibility with neurological disease, such as demonstrating that physical signs elicited through one examination method are no longer positive when tested a different way. For example, a patient may show marked weakness in the ability to downward flex the ankle when tested in bed but can walk normally on tiptoes, a movement that requires normal ankle flexion; or a patient may present with a tremor in one hand that changes or disappears when the patient is distracted. It is important to recognize that although the neurological symptoms in Functional Neurological Symptom Disorder are not genuine (in the sense of being indicative of a known neurological condition), individuals with Functional Neurological Symptom Disorder are not consciously faking these symptoms. To the patient with Functional Neurological Symptom Disorder, the experience of paralysis, blindness, or seizures is real. This experience is in marked contrast to the experience of an individual who is Malingering—that is, intentionally producing false or greatly exaggerated physical symptoms, motivated by external incentives such as avoiding military duty or work or obtaining financial compensation.

Although transient functional neurological symptoms may be relatively common, the incidence of persistent functional neurological symptoms in the general population is rare, estimated to be 2–5/100,000 per year. Functional Neurological Symptom Disorder is much more common among populations of neurological patients; among patients referred to neurology clinics, between 5% and 15% meet criteria for this disorder. Functional Neurological Symptom Disorder is more common in cultures that emphasize religious and spiritual healings. Functional Neurological Symptom Disorder is two to three times more common in women than in men.

Fits

A 26-year-old married woman, Pari Chatterjee, attends a clinic in New Delhi, India, with complaints of having had "fits" for the past 4 years. The fits are always sudden in onset and usually last 30–60 minutes. A few minutes before a fit begins, she knows that it is imminent, and she usually goes to bed. During the fits, she becomes unresponsive and rigid throughout her body, with bizarre and thrashing movements of her extremities. Her eyes close and her jaw is clenched and she froths at the mouth. She frequently cries and sometimes shouts abusive language. She is never incontinent of urine or feces, and she never bites her tongue. After a fit, she claims to have no memory of it.

These episodes recur about once or twice a month. Mrs. Chatterjee functions well between the episodes and reports no prominent depressive or anxiety symptoms.

Both Mrs. Chatterjee and her family believe that her fits are evidence of a physical illness and are not under her control. However, they recognize that the fits often occur following some stressor, such as arguments with family members or friends.

Mrs. Chatterjee comes from an urban middle-class family. She has been married for 5 years to a clerk in a government office. They have two children. Her husband's parents live with them, and this arrangement has sometimes led to conflicts.

She is described by her family as somewhat immature but "quite social" and good company. Her family also reports that she is self-centered, that she craves attention from others, and that she often reacts with irritability and anger if her wishes are not immediately fulfilled. She handles routine household tasks well.

On physical examination, Mrs. Chatterjee was found to have mild anemia but to be otherwise healthy. A mental status examination did not reveal any abnormality in her speech, thought processes or content, orientation, perception, or intellectual functions. She did not display any sustained mood change, and her memory was normal. A routine electroencephalogram (EEG) done in the clinic office (but not during a seizure) showed no seizure activity. A skull X-ray was also normal. An ambulatory EEG study, in which a portable EEG device is worn while the patient engages in daily life activities, was conducted to measure brain wave activity during one of her fits. Mrs. Chatterjee was instructed to wear the device for 3 days and to record any seizure activity in a detailed diary. She reported that on the morning of the third day of monitoring, she had one of her usual fits, which was witnessed by her husband. Examination of the EEG record during the fit showed no abnormal changes in the EEG, confirming the absence of a neurological cause for her fits.

Over the next 2 months, Mrs. Chatterjee was treated, with her husband, in family sessions. The couple was taught that Mrs. Chatterjee's fits were not evidence of a serious physical illness. In addition, the husband was urged to take a more active role in handling problems that arose between the patient and her in-laws and to pay more attention to the patient in general, but not during her fits. The couple stopped therapy after 2 months, during which time the patient had no more fits.

Discussion of "Fits"

Mrs. Chatterjee's predominant symptom resembles an epileptic seizure; however, the absence of typical features of neurological seizures, such as incontinence and biting of the tongue, strongly suggests that a neurological condition or nonpsychiatric medical condition cannot explain the seizures. The pseudo-neurological nature of the seizure presentation is confirmed by the ambulatory EEG: the absence of concurrent seizure activity in the brain during the seizure-like behavior is inconsistent with what would be expected in true epilepsy, and therefore indicates a DSM-5-TR diagnosis of Functional Neurological Symptom Disorder, With Attacks or Seizures (DSM-5-TR, p. 360).

Mrs. Chatterjee also has histrionic and narcissistic personality traits ("she is self-centered, craves attention from others, and often reacts with irritability and anger if her wishes are not immediately fulfilled"), which is notable given that maladaptive personality traits are commonly associated with Functional Neurological Symptom Disorder.

9.4
Psychological Factors Affecting Other Medical Conditions

The DSM-5-TR diagnosis Psychological Factors Affecting Other Medical Conditions is reserved for situations in which psychological or behavioral factors adversely affect the course or outcome of an existing nonpsychiatric medical condition (e.g., diabetes mellitus, heart disease) or symptom (e.g., pain). The influence of psychological factors on a medical condition can be demonstrated in a number of ways. There could be a close temporal association between the psychological factors and the development or exacerbation of, or delayed recovery from, the medical condition. The factors might interfere with the treatment of a medical condition, as when a patient's denial of the significance or severity of medical symptoms leads to poor adherence to prescribed testing or treatment. Finally, the factors could constitute a well-established health risk for the individual, such as chronic occupational stress that increases the patient's risk for hypertension.

Common clinical examples of this condition include asthma exacerbated by anxiety, denial of the need for treatment in a patient with cancer, and manipulation of insulin by an individual with diabetes in an effort to lose weight. Many different types of psychological factors—for example, symptoms of depression or anxiety, stressful life events, personality traits, and coping styles—have been shown to adversely influence medical conditions. The adverse effects can range from acute, with immediate medical consequences (e.g., refusal to seek care during an acute myocardial infarction), to chronic, occurring over a long period of time (e.g., stress leading to overeating and obesity).

Ulcers

Eileen Cameron, a 42-year-old trial lawyer who is married and the mother of two children, is referred to a psychologist for consultation by her gastroenterologist following her third episode of duodenal ulcer disease. Her ulcer disease was first diagnosed 4 years ago. At that time she completed a course of antibiotics for *Helicobacter pylori* (the bacterium discovered to play an important role in the development of peptic ulcer disease) and was advised to avoid taking nonsteroidal anti-inflammatory drugs (NSAIDs) and to limit alcohol consumption. The gastroenterologist has requested the consultation because he wonders if stress may be contributing to her condition.

Mrs. Cameron appears exactly on time for her appointment; she is neatly and conservatively dressed. She presents an organized, coherent account of her medical problem and denies any past or immediate family history of significant mental disorder. She states, "Ulcers are supposed to be related to stress, and that just isn't true with me." During the last 4 years, her workload has increased considerably after having been assigned to work on several dramatic and highly taxing court cases, which she said she won although the credit was taken by the senior partner in the firm. She married a law school classmate, who is also quite successful. Their marriage is strained because she feels he leaves most responsibilities involving the household and children for her to handle. Last year one of the children was hospitalized after an anaphylactic reaction to peanuts.

The psychologist reflected back to the patient that she did indeed have a great deal of stress in her life and wondered how she managed to handle it all so capably. Mrs. Cameron paused and replied, "I get done what has to be done, and don't think about the rest." The psychologist suggested that exploring alternative ways to cope would likely make her feel better, and might even reduce risk of another ulcer, and Mrs. Cameron agreed.

Discussion of "Ulcers"

In the past, certain disorders such as duodenal ulcer were assumed to be caused by emotional factors (a very early edition of DSM classified it as a Psychophysiological Disorder). Now, however, these disorders are understood to be multifactorial in etiology, involving biological, social, and psychological factors. Peptic ulcer disease is highly associated with infection with *H. pylori* and/or with taking NSAIDs, but many people who have *H. pylori* infections or who take NSAIDs do not develop peptic ulcer disease. The incidence of peptic ulcer disease has been shown to be increased with disasters, job stress, family conflict, depression, and hostility. As is typical in these kinds of cases, it is difficult to establish the strength of the relationship between the stressors and the patient's recurrent ulcer disease. However, the observation that Mrs. Cameron's ulcer disease has grown worse coincident with her increased stress at work and at home is highly suggestive of the possibility that stress is exacerbating her peptic ulcer disease, justifying the DSM-5-TR diagnosis of Psychological Factors Affecting Other Medical Condition (DSM-5-TR, p. 364).

9.5
Factitious Disorder

Factitious Disorder is characterized by the individual's falsification of medical or psychological signs and symptoms in self or others. The word *factitious* comes from the Latin word for "artificial." Most symptoms in people with this disorder are related to physical illness—symptoms such as chest pain, stomach problems, or fever—rather than a mental disorder.

The diagnosis requires demonstrating that the individual is misrepresenting, simulating, or causing signs or symptoms of illness or injury. For example, individuals with Factitious Disorder might report feelings of depression and suicidality related to the death of a spouse—even though a death did not occur or the individual did not even have a spouse; deceptively report episodes of neurological symptoms (e.g., seizures, dizziness, blacking out); manipulate a laboratory test (e.g., by adding blood to urine) to falsely indicate an abnormality; falsify medical records to indicate an illness; ingest a substance (e.g., insulin) to induce an abnormal laboratory result such as low blood sugar; or physically injure themselves or induce illness in themselves or another person (e.g., by injecting fecal material to produce an abscess or to induce a blood infection).

Factitious Disorder comes in two forms. The more common form of this rare condition is Factitious Disorder Imposed on Self, in which the individual presents themself as ill, impaired, or injured. It has been hypothesized that the motivation for the deceptive behavior in Factitious Disorder is a desire to assume the sick role to obtain the sympathy and special attention given to people who are truly ill. In Factitious Disorder Imposed on Another (formerly called Factious Disorder by Proxy), the individual produces or fabricates symptoms of illness in a dependent (e.g., child, elderly adult, disabled person, pet) and then takes the victim for medical care while denying any knowledge about the cause of the problem. In such cases, the diagnosis of Factitious Disorder is not given to the individual presenting with the apparent medical problems, who is the victim of abuse, but rather to the perpetrator, who is the one with the mental disorder.

The diagnosis should not be made if there are obvious external rewards to be obtained by appearing to be sick or injured, such as collecting insurance money as a compensation for an "injury," qualifying for medical disability, or evading criminal responsibility or military service. In such cases, the person is considered to be Malingering, which is not considered to be a mental disorder but is included in the DSM-5-TR chapter "Other Conditions That May Be a Focus of Clinical Attention" (DSM-5-TR, p. 835).

There are no reliable statistics regarding the number of people who have Factitious Disorder, given that obtaining accurate statistics is difficult because dishonesty is a core feature of this disorder. In addition, people with Factitious Disorder tend to seek treatment at many different health care facilities, resulting in statistics that are misleading because the same patient may be counted multiple times. It is estimated that about 1% of individuals admitted to hospitals may have Factitious Disorder.

Fraulein von Willebrand

Jane Powell, a 29-year-old laboratory technician, was admitted to the medical service via the emergency room because of blood in her urine. Ms. Powell said that she was being treated for systemic lupus erythematosus (SLE; an autoimmune disease characterized by acute and chronic inflammation of various tissues of the body) by a physician located in a different city. She also mentioned having had von Willebrand disease (a rare hereditary blood disorder that can cause extended or excessive bleeding) as a child. On the third day of her hospitalization, a medical student mentioned to the resident that she had seen this patient several weeks earlier at a different hospital in the area, where the patient had been admitted for the same problem but had left that hospital suddenly before the workup could be completed. The fact that she neglected to report such a recent prior hospitalization raised suspicions among the hospital staff and prompted a search of the patient's belongings, which revealed a cache of anticoagulant medication. When confronted with this information, Ms. Powell refused to discuss the matter and hurriedly signed out of the hospital against medical advice.

Discussion of "Fraulein von Willebrand"

Ms. Powell presented to the emergency room with blood in her urine, a symptom that is easily confirmed on urinalysis and might be expected in someone with a history of a hereditary bleeding disorder combined with SLE. One of the more serious complications of SLE is lupus nephritis, in which the immune system attacks the part of the kidneys that filter the blood for waste products. The combination of blood in the urine plus a history of both SLE and von Willebrand disease prompted admission to the hospital for a full workup for blood in the urine. However, the discovery that Ms. Powell had neglected to inform the medical staff that she had recently been in the hospital for the same problem, combined with the fact that she had anticoagulant medication in her belongings, strongly suggested that the blood in her urine was not a symptom of a bona fide medical illness but instead was a consequence of her taking unprescribed anticoagulant medication. She presumably brought a cache of this medication with her so she could continue to induce urinary tract bleeding during her hospital stay in order to keep up the charade. As is often typical with such patients, as soon as attempts were made to confront her about her deception, she discharged herself from the hospital.

In the face of this likely deception, the only diagnostic issue is whether Ms. Powell's behavior is explained by a mental illness (i.e., Factitious Disorder) or whether it represents Malingering. The absence of apparent external rewards for her behavior, such as attempting to get disability payments, points toward the diagnosis of Factitious Disorder Imposed on Self (DSM-5-TR, p. 367). It has been suggested that one way to prevent patients from getting unnecessary tests and treatments for their feigned conditions is for hospitals to maintain a registry of such patients once they are identified as having Factitious Disorder, something that would have potentially identified Ms. Powell in the emergency room.

Take Me Seriously

Clara Beaumont was a 56-year-old unmarried woman who presented to an outpatient mental health care clinic for help in refuting a diagnosis of Factitious Disorder that had been suggested to her by a medical provider (although he did not feel comfortable documenting this in her medical chart). Her initial reason for seeking therapy was to have an expert in Factitious Disorder provide written documentation that she did not have Factitious Disorder so that her doctors would take her medical complaints seriously and provide the treatment that she felt she required.

She reported a long history of medical problems, including osteonecrosis (bone death caused by poor blood supply) that necessitated previous shoulder and knee joint replacements; current chronic obstructive pulmonary disease (COPD) requiring supplemental oxygen; ovarian cancer, which was in remission at the time she was seen; and a host of other medical illnesses and injuries. At the initial interview, she appeared 10 years older than her stated age, was very frail, and was unable to walk without the assistance of a wheelchair. The few medical records that were obtained included compelling X-ray verification of the osteonecrosis and the COPD, but no evidence of the other illnesses or injuries. They also contained indicators of medical deception, such as her reporting exaggerated symptoms (e.g., a 3-week period of constant diarrhea and vomiting that did not require hospitalization for hydration) and patently false or improbable information about her prior medical history (e.g., fever of 108° F). She was selective in providing consent for the clinic to obtain her past medical records and insisted that some records had been lost or destroyed in Hurricane Katrina. In telephone conversations, her primary care physician refuted numerous diagnoses and recommendations that Ms. Beaumont had attributed to him, including her need for a wheelchair, a recommendation that she enter hospice care, and video EEG confirmation of a seizure disorder.

Over the course of three extended diagnostic interview sessions, Ms. Beaumont reported a medical and social history that became increasingly fantastic, and the telling of her story became increasingly dramatic. In addition to her dubious medical history, she claimed to have been married to a man who developed a brain tumor that caused him to go missing for months and who later turned up dead; she stated that she was a successful child actor and a champion junior golfer; and she claimed that she and her husband were forced to flee their home and jobs when they uncovered an illegal drug operation. The majority of the claims she made could not be verified, and when asked to provide documentation, she provided equally fantastic explanations for why the documentation could not be obtained (e.g., a house fire in which family photos were all destroyed). Despite the questionably delusional quality of her representations, there was no evidence of disorganized thinking (which would be characteristic of Schizophrenia), and her results on the Minnesota Multiphasic Personality Inventory suggested no evidence of a Psychotic Disorder but did show indicators of interpersonal insecurity consistent with Borderline Personality Disorder.

Ms. Beaumont lived in abject poverty. She had no source of income and no living family members or friends. She lived with a man with a chronic mental disorder, sharing his Social Security disability benefits. He served as her caregiver. Beyond this man, her social support network comprised only people who were involved in her life on the basis of her status as a medical patient. She used her representations of her medical problems to solicit caring and kindness from local civic and church groups that helped her with clothes, food, and temporary lodging.

Pharmacy records indicated that Ms. Beaumont had successfully used a large roster of medical providers, who appear to have been unaware of one another, to obtain narcotic analgesic medicine. She had several hospitalizations that appeared to be related to drug overdoses, but she denied that characterization.

The results of her initial diagnostic evaluation, a review of her available medical records, and discussions with her general practitioner indicated that she did indeed have Factitious Disorder. In more than 50 subsequent treatment sessions, an attempt was made to help her minimize her factitious illness behavior and improve her communication with her doctors so that she could secure effective medical care.

Ms. Beaumont died of respiratory arrest not long after she discontinued treatment. No autopsy was performed, so the exact cause of her respiratory arrest is unknown. However, her caregiver admitted to improvising with her medicines to help her achieve pain relief.

Discussion of "Take Me Seriously"

In contrast to the previous case of Factitious Disorder ("Fraulein von Willebrand"), in which the patient created what at first appeared to be legitimate medical symptoms by deceptively self-administering unprescribed anticoagulant medication, this case is about a patient whose deceptive behavior involves lying about symptoms and her past medical history. In this case, however, the diagnosis of Factitious Disorder is complicated by the presence of 1) verified medical illnesses (i.e., osteonecrosis and COPD) and 2) multiple external incentives that might account for exaggerated illness behavior and suggest the presence of Malingering (i.e., her opioid-seeking behavior and her use of representations of her medical problems to solicit caring and kindness from civic and church groups). Despite these complicating factors, it was clear that Ms. Beaumont's dramatic and exaggerated representations of her medical conditions were deceptive in nature and were not used solely to leverage requests for narcotic medication or material support. Thus, the diagnosis is Factitious Disorder Imposed on Self (DSM-5-TR, p. 367).

Ms. Beaumont's presentation conforms to Munchausen syndrome, a particularly severe and chronic form of Factitious Disorder with physical symptoms first identified in 1851. This syndrome was named for Baron von Münchhausen, an eighteenth-century German officer who was renowned for embellishing his stories of his life and experiences. Although the term "Munchausen syndrome" is widely used interchangeably with Factitious Disorder, it is in fact a distinct type with three components: feigning illness, wandering from place to place (usually from hospital to hospital), and pathological lying. Ms. Beaumont has no family or social ties, no work or professional identity, and no permanent place of residence, living an itinerant life that was singularly defined by her status as a medical patient. Ms. Beaumont's fantastic tales of accomplishments, high status, and persecution are evidence of her tendency toward pathological lying. Moreover, the presence of pathological lying can aid in differentiating Factitious Disorder from the behavior of Malingering. Whereas people who malinger typically use only the minimal deception and attention seeking required to achieve their goals, patients with Factitious Disorder, for whom attention is usually the primary aim, engage in audacious deceptions that go well beyond what is necessary to achieve instrumental gains.

Although Ms. Beaumont's excessive illness behaviors cannot be adequately accounted for as solely drug-seeking behaviors, there is no doubt that she also had an opioid addiction. Also, she had a genuine pain-related condition (i.e., osteonecrosis) for which opioid medication was a reasonable management strategy. In this case, however, Ms. Beaumont's excessive and dramatic illness enactments understandably caused her doctors to be reluctant to treat her bone pain as they might in a patient without Factitious Disorder. Although understandable, failure to adequately treat Ms. Beaumont's pain is a medical error, as is succumbing to her requests for unnecessary assessments and treatments. Indeed, any departures from standards of care—both overtreatment and undertreatment—are hallmarks of Factitious Disorder cases.

It is also important to guard against hasty conclusions that a link between illness behavior and external material benefits supports the identification of Malingering behavior. Patients seeking material support from family, friends, and community groups may not be motivated by financial gain, but instead may be soliciting such support as evidence that they are loved, cared for, and appreciated.

Medical Miscreant

Chris, an 11-year-old boy, is brought in by his mother for examination. His medical problems had emerged after he suffered a nasty fall from a spiral staircase while at a party with his family when he was 6 years old. Despite a complete recovery within days of the accident, he has continued to receive medical attention for a bewildering array of problems, many unrelated to his fall. At the insistence of his mother, a 41-year-old hospital clerk, Chris has been assessed by neurologists in California for seizures, visual deficits, and severe headaches suggestive of fluid buildup in the brain. His mother has taken him to out-of-state hospitals for investigation of vocal cord dysfunction, thyroiditis (inflammation of the thyroid gland), difficulty eating and drinking, excessive urination, and autoimmune disease. Chris has even been examined by psychiatrists for amnesia, autism, posttraumatic stress symptoms, and Attention-Deficit/Hyperactivity Disorder (ADHD), following reports from his mother of poor behavioral control and difficulty concentrating. However, at no point during these extensive workups have any objective signs of illness been found, and in the current examination, Chris has generally appeared to be a normal, healthy boy. In fact, when interviewed, Chris has been unable to describe any of his symptoms, much to the amazement of the care team, who are under the impression that he suffers from a host of chronic and severe disorders. This confusion is due to the false medical history provided to them by his mother, who knows perfectly well that Chris is not sick.

Faced with a confusing clinical picture and unrelenting pressure from a child's mother, many clinicians have been convinced to pursue aggressive diagnostic studies or treatments. At times, Chris's mother has supplemented her child's fabricated history with additional false information, claiming variously to be a registered nurse with pediatric expertise, to have medical documents that confirm the findings of serious illnesses, or to have witnessed the negligence of staff members formerly involved in Chris's care. The medical history she relates on her son's behalf is often inconsistent and occasionally outright nonsensical. Sometimes, Chris's "symptoms" take the form of illnesses his mother herself has falsely claimed to have, including ADHD and autoimmune disease. When she has been unable to gain the support of a doctor, she has sought an alternative opinion or traveled to another hospital.

In the course of his mother's deception, Chris has undergone a disturbing series of procedures. His mother has welcomed, if not actively solicited, even very uncomfortable procedures for her son. Remarkably, these interventions have included a period of water deprivation to investigate his alleged excessive urination and the installation of a feeding tube. For 5 years, no specialist or subspecialist has been able to bring about the slightest improvement of his "symptoms." In fact, in combination with a heavy medication regimen, these treatments have resulted in considerable disability for Chris. His impairments, both real and falsified, have made his family eligible for state financial support. While Chris has been deprived of a social life of his own, his mother has thrived on the opportunity to present herself to her peers as the heroic, if not indefatigable, caregiver of a sick child.

Chris was subsequently removed from his mother's care, following a report filed with Child Protective Services by a teacher concerned that he had needlessly been enrolled by his mother in a school for autistic children. His health has since improved, and he has been weaned successfully from most of the medications he had been taking. His mother was arrested and charged with child endangerment.

Discussion of "Medical Miscreant"

The essential feature of Factitious Disorder Imposed on Another (DSM-5-TR, p. 367) is the falsification of medical or psychological signs and symptoms in another person, associated with deceptive behavior. Chris's mother shows a clear and persistent desire to manipulate the medical system, with a psychological need for her son to be viewed as severely ill, if not incapacitated. Although there was a financial incentive for her illness deception, Chris's "symptoms" far exceeded the threshold for state financial support, and therefore this incentive cannot be seen as the primary motivation for her behavior.

Of significant concern in this case was the willingness of numerous health professionals to subject Chris to painful procedures with a high risk of harm in response to reports made by his mother rather than on the basis of objective clinical evidence. When diagnostic studies had normal results or when clinicians expressed doubts concerning the "symptoms" under review, Chris's mother refused to comply with medical recommendations and habitually attempted to discredit the clinicians involved. Doctors were accused, sometimes publicly, of not being advocates for her child. Chris's mother also falsely claimed to have worked in pediatric care to enhance the credibility of her claims. This campaign of intimidation and deception impelled clinicians to act on a clinical picture that was highly suspicious.

The motivations underlying Factitious Disorder Imposed on Another are often unclear. Because perpetrators desire sympathy and attention, they manipulate both their victim and the health care system. The fact that Chris's mother herself had a history of Factitious Disorder also raises questions regarding her attitudes toward illness. Unchecked, her actions could have resulted in Chris's permanent disability or even death. This case highlights the need for health care professionals to consider Factitious Disorder Imposed on Another when presented with children whose signs and symptoms do not make medical sense or lack corroborative clinical evidence. Improvement of the child while separated from the suspected parent is a strong indicator of medical deception.

CHAPTER 10

Feeding and Eating Disorders

Changes in eating and eating-related behavior may be a feature of various mental disorders (e.g., losing weight during a depression because the individual does not have an appetite); thus, eating disturbances in and of themselves do not indicate that a Feeding and Eating Disorder is present. However, the disorders classified in the DSM-5-TR chapter "Feeding and Eating Disorders" are those whose primary manifestations are persistent disturbances in "eating or eating-related behavior that results in the altered consumption or absorption of food and that significantly impairs physical health or psychosocial functioning" (DSM-5-TR, p. 371). With these disorders, a person's eating can be disturbed in any of several ways, including by persistently eating things that are not normally considered food (Pica), repeatedly regurgitating food before it has been absorbed in the gastrointestinal tract (Rumination Disorder), not eating enough food for a variety of reasons other than to be thin (Avoidant/Restrictive Food Intake Disorder; ARFID), starving themselves in order to be extremely thin (Anorexia Nervosa), binge eating and purging (Bulimia Nervosa), and binge eating without purging (Binge-Eating Disorder). (Table 10–1 lists characteristic features of these Feeding and Eating Disorders.)

Anorexia Nervosa, Bulimia Nervosa, and Binge-Eating Disorder are mutually exclusive for a given episode of illness, so only one diagnosis can be given at a time. The reason for this diagnostic convention is that although these disorders share some behavioral and psychological features, they have different longitudinal courses, outcomes, and treatment needs.

TABLE 10–1. **Characteristic features of Feeding and Eating Disorders**

Disorder	Key characteristics
Pica	Eating of nonnutritive, nonfood substances
Rumination Disorder	Regurgitation of food
Avoidant/Restrictive Food Intake Disorder	Avoidance or restriction of food intake associated with significant weight loss, nutritional deficiency, dependence on nutritional supplements, or interference with psychosocial functioning
Anorexia Nervosa	Restriction of energy intake, leading to significantly low body weight
	Intense fear of gaining weight or of becoming fat
	Disturbance in how one's body weight or shape is experienced
Bulimia Nervosa	Binge eating
	Inappropriate compensatory behaviors to prevent weight gain
	Self-evaluation unduly influenced by body shape and weight
Binge-Eating Disorder	Binge eating
	No inappropriate compensatory behaviors to prevent weight gain
	Binge eating not exclusively during course of Bulimia Nervosa or Anorexia Nervosa

10.1
Pica

Pica is characterized by the persistent eating of nonnutritive, nonfood substances. Typical substances that may be consumed include "paper, soap, cloth, hair, string, wool, soil, chalk, talcum powder, paint, gum, metal, pebbles, charcoal or coal, ash, clay, starch, or ice" (DSM-5-TR, p. 372). A diagnosis of Pica does not apply when infants accidentally ingest something that they are mouthing, as they commonly do.

Pica may occur at any age, although it is most common in children. Its prevalence among school-age children is estimated at about 5%. Pica occurs in both sexes, but it is most prevalent (28%) among pregnant and postpartum women, particularly those with food insecurity. Pregnant women who have cravings for nonnutritive, nonfood substances, such as chalk, are not given a diagnosis of Pica unless the behavior causes or poses a risk for medical problems. In children, Autism Spectrum Disorder and Intellectual Developmental Disorder commonly co-occur with Pica. In older individuals, Pica is most often associated with Schizophrenia, Obsessive-Compulsive Disorder, Trichotillomania, or Excoriation Disorder. Pica can be a chronic and serious disorder because it may lead to medical emergencies (e.g., intestinal obstruction, poisoning) or to nutritional deficiencies.

Omnivorous George

George, a thin, pale 5-year-old, was admitted to the hospital for nutritional anemia (a condition in which a person has fewer red blood cells than normal and feels very weak and tired) that seemed to be due to his ingestion of paint, plaster, dirt, wood, and paste. He had had numerous hospitalizations under similar circumstances, beginning at age 19 months, when he had ingested lighter fluid.

George's parents subsisted on welfare and were described as immature and passive. He was the product of an unplanned but normal pregnancy. His mother began eating dirt when she was pregnant, at age 16 years. His father periodically abused drugs and alcohol.

Discussion of "Omnivorous George"

Eating of nonnutritive substances may be developmentally appropriate for an infant, but its persistence up to age 5 warrants a diagnosis of Pica (DSM-5-TR, p. 371). As in this case, it is commonly associated with a similar history in the mother during pregnancy and with low socioeconomic status.

In some cultural settings, the eating of nonnutritive substances, such as clay, may be a sanctioned practice, in which case the diagnosis would not apply, but that certainly is not true for George. In other cases, the disturbance may be associated with other disorders, such as Intellectual Developmental Disorder, Autism Spectrum Disorder, Schizophrenia, or the neurological disorder Kleine-Levin syndrome.

10.2
Rumination Disorder

Rumination Disorder is characterized by "repeated regurgitation of food occurring after feeding or eating" (DSM-5-TR, p. 374). The regurgitated food may be partially digested and may be re-chewed, re-swallowed, or spit out. The regurgitation is not caused by a gastrointestinal condition, such as gastroesophageal reflux (in which food from the stomach reenters the esophagus and potentially the mouth because of a relaxation of the esophageal sphincter) or pyloric stenosis (a narrowing of the exit from the stomach into the small intestine). Individuals with Anorexia Nervosa (see Section 10.4) or Bulimia Nervosa (see Section 10.5) may regurgitate and spit out food as a means of getting rid of ingested calories and controlling weight gain. If the eating disturbance is considered a symptom of one of these other Eating Disorders, a diagnosis of Rumination Disorder is not made. If rumination occurs in the context of another mental disorder, such as Intellectual Developmental Disorder, the diagnosis of Rumination Disorder is made only if symptoms are severe enough to warrant special clinical attention.

Rumination Disorder can occur in infancy, childhood, adolescence, or adulthood. It is most common among infants between ages 3 and 12 months. It can be a serious disorder because it can lead to malnutrition, growth delay, and developmental and learning problems. It can be fatal in infants.

Baby Olivia

Olivia was taken to the hospital at age 6 months by an aunt, for evaluation of failure to gain weight. She had been born into an impoverished family after an unplanned, uncomplicated pregnancy. During the first 4 months of her life, Olivia gained weight steadily. Regurgitation was first noted during the fifth month, and then it increased in severity to the point where she was regurgitating after every feeding. After each feeding, Olivia would engage in one of two behaviors: 1) she would open her mouth, elevate her tongue, and rapidly thrust it back and forward, after which milk would appear at the back of her mouth and slowly trickle out, or 2) she would vigorously suck her thumb and place fingers in her mouth, following which milk would slowly flow out of the corner of her mouth.

In the past 2 months, Olivia had been cared for by a number of people, including her aunt and paternal grandmother. Her parents were making a marginal marital adjustment and often talked about separation or divorce. Nevertheless, Olivia often smiles and is responsive to all of her caregivers.

Discussion of "Baby Olivia"

In an infant for whom nonpsychiatric medical conditions have been ruled out, weight loss or failure to gain weight suggests Rumination Disorder, ARFID (see "Bottle Baby" in Section 10.3), or Reactive Attachment Disorder (see "Grandma's Child" in Section 7.1). It is clear in this case that Olivia is not gaining weight because of the regurgitation of food after each feeding, indicating the presence of Rumination Disorder (DSM-5-TR, p. 374). Typically, a child with this disorder strains and arches their back and makes sucking movements with their tongue. The food is ejected from their mouth or re-chewed and re-swallowed. The child often gives the impression of gaining considerable satisfaction from the activity. As in this case, the disorder usually appears between 3 and 12 months of age.

There is a suggestion in Olivia's case that the quality of parental care may have been inadequate. However, the absence of any evidence of inappropriate social relatedness on Olivia's part rules out the diagnosis of Reactive Attachment Disorder. Also, because the cause of the weight loss is the regurgitation and not a lack of interest in eating or food, or avoidance of food because of its sensory characteristics, the diagnosis of ARFID (see Section 10.3) would not apply.

10.3
Avoidant/Restrictive
Food Intake Disorder

ARFID is characterized by "avoidance or restriction of food intake" (DSM-5-TR, p. 376) associated with a lack of interest in eating or food, food avoidance based on extreme sensitivity to the sensory (e.g., color, smell, texture, temperature, taste) characteristics of food, or concern about negative consequences of eating (e.g., choking, vomiting). The eating disturbance results in weight loss or failure to gain weight (in children), nutritional deficiency, the need for food supplements, or impairment in psychosocial (school, work, and social) functioning.

Although ARFID occurs most frequently in infancy and early childhood (when it is commonly known as "failure to thrive"), in DSM-5-TR, the diagnostic concept has been expanded to include food avoidance or restriction that occurs in individuals of any age. ARFID thus subsumes "choosy eating" or "chronic food refusal" that is not related to Anorexia Nervosa (see Section 10.4) or Bulimia Nervosa (see Section 10.5), is not attributable to a concurrent nonpsychiatric medical condition, and is not better explained by another mental disorder. ARFID may occur in association with other mental disorders, such as Anxiety Disorders, Obsessive-Compulsive Disorder, Autism Spectrum Disorder, Intellectual Developmental Disorder, or Attention-Deficit/Hyperactivity Disorder. In such cases, ARFID is diagnosed in addition to the other disorder if the food avoidance is particularly severe or requires special clinical attention. If gastrointestinal problems (e.g., gastroesophageal reflux) are the cause of the patient's food avoidance, a diagnosis of ARFID is not warranted.

Bottle Baby

Six-month-old Roberto was admitted to a hospital for evaluation of his failure to gain weight when, at 15 pounds, he fell below the 15th percentile for weight for his age. He was the second of two children born to working-class parents following an unplanned but normal pregnancy. He weighed almost 9 pounds at birth.

Although Roberto, as the only son, was the apple of his father's eye, Roberto's mother had had continual difficulties with the infant. He was bottle-fed, and his mother reported that he had severe colic (i.e., recurrent episodes of prolonged crying and irritability). His pediatrician made several formula changes and suggested other treatments for colic, but Roberto continued to fail to gain weight.

In the hospital, nurses watched his mother attempt to feed him. There was poor synchrony between the mother and baby around feeding, in that his mother often did not seem to know when Roberto was hungry, when he needed to be burped, and when he was finished eating. Consequently, Roberto seemed often disinterested in feeding, which became a distressing experience for both mother and child. However, the nurses and aides were able to feed Roberto without any difficulty. Various medical investigations failed to disclose any specific medical condition that might account for the baby's difficulties. Discussion with the mother gradually revealed that she had been depressed throughout the pregnancy and resented the baby's demands. Treatment of her depression and the underlying marital problems, as well as focused instruction on feeding, facilitated the mother's adjustment. Roberto's feeding difficulties gradually diminished, and within a few weeks he gained several pounds.

Discussion of "Bottle Baby"

ARFID (DSM-5-TR, p. 376) is diagnosed when a child fails to eat adequately, which results in a significant failure to gain weight or a significant weight loss, and when the condition, as in this case, cannot be better accounted for by a nonpsychiatric medical condition (e.g., gastroesophageal reflux), by simple absence of available food, or by Rumination Disorder (see "Baby Olivia" in Section 10.2). In Rumination Disorder, weight loss is sometimes observed, but it is accompanied by characteristic regurgitation and re-chewing or spitting out of food.

In this case, marital problems and maternal depression probably contributed to the mother's difficulties in feeding Roberto. Problems in parent-child interactions are known to contribute to the infant's feeding problems in some instances.

Picky Eater

Nicole is a 14-year-old ninth grader whose mother brought her to treatment because of concerns about Nicole's ability to socialize with peers outside of school and her timidity in approaching new situations.

Nicole states that she prefers to be alone and finds going to parties or any new places difficult. She avoids eating in public, when possible, but she will eat a limited amount at school lunch because she is unable to go the whole school day without eating. She takes a grilled cheese sandwich to school daily for lunch and is embarrassed that her friends notice that she eats the same thing every day and does not eat very much. She refuses to go to restaurants or to any parties where food is served.

Nicole has limited preferred foods: white bread and butter, crepes, grilled cheese, pizza, yogurt drinks, milk, and one brand of juice. She does not eat fruits, vegetables, meat, or chicken. She avoids trying new foods because she does not like new textures and worries about experiencing abdominal pain after trying new foods. Although Nicole does not focus on any particular experience when abdominal pain has caused her problems, she limits both the quantity and the type of food to minimize the risk of stomach upset. It is notable that Nicole's preferred foods are all soft, bland, and generally colorless with the exception of pizza.

Nicole worries about evaluation by others in situations beyond eating or meals, including giving presentations in class, speaking when the teacher calls on her, or introducing herself to a new person. She reports having many friends but not a best friend.

Nicole has always been below the normal curve for weight on a growth chart. She recently has grown significantly in height so that she is now below the 1st percentile for weight (73 pounds) but is in the 90th percentile for height (5'7"); therefore, she has become even more significantly underweight. Nicole has not started menstruating, which may be attributable to low weight/body fat; in contrast, her mother's menarche was at age 11. Nicole acknowledges that she is tall and lanky. She denies any concerns about her appearance. She understands that she may be too thin to begin menstruating and she wants to avoid having any medical problems. She denies any concern about how she would look if she gained weight (to a medically healthy weight that allows menarche), but she is overwhelmed about the prospect of needing to eat more food or different foods that may provide more nutritional value.

Nicole's developmental history is remarkable for early feeding concerns. She was started on formula because of a suspected milk allergy, but she refused to drink soy-based formula and ultimately had to be switched to a milk-based formula, which she tolerated. Her mother recalls that when introduced to solid foods, Nicole often threw new foods on the floor and refused to try them even after they were offered on multiple occasions (as recommended by the pediatrician). Her mother states that Nicole ate a slightly larger variety of foods at a young age but never ate fruits, vegetables, or proteins beyond dairy. Otherwise, she met developmental milestones within normal time frames and has done well in school academically. Because of Nicole's feeding difficulties, her mother once requested a medical assessment and a barium swallow study of Nicole's gastrointestinal tract, which showed no abnormalities.

Nicole's treatment was informed by the evidence-based treatments used in Eating and Anxiety Disorders. Her comorbid social anxiety symptoms caused significant impairment; therefore, the severity of her anxiety was considered to be in the moderate to severe range, for which the recommended treatment is a combination of medication (a selective serotonin reuptake inhibitor; SSRI) and cognitive-behavioral therapy (CBT). Fluoxetine was initiated, as well as weekly CBT. The reasoning underlying these treatments is that a lowered anxiety level allows for less rigidity overall, which extends into the realm of feeding and eating behavior, and/or that anxiety underlies avoidant and restrictive eating, in which case the SSRI is more directly therapeutic. Treatment goals to increase Nicole's ability to eat in different settings were incorporated into her social anxiety hierarchy. A separate hierarchy was established with feared foods to expand her food variety, and parent management strategies informed by family-based treatment used for Anorexia Nervosa were implemented to increase Nicole's food intake. Additionally, phobia exposure work was used to target Nicole's concerns about abdominal pain.

Discussion of "Picky Eater"

Several disorders need to be considered as possible explanations for Nicole's restricted repertoire of eating. If she had a disturbance in the way she experienced her body weight and shape and an intense fear of gaining weight or becoming fat, she might be diagnosed as having Anorexia Nervosa (see "Sixty-Seven Pound Weakling" in Section 10.4). However, she acknowledges that she is tall and lanky, and she denies any concerns about her appearance or how she would look if she gained weight, so the diagnosis of Anorexia Nervosa does not apply. Nicole also reports embarrassment in situations in which she is eating the same thing every day at school and has some social anxiety that extends beyond her eating behavior to making presentations in class, answering teacher questions, meeting new people, and trying new activities. These concerns may warrant a diagnosis of Social Anxiety Disorder (see "Mail Sorter" in Section 5.4), but embarrassment about eating in public does not appear to capture the essence of her eating problems. When a person experiences significant weight loss or fails to gain expected weight for their age because of food restriction based on the sensory characteristics of certain foods (she eats only soft, bland, and colorless food) and/or the potentially aversive consequences of eating (she worries about developing abdominal pain), the diagnosis is ARFID (DSM-5-TR, p. 376).

This case illustrates that ARFID usually manifests in childhood, but it can persist into adolescence (and beyond). Also, even though Nicole does not have Anorexia Nervosa, some of the same treatment techniques that are used with such patients to encourage healthy eating and healthy portions can also be useful in ARFID. Treatments for mental disorders are often symptom or problem focused rather than diagnosis specific.

10.4
Anorexia Nervosa

Anorexia Nervosa is characterized by 1) persistent refusal to maintain body weight; 2) fears of gaining weight or becoming fat, or behavior that interferes with weight gain; and 3) a disturbance in self-perceived weight or shape (DSM-5-TR, p. 381). A person with Anorexia Nervosa maintains a weight that is significantly below normal for the person's age, sex, developmental stage, and physical health. The individual has lost a significant amount of weight or failed to make expected weight gains (in the case of a child or adolescent), either as a result of dieting, fasting, or excessive exercise (noted with the subtype Restricting Type) or, if also engaging in eating binges, as a result of self-induced vomiting or misuse of laxatives, diuretics, or enemas (noted with the subtype Binge-Eating/Purging Type). The fear of gaining weight or of becoming fat often persists, or even increases, as weight is lost. Some individuals with Anorexia Nervosa deny a fear of becoming fat but do things to interfere with maintaining their weight, such as engaging in self-starvation. Some people with Anorexia Nervosa feel fat all over, whereas others focus on specific parts of their bodies—commonly their abdomens, buttocks, or thighs—which they insist are "fat," and they are constantly weighing and measuring themselves and checking their appearance in a mirror. Weight loss is perceived as a sign of self-control; weight gain is a failure. Those who acknowledge that they are thin often deny the medical seriousness of their condition.

Although laboratory findings are not used as diagnostic criteria for Anorexia Nervosa, a number of laboratory abnormalities can be observed that can increase confidence in the diagnosis. Such findings may include a low white blood cell count, elevated blood urea nitrogen (indicative of dehydration), elevated liver enzymes, low levels of thyroid and sex hormones, low blood pressure, slow heart rate, low bone density, and abnormal electroencephalogram. Physical signs of Anorexia Nervosa may include emaciation, amenorrhea (not menstruating), delayed menarche (if pre-pubertal), peripheral edema (swelling of the legs), increased size of the salivary glands (in persons who self-induce vomiting), and dental enamel erosion.

In the United States, the 12-month prevalence of Anorexia Nervosa ranges from 0.00% to 0.05%, with much higher rates in women (0.0%–0.8%) than in men (0.0%–0.1%). The lifetime prevalence if the disorder ranges from 0.60% to 0.80%, with women outnumbering men by about 5–7:1. Anorexia Nervosa usually begins during adolescence or young adulthood. It is an extremely serious condition and can be life-threatening because malnutrition negatively affects many of the body's major organ systems. Obsessive-compulsive behaviors surrounding food and other issues are common. A diagnosis of Obsessive-Compulsive Disorder (see "Thin Tim," later in this section) is made if the obsessions and compulsions are not related to food, body shape, or weight. Cultural values of "thinness," and occupations and avocations that encourage thinness, such as modeling and some athletics, may increase the risk for Anorexia Nervosa.

The course of Anorexia Nervosa is variable, with some individuals having only a single episode, some having remissions and relapses, and some having a chronic course. Hospitalizations may be necessitated by medical complications. Most individuals with Anorexia Nervosa experience symptom remission within 5 years of the initial diagnosis. Suicide risk is elevated in Anorexia Nervosa, with rates estimated at 18 times greater than in gender- and age-matched comparison subjects. Suicide is the second leading cause of death in Anorexia Nervosa (medical complications of the disorder are the first). Bipolar, Depressive, and Anxiety Disorders commonly co-occur with Anorexia Nervosa. Obsessive-Compulsive Disorder is described in some individuals with Anorexia Nervosa, especially those with the Restricting Type.

Sixty-Seven Pound Weakling

When Peggy Sims was first evaluated for admission to an inpatient eating disorders program, she was a 20-year-old woman who had difficulty supporting her 5'3" body with a weight of only 67 pounds. She had begun to lose weight 4 years earlier, initially dieting to lose an unwanted 6 pounds. Encouraged by compliments on her new body, she proceeded to lose 8 more pounds. Over the next 2 years, Ms. Sims continued to lose weight and increased her physical activity until her weight reached a low of 64 pounds; she stopped menstruating. She was admitted to a medical unit, treated for peptic ulcer disease, and discharged, only to be admitted 3 months later to the psychiatric unit of a general hospital. During that 8-week hospitalization, her weight increased from 84 to 100 pounds. She did well until she went off to college, where, with increased academic and social demands, she again began to diet until she weighed only 67 pounds. She reported that she had become troubled by changes in her body when she was heavier, and she became increasingly anxious as her figure developed. Her eating habits were ritualized: she cut food into very small pieces, moved it around on the plate, and ate very slowly. She resisted eating foods with high fat and carbohydrate content. She was forced to drop out of school and to accept another hospitalization.

Ms. Sims was motivated to comply with treatment, but her fears of gaining weight and becoming obese affected her progress. She was expected to gain a minimum of 2 pounds every week, and she was restricted to bed rest if she failed to gain sufficient weight. In psychotherapy, Ms. Sims was gradually guided to discuss her feelings and to actually look at herself in the mirror. She was initially instructed to look at one part of her body for a minimum of 10 seconds, and the time was progressively increased until she could look at her whole body without any anxiety. Her menses returned at a weight of 93 pounds. After 7 months of individual and family treatment, she was discharged at a weight of 100 pounds. Ms. Sims returned to college while working part time and living with her parents.

Over the next 10 years, Ms. Sims graduated from college with a degree in nutrition and was selected to do an internship with a major corporation. She has excelled in her work, receiving several promotions. She married, but the relationship deteriorated as her husband became physically abusive. She moved out, obtained a court order of protection, and eventually was divorced. Her most recent correspondence told of her return to graduate school (with all expenses paid plus full salary from her employer), a new romance, and success in a marathon (third place in a 26-mile race). She has maintained her weight at around 116 pounds and menstruates normally. She did seek counseling to sort out issues related to her broken marriage and her estrangement from her sister (which has since been resolved). She describes her life now as full and satisfying.

Discussion of "Sixty-Seven Pound Weakling"

As is usually the case with Anorexia Nervosa (DSM-5-TR, p. 381), the characteristic signs and symptoms leave little doubt as to the correct diagnosis. Ms. Sims has all of the salient features of Anorexia Nervosa, including refusal to maintain body weight at or above a minimally normal weight for age and height, intense fear of gaining weight or of becoming fat despite being underweight, and disturbance in the way in which her body weight or shape is experienced (anxiety when viewing her body). She also has the common but not universal sign (in postmenarcheal females) of amenorrhea. Amenorrhea in Anorexia Nervosa is believed to be caused by underactivity of hypothalamic and pituitary gland hormones due to stress or nutritional factors, which in turn leads to underactivity of the ovarian hormones responsible for the menstrual cycle. Because Ms. Sims's method of losing weight has never involved purging (self-induced vomiting or use of laxatives or diuretics) and she has never engaged in binge eating (consumption of large amounts of food with a sense of loss of control), the subtype is the Restricting Type.

Ms. Sims exhibited compulsive ritualistic behavior surrounding food (e.g., cutting her food into very small pieces and moving it around on her plate before eating it), a feature commonly seen in patients with Anorexia Nervosa. Although her compulsive eating behavior might suggest the possible additional diagnosis of Obsessive-Compulsive Disorder (see "Lady Macbeth" in Section 6.1), a separate diagnosis is not given because her compulsive behavior only involves food and is thus explained by the diagnosis of Anorexia Nervosa.

Anorexia Nervosa is a serious and often life-threatening disorder. This case illustrates that with expert treatment, a good outcome is possible.

Close to the Bone[1]

A 23-year-old woman from Arkansas wrote a letter to the head of a New York research group after seeing a television program in which he described his work with patients with unusual eating patterns. In the letter, which requested that she be accepted into his program, the woman described her problems as follows:

Several years ago, in college, I started using laxatives to lose weight. I started with a few and increased the number as they became ineffective. After 2 years I was taking 250–300 Ex-Lax pills at one time with a glass of water, 20 per gulp. I would lose as much as 20 pounds in a 24-hour period, mostly water and some food, so dehydrated that I couldn't stand, and could barely talk. I ended up in the university infirmary several times with diagnoses of food poisoning, severe gastrointestinal flu, etc., with bland di-

---

[1]Reprinted from Spitzer RL, Skodol AE, Gibbon M, Williams, JBW: *Psychopathology: A Case Book*. New York, McGraw-Hill, 1983, pp. 224-228. Copyright © 1983 Spitzer RL, Skodol AE, Gibbon M, Williams, JBW. Used with permission.

ets and medications. I was released within a day or two. A small duodenal ulcer appeared and disappeared on X-rays in 1975.

I would not eat for days, then would eat something, and, overcome by guilt at eating, and hunger, would eat-eat-eat. A girl on my dorm floor told me that she occasionally forced herself to vomit so that she wouldn't gain weight. I did this every once in a while and discovered that I could consume large amounts of food, vomit, and still lose weight. This was spring of 1975. I lost nearly 50 pounds over a few months, to 90 pounds. My hair started coming out in handfuls, and my teeth were loose.

I never felt lovelier or more confident about my appearance: physically liberated, streamlined, close to the bone. I was flat everywhere except my stomach when I binged, when I would be full-blown and distended. When I bent over, each rib and back vertebra was outlined. After vomiting, my stomach was once more flat, empty. The more I lost, the more I was afraid of getting fat. I was afraid to drink water for days at a time because it would add pounds on the scale and make me miserable. Yet I drank (or drink; perhaps I should be writing this all in the present tense) easily a half-gallon of milk and other liquids at once when bingeing. I didn't need the laxatives as much to get rid of food and eventually stopped using them altogether (although I am still chronically constipated, I become nauseous whenever I see them in the drugstore).

I exercised for hours each day to tone my figure from the weight fluctuations and joined the university track team. I wore track shoes all the time and ran to classes and around town, stick-legs pumping. I went to track practice daily after being sick, until I was forced to quit; a single lap would make me dizzy, with cramps in my stomach and legs.

At some point during my last semester before dropping out I came across an article on Anorexia Nervosa. It frightened me; my own personal obsession with food and body weight was shared by other people. I had not menstruated in 2 years. So, I forced myself to eat and digest healthy food. Hated it. I studied nutrition and gradually forced myself to accept a new attitude toward food—vitalizing—something needed for life. I gained weight, fighting panic. In a rigid, controlled way I have maintained myself nutritionally ever since: 105–115 pounds at 5'6". I know what I need to survive, and I eat it—a balanced diet with the fewest possible calories, mostly vegetables, fruits, fish, fowl, whole grain products, etc. In 5 years, I have not eaten anything like pizza, pastas or pork, sweets, or anything fattening, fried, or rich without being very sick. Once I allowed myself an ice cream cone. But I am usually sick if I deviate as much as one bite.

It was difficult for me to face people at school, and I dropped courses each semester, collecting incompletes but finishing well in the few classes I stayed with. The absurdity of my reclusiveness was even evident to me during my last semester when I signed up for correspondence courses, while living only two blocks from the correspondence university building on campus. I felt I would only be able to face people when I lost "just a few more pounds."

Fat. I cannot stand it. This feeling is stronger and more desperate than any horror at what I am doing to myself. If I gain a few pounds I hate to leave the house and let people see me. Yet I am sad to see how I have pushed aside the friends, activities, and state of energized health that once rounded my life.

For all of this hiding, it will surprise you to know that I am by profession a model. Last year when I was more in control of my eating-vomiting I enjoyed working in front of a camera, and I was doing well. Lately I've been sick too much and feel out-of-shape and physically un-self-confident for the discipline involved. I keep myself supported during this time with part-time secretarial work, and whatever unsolicited photo bookings my past clients give me. For the most part I do the secretarial work. And I can't seem to stop being sick all of the time.

The more I threw up when I was in college, the longer it took, and the harder it became. I needed to use different instruments to induce vomiting. Now I double two electrical cords and shove them several feet down into my throat. This is preceded by 6–10 doses of ipecac [an emetic]. My knees are calloused from the time spent kneeling sick. The eating-vomiting process takes usually 2–3 hours, sometimes as long as 8. I dread the gagging and pain and sometimes my throat is very sore, and I procrastinate using the ipecac and cords. I sit on the floor, biting my nails, and pulling the skin off around my nails with tweezers. Usually, I wear rubber gloves to prevent this somewhat.

After emptying my stomach completely, I wash thoroughly. In a little while I will hydrate myself with a bottle of diet pop and take a handful of Lasix 40 mg [a diuretic] (which I have numerous prescriptions for). Sometimes I am faint, very cold. I splash cool water on my face, smooth my hair, but my hands are shaking some. I will take aspirin if my hands hurt sharply…so I can sleep later. My lips and fingers are bluish and cold. I see in the mirror that blood vessels are broken. There are red spots over my eyes. They always fade in a day or two. There is a certain relief when it is over, that the food is gone, and I am not horribly fat from it. And I cry often…for some rest, some calm. It is foolish for me to cry for someone, someone to help me, when it is only me who is hiding and hurting myself.

Now there is a funny new split in my behavior, this honesty about my illness. Hopefully it will bring me more help than humiliation. Sometimes I feel hypocrisy in my actions, and in the frightened, well-ordered attempts to seek out help. All the while I am still sick, night after night after night. And often days as well.

Two sets of logic seem to be operating against each other, each determined, each half-canceling the effects of the other. It is the part of me which forced me to eat that I'm talking about…which cools my throat with water after hours of heaving, which takes potassium supplements to counteract diuretics, and aspirin for torn hands. It is this part of me, which walks into a psychiatrist's office twice weekly and sees the liability of hurting myself seriously, which makes constant small efforts to repair the tearing-down.

It almost sounds as if I am being brutalized by some unrelenting force. Ridiculous to feel this way, or to stand and cry, because the hands that cool my throat and try to make small repairs only just punched lengths of cord into my stomach. No demons, only me.

For your consideration, I am

Gratefully yours,

Nancy Lee Duval

Ms. Duval was admitted to the research ward for study. Additional history revealed that her eating problems began gradually during her adolescence and had been severe for the past 3–4 years. At age 14, she weighed 128 pounds and had reached her adult height of 5'6". She felt "terribly fat" and began to diet without great success. At age 17 she weighed 165 pounds and began to diet more seriously for fear that she would be ridiculed and went down to 130 pounds over the next year. She recalled feeling very depressed, overwhelmed, and insignificant. She began to avoid difficult classes so that she would never get less than straight As and began to lie about her school and grade performance for fear of being humiliated. She had great social anxiety in dealing with boys, which culminated in her transferring to a girls' school for the last year of high school.

When she left for college, her difficulties increased. She had trouble deciding how to organize her time, whether to study, to date, or to see friends. She became more desperate to lose weight and began to use laxatives, as she describes in her letter. At age 20, in her sophomore year of college, she reached her lowest weight of 88 pounds (70% of ideal body weight) and stopped menstruating.

As Ms. Duval describes in her letter, she recognized that there was a problem and eventually forced herself to gain weight. Nonetheless, the overeating and vomiting she had begun the previous year worsened. Because of her preoccupation with her weight and her eating, her academic performance suffered, and she dropped out of school midway through college at age 21.

Ms. Duval is the second of four children and the only girl. She comes from an upper-middle-class professional family. From the patient's description, it sounds as though the father has a history of alcoholism. There are clear indications of difficulties between the mother and the father, and between the boys and the parents, but no other family member has ever had psychiatric treatment.

Ms. Duval remained on the research ward for several weeks, during which time she participated in research studies and, under the structure of the hospital setting, was able to give up her abuse of laxatives and diuretics. After her return home, she continued in treatment with a psychiatrist in psychoanalytically oriented psychotherapy two times a week, which she had begun 6 months previously. That therapy continued for approximately another 6 months, when her family refused to support it. The patient also felt that while she had gained some insight into her difficulties, she had been unable to change her behavior.

Two years after leaving the hospital, she wrote that she was "doing much better." She had reenrolled in college and was completing her course work satisfactorily. She had seen a nutritionist and felt that form of treatment was useful for her in learning what a normal diet was and how to maintain a normal weight. She was also receiving counseling from the school guidance counselors, but she did not directly relate that to her eating difficulties. Her weight was normal, and she was menstruating regularly. She continued to have intermittent difficulty with binge eating and vomiting, but the frequency and severity of these problems were much reduced. She no longer abused diuretics or laxatives.

Discussion of "Close to the Bone"

Ms. Duval has Anorexia Nervosa (DSM-5-TR, p. 381), a disorder that was first described 300 years ago and given its current name in 1868. Although theories about the cause of the disorder have come and gone, the essential features have remained unchanged. Ms. Duval poignantly describes these features.

She had an intense and irrational fear of becoming obese, even when she was emaciated. Her body image was disturbed in that she perceived herself as fat when her weight was average and that she "never felt lovelier" when, to others, she must have appeared grotesquely thin. She lost about 30% of her body weight through relentless dieting and exercising, self-induced vomiting, and use of cathartics and diuretics. She had not menstruated for the past 3 years.

Significantly, Ms. Duval's dieting takes place despite persistent hunger; thus, the word *anorexia* (meaning "loss of appetite") makes the name of the disorder a misnomer. In fact, she also has recurrent episodes of binge eating—that is, rapid, uncontrolled consumption of high-caloric foods. These binges are followed by vomiting and remorse. This pattern of recurrent binge eating and purging, if it occurred by itself, would warrant the diagnosis of Bulimia Nervosa (see Section 10.5). However, when this pattern occurs during the course of Anorexia Nervosa, the appropriate diagnosis is Anorexia Nervosa, Binge-Eating/Purging Type. Thus, Ms. Duval's condition differs from that of the previous case of Ms. Sims in this section (see "Sixty-Seven Pound Weakling"), because Ms. Duval periodically went on eating binges (would "eat-eat-eat") and engaged in compensatory purging behaviors to try to lose weight, whereas Ms. Sims tried to lose weight strictly by reducing her intake of food.

When an emaciated patient with Anorexia Nervosa insists that she is fat, this suggests the presence of a somatic delusion, as might be seen in a Delusional Disorder (see "Fleas" in Section 2.4) or Major Depressive Disorder (see "Stonemason" in Section 4.2). However, patients with Anorexia Nervosa are generally not considered to have a delusion because they are describing how they experience themself rather than disputing the facts of their weight.

Thin Tim

Eight-year-old Tim was referred by a pediatrician who asked for an emergency evaluation because of serious weight loss during the past year for which the pediatrician could find no medical cause. Tim is extremely concerned about his weight and weighs himself daily. He complains that he is too fat, and if he does not lose weight, he cuts back on food. He has lost 10 pounds in the past year and still feels that he is too fat, although it is clear that he is underweight. In desperation, his parents have removed the scales from the house; as a result, Tim is keeping a record of the calories that he eats daily. He spends a lot of time on this task, checking and rechecking that he has done it just right.

In addition, Tim is described as being obsessed with cleanliness and neatness. Currently, he has no friends because he refuses to visit them, feeling that their houses are "dirty"; he gets upset when another child touches him. He is always checking whether he is doing things the way they "should" be done. He becomes very agitated and anxious about this. He has to get up at least 2 hours before leaving for school each day to give himself time to get ready. Recently, he woke up at 1:30 in the morning to prepare for school.

Discussion of "Thin Tim"

The emergency evaluation is because of Tim's recent weight loss. He has lost 10 pounds in the last year, during which time a boy of his age might have been expected to gain about that amount. This means he is likely 20 pounds below the expected weight for his age. Although Anorexia Nervosa is unusual in a male and in one so young, Tim's refusal to maintain a normal weight suggests this diagnosis (DSM-5-TR, p. 381). Tim also has the other characteristic features of the disorder: fear of becoming fat and feeling fat even when obviously underweight. Because Tim loses weight exclusively by restricting his food intake (i.e., by dieting) and he does not engage in binge eating or purging behavior, his Anorexia Nervosa would be the Restricting Type.

Although not the focus of attention, Tim's preoccupation with various recurrent thoughts concerning dirtiness causes him considerable distress. Moreover, he has to check whether he is doing things the way they "should" be done, and such activities apparently interfere with his normal functioning (he has to get up several hours before school to get ready on time). It is reasonable to assume that the thoughts intrude into his consciousness and are beyond his control, and that his lengthy "getting ready" routines are performed in response to these thoughts. Thus, they represent true obsessions and compulsions. Because the content of these obsessions and compulsions is unrelated to Tim's eating disorder, an additional diagnosis of Obsessive-Compulsive Disorder (DSM-5-TR, p. 265) is made but is considered secondary because the initial focus of attention is the eating disorder.

10.5
Bulimia Nervosa

The characteristic features of Bulimia Nervosa are 1) recurrent episodes of binge eating, 2) recurrent inappropriate behaviors to compensate for binge eating in order to prevent weight gain, and 3) a self-evaluation that overemphasizes body shape and weight. Binge eating and engaging in compensatory behaviors must be regularly occurring (i.e., at least once per week) and relatively persistent (i.e., over at least a 3-month period). An episode of binge eating is defined as "eating, in a discrete period of time, an amount of food that is definitely larger than most individuals would eat in a similar period of time under similar circumstances" (DSM-5-TR, p. 388). For example, an individual might eat several quarts of ice cream or several large pizzas at one sitting. The technical use of the term *eating binge* would not ordinarily apply, however, to culturally sanctioned "overeating," such as occurs at weddings or family Thanksgiving meals (although binge eating can occur at such events; see "A Visit to Food Hell," later in this section). An eating binge is typically associated with a feeling of a loss of control over eating, such that the individual cannot stop eating once started. Some people report feeling "dissociated" (i.e., split off from conscious awareness of their behavior) when bingeing. Sometimes, people will report that they have completely given up trying to control their eating behavior. People will typically feel embarrassed about bingeing and will often eat in secrecy. Binges are often triggered by psychosocial stress, feelings of depression, or anxiety.

Compensatory behaviors in Bulimia Nervosa are colloquially called *purge behaviors* or *purging* and include self-induced vomiting (most common) and misuse of laxatives, diuretics, or enemas. Some people with the disorder do not purge but rather compensate for overeating with fasting or excessive exercise (e.g., spending hours each day at the gym). Individuals with Bulimia Nervosa are also very concerned about their body shape and weight as sources of self-esteem. In this respect, they are similar to people with Anorexia Nervosa (see Section 10.4); however, they do not have the low body weight caused by food restriction. Bulimia Nervosa is not diagnosed when a person has Anorexia Nervosa. People with Bulimia Nervosa are most commonly either normal weight or overweight. Serious medical complications can result from purging behaviors, including fluid and electrolyte imbalances, tears of the esophagus or rupture of the stomach (from vomiting), and cardiac arrhythmias (an alteration in the rhythm of the heartbeat in timing or force).

The 12-month prevalence of Bulimia Nervosa in the United States ranges from 0.14% to 0.3%, with much higher rates in women (0.22%–0.5%) than in men (0.05%–0.10%). The lifetime prevalence ranges from 0.28% to 1.0%. In the United States, the disorder is equally common across ethnoracial groups. The prevalence of Bulimia Nervosa is highest in high-income industrialized countries, such as the United States, Canada, Australia, New Zealand, and many European countries.

Bulimia Nervosa typically begins during late adolescence or early adulthood. The clinical course may be chronic or intermittent; the symptoms may also diminish with time, with or without treatment, although treatment clearly leads to better outcomes. People with Bulimia Nervosa have impaired social functioning in some cases (e.g., they may spend all of their "free time" bingeing and purging, instead of seeing friends or family, or they may avoid going out to restaurants because of a fear of engaging in an eating binge). People with this disorder are at increased risk for suicide. Most individuals with Bulimia Nervosa have at least one other mental disorder, most commonly a Depressive Disorder, a Substance Use Disorder, or a Personality Disorder (e.g., Borderline Personality Disorder).

A Visit to Food Hell

Abby Thurmond, age 42, had not had a food binge for more than 2 years when she flew from Miami to Chicago to attend the wedding of her friend's daughter. Single, independent, and devoted to her work, Ms. Thurmond had just sold her first screenplay. She was pleased, but she was also experiencing the "postpartum" letdown that always occurred when she finished a major project.

Ms. Thurmond knew from her 2 years in Overeaters Anonymous (OA; a self-help group program similar to Alcoholics Anonymous) that she needed to keep a safe distance from food, especially during emotionally hard times. Nevertheless, Ms. Thurmond spent the entire day of the wedding rehearsal party in close proximity to food. She stood in her friend's kitchen for hours—cutting, chopping, sorting, arranging, and eventually picking at the food.

That night, when the guests arrived, the flurry of activity made it easy for Ms. Thurmond to disappear—physically and emotionally—into a binge. She started with a plate of what would have been an "abstinent" meal (an OA concept for whatever is included on an individual's meal plan): pasta salad, green salad, cold cuts, and a roll. Although the portions were generous, she wanted more. She spent the next 5 hours eating, at first trying to graze among the guests, but then, when shame set in, retreating to dark corners of the room to take frantic, stolen bites.

Ms. Thurmond stuffed herself with crackers, cheeses, breads, chicken, turkey, pasta, and salads, but all that was a prelude to what she really wanted—sugar. She had been waiting for the guests to leave the dining room, where the desserts were. When they finally did, she cut herself two pieces of cake, then two more, and then ate directly from the serving tray, shoveling the food into her mouth. She reached for cookies, more cake, and cookies again. Heart racing, terrified of being discovered, she finally tore herself away and slipped out onto the terrace.

At this point, in what she thought of as a "food trance," Ms. Thurmond piled her plate with bread, onto which she smeared some unidentifiable spread. Although the food tasted like mud, she kept eating. Soon, other guests came out to the terrace, leaving Ms. Thurmond feeling she had to move again, which she did, stepping into the kitchen—and the light. When she glanced down at her plate, she was horrified; ants were crawling all over it. Instead of reflexively spitting out the food, Ms. Thurmond, overcome by shame, could only swallow. Then her eyes began to search the debris on her plate for uncontaminated morsels. Witnessing her own madness, Ms. Thurmond began to cry. She flung the plate into the trash and ran to her room.

That event marked the beginning of a 6-month relapse into binge eating—Ms. Thurmond's worst experience with binge eating since the problem began 15 years earlier. During the relapse, she binged on sugar foods and refined carbohydrates, returned to cigarette smoking to control the binge eating, and once again was driven to "get rid" of the calories by incessant exercise after each binge, walking 4–5 hours at a time, dragging her bicycle up and down six flights of stairs, and biking miles after dark in a dangerous city park.

Throughout the relapse, Ms. Thurmond went to therapy and to OA. However, the binge eating worsened, as did the accompanying isolation and depression, which kept her awake, often crying uncontrollably, until the early morning hours. Finally, her therapist, a social worker, referred her to a psychiatrist, who prescribed an antidepressant medication that has been used to control binge eating, as well as a structured food plan that excluded refined sugars, breads, crackers, and similar carbohydrates. Within a few weeks, she was able to stop binge eating, come out of the depression, and resume her life. After 2 years of taking the medication, during which time she had no binges and gradually reintroduced breads and related carbohydrates to her diet, Ms. Thurmond was able to discontinue the antidepressant without depression or a return to binge eating. She continues to be active in OA.

Discussion of "A Visit to Food Hell"

The term *eating binge* is often used by people to describe an occasion on which they ate more food than they should have. However, Ms. Thurmond's description of the amount of food she consumed in her eating episode at the wedding rehearsal leaves little doubt that her episodes of binge eating, during which she lacks a sense of control over how much she eats, represent a serious symptom. When a clinician is diagnosing an individual with recurrent eating binges, the first question is whether the individual regularly compensates for the overeating by some drastic inappropriate behavior. If the answer is no, the diagnosis is probably Binge-Eating Disorder (see "Eating Until It Hurts" in Section 10.6). If the answer is yes and the person's self-evaluation is unduly influenced by body shape and weight (as usually occurs), the diagnosis is Bulimia Nervosa. Most patients with Bulimia Nervosa compensate for the binge eating by some method of purging—either self-induced vomiting (most common) or the use of diuretics or laxatives. Ms. Thurmond's case is an example of the relatively less common diagnosis of Bulimia Nervosa (DSM-5-TR, p. 387) in which the patient uses excessive exercise (her method) or fasting (in other cases) instead of purging.

The Fat Man

Gregory James, a 43-year-old theater manager, was evaluated at an eating disorders clinic in San Francisco. Although he had lost 58 pounds in the previous 5 months, dropping from 250 to 192 pounds on a 6'1" frame, he was still terrified of getting fat.

Mr. James first began to diet 5 months earlier when his wife told him he was "a fat slob" and implied that she might be considering a divorce. This encounter terrified him and started him on a strict dietary regimen: an omelet and bran for breakfast, coffee for lunch, and salad and shrimp or chicken for dinner. His original goal was to lose about 50 pounds. When dieting did not result in sufficiently rapid loss of weight, he started sticking his finger down his throat to induce vomiting after meals.

Mr. James is now "obsessed" with food. Before he goes to a restaurant, he worries about what he will order. He has done a study of what he eats in terms of what is easiest to purge, and he knows all the bathrooms in the areas he frequents. He cannot bear feeling full after eating and worries that his stomach is "fat." Three or four times a week he is unable to resist the urge to "binge." At those times he feels that his eating is out of control, and he may gobble down as much as three hamburgers, two orders of French fries, a pint of ice cream, and two packages of Oreo cookies. He always induces vomiting after a binge. He has never used laxatives, diuretics, or diet pills to lose weight.

Mr. James is also preoccupied with becoming thin. He has progressively revised downward his original weight goal, first to 190 and then to 185 pounds. He has begun to exercise, walking at least an hour a day and, more recently, working out with weights several times a week. He believes that women look at him differently now: when he was heavy, they glanced at him casually, whereas now their response is "admiring."

Mr. James has always been somewhat heavy, turning to food in times of stress, but he never worried about his weight until his wife criticized his appearance. He can no longer enjoy any meals and feels he has lost control of this area of his life because he cannot stop dieting, even though his wife has told him he is now too thin. He therefore recently saw his internist, who found no physical problems and referred him for psychiatric evaluation.

Discussion of "The Fat Man"

Mr. James's eating disorder began, as is often the case, with a reasonable attempt to lose some weight. He soon became preoccupied with losing weight and continued to view his body as "fat" even though others did not. His preoccupation with losing weight and distorted body image suggest Anorexia Nervosa, but this diagnosis is not made because he has not lost so much weight that he has significantly low body weight in the context of his age, sex, developmental trajectory, and physical health.

Mr. James's binges (recurrently eating a large amount of food with a sense of loss of control), his recurrent inappropriate compensatory behavior to avoid weight gain (in his case, by self-induced vomiting), and his overconcern with weight and shape indicate Bulimia Nervosa (DSM-5-TR, p. 387). Mr. James uses vomiting, the most common method for avoiding weight gain among individuals with Bulimia Nervosa. Less common methods for avoiding weight gain are misuse of laxatives or diuretics, fasting, and excessive exercise (see the previous case in this section, "A Visit to Food Hell").

Mr. James's case of Bulimia Nervosa is unusual in that he is a man (the disorder is at least five times more common among women) and the onset of his disorder occurred relatively later in life (onset is usually during adolescence or early adulthood, and new onset is uncommon after age 40).

10.6
Binge-Eating Disorder

The characteristic features of Binge-Eating Disorder are recurrent episodes of binge eating but no inappropriate compensatory behaviors, as occur in Bulimia Nervosa. The eating binges are identical to those in Bulimia Nervosa—that is, they involve discrete episodes of eating amounts of food that are larger than most people would eat over the same time period and under similar circumstances, and they are associated with a sense of lack of control over eating. In addition, eating binges in Binge-Eating Disorder are often characterized by eating much more rapidly than normal, eating until uncomfortably full, eating large amounts of food when not hungry, eating alone because of embarrassment over how much one is eating, and feeling disgusted with oneself, depressed, or guilty afterward. The eating binges occur regularly (i.e., at least once per week) and are relatively persistent (i.e., occurring over at least a 3-month period).

Binge-Eating Disorder occurs in normal-weight, overweight, and obese individuals. The 12-month prevalence in the United States ranges from 0.44% to 1.2%, with prevalence rates two to three times higher in women (0.6%–1.6%) than in men (0.26%–0.8%). The lifetime prevalence ranges from 0.85% to 2.8%. Binge-Eating Disorder appears to have a comparable prevalence across U.S. ethnoracial groups. The disorder has a similar prevalence across most high-income countries of the world, including the United States, Canada, Australia, New Zealand, and many European countries. Binge eating can occur in children, and it is common in adolescents and college-age people. Typically, its onset is in adolescence or early adulthood. Remission rates are higher for Binge-Eating Disorder than for either Bulimia Nervosa or Anorexia Nervosa, whether treated or not.

Binge-Eating Disorder can be associated with poor social adjustment, impaired health-related quality of life, increased medical morbidity and mortality, and increased health care utilization. Suicidal ideation has been reported in a minority of cases. The most common co-occurring mental disorders are Major Depressive Disorder and Alcohol Use Disorder.

Eating Until It Hurts

Andrea Simpson, age 35, weighed 230 pounds when she returned to her therapist to get help for the eating and weight problems that had caused her grief since she was a child. She was again having uncontrollable eating binges and had gained more than 50 pounds in 6 months.

Ms. Simpson remembered being called "fatty" by her schoolmates in early elementary school and having frequent arguments with her mother about her excessive eating and weight throughout childhood and adolescence. During high school she nibbled throughout the day. After each bite she vowed to herself that this bite would be her last, and she would go on a diet, but she was never able to keep this vow. She felt very ashamed of her weight, but she gradually gained more. She did most of her eating in private so that others would not see. At graduation from high school, with a height of 5'5", she weighed 203 pounds.

Ms. Simpson believes that her binge eating began in college. She lost about 40 pounds by dieting when she began college, and then she began to alternate between periods of dieting and overeating, lasting several weeks to several months. During periods of overeating, she often ate a large breakfast (e.g., several eggs with cheese, two or three slices of toast, and two large glasses of orange juice) in the university cafeteria. She would then take large quantities of food back to her dorm room (e.g., two or three peanut butter sandwiches, two or three dozen cookies, potato chips, cheese), which she ate over the next few hours. She ate until she felt physically uncomfortable and then fell asleep. She felt very depressed and ashamed about her weight during this time. She does not recall feeling out of control during the eating because she always believed that she would stop when she had finished whatever piece of food she was eating, although this seldom happened. She had a number of weight fluctuations in college; her weight ranged from 170 to 230 pounds.

Ms. Simpson got down to a normal weight in her last year of college and got married after graduation. She began to overeat again on her honeymoon. Her husband was angry about the eating and weight gain. They argued a great deal about this issue and about her dishonesty concerning her eating (motivated largely by shame about what she had eaten). She feels that her eating problems contributed significantly to her subsequent divorce.

Over the next several years, Ms. Simpson continued to struggle with her weight and eating. She went to Weight Watchers several times, tried numerous diets in magazines, used prescribed and illicit amphetamines to decrease her appetite, and spoke to internists about her weight and tried diets they gave her. However, she continued to be overweight with marked weight fluctuations. During periods of dieting, she was preoccupied with food and urges to eat.

Ms. Simpson was in psychotherapy in her mid-20s for issues related to her divorce and family. Although she tried to discuss her weight and eating problems, the therapy was ineffective for these issues because the therapist's interventions were largely limited to suggesting diets.

Ms. Simpson describes the periods of binge eating as "a nightmare," during which she is preoccupied with fighting the urge to eat, planning additional eating, and feeling guilty and ashamed about her eating and the inevitable weight gain that will follow. Her worst period of daily binge eating, lasting about 10 months, occurred approximately 2 years ago. She ate boxes of cookies, ice cream, and other sweets; large amounts of peanut butter and bread; and many bowls of cereal when nothing else was in the house. She felt out of control of her eating and desperate about her inability to stop binge eating. She often ate until she had stomach pain, never felt hungry because she was always eating so much, essentially lost all semblance of a meal structure, avoided eating in front of others because she was ashamed of the eating, and constantly felt depressed. She gained 90 pounds during this period of binge eating.

When she returned to her therapist at age 35, she was encouraged to join OA. She found the combination of OA and psychotherapy helpful. She lost about 80 pounds, without rigid or restrictive dieting, and has kept off 60 of these pounds for about 5 years. She is pleased that she does not often feel preoccupied with food or urges to eat between meals, although she continues to have trouble controlling the size of her meals. She feels quite sure that she will never be entirely free of her eating problem and could begin binge eating again at some unpredictable future time. For this reason, she continues to attend OA meetings.

Discussion of "Eating Until It Hurts"

Many individuals who binge eat are concerned about their overeating and inability to maintain a normal weight. They may try a variety of diets and weight maintenance programs. A minority of those with the disorder engage in recurrent eating binges during which they eat large amounts of food and feel that their eating is out of control. When a pattern emerges of binge eating more than once a week for longer than 3 months, as occurred in Ms. Simpson's case, the diagnosis is Binge-Eating Disorder (DSM-5-TR, p. 392). This diagnosis is not made if the individual additionally engages in the inappropriate compensatory behavior that characterizes Bulimia Nervosa (e.g., self-induced vomiting or excessive exercise; see Section 10.5).

CHAPTER 11

Elimination Disorders

A child usually becomes interested in mastering elimination of body waste during the toddler phase (ages 1–3 years), and by age 4 years, most children have achieved bowel and bladder continence, in the following order of success: nighttime bowel control, daytime bowel control, daytime bladder control, and nighttime bladder control. Elimination Disorders involve the inappropriate elimination of urine or feces and usually affect children older than 4 years who have already been toilet trained. This diagnostic class includes two disorders: Enuresis (more commonly known as wetting), which is the repeated voiding of urine into inappropriate places, and Encopresis (soiling), which is the repeated passage of feces into inappropriate places. The minimum age requirements for diagnosis of both disorders are based on developmental age—that is, age as determined by degree of emotional, mental, anatomical, and physiological maturation—and not solely on chronological age. (Table 11–1 lists characteristic features of the Elimination Disorders.) Both Enuresis and Encopresis may be voluntary or involuntary. Although these disorders typically occur separately, co-occurrence may also be observed.

TABLE 11–1. **Characteristic features of Elimination Disorders**

Disorder	Key characteristics
Enuresis	Repeated voiding of urine into bed or clothes
	Chronological age of at least 5 years or equivalent developmental level
Encopresis	Repeated passage of feces into inappropriate places
	Chronological age of at least 4 years or equivalent developmental level

11.1
Enuresis

Enuresis involves the individual's repeated voiding of urine during the day or at night into their bed or clothes. Most often the voiding of urine is not under the person's control, but occasionally it may be intentional. Occasional episodes are not sufficient to justify a diagnosis of Enuresis. DSM-5-TR sets a minimum frequency of at least twice a week for at least 3 consecutive months for the diagnosis. Alternatively, the diagnosis can be given if a lower frequency of occurrences causes clinically significant distress or impairment in social, academic (occupational), or other important areas of functioning, such as limiting a child's social activities by making them ineligible for sleepaway camp or resulting in social ostracism by peers. Moreover, to qualify for the diagnosis, the child must have reached an age at which continence is expected, which is a chronological or mental age of at least 5 years. Finally, the diagnosis cannot be given if the incontinence is due to the physiological effects of a substance or medication such as a diuretic (a medication used to increase urination so as to eliminate excess fluid from the body) or an antipsychotic, or if the incontinence is due to a nonpsychiatric medical condition such as diabetes, spina bifida (a condition in which the spine does not develop completely and does not completely cover the spinal cord), or a seizure disorder (urinary incontinence during a seizure).

In the most common form of Enuresis, sometimes referred to as *monosymptomatic enuresis*, the urinary incontinence occurs only during nighttime sleep (Nocturnal Only subtype), typically during the first one-third of the night. The less common form, referred to as *urinary incontinence* (Diurnal Only subtype), involves urinary voiding only during waking hours. Individuals with this type can be divided into two groups: those with "urge incontinence" have sudden urges to urinate quickly followed by involuntary voiding, and those with "voiding postponement" consciously defer urges to void urine until incontinence results. Finally, some individuals have urinary incontinence during both daytime and nighttime (Nocturnal and Diurnal subtypes), a form of Enuresis known as *nonmonosymptomatic enuresis*.

The prevalence of daytime urinary incontinence ranges from 3% to 9% in 7-year-olds, from 1% to 4% in 11- to 13-year-olds, and from 1% to 3% in adolescents ages 15–17 years. The prevalence of Nocturnal Enuresis is 5%–10% among 5-year-olds, 3%–5% among 10-year-olds, and about 1% for individuals age 15 years or older. Enuresis may also have a higher prevalence among youth with learning disabilities or Attention-Deficit/Hyperactivity Disorder. Nocturnal Enuresis is twice as common in boys as in girls, whereas diurnal incontinence is more common in girls.

Never Dry

Angelo, who is 7 years old, was referred to the clinic by his parents because of wetting himself at night and during the day. His parents were also concerned about his temper tantrums and other behavior problems.

Angelo has never been consistently dry. He is now wet most nights, often several times each night, although he is usually dry for a few days when sleeping over at his grandparents' house. The longest period during which he has been continuously dry at night was for 2 weeks when, 2 years ago, he was in a hospital because of a fractured leg.

Angelo has never been dry through the day. Since starting at a new school 3 months ago, he has managed to be dry during school hours. However, he invariably wets himself once he returns home from school and again before bedtime.

His parents have tried a variety of methods to stop the wetting. They have praised Angelo, offered him rewards if he would stay dry, "told him off" in private and in public, and, on one occasion, even gave him a mild spanking. He has received various forms of medication from his pediatrician but has never continued with them for very long; his parents feel that the medication has never been very helpful. His parents have tried waking him up to urinate after he has gone to sleep and before they go to bed, but this practice has not had a predictable effect on whether he will be wet later at night.

Before wetting himself during the daytime, Angelo often seems to become agitated, crosses his legs, and hops up and down. If his parents notice him doing this and tell him to go to the toilet, they feel that they can avert his wetting. During family outings in an automobile, Angelo seems to need to urinate more often than other children of his mother's acquaintance.

The boy has been evaluated by a urologist, who found no urinary infection or other genitourinary abnormality.

His mother describes Angelo as having frequent temper tantrums at home. These occur two to three times a week and are precipitated by only minor frustrations. For example, the day before his first attendance at the clinic, he had a temper tantrum when he could not find his jacket before going outside in the cold weather. At such times, he jumps up and down and shrieks, or sits or lies down and kicks his legs. The tantrums last up to 10 minutes, and then everything seems to be forgotten. Angelo's parents describe him as also being generally stubborn and very persistent in trying to get something he wants. He often is oppositional and refuses to do as he is told: "He always thinks he knows best." The mother notes, however, that the temper tantrums have only occurred at home and never at school.

In other ways Angelo's behavior is essentially normal. He eats and sleeps well, enjoys going to school, and has many friends, although his friendships often are short-lived. He rarely gets into a fight. His teachers regard him as being precocious in his ability to talk about grown-up things.

He is very close to his mother and spends a lot of time telling her every-thing that he has been doing during the day. He also enjoys his father's com-pany. He ignores his 11-year-old sister, whom he regards as a nuisance.

Angelo had normal developmental motor milestones, sitting at 7 months and walking at 1 year. His parents believe that he was slow to speak and recall that he only started to say single words at 16 months and was not putting sen-tences together until at least age 2 years. He stopped soiling himself (with fe-ces) during the day at age 3 years.

On examination, Angelo was a slim, pleasant-looking boy with no physical abnormalities. His intravenous pyelogram (an X-ray study of the kidneys and urinary tract) was reviewed and found to be normal. His IQ had previously been tested, and he was known to have a full-scale IQ of 110 (above aver-age), with verbal and performance scores close to that. The psychologist who tested him reported that Angelo was anxious about his performance and eas-ily became distressed if he could not do an item or feared that he might have done it wrong.

During the interview, Angelo was active in exploring the room, talked read-ily, and had good rapport with the interviewer. He seemed confident and ma-ture for his age and discussed his bed-wetting without seeming concerned. He often approached aggressive themes during play but very rarely followed through on them.

Discussion of "Never Dry"

Persistent Enuresis at age 7 is clearly abnormal. The absence of any physical explanation for Angelo's wetting suggests the diagnosis of Enuresis (DSM-5-TR, p. 399). Because his Enuresis occurs both during waking hours and over-night, the subtype Nocturnal and Diurnal would also apply. Several of An-gelo's behaviors—frequent temper tantrums, stubbornness, and frequent refusal to do as he is told—might be indicative of Oppositional Defiant Disor-der (see "No Brakes" in Section 15.1), but in the absence of evidence that his oppositional behavior is pervasive (e.g., also seen at school and with other au-thority figures), the clinician would be reluctant to give an additional diagno-sis of Oppositional Defiant Disorder, although it would need to be ruled out.

11.2
Encopresis

Encopresis involves the repeated passage of feces into inappropriate places, such as in clothing or on the floor. Most often this behavior is involuntary, but occasionally it may be intentional. For the behavior to qualify for the DSM-5-TR diagnosis of Encopresis, the passage of feces must occur at least once a month for at least 3 months. Moreover, to qualify for the diagnosis, the child must have a chronological or mental age of at least 4 years. Finally, the fecal incontinence must not be exclusively attributable to the effects of medications (e.g., laxatives) or to a nonpsychiatric medical condition that causes incontinence, such as chronic diarrhea, spina bifida, or an anal fissure.

When the passage of feces is involuntary rather than intentional, it is often related to constipation, impaction, and retention with subsequent overflow, warranting the DSM-5-TR subtype With Constipation and Overflow Incontinence. The constipation may develop for psychological reasons (e.g., anxiety about defecating in a particular place, a more general pattern of anxious or oppositional behavior), leading to avoidance of defecation, or for physical reasons (e.g., from dehydration associated with a febrile illness, hypothyroidism, or a medication side effect). In the subtype Without Constipation and Overflow Incontinence, feces may be deposited in a prominent location, and it is usually associated with the presence of Oppositional Defiant Disorder (see Section 15.1) or Conduct Disorder (see Section 15.3). Soiling without constipation appears to be less common than soiling with constipation.

Encopresis affects 1%–4% of children in high-income countries and is more prevalent among children ages 4–6 years (>4%) than among children ages 10–12 years (<2%). Among children younger than 5 years, the gender ratio appears to be equal; among older children, Encopresis tends to be more common in boys than in girls.

Soiled Again

Lucas, a 6-year-old in first grade, was referred to the clinic by his pediatrician because of persistent soiling. A medical workup did not reveal any nonpsychiatric medical condition that would account for this symptom.

Lucas had never gained control of his bowel habits. He was not constipated as an infant, but after a febrile illness at age 2, he had become constipated. Six months after the illness (at age 2½), he had impacted feces and was seen by a surgeon, who prescribed laxatives and suppositories. Following this episode, there was a pattern of alternating constipation, when Lucas did not go to the toilet for several days, and runny diarrhea, when he soiled his pants many times a day. At age 4, Lucas took laxatives regularly, and his stool became softer and more regular. At about the same time, his mother first attempted to toilet train him. He was made to sit on the toilet every evening until he "performed." Although he usually managed this, producing a tiny amount or, rarely, a normal stool, he continued to soil his pants frequently during the day. His mother said that within 30 minutes of changing his pants, he would be soiled again, and this pattern has continued until the present time.

Lucas himself has been distressed about the soiling since starting school. He hates taking his clothes off for gym or at the beach. He worries that people will notice if, as occasionally happens, feces drop out of his pants. He is anxious when sitting on the toilet in the evenings, and at first would do so only if bribed. Now he insists that his mother stay in the bathroom with him.

Lucas is also enuretic at night. He became dry by day at age 3½ but has continued to wet at night. Because waking him at night has not prevented his wetting, Lucas still wears pull-on diapers.

For the past month, since seeing a puppet show, Lucas has awakened frequently with nightmares about witches. He often asks about witches, and his mother has tried to assure him that they do not exist. He has had a light on all night in his room for the past month. He never goes into his parents' bed, which they do not allow because of his potentially being wet.

His mother says that Lucas has seemed rather preoccupied with death. He often asks why people have to die and if he or his parents will die first. He then works out how old he might be when his parents die. He has said that he does not want to be buried because then people would walk over him.

Apart from her son's problems of soiling and wetting, Lucas's mother feels that he is a normal little boy who is happy and outgoing. He is very affectionate with his mother and likes to receive lots of kisses and hugs. His mother implied that this demonstrativeness might be excessive for a boy. He is attached to his father, but not as much as to his mother. He likes to play and go out with his father, but with his mother he is clinging and likes to stay close to her.

Until age 4, Lucas had worried his parents because of seeming rather effeminate. He liked to dress in girls' clothes and talked of "when I grow up to be a girl." Now when playing, he likes to take more traditionally male roles, such as a policeman or bus conductor.

There was initially some difficulty in Lucas's adjustment at school. He used to scream when his mother left him, and he was reported to be very timid and afraid of other children. This behavior lasted for most of the first term, but he eventually began "to stand up for himself" and has been quite happy at school since then. He has several friends there, and the school is satisfied with his progress.

Lucas's developmental milestones were all a little behind those of his two older sisters, but his mother could not recall them exactly. He sat at about 6 months, shuffled about on his bottom and did not crawl, and walked at about 18 months, which are within the normal range. He also spoke his first words at about 18 months.

Lucas's mother is a smartly dressed, 35-year-old laboratory technician who seems timid and speaks quietly, but at the same time is quite forceful and articulate in what she says. She seems to feel unsure of herself with Lucas and says she thinks that bringing up a boy is much more difficult than bringing up her daughters. She is embarrassed, as a professional person, not to have sought help earlier. She recalls that in childhood, she also had hated to use lavatories away from home.

Lucas's father is a 40-year-old general contractor. An intelligent, distinguished-looking man, he was reticent during the interview. He readily admitted that he did not take an active part in the rearing of the children, although he enjoyed them and was very fond of them. He explained that he was rather disgusted by the soiling and tried to keep out of the situation for fear of being too punitive.

In the interview, Lucas appeared rather small for his age and had a baby-ish, full face. At first, he was very timid and shy and clung to his mother; how-ever, he did allow his mother to leave the room after a short period and became much more assertive and outgoing once she had left. He played with family figures in the dollhouse and soon had the little boy figure on the toilet and all the other members of the family watching him. His speech was imma-ture and difficult to understand, but his vocabulary was extensive.

Lucas was also seen by a pediatrician. On physical examination, a fecal mass the size of a small melon could be palpated in the lower abdomen, and soft feces could be felt in his rectum.

Discussion of "Soiled Again"

Because Lucas's fecal incontinence has been persistent and because medical causes for the incontinence have been ruled out, the diagnosis is Encopresis (DSM-5-TR, p. 402). Because his fecal incontinence is apparently associated with constipation and overflow incontinence, the subtype With Constipation and Overflow Incontinence would also be noted. Also, Lucas continues to have nighttime wetting, warranting an additional diagnosis of Enuresis, Noc-turnal Only (DSM-5-TR, p. 399).

Lucas apparently went through a phase during which he showed some signs of possible disturbance in gender identity (see "Dolls" in Section 14.1), but he now seems to have a clear sense of himself as a male. He also showed some signs of separation anxiety when he began school, although he had in-sufficient symptoms for a diagnosis of Separation Anxiety Disorder (see "Tiny Tina" in Section 5.1).

CHAPTER 12

Sleep-Wake Disorders

Most people have experienced trouble sleeping at one time or another. Occasional difficulty sleeping is normal and usually temporary, due to stress or other outside factors. When sleep problems are a regular occurrence and interfere with daily functioning, a DSM-5-TR diagnosis of a Sleep-Wake Disorder may be appropriate. Individuals with a Sleep-Wake Disorder typically present with sleep-wake complaints of dissatisfaction regarding the quality, timing, and amount of sleep. Resulting daytime distress and impairment are core features shared by all of the DSM-5-TR Sleep-Wake Disorders.

The four distinct stages of sleep—rapid eye movement (REM) sleep and three stages of non–rapid eye movement (NREM) sleep—can be characterized as follows:

- REM sleep, during which the majority of typical storylike dreams occur, occupies approximately 20%–25% of sleep time. REM sleep occurs cyclically throughout the night, alternating with NREM sleep every 80–100 minutes, and increases in duration toward the morning.
- NREM sleep stage 1 (N1) occurs during the transition from wakefulness to sleep and occupies about 5% of the time spent asleep in healthy adults.
- NREM sleep stage 2 (N2) takes up about 50% of the sleep time.
- NREM sleep stage 3 (N3) is the deepest level of sleep, occupies about 20% of the time spent asleep, tends to occur during the first one-third to one-half of the night, and increases in duration in response to sleep deprivation.

The characteristics of an individual patient's sleep stages can be measured by polysomnography, a type of sleep study that measures brain waves, blood oxygen level, heart rate and breathing, and eye and leg movements during sleep. Some of the DSM-5-TR Sleep-Wake Disorders affect specific stages of sleep (e.g., REM Sleep Behavior Disorder, which involves episodes of arousal during REM sleep).

Ten specific DSM-5-TR Sleep-Wake Disorders are covered in this chapter (see Table 12–1 for characteristic features). These disorders differ according to the nature of their symptoms, their timing, and their association with certain nonpsychiatric medical conditions and substance use:

TABLE 12–1. **Characteristic features of Sleep-Wake Disorders**

Disorder	Key characteristics
Insomnia Disorder	Dissatisfaction with sleep quantity or quality, associated with difficulty initiating or maintaining sleep or early-morning awakening with inability to return to sleep
Hypersomnolence Disorder	Excessive sleepiness associated with recurrent periods of sleep or lapses into sleep, unrefreshing prolonged main sleep episodes, or difficulty being awake after abrupt awakening
Narcolepsy	Recurrent periods of an irrepressible need to sleep, lapsing into sleep, or napping occurring within the same day
	Cataplexy (bilateral loss of muscle tone) or abnormal laboratory test findings (hypocretin deficiency) or polysomnography abnormalities
Obstructive Sleep Apnea Hypopnea[a]	Laboratory evidence of at least five obstructive apneas or hypopneas per hour of sleep, possibly with nighttime breathing disturbances or daytime fatigue
Circadian Rhythm Sleep-Wake Disorders	Sleep disruption due to alteration of circadian system or misalignment between circadian rhythm and sleep-wake schedule
Non–Rapid Eye Movement Sleep Arousal Disorders[b]	Recurrent episodes of incomplete awakening from sleep, accompanied by either sleepwalking (rising from bed during sleep) or sleep terrors (abrupt terror arousals from sleep)
	Amnesia for the episodes
Nightmare Disorder[b]	Extended dysphoric and well-remembered dreams that cause significant distress or impairment
Rapid Eye Movement (REM) Sleep Behavior Disorder[b]	Arousals during REM sleep that are associated with vocalizations or complex motor behavior
Restless Legs Syndrome	Urge to move the legs, often accompanied by or in response to uncomfortable sensations in the legs
Substance/Medication-Induced Sleep Disorder	Persistent and severe sleep disturbance due to the direct effects of a substance or medication on the central nervous system

[a]Grouped with the Breathing-Related Sleep Disorders, which also include Central Sleep Apnea and Sleep-Related Hypoventilation.
[b]Grouped with the Parasomnias.

- Insomnia Disorder and Hypersomnolence Disorder are diagnosed when individuals' primary complaints are inability to sleep and excessive daytime sleepiness, respectively.
- Narcolepsy (a neurological condition involving loss of the brain's ability to regulate sleep-wake cycles normally) and the Breathing-Related Sleep Disorders (conditions involving sleep disruption caused by episodes of abnormal breathing during sleep; consist of Obstructive Sleep Apnea Hypopnea, Central Sleep Apnea, and Sleep-Related Hypoventilation) are included in the DSM-5-TR Sleep-Wake Disorders because these conditions must be considered and ruled out when a per-

son presents with excessive daytime sleepiness. (Because it is by far the most common type of Breathing-Related Sleep Disorder, Obstructive Sleep Apnea Hypopnea is the only Breathing-Related Sleep Disorder covered in this book.)

- Circadian Rhythm Sleep-Wake Disorders are characterized by a problem with the timing of sleep in which individuals are unable to sleep and wake up at the times required for normal work, school, and social needs.
- The set of DSM-5-TR Sleep-Wake Disorders referred to as the Parasomnias involve abnormal movements, behaviors, emotions, perceptions, and dreams that occur while falling asleep, while asleep, between sleep stages, or during arousals from sleep. These conditions include NREM Sleep Arousal Disorders (encompassing sleepwalking and sleep terrors during the night), Nightmare Disorder, and REM Sleep Behavior Disorder.
- Restless Legs Syndrome is a neurological disorder characterized by unpleasant sensations in the legs that occur primarily at night.
- Substance/Medication-Induced Sleep Disorder is diagnosed when there are clinically significant sleep disturbances caused by substance or medication use.

12.1
Insomnia Disorder

The predominant complaint in Insomnia Disorder is dissatisfaction with the amount or quality of sleep. Manifestations of insomnia can occur at different times of the sleep period. A person can have trouble initiating sleep at bedtime (called *initial insomnia*), staying asleep throughout the night with frequent or prolonged middle-of-the-night awakenings (*middle insomnia*), or waking up early in the morning with an inability to return to sleep (*late insomnia*). DSM-5-TR sets a minimum frequency requirement of the symptoms occurring for at least 3 nights a week and a minimum duration requirement of at least 3 months. Moreover, to qualify for a DSM-5-TR diagnosis of Insomnia Disorder, the sleep complaints have to be sufficiently severe to cause clinically significant distress or impairment in social, occupational, or other important areas of functioning. Although the difficulty sleeping may occur on its own in the absence of any other condition, difficulty sleeping may also be a symptom of another sleep disorder, such as a Breathing-Related Sleep Disorder; a symptom of another mental disorder, such as Major Depressive Disorder; or a consequence of a nonpsychiatric medical condition, such as chronic pain. In such cases, a separate diagnosis of Insomnia Disorder (in addition to the other sleep disorder, mental disorder, or nonpsychiatric medical condition) is given only if the sleep problems are severe enough to warrant clinical attention in their own right.

In addition to having nighttime sleep difficulties, people with Insomnia Disorder have daytime impairments. These include fatigue or daytime sleepiness, as well as impairment in cognitive performance that can include difficulties with attention, concentration, and memory, and even with performing simple manual tasks. Associated mood disturbances include irritability or mood lability and, less commonly, depressive or anxiety symptoms.

Symptoms of insomnia are common in the general population, with about one-third of adults reporting problems with insomnia. About 10%–15% experience daytime impairment as a result of their insomnia symptoms. It is estimated, however, that only 10% have insomnia symptoms that meet criteria for the DSM-5-TR diagnosis of Insomnia Disorder, in terms of meeting the minimum frequency and duration requirements, as well as the requirement that the symptoms cause clinically significant distress or impairment. Insomnia complaints are most prevalent among middle-age and older adults. The type of sleep complaint changes as a function of age, with difficulties falling asleep reported more frequently among young adults and problems maintaining sleep reported more frequently among middle-age and older adults. Insomnia complaints are more common in women than in men, with a gender ratio of approximately 1.3 to 1. Insomnia commonly co-occurs with a variety of non-psychiatric medical conditions, such as cancer, diabetes, coronary heart disease, chronic obstructive pulmonary disease, arthritis and other chronic pain conditions, and degenerative brain diseases (e.g., Alzheimer's disease).

High-Strung

Mia Harrington, a 36-year-old vice president of a Detroit department store, responded to an advertisement describing a new clinic specializing in the treatment of sleep problems. Ever since starting college, she has had difficulty falling asleep most nights. She feels "mentally hyperactive" at bedtime and is unable to stop thinking about significant experiences of the day, particularly her interactions with dissatisfied customers. When she feels she has accomplished too little during a particular day, she feels she does not "deserve" to go to bed. Any evening excitement, such as an interesting movie or a lively party, leaves her unable to simmer down for hours afterward. Occasionally, in the middle of the night, she awakens feeling wide awake and again finds herself ruminating about the day's events. When she sleeps poorly, she feels "high strung" and tense the following day. The insomnia has worsened during the past year, coincident with more stress at work.

Ms. Harrington's business involves occasionally "wining and dining" other executives, but she finds that late meals or alcohol intake aggravate her insomnia. She has noticed that on days when she has cocktails with dinner, she invariably awakens in the middle of the night, feeling wide awake and slightly sweaty. Business travel also worsens her sleep. She finds herself in a state of unrelieved overstimulation when her job requires "running from city to city" for extended periods.

Ms. Harrington was divorced 3 years ago after 10 years of marriage. She has a wide circle of friends and enjoys socializing with them. Relaxing alone, however, has long been considered "dead time." Both of her parents and a sister have had problems with alcohol. She is the only one in her family to be steadily employed. During the last year she has been in once-a-week psychotherapy to try to understand "why I am so driven." The therapy has not helped her insomnia. She has also tried sleeping pills, which leave her "hungover" the following day.

Discussion of "High-Strung"

Ms. Harrington has long-standing problems with falling asleep at night, frequently awakening during the night, and being unable to return to sleep. The frequency and severity of the sleep difficulty and resulting daytime fatigue are clearly clinically significant, justifying a DSM-5-TR diagnosis of Insomnia Disorder (DSM-5-TR, p. 409). Although a number of factors, such as workday stressors and late-night alcohol intake, are likely contributing to her sleep difficulties, the descriptive diagnosis of Insomnia Disorder still applies given that her sleep problems meet the duration, frequency, and clinical significance requirements of the DSM-5-TR diagnosis.

12.2
Hypersomnolence Disorder

Individuals with Hypersomnolence Disorder experience excessive sleepiness despite having had an adequate amount of nighttime sleep (i.e., at least 7 hours). The symptom of excessive sleepiness can manifest in a number of ways. The person may feel compelled to nap throughout the day at inappropriate times, such as at work, while eating a meal, during a conversation, or while driving a car. Daytime naps usually provide no relief from symptoms. The individual may also report not feeling refreshed after awakening in the morning despite having slept for a long period of time (e.g., 9 hours or longer). The person may also experience what is known as *sleep inertia* or *sleep drunkenness*, which is defined as a period of impaired performance and reduced vigilance following awakening from a regular sleep episode or from a nap. DSM-5-TR requires a minimum frequency of at least three times per week of hypersomnolence symptoms and a minimum duration of 3 months, and also requires that the symptoms be sufficiently severe to cause clinically significant distress or impairment in social, occupational, or other important areas of functioning.

Although excessive daytime sleepiness may occur on its own in the absence of any other condition, it more often is a symptom of another sleep disorder, such as a Breathing-Related Sleep Disorder or Narcolepsy; a symptom of another mental disorder, such as Major Depressive Disorder; or a consequence of a nonpsychiatric medical condition, such as chronic pain. In such situations, a separate additional diagnosis of Hypersomnolence Disorder is given only if the hypersomnolence symptoms are a particular focus of clinical attention.

The persistent need for sleep can lead to automatic behavior that the person carries out with little or no subsequent recall of what they had been doing. For example, a person may find themselves having driven several miles from where they thought they were located, unaware of the "automatic" driving they did in the preceding minutes. Other symptoms may include anxiety, increased irritation, decreased energy, restlessness, slow thinking, slow speech, loss of appetite, hallucinations, and memory difficulty.

Approximately 5%–10% of individuals who seek consultation in sleep disorder clinics with complaints of daytime sleepiness receive a diagnosis of Hypersomnolence Disorder. Hypersomnolence occurs with relatively equal frequency in men and women.

Sleepy

Jerome Coopersmith, a 55-year-old businessman, has had excessive sleepiness since age 21. When he described this history to his new family physician, Mr. Coopersmith was referred to a sleep specialist. He typically sleeps from 10:15 P.M. to 7:30 A.M. He also takes half-hour to three-quarter-hour naps between 9:00 and 10:15 A.M. and between 1:30 and 2:00 P.M. and naps irregularly between 4:30 and 8:30 P.M. When napping at work, on his office floor, he sets incoming phone calls to automatically go to voicemail. He awakens temporarily refreshed. Delaying his naps causes overwhelming fatigue. He has no sudden loss of muscle tone (as in *cataplexy*, defined as episodes of loss of muscle tone and episodes of falling, often in association with intense emotions, such as laughter, anger, or fear) or other symptoms suggesting Narcolepsy, and neither snores nor has any other symptoms suggesting a Breathing-Related Sleep Disorder.

Although Mr. Coopersmith owns a TV station in Birmingham, Alabama, he is spared obligatory hard work because his staff can run the operation. Nevertheless, he is an organized, motivated person. He is in good health and jogs 4–5 miles daily. He lives with his wife and youngest son. He enjoys socializing with his married children and their families and dabbling in local politics. He takes a longer afternoon nap in anticipation of any evening activity, which he always leaves early in favor of his regular bedtime.

Mr. Coopersmith's father had taken a nap daily after lunch, and his paternal grandfather had also been excessively sleepy. During childhood, Mr. Coopersmith had had some nightmares but no other sleep problems.

During the interview, Mr. Coopersmith was friendly, informative, and self-assured. He denied depressed mood or loss of interest or pleasure. He regarded his sleepiness as a difficulty with which he had come to terms but would be grateful for further relief.

Tests of daytime vigilance indicated impaired arousal. During five polysomnographically recorded naps, his average time interval to sleep onset was

11 minutes, which is within the normal range. During a nighttime polysomno-graphic recording, he had normal-appearing sleep that continued uninter-rupted for 9½ hours until he had to be awakened.

Discussion of "Sleepy"

Mr. Coopersmith comes to his physician complaining of excessive daytime sleepiness, occurring every day for more than 30 years, and he presents with the typical symptoms of Hypersomnolence Disorder: he experiences daytime sleepiness even when sleeping for at least 9 hours at night, he takes multiple naps during the day, and he experiences extreme fatigue if he puts off napping. Although he is still able to function (albeit with accommodations like having his staff run the TV station he owns), he is clearly sufficiently distressed by this problem to follow through with his family physician's referral for help at a sleep center. Because excessive daytime sleepiness is often a feature of another sleep disorder (e.g., Narcolepsy or a Breathing-Related Sleep Disorder), an-other mental disorder (e.g., depression), or a nonpsychiatric medical condi-tion, or may be a side effect of a medication, the first step in the evaluation of excessive daytime sleepiness is to rule out these other causes, each of which has its own specific treatment. Given that Mr. Coopersmith is medically healthy and is not taking any medication, is not drinking or using substances, and has reported no signs or symptoms suggestive of a mental disorder or other sleep disorder, a specific cause for the hypersomnolence seems unlikely.

Both daytime polysomnography (to measure the extent of daytime sleepi-ness) and overnight polysomnography were done to rule out other sleep disor-ders, such as Narcolepsy, Breathing-Related Sleep Disorders, or Restless Legs Syndrome, as is typically done in cases of excessive daytime sleepiness evalu-ated at a sleep center. The Multiple Sleep Latency Test, performed during the daytime polysomnographic evaluation, measured how quickly Mr. Coopersmith fell asleep when asked to lie down in a darkened room. An average time to fall asleep of less than 8 minutes across four trials is considered objective ev-idence of excessive sleepiness. Mr. Coopersmith fell asleep in 11 minutes, which is within the normal adult range of 10 to 20 minutes. No sleep abnormalities were found on the overnight sleep study. Thus, the DSM-5-TR diagnosis in this case would be Hypersomnolence Disorder (DSM-5-TR, p. 417) occurring in the absence of other associated conditions.

Cry Me a River

Aliyssa Campbell, a 38-year-old clerical worker, presents to a psychiatrist describing how she has been suffering from a disabling sleep problem for 1½ years. She usually goes to bed at 6:00 P.M. and sleeps straight through until 7:00 A.M. The reason that she comes for help now is that last month her driver's license was suspended after she fell asleep while driving her car out of a parking lot and hit a telephone pole. As a result, she now has to get up at 6:00 A.M. to use public transportation to arrive in time for work at 8:15 A.M. On arising, Ms. Campbell typically feels groggy and "out of it." During the day, she remains sleepy. She frequently falls asleep on buses, missing her stop. In an attempt to remain on her feet at least some of the time that she is away from her office job, she recently took a sales job after her daytime job, which requires her to work from 6:00 P.M. to 10:00 P.M. 2 nights a week. On most weekends, Ms. Campbell remains in bed, asleep all day, arising only to go to the toilet or for meals, except on an occasional Saturday when she does her routine chores.

When asked by the psychiatrist during the evaluation about other sleep-related symptoms, Ms. Campbell reported that she does not believe she snores during sleep, as would be likely in sleep apnea, and she denies nightmares, sleepwalking, or sudden losses of muscle tone (cataplexy) or feelings of paralysis on awakening, which are both symptoms of Narcolepsy.

Before the onset of her sleep problem 1½ years ago, Ms. Campbell generally required only 6–7 hours of sleep a night. During the first year of her "sleepiness," she began to treat herself with caffeine, drinking up to 10 cups of coffee and 1–2 liters of cola daily in an attempt to stay awake.

When the psychiatrist asked whether she has had any psychiatric problems, Ms. Campbell reported that in addition to the sleepiness, she has had severe, recurrent periods of depression since approximately age 13. For several months before the evaluation, she was having crying spells in her office. These sometimes would come on so suddenly that she had no time to run to the restroom to hide. She acknowledged trouble concentrating on her job and noted that she was getting little pleasure from her work, something she used to enjoy. She had been harboring angry and pessimistic feelings for the past several years, and noted that these were more severe recently because she had allowed her diabetes and weight to get out of control. She felt guilty that she was physically damaging herself and slowly dying in this way. She sometimes thought that she deserved to be dead.

She had been treated from age 18 to age 33 with psychotherapy, during which time her depression gradually worsened. More recently, she had been given trials of several different antidepressants, each of which had made improvements in mood and wakefulness that lasted several months. She tended to fall asleep during evening group psychotherapy sessions.

Ms. Campbell had done poorly in high school, and she had gone to business school for 4 years but had failed to graduate. Despite entertaining hopes for a romantic relationship, she had never had a steady boyfriend. She lives at home with her mother and has no close friends outside her family. On close questioning, it became apparent that the onset of her sleep problems and the beginning of her most recent period of depression had coincided.

As she described her problem to the psychiatrist, she gazed continually downward and spoke in a low monotone. She answered questions dutifully but without elaboration. She shed copious tears.

Discussion of "Cry Me a River"

Ms. Campbell experiences recurrent periods of depression, although her predominant complaints are of disabling excessive daytime sleepiness that has persisted for the past 1½ years. She lapses into sleep throughout the day (e.g., she fell asleep while driving her car, she falls asleep on buses and misses her stop), remains in bed asleep all day on weekends, and has symptoms of sleep inertia, feeling groggy and "out of it" on awakening.

As in all cases in which a person presents with excessive daytime sleepiness, it is important to first determine whether there are any accompanying conditions that might explain the symptoms. In Ms. Campbell's case, there is no evidence that her excessive daytime sleepiness is entirely explained by another sleep disorder, such as a Breathing-Related Sleep Disorder or Narcolepsy, or that it is due to substance use or is a side effect of a medication. However, Ms. Campbell has recurrent depression, and her sleep problems developed in the midst of her latest depressive episode. Given that hypersomnia is a common symptom of depression, it is fairly clear that her excessive daytime sleepiness is not an independent sleep problem but instead is part of the presentation of Major Depressive Disorder. The DSM-5-TR criteria for Hypersomnolence Disorder (DSM-5-TR, p. 417) allow the diagnosis to be given in addition to a preexisting mental disorder diagnosis only if the mental disorder (in this case, Major Depressive Disorder) does not adequately explain the complaint of hypersomnolence. In Ms. Campbell's case, the onset of her sleep problem coincided with the onset of her current episode of depression; therefore, the diagnosis of Hypersomnolence Disorder would not be appropriate. If, however, Ms. Campbell were to experience hypersomnolence at times other than when she was depressed, an additional diagnosis of Hypersomnolence Disorder would be warranted.

12.3
Narcolepsy

Narcolepsy is a chronic neurological disorder involving poor control of the sleep-wake cycle. It is included in DSM-5-TR because it is one of the conditions a clinician needs to rule out when a patient presents with excessive daytime sleepiness. Individuals with Narcolepsy experience daytime sleepiness accompanied by intermittent uncontrollable bouts of falling asleep during the daytime that usually last a few seconds to several minutes. These "sleep attacks" can greatly affect daily functioning, because people may unwillingly fall asleep at work, at school, in the middle of a conversation, while eating a meal, or most dangerously, while driving a car or operating other types of machinery. Most individuals with Narcolepsy experience episodes of *cataplexy,* a phenomenon that involves a sudden loss of voluntary muscle tone lasting from seconds to minutes that is precipitated by emotional reactions such as laughter, anger, surprise, or fear. Muscles affected in cataplexy may include those of the neck, jaw, arms, legs, or whole body, resulting in head bobbing, jaw dropping, or complete falls.

A DSM-5-TR diagnosis of Narcolepsy applies to individuals who have had at least three lapses into sleep per week over the past 3 months, plus at least a few episodes per month of cataplexy. For those individuals with bouts of lapsing into sleep who do not have cataplexy, the Narcolepsy diagnosis can still be made if there is either evidence of hypocretin deficiency or evidence from polysomnography of a shortened period of time from the onset of sleep to the start of the first REM sleep period (REM latency). The neurotransmitter hypocretin, which is measured in cerebrospinal fluid obtained from a spinal tap, is reduced in patients with Narcolepsy, reflecting the loss of hypocretin-producing cells in the hypothalamus (a region of the brain responsible for the production of many of the body's essential hormones), which appears to be the cause of most cases of Narcolepsy. The shortened REM latency time seen on polysomnography is also a hallmark of Narcolepsy. In a normal sleep cycle, REM sleep does not start until at least 60–90 minutes after a person falls asleep. In individuals with Narcolepsy, however, REM sleep occurs within minutes of falling asleep.

Other symptoms that commonly occur in Narcolepsy include sleep paralysis and vivid hallucinations. Sleep paralysis involves the temporary inability to talk or move on awakening or when falling asleep, lasting from a few seconds to minutes. It is a normal brain mechanism occurring during REM sleep and is what prevents a person from acting out dream content while in the midst of a dream. In Narcolepsy, it also occurs during transitions from wakefulness to sleep. Visual hallucinations (see introduction to Chapter 2, "Schizophrenia Spectrum and Other Psychotic Disorders") may accompany sleep paralysis and occur when the person is falling asleep or awakening. Referred to as *hypnagogic hallucinations* when they occur during sleep onset and *hypnopompic hallucinations* when occurring during the transition from sleep to wakefulness, these images are unusually vivid, seem real, and can be quite frightening.

Narcolepsy typically starts in childhood, adolescence, or young adulthood. Narcolepsy is quite rare, affecting less than 0.05% of the general population.

Catnaps

Nora Thompson, a 24-year-old graduate student, complained to her primary care doctor of episodes of severe daytime sleepiness that force her to take naps. Sometimes, when she attempts to stay awake, she is unable to do so, and she has fallen asleep at the dinner table and even when walking. She has trouble staying alert enough to get off at the right bus stop. In fact, she is unable to remain seated without becoming sleepy. She slept through classes and failed her courses in graduate school.

Ms. Thompson is also bothered by frequent episodes of cataplexy, in which she becomes limp and briefly unable to move after sudden emotional arousal—for example, after discovering that her cat had urinated on her rug, and after becoming enraged with her roommate. On another occasion, she nearly had a car accident when another driver did something that annoyed her and she almost lost control of the car.

As she falls asleep at night, Ms. Thompson sees vivid scenes that seem real and she feels that someone else is in the room with her. She still feels awake, however, and knows that there really is no one else there. Her sleep is frequently punctuated by nightmares. She then wakes up feeling very hungry and has a snack.

Extremely bothersome to Ms. Thompson is her continual "automatic behavior," in which she suddenly discovers that she has accomplished very little after a lengthy period of work on a task. For example, she spent 2 hours unsuccessfully trying to fix her glasses and was unaware of this until her roommate interrupted her and pointed it out. The automatic behavior makes it difficult for her to change from one task to another, so it sometimes takes her 2 hours to get out of the house in the morning or to get ready for bed at night. Delays in getting to bed prevent her from getting a good night's sleep, which further aggravates her daytime sleepiness. Her roommate grew weary of her undependability, and she had to move back to her parents' home.

Ms. Thompson was referred to a sleep center, where she was instructed to keep records of her in-bed times, nap times, cataplexy attacks, episodes of night eating, and automatic behaviors. At the time of her evaluation, she was on a drug regimen from her primary care doctor consisting of nortriptyline, an antidepressant; dextroamphetamine, a stimulant; and zolpidem, a sleeping pill. Psychotherapy was started, which focused on examining those behaviors that worsened her situation, such as her failure to adhere to prescribed bedtimes and forgetting to take medication. The zolpidem was tapered and discontinued, and the dosages of nortriptyline and dextroamphetamine were empirically adjusted on the basis of the records she kept of her behavior.

Ms. Thompson's symptoms gradually disappeared, and she was able to move out of her parents' house, get a job, reestablish a social life, and return to graduate school.

Discussion of "Catnaps"

Ms. Thompson's symptomatic presentation is characteristic of Narcolepsy. She has recurrent periods of an irrepressible need for sleep (e.g., she has fallen asleep at the dinner table and has missed her bus stop because of inability to stay awake), as well as episodes of cataplexy, such as when she nearly had a car accident when another driver did something that annoyed her and she almost lost control of her car. Although polysomnographic evidence of shortened REM latency or hypocretin deficiency as measured by a spinal tap are also indicative of Narcolepsy, the presence of frequent lapses into sleep accompanied by episodes of cataplexy are sufficient for Ms. Thompson's presentation to meet the DSM-5-TR definitional requirements for Narcolepsy (DSM-5-TR, p. 422). Many of the other symptoms that she has experienced, such as vivid visual hallucinations that occur as she is falling asleep and automatic behaviors, in which she continues her activities in a semiautomatic haze-like fashion without memory or consciousness, are commonly associated with, although not diagnostic of, Narcolepsy.

12.4
Obstructive Sleep Apnea Hypopnea

DSM-5-TR includes a Breathing-Related Sleep Disorders subgroup of conditions that involve difficulty breathing during sleep. The most common breathing-related sleep disorder, Obstructive Sleep Apnea Hypopnea, is characterized by repeated episodes in which the person's breathing is interrupted by a physical block to airflow during sleep. If there is a total absence of airflow, these episodes are called *apneas*; if there is a reduction in airflow, they are referred to as *hypopneas*. These periods of absence of or reduction in breathing last at least 10 seconds and are associated with reduced blood oxygen saturation. The chronic reduction of overnight blood oxygen can have a number of long-term, adverse medical consequences, including high blood pressure, heart disease, stroke, diabetes, and depression. Individuals with Obstructive Sleep Apnea Hypopnea are rarely aware of having difficulty breathing at night, even on awakening, but typically experience daytime sleepiness and fatigue, morning headaches, and moodiness. The nighttime breathing difficulties are usually first recognized as a problem by bed partners who witness the episodes of not breathing.

Obstructive Sleep Apnea Hypopnea is diagnosed on the basis of polysomnographic findings and symptoms. A definitive diagnosis requires an overnight stay in a sleep lab. Diagnosis can be made if the patient is found through polysomnography to have five or more obstructive apneas or hypopneas per hour of sleep plus either of the following symptoms: 1) sleep-related breathing disturbances, such as snoring, snorting/gasping, and breathing pauses during sleep, or 2) complaints of daytime sleepiness, fatigue, or unrefreshing sleep despite sufficient opportunities to sleep. Alternatively, the diagnosis can be made in the absence of symptoms if more than 15 apneas or hypopneas per hour are detected during polysomnography.

The two other breathing-related sleep disorders included in DSM-5-TR, Central Sleep Apnea and Sleep-Related Hypoventilation, are characterized by insufficient sleep-related ventilation not caused by airway obstruction. Central Sleep Apnea is characterized by repeated episodes of apneas and hypopneas during sleep caused by variability in respiratory effort; the disorder may be due to a nonpsychiatric medical condition, such as heart failure, stroke, and renal failure, or it may occur as a side effect of a long-acting opioid (e.g., methadone) or after ascending to a high altitude (generally above 8,000 feet). In Sleep-Related Hypoventilation, the episodes of insufficient sleep-related breathing are more sustained than those in Central Sleep Apnea and are typically related to a nonpsychiatric medical condition (e.g., chronic obstructive pulmonary disease, kyphoscoliosis, obesity) or to the use of central nervous system depressants (e.g., alcohol, benzodiazepines, opioids).

Obstructive Sleep Apnea Hypopnea is a common disorder. In the United States, 13% of men and 6% of women have polysomnographic evidence of 15 or more obstructive apneas or hypopneas per hour of sleep, and 14% of men and 5% of women have polysomnographic evidence of more than 5 obstructive apneas or hypopneas per hour, plus symptoms of daytime sleepiness. In adults, the male-to-female ratio ranges from 2:1 to 4:1. Obstructive Sleep Apnea Hypopnea is also associated with obesity. It is believed that the airway of an obese individual becomes blocked by large tonsils, an enlarged tongue, and increased fat in the neck. However, the common assumption that Obstructive Sleep Apnea Hypopnea affects only older, overweight men is wrong; anyone can have sleep apnea, regardless of gender, age, or body type.

Food for Thought

Thomas Grim is a 46-year-old advertising salesman and writer for a small magazine. During 15 years of marriage, his wife has noticed loud snoring and episodes, lasting 10–15 seconds, during which Mr. Grim does not breathe. According to his wife, "then he takes a giant breath, exhales, inhales one to four or five times, then he stops breathing for another one of these silences." During longer "not-breathing" periods, as she refers to them, "he is very restless. He can dish out quite a kick or punch if I haven't moved far enough out of the way." After nights full of such events, Mr. Grim groggily drags himself out of bed in the morning with a severe headache.

Mr. Grim is usually sleepy during the day, especially while driving the turnpikes around New England, as required for his work. To remain vigilant, he munches on fast-food hamburgers, washed down by gallons of Mountain Dew. Any alcoholic beverages make him want to fall asleep.

As a result of his snacks, Mr. Grim has 280 pounds packed onto his 5'8" frame. He is able to diet and lose weight only temporarily. Recently, he has developed a hiatal hernia (a protrusion of the upper part of the stomach into the chest through a weakness in the diaphragm) associated with stomach pain and indigestion, mild diabetes, and high blood pressure, all complications of the obesity.

When Mr. Grim was a child, his mother constantly berated him for being too fat, and he feared she would starve him. It was then that he developed a habit of stopping for food whenever he was out of the house.

Nasal stuffiness during hay fever season (generally in the early autumn months) worsens his snoring, the nocturnal "struggles," and the morning headaches. Just before his first interview with a physician at a sleep disorders clinic about his sleep problems, Mr. Grim had cleaned out an old barn and attic, both full of dust and pigeon droppings, and had experienced a severe allergy attack.

Physical examination disclosed a deviated nasal septum, enlargement and thickening of the pharyngeal (throat) structures, and collapse of his pharyngeal walls into the airway on taking a deep breath with his nose blocked.

A daytime Continuous Performance Test was then administered to assess Mr. Grim's ability to maintain a consistent focus on a continuous activity, which can be an indicator of daytime impairment. During the test, in which letters were presented at a rate of 1 per second, Mr. Grim was instructed to push a button whenever he saw certain letters. He scored 44% correct, compared with a normal rate of 66%–78%, indicating moderate impairment in concentration, which was worse in the morning. Laboratory sleep monitoring revealed the occurrence of more than 30 episodes per hour of 15- to 60-second periods of not breathing (sleep apnea). Each episode was associated with 1) decreased oxygen saturation (levels frequently below 50%, where 90% is considered normal during sleep) and 2) a decreased heart rate (50–55 beats per minute) followed by an increased heart rate (to about 90 beats per minute). No normal periods of deep sleep were recorded on the polysomnogram. These findings indicated severe sleep apnea, which interfered with the quality of Mr. Grim's nocturnal sleep and caused his daytime sleepiness and impaired daytime arousal. The clinician decided that Mr. Grim's obesity and the structural and functional impairment of his upper airway were the causes of the apnea.

Treatment of the sleep apnea was by continuous positive airway pressure (CPAP), a technique in which the pressure of the inspired air is increased by a machine connected to the patient with a face mask and tube at night, which helps overcome the airway obstruction. Mr. Grim's snoring and sleepiness were rapidly relieved, and he became motivated, for the first time in his life, to stay on a diet. Within 6 months, he had lost 80 pounds. He said he felt "like I have gotten my youth back."

Discussion of "Food for Thought"

Mr. Grim's primary problem is chronic excessive daytime sleepiness due to recurrent periods of sleep apnea. Although his sleep is adequate in amount, it is not restful. As is typical for this disorder, the patient himself was not aware of his nocturnal breathing pauses; it was only evident on collateral reporting by his wife. Polysomnography indicated more than 30 episodes per hour, which far exceeded the minimum requirement of 5 per hour in someone who has daytime sleepiness, confirming the diagnosis of Obstructive Sleep Apnea Hypopnea (DSM-5-TR, p. 429). The CPAP device was successful in treating Mr. Grim's condition, resulting in relief of both his nighttime breathing difficulties and his daytime sleepiness. Although CPAP has a nearly 100% success rate, it is often difficult to get patients to comply with the nighttime treatment because many find the device uncomfortable to use regularly. Perhaps Mr. Grim's newfound motivation to stay on a diet will allow him to lose enough weight to reduce or eliminate his sleep apnea.

12.5
Circadian Rhythm
Sleep-Wake Disorders

Humans, like most living organisms, have biological rhythms known as circadian rhythms, which are controlled by an internal body clock in a control center of the brain known as the suprachiasmatic nucleus, which is located in the hypothalamus. The primary circadian rhythm that this body clock controls is the sleep-wake cycle. Because of the circadian clock, sleepiness does not continuously increase as time passes. A person's desire and ability to fall asleep is influenced both by the length of time elapsed since the person last woke from an adequate sleep and by internal circadian rhythms. Thus, the body is ready for sleep and for wakefulness at different times of the day. The circadian clock functions in a cycle that lasts a little longer than 24 hours and is set primarily by visual cues of light and darkness, which keep the clock synchronized to the 24-hour day.

Circadian Rhythm Sleep-Wake Disorders include a variety of subtypes in which there is a continuous or occasional disruption of sleep patterns. The disruption results from either a malfunction in the internal body clock or a mismatch between the internal body clock and the demands of the external environment regarding the timing and duration of sleep. As a result of the circadian mismatch, individuals with these disorders usually complain of insomnia at certain times and excessive sleepiness at other times of the day, resulting in work, school, or social impairments. They are generally able to get enough sleep, however, if allowed to sleep and wake at the times dictated by their body clocks. Unless they also have another sleep disorder, the quality of their sleep is usually normal.

DSM-5-TR includes five specific subtypes of Circadian Rhythm Sleep-Wake Disorders. For contrast, a person with a normal circadian rhythm will regularly experience sleepiness in the latter part of the evening (around 10 P.M.). For a person with the Delayed Sleep Phase Type (a so-called night owl), the tendency to feel sleepy at night is delayed relative to conventional bedtimes, with the person typically feeling sleepy around 2:00 A.M. or later and waking up later in the morning. A person with the Advanced Sleep Phase Type (a so-called lark) will regularly feel sleepy several hours earlier in the evening than is normal, between 6:00 P.M. and 9:00 P.M., and wake up between 2:00 A.M. and 5:00 A.M. In the Irregular Sleep-Wake Type, there is a lack of discernible circadian rhythm, such that the timing of sleep and wake periods is variable throughout the 24-hour period. In the Non-24-Hour Sleep-Wake Type, there is a pattern of sleep-wake cycles that is not synchronized to the 24-hour environment, with a consistent daily drift (usually to later and later times) of sleep onset and wake times. Shift Work Type affects people who frequently rotate shifts or work at night and have particular difficulty adjusting to the change.

Although the prevalence of Circadian Rhythm Sleep-Wake Disorders in general is unknown, some of the subtypes occur more frequently among specific population groups. The Delayed Sleep Phase Type is most common in teens and young adults, with a prevalence of about 4% in this age group. The Advanced Sleep Phase Type becomes more common with increased age, with a prevalence of about 1% of middle-age and older adults. The Non-24-Hour Sleep-Wake Type is estimated to occur in about half of blind individuals. The Shift Work Type is estimated to affect 5%–10% of the night worker population.

The Director

Joe Neeley, a 36-year-old film director, has had frequent difficulty falling asleep since early childhood. He typically goes to bed between 11:30 P.M. and 3:30 A.M. and gets up at irregular times before 1:00 P.M. His sleep is lighter at the beginning of the night, when he is easily disturbed by random noises or his wife's shifting in bed. Later in the night he sleeps more soundly, and he feels that his deepest sleep occurs at about 8:00 A.M. He feels groggy for half an hour or longer on first arising and is not able to function well in the early part of the day.

Mr. Neeley is currently free of scheduled work obligations except a morning meeting once a week. This has further lessened his motivation to get out of bed in the morning. In the evening, however, he experiences a surge of productive energy. His mind is enjoyably active, and he delays bedtimes to capitalize on his high work capacity. When on fishing trips, he arises at 5:00 A.M. and takes a nap at 9:00 A.M. The discrepancy between his and others' sleep schedules on weekends and other social inconveniences caused by his sleep schedule have motivated him to seek help.

Mr. Neeley drinks 2–5 cups of coffee daily, more during occasional work crises. He has had a frequently stuffy nose, and occasionally uses the over-the-counter cold medication pseudoephedrine for stimulation, as well as a nasal decongestant (such medications often have long-lasting stimulant effects).

At the time of the evaluation, Mr. Neeley was casually dressed, ingratiating, and friendly. Despite professions of self-doubt, he was forward, frank, and engaging. The psychiatrist recommended that he keep a sleep chart for 1 month. The sleep chart revealed bedtimes that were progressively delayed from 9:00 or 10:00 P.M. until about 3:15 A.M. over 5- to 7-day cycles. Arising times were even less regular in pattern, generally becoming later at the end of three cycles. Usually, some obligation required him to get up even after a late bedtime, causing him to take an afternoon nap or to go to sleep for the evening at around 10:00 P.M. Thereafter, he would fail to fall asleep for some hours. After 1 or 2 such days, the cycle would begin again.

Discussion of "The Director"

Mr. Neeley shows the characteristic features of Circadian Rhythm Sleep-Wake Disorder, Delayed Sleep Phase Type (DSM-5-TR, p. 443). There is a mismatch between his normal circadian sleep-wake pattern and the sleep-wake schedule for his environment. The mismatch is that his preferred sleep onset and offset are several hours later than those of people he works and socializes with; that is, his sleep schedule is *delayed* relative to the conventional societal sleep-wake schedule.

The lack of regular work hours, the "night-person" pattern of greater evening productivity, and the subjectively deeper sleep later in the night are all typical of individuals with the Delayed Sleep Phase Type of Circadian Rhythm Sleep-Wake Disorder. The lack of scheduled work obligations removed an important pacemaker for Mr. Neeley's sleep-wake schedule, unmasking the delaying tendency. Mr. Neeley's use of stimulants contributed to his evening productivity and to his difficulty in falling asleep earlier.

Evening Shift

Richard Symanski, a 30-year-old warehouse worker, sought medical help for his sleep problem. He reported that he had experienced episodes of poor sleep for the preceding 5 years whenever he had to work the evening shift. Every 2 weeks he alternated between working evenings (3:00 P.M. to 11:00 P.M.) and working the day shift (7:00 A.M. to 3:00 P.M.). When he worked the evening shift, he would go to bed about 2 hours after work, around 1:00 A.M. About half the time, it would take him 1–2 hours to fall asleep. When this happened, he typically would awaken at 5:00 A.M., his normal time for getting up to go to work for the day shift. He would have a snack and then return to bed and drift in and out of sleep until arising between 8:30 A.M. and 11:00 A.M. On weekends and holidays, however, he would revert to his normal bedtime, approximately 10:00 P.M., when he would fall into bed exhausted.

When Mr. Symanski slept poorly at night, he felt sleepy the next day; if he slept well, he felt alert. When he worked the day shift and when on vacations, he slept well and felt alert the next day.

The physician advised Mr. Symanski to gradually discontinue eating at night to stop reinforcing his nocturnal appetite and wakefulness. In addition, Mr. Symanski was advised to arise at 8:30 A.M. when he worked the evening shift, no matter how tired he felt. The hope was that he would feel tired enough at 1:00 A.M. to fall asleep immediately and then have a full night's sleep.

After trying the program, the patient reported that he could not stick to the recommended plan. He said he became "like a madman" during the night, searching everywhere for his favorite snacks after his wife, with his consent, had hidden them. Nor could he remain awake until 1:00 A.M. on the weekend between the 2 weeks of the evening shift.

Mr. Symanski did not return for another appointment, but he called several months later to report that he had been able to convince his employer to take him off the evening work shift permanently, which completely relieved his sleep problem.

Discussion of "Evening Shift"

Mr. Symanski's sleep rhythm induced by daytime work persists when he works the evening shift. The mismatch between his circadian rhythm and the demands of his evening work schedule result in insomnia (trouble falling asleep and staying asleep). His biological clock causes sleepiness at 10:00 P.M. and awakening at about 5:00 A.M. When he works the evening shift, he is forced to stay awake for hours beyond his usual bedtime, and he initially awakens at his usual arising time. Given that his disrupted sleep is primarily due to a misalignment between his endogenous circadian rhythm and the schedule required by his shift work, the DSM-5-TR diagnosis is Circadian Rhythm Sleep-Wake Disorder, Shift Work Type (DSM-5-TR, p. 444).

If Mr. Symanski were able to stay on the evening shift for several months and maintain the same sleep times, his biological clock would gradually be reset so that his sleep schedule would harmonize with the hours of his workday. In his case, because the hours of his shift kept changing, and he was apparently particularly intolerant of the mismatch between his circadian rhythm and his daily work schedule, he could not sleep during desirable hours.

12.6
Non–Rapid Eye Movement Sleep Arousal Disorders

NREM Sleep Arousal Disorders are characterized by the repeated occurrence of incomplete awakening from periods of deep non-REM sleep (usually stage 3) and can involve either sleepwalking (diagnosed as Sleepwalking Type) or sleep terrors (diagnosed as Sleep Terror Type). Given that the amount of time spent in non-REM sleep is greater early in the night, sleepwalking and sleep terrors usually occur during the first third of the major sleep episode.

Sleepwalking may involve sitting up and looking awake, getting up, and walking around when the individual is actually asleep. While sleepwalking, the person has a blank staring face, is relatively unresponsive to the efforts of others to communicate with them, and can be awakened only with great difficulty. Although the majority of sleepwalking episodes involve benign behaviors such as walking and talking, some individuals engage in sexual activity or sleep eating. Sleepwalking is much more common in children than in adults and is more likely to occur if a person is sleep-deprived.

Sleep terrors (also known as night terrors) are recurrent episodes of abrupt physiological arousal that partially awaken the person in a state of fear, and usually begin with a panicky scream. During a typical episode of sleep terror, the individual abruptly sits up in bed screaming or crying, with a frightened expression and physical signs of intense anxiety (e.g., rapid heartbeat, rapid breathing, sweating, pupil dilation). The person may be inconsolable and is usually unresponsive to the efforts of others to awaken or comfort them.

Given that these episodes occur during non-REM sleep, the individual recalls little or no dream imagery on awakening. Moreover, the person is unable to remember the sleepwalking or sleep terror episodes immediately afterward or the next morning.

Isolated or occasional episodes of sleepwalking or sleep terrors are very common in the general population. Between 10% and 30% of children have had at least one episode of sleepwalking, and the 12-month prevalence rate in children is about 5%. In adults, the lifetime prevalence of sleepwalking episodes ranges from 7% to 29% around the world, with a past-year prevalence of 1.5%–4%. Note that occasional sleep terror episodes should not be confused with the Sleep Terror Type of NREM Sleep Arousal Disorder, in which there is recurrence and distress or impairment. The prevalence of occasional sleep terror episodes is approximately 35% in children 18 months of age, 20% in those 30 months of age, and 2% in adults.

Zombie

Meghan, an 11-year-old girl, told her mother that she was afraid she might be "going crazy," and her mother has brought her to a psychiatrist. Several times during the last 2 months Meghan has awakened confused about where she is, until she realizes she is on the living room couch or in her little sister's bed, even though she went to bed in her own room. When she recently woke up in her older brother's bedroom, she became very concerned and felt quite guilty about it. Her younger sister says that she has seen Meghan walking during the night, looking like a "zombie"; that Meghan did not answer when called; and that Meghan has done that several times but usually goes back to her bed. Meghan fears she may have "amnesia" because she has no memory of anything happening during the night.

Meghan has never had a seizure or experienced similar episodes during the day. An electroencephalogram (EEG) and physical examination are normal. Meghan's mental status is unremarkable except for some anxiety about her symptom and the usual early-adolescence concerns about fitting in with her friends. Her school and family functioning are excellent.

Discussion of "Zombie"

Meghan is not "going crazy" but rather is experiencing the characteristic features of the Sleepwalking Type of NREM Sleep Arousal Disorder (DSM-5-TR,

p. 452): episodes of arising from bed during sleep and walking about, appearing unresponsive during the episodes, experiencing amnesia for the episodes on awakening, and exhibiting no evidence of impairment in consciousness several minutes after awakening. Psychomotor epileptic seizures are ruled out by the normal EEG and the absence of any seizure-like behavior during the waking state.

Goose Pimples

Matthew, an 8-year-old boy, was taken by his parents to the pediatric emergency room one night at 12:30 A.M. The parents were very concerned because he woke them up with a sudden, intense, bloodcurdling scream. They went to his room and found him sitting up in bed perspiring copiously, anxious and trembling, with rapid breathing and "goose pimples." He kept putting his forefinger in his nose (an unusual gesture for him) and was quite disoriented and anxious, as if something terrible were about to happen. His speech was not intelligible. He remained in this state for about 10 minutes, despite his parents' efforts to calm him. Once in the car on the way to the hospital, he calmed down and became quite sleepy again.

When first seen in the emergency room, Matthew was asleep, but after being awakened, he resisted being examined. His physical examination was negative except he had a pulse rate of 110 beats per minute and mildly damp pajamas (because of excessive sweating).

Matthew's mother is afraid he may have epilepsy, as an uncle of hers had, but she noticed that her son, unlike her uncle, had not bitten his tongue or wet himself during the episode. Matthew has no history of seizures or febrile convulsions. When he was about 4½, he had occasional nightmares for a few months, but his mother thinks that the current incident "is different."

Discussion of "Goose Pimples"

Matthew's mother is probably correct in ruling out epilepsy. In fact, what Matthew appears to have experienced are the characteristic features of an episode of sleep terrors, described in NREM Sleep Arousal Disorder, Sleep Terror Type (DSM-5-TR, p. 452): abrupt awakening from sleep without a dream and with a scream; intense anxiety during the episode, with sweating, rapid breathing, and piloerection ("goose pimples"); relative unresponsiveness to efforts of others to comfort him; and disorientation, confusion, and perseverative motor movements (he kept putting his forefinger in his nose). Because the DSM-5-TR criteria require "recurrent" sleep terror episodes to justify a diagnosis, no diagnosis would be given to Matthew at this point in time. If these episodes become frequent and cause him problems (e.g., avoiding sleepaway camp), a diagnosis may eventually become warranted.

12.7
Nightmare Disorder

Nightmare Disorder is characterized by repeated awakenings from the major sleep period or from naps, with detailed recall of extended and extremely frightening dreams, usually involving threats to survival, security, or self-esteem. On awakening from the frightening dreams, the person rapidly becomes oriented and alert (in contrast to the confusion and disorientation seen when a person is awakened from a sleep terror or sleepwalking).

Nightmares generally occur during periods of REM sleep. Given that the REM sleep stages lengthen throughout the night, starting from several minutes long in the first cycle and extending to up to an hour in the last cycle, nightmares are more likely to occur in the second half of the major sleep period. Nightmares often begin between ages 3 and 6 years but are most common and severe in late adolescence or early adulthood. In a minority of people, frequent nightmares persist into adulthood, becoming virtually a lifelong disturbance.

The prevalence of nightmares during childhood is approximately 1%–5%. The prevalence of nightmares occurring at least once a month in adults is 6%. A DSM-5-TR diagnosis of Nightmare Disorder is reserved for individuals whose nightmares cause significant distress or impairment in functioning, such as might occur if the awakenings are frequent or result in avoidance of sleep, which can lead to excessive daytime sleepiness, poor concentration, depression, anxiety, and irritability.

Bad Dreamer

Mayra Sanchez, a 35-year-old married woman with a young daughter, has experienced nightmares every night since her early teenage years. She comes to a sleep specialist at the insistence of her husband, who is fed up with her behavior, both while sleeping and while awake. One to four times a night, she awakens out of a dream, the content of which is always disturbing. She often dreams of yelling at other people or of menacing confrontations. In the dreams, she feels angry and frustrated. Typically, she awakens from the dreams feeling extremely tense.

She denies having sudden, irresistible attacks of sleepiness, cataplexy (sudden loss of motor power), hypnopompic hallucinations (hallucinations that occur while waking up), or sleep paralysis (motor weakness and brief inability to move on sudden awakening), all of which are characteristic of Narcolepsy. She denies feeling confused or disoriented when she awakens from her dreams (as might occur in impaired arousal states, such as in episodes associated with temporal lobe dysfunction). Mrs. Sanchez is not currently taking any medication and denies use of alcohol or any recreational drugs.

At the initial evaluation, Mrs. Sanchez appeared downcast but did not cry. She was organized and informative. She made three mistakes on serial 7s (a test of cognitive functioning in which a person is asked to count backward from 100 by 7s), but her cognitive functioning was otherwise intact. She spoke of her work as a registrar in a small college, a job that she considers enjoyable and her "salvation." Her 4-year-old daughter is bright and well. Mrs. Sanchez denied any past history of trauma exposure.

Mrs. Sanchez has smoked a pack of cigarettes a day for 20 years, and drinks a cup of coffee and 48 ounces of cola beverages daily. She drinks alcohol only a few times each year.

All-night sleep recording revealed 9 hours of continuous sleep. REM sleep latency (the time spent before the initial appearance of REM sleep), density, and amount were normal, and other stages of sleep were of normal pattern and percentage. However, there were no reports of nightmares during the night.

Treatment has included psychotherapy, attempts to control dream content through a lucid dreaming routine (in which the dreamer directs the events of the dream or attempts to converse with the characters in it), and trials of an antidepressant medication and of an anticonvulsant medication.

Discussion of "Bad Dreamer"

Mrs. Sanchez's predominant complaint is recurrent nightmares that are distressing to both her and her husband. There is no evidence of any specific cause for her nightmares, such as another sleep disorder (e.g., REM Sleep Behavior Disorder [see Section 12.8]) that may be responsible for the nightmares; a medication that is known to cause nightmares, such as an antidepressant or blood pressure medication; cocaine or amphetamine use; withdrawal from alcohol or sleeping pills; or Posttraumatic Stress Disorder (see "The Singer" in Section 7.3), which is often associated with nightmares involving the traumatic event. Thus, the DSM-5-TR diagnosis for Mrs. Sanchez would be Nightmare Disorder (DSM-5-TR, p. 457).

12.8
Rapid Eye Movement
Sleep Behavior Disorder

In a person with REM Sleep Behavior Disorder, the muscle paralysis that normally occurs during REM sleep is incomplete or absent, allowing the person to "act out" their dreams. These behaviors often reflect motor enactments of or responses to the content of action-filled or violent dreams of being attacked or trying to escape from a threatening situation. Vocalizations occur, which are often loud, emotion filled, and profane. These behaviors may be very bothersome to the individual and their bed partner and may result in significant injury (e.g., falling, jumping, or flying out of bed; running; punching; thrusting; hitting; kicking). On awakening, the individual is immediately awake, alert, and oriented to where they are and the general time of day, and is often able to recall dream content, which closely correlates with the observed behavior.

REM Sleep Behavior Disorder can be confused with the NREM Sleep Arousal Disorders, which are also characterized by behaviors occurring during sleep (i.e., sleepwalking or sleep terrors; see Section 12.6). In these latter disorders, which occur during NREM stages of deep sleep, the sleeper is usually confused on awakening; they do not become rapidly alert. In contrast, it is normally easy to wake a person with REM Sleep Behavior Disorder who is acting out a dream.

REM Sleep Behavior Disorder can be caused by adverse reactions to certain drugs or can occur during drug withdrawal; however, it is most often associated with older age and with neurodegenerative disorders such as Parkinson's disease and Lewy body dementia (a type of dementia associated with abnormal deposits of a protein called alpha-synuclein in the brain). The prevalence of REM Sleep Behavior Disorder is 1%–2% in middle- to older-age individuals in the general population. REM Sleep Behavior Disorder is present concurrently in 30% of patients with Narcolepsy. The majority of people with REM Sleep Behavior Disorder are men, and the disorder usually affects individuals who are older than 50 years. Increasingly, the disorder is being found in women and younger people.

Falling Out of Bed

Ethan Bonner is a 65-year-old married English professor whose wife had encouraged him to seek medical attention after he had fallen out of bed, sustaining a head injury without loss of consciousness but incurring a scalp laceration requiring sutures. He reported that at the time of the fall, he had been dreaming that he was being chased by dogs and jumped over a small stream, at which time he awakened as his head hit the floor.

Mr. Bonner's wife, who had been asked to accompany him to the clinic visit, reported that over the past 4–5 years, her husband's sleep had become progressively disturbed—interrupted by vocalizations (often profane), shouting, and screaming and by increased motor behaviors that began as only minor twitching, but progressed over time to arm and leg flailing, pounding the mattress or his pillow, running or boxing movements, and occasionally punching or hitting his wife. If his wife awakened him during one of these episodes, he often reported dream content that exactly mirrored the vocal or motor activity. Over the course of the past few years, the nature of his dreaming had become more action-packed (being attacked or chased by people or animals), in concert with the occurrence of more frequent and dramatic vocalizations and behaviors. He and his wife had searched the internet for "sleep-related violent behavior" and had become aware of the possible association between complex sleep-related behaviors and Parkinson's disease; in fact, they admitted that they had sought medical attention more because of concerns about the possibility of Parkinson's disease than because of the sleep-related behaviors themselves.

The family history was remarkable only for Parkinson's disease in a maternal grandfather. Mr. Bonner was taking no medications.

The neurological history was completely unremarkable, with the exception of gradually worsening constipation and a diminution in the sense of smell (often early nonmotor manifestations of Parkinson's disease) over the past couple of years. The neurological examination was unremarkable with the exception of very mild postural instability on rapid turning while walking. Specifically, he had no signs of Parkinson's disease, such as tremor, rigidity, or bradykinesia (slowness of motor movement).

Mr. Bonner underwent a formal polysomnographic study with brain wave activity monitoring for seizure activity and extensive muscle activity during sleep. The study revealed a striking persistence of intermittent muscle activity during REM sleep, which was occasionally associated with extremity twitching and minor vocalizations. There was no seizure activity on the EEG that could possibly explain the clinical behaviors.

Because of the risk that Mr. Bonner might become injured during these episodes, the clinician recommended that the couple put heavy draperies over the bedroom windows and remove all bedside furniture. She also suggested that they may want to consider sleeping on a futon on the floor, given that Mr. Bonner has fallen out of bed. An infrared alarm for the bedroom door was also suggested. If Mr. Bonner tries to leave the bedroom, the infrared beam across the open door will be broken, sounding an alarm that would awaken him or his wife. Mr. Bonner was initially treated with clonazepam, a long-acting benzodiazepine drug, 1 hour before bedtime, which resulted in definite but incomplete improvement. Melatonin, 6 mg per night, was added, with nearly complete resolution of the dream-enacting behaviors and a marked reduction in the action-packed nature of his dreams.

At the 1-year routine follow-up visit, Mr. Bonner reported that he continued to have very few sleep-related symptoms. However, on examination, early Parkinson's disease was evidenced by bradykinesia, an intermittent resting tremor, and some muscular rigidity. At that time, the medications clonazepam and melatonin were continued, and Mr. Bonner was referred to a Parkinson's disease clinic.

Discussion of "Falling Out of Bed"

Mr. Bonner's episodes of complex motor behavior and vocalizations during sleep could be attributable to a nocturnal seizure disorder, an NREM Sleep Arousal Disorder such as sleepwalking, or REM Sleep Behavior Disorder. Several aspects of Mr. Bonner's sleep-wake behavior are particularly suggestive of REM Sleep Behavior Disorder. When Mr. Bonner was awakened from these episodes, he would recall dream content that exactly mirrored the vocal and motor activity in bed, strongly suggesting that the behavior constituted dream enactment. Also, the lack of confusion or disorientation on awakening from these episodes is uncharacteristic of either NREM Sleep Arousal Disorders or seizure activity. The polysomnographic results clinch the diagnosis of REM Sleep Behavior Disorder (DSM-5-TR, p. 461). Mr. Bonner lacked the usual paralysis of muscles (other than those used to breathe) that occurs during REM sleep, which serves to protect a person from injury while dreaming. The absence of muscle atonia is a cardinal feature of REM Sleep Behavior Disorder and allows for the complex and sometimes dangerous behaviors observed.

As noted in the case description, the issue that brought Mr. Bonner to clinical attention was not the sleep behavior itself but rather the couple's concern that the behavior might be indicative of Parkinson's disease. Although none of the typical manifestations of Parkinson's disease, such as tremor or muscular rigidity, could be elicited during the initial physical examination, the diminution in Mr. Bonner's sense of smell (typically tested by asking the patient to sniff ground coffee) suggested that he might develop full-blown Parkinson's disease in the future. Indeed, within a year, the first signs of Parkinson's disease were evident.

12.9
Restless Legs Syndrome

Restless Legs Syndrome (RLS) is a neurological disorder characterized by throbbing, pulling, creeping, or other unpleasant sensations in the legs and an uncontrollable, and sometimes overwhelming, urge to move them. Symptoms occur primarily at night when a person is relaxing or at rest and can increase in severity during the night. Moving the legs partially or totally relieves the discomfort. The disorder most commonly affects the legs, but can affect the arms, torso, head, and even phantom limbs (the sensation that an amputated or missing limb is still attached to the body and is moving appropriately with other body parts). The most distinctive or unusual aspect of the condition is that lying down and trying to relax activates the symptoms. Most people with RLS have difficulty falling asleep and staying asleep. Left untreated, the condition causes exhaustion and daytime fatigue. Many people with RLS report that their job, personal relations, and activities of daily living are strongly affected as a result of sleep deprivation. They are often unable to concentrate, have impaired memory, or fail to accomplish daily tasks. The disorder also can make traveling difficult and can cause depression.

The prevalence of DSM-5-TR-defined RLS (i.e., symptom frequency of at least three times a week with at least moderate distress) is estimated to be 1.6%. RLS is about twice as common in women as in men. RLS may begin at any age; however, many individuals who are severely affected are middle age and older, and the symptoms typically become more frequent and last longer with age. Up to 90% of people with RLS also experience a more common condition known as periodic limb movements in sleep (PLMS), which is characterized by involuntary leg twitching or jerking movements during sleep that typically occur every 15 to 40 seconds, sometimes throughout the night. RLS is associated with higher rates of depression, Generalized Anxiety Disorder, Panic Disorder, Posttraumatic Stress Disorder, cardiovascular disease, and other sleep disorders.

Bugs Crawling

Lisa Bianchi, a 45-year-old married businesswoman, was referred by her primary care physician to see a psychiatrist for depression and anxiety. Initially, Mrs. Bianchi's primary care physician prescribed a 10-mg dose of escitalopram—a selective serotonin reuptake inhibitor (SSRI) antidepressant, for treatment of her depression and anxiety—and told her to take a 50-mg dose of diphenhydramine, a sedating antihistamine, at bedtime on an as-needed basis to promote sleep. However, 3 days later—after staying up nearly all night—Mrs. Bianchi called her primary care physician in despair and complained of worsening insomnia along with worsening depression and anxiety. Urgent referral was made to a psychiatrist for further evaluation.

During the psychiatric evaluation, Mrs. Bianchi endorsed several depressive symptoms, such as difficulty falling asleep, low mood, difficulty with concentration, poor appetite, and low energy. Among her depressive symptoms, her inability to fall asleep is the most bothersome to her. Her job performance is compromised by her daytime fatigue and difficulty concentrating. On more detailed questioning about her insomnia symptoms, Mrs. Bianchi revealed difficulty falling asleep 3–4 nights per week for the past several years because of an irresistible urge to pace and an uncomfortable sensation—not exactly a pain—in her legs. Mrs. Bianchi described this deep uncomfortable sensation in her legs as "bugs crawling in her legs."

Usually, the urge to move her legs starts in the late evening and goes away after she walks around her house for a while, but when she lies down in her bed to sleep, the uncomfortable sensation in her legs returns. Although not painful, the leg discomfort sometimes prevents her from relaxing and watching TV in her bed because she just "has to move" her legs. The uncomfortable urge to move her legs waxes and wanes and varies from day to day. Moreover, the alcohol that she often drinks before going to bed, after having an initial sedative effect, causes her to sleep more lightly, with more frequent episodes of wakefulness. At times, the urge to move her legs has been so irresistible that she rides her exercise bike for 1–2 hours until the discomfort subsides.

Mrs. Bianchi was accompanied by her husband at the psychiatric evaluation. He shares a bed with her and reported that he observed her having jerky movements in her legs during the nights. For several days after she began taking the escitalopram, Mrs. Bianchi's leg discomfort became more intense and lasted most of the night. Unlike drug-induced akathisia (a feeling of inner restlessness and a compelling need to be in constant motion that is a side effect of certain medications, especially antipsychotic drugs), her urges to move her legs occur nightly, starting in the evening and subsiding in the early morning. Moreover, the feeling is more focused in her legs than any other parts of her body. She also revealed that her mother experienced similar nighttime leg restlessness but never received treatment for it.

The antidepressant medication was stopped, and her symptoms subsided after treatment with gabapentin, an anticonvulsant medication that is also used to treat nerve pain.

Discussion of "Bugs Crawling"

Although Mrs. Bianchi sought treatment for depression and anxiety, the SSRI prescribed by her primary care physician caused a number of side effects, including exacerbation of a preexisting sleep-related movement disorder that she had been experiencing for the past several years. Her nighttime urge to move her legs meets all of the DSM-5-TR definitional criteria for RLS: the urge starts in the late evening, the urge is relieved by movement ("[it] goes away after she walks around her house for a while") and worsens during periods of rest or inactivity ("when she lies down in her bed to sleep, the uncomfortable sensation in her legs returns"), the urges have occurred at least three times a week and have persisted for at least 3 months, and the symptoms are accompanied by distress or impairment in functioning ("her job performance is compromised"). Finally, DSM-5-TR requires that the symptoms not be attributable to another mental disorder or a nonpsychiatric medical condition and not be due to the physiological effects of a drug of abuse or a medication. Although Mrs. Bianchi's symptoms clearly worsened when she started taking the SSRI antidepressant, and such medications are known to induce or aggravate symptoms in susceptible individuals, the fact that her RLS symptoms predated her use of antidepressants means that the symptoms cannot be attributed to the medication. Therefore, the DSM-5-TR diagnosis is Restless Legs Syndrome (DSM-5-TR, p. 464). Moreover, as reported by her husband, Mrs. Bianchi also experiences PLMS, which commonly accompanies RLS.

12.10
Substance/Medication-Induced Sleep Disorder

Many medications and substances of abuse have the potential to cause sleep problems, including insomnia, daytime sleepiness, and abnormal behaviors during sleep (e.g., sleepwalking). Substance/Medication-Induced Sleep Disorder is diagnosed when an individual has a prominent sleep disturbance that is judged to be the direct physiological effect of a medication or a drug of abuse. Prominent and severe sleep disturbances can occur in association with intoxication or withdrawal from alcohol; caffeine; cannabis; opioids; sedatives, hypnotics, or anxiolytics; and stimulants (including cocaine). Withdrawal from tobacco can also cause sleep disturbance. Among the many medications that can invoke sleep disturbances are adrenergic agonists (e.g., pseudoephedrine) and antagonists (e.g., beta-blockers), dopamine agonists (e.g., medications used to treat Parkinson's disease) and antagonists (e.g., antipsychotic medications), cholinergic agonists (e.g., medications used to increase salivation) and antagonists (e.g., medications used to treat motion sickness), serotonergic agonists (e.g., medications used to prevent migraines) and antagonists (e.g., medications used to treat nausea), antihistamines, and corticosteroids.

The clinician can indicate the specific symptomatic presentation by using one of the various subtypes. Insomnia Type is for presentations in which the person has difficulty falling asleep or maintaining sleep, frequent awakenings during the night, or nonrestorative sleep. Daytime Sleepiness Type is for presentations in which the person experiences excessive sleepiness or fatigue during daytime hours. Parasomnia Type is for abnormal behavior occurring during sleep such as nightmares.

Mystery Mastery

Donna Lazarus, a 28-year-old lawyer, described her problems to a psychiatrist. She frequently felt anxious and upset around bedtime. On these nights, it would take her an hour or more to fall asleep. She dreaded going to bed and would engross herself in reading murder mysteries until late hours. Her bedtimes varied from 7:00 P.M. to 2:00 A.M. On awakening in the morning, she felt groggy and incapacitated, hardly able to crawl out of bed. Some mornings, she missed work completely. She slept until noon on weekends. Worry about her tardiness getting to work motivated her to seek a consultation.

Ms. Lazarus was diagnosed with bronchial asthma at age 18 months. Her mother had constantly worried that her daughter would die during the night. As a teenager, Ms. Lazarus used epinephrine (a stimulant) inhalers to remain awake reading until 1:00–3:00 A.M. She remembers her father screaming at her to turn out the lights. She always considered the late-night hours, when everyone else was asleep, a "safe time," free from interference by others.

Ms. Lazarus was particularly prone to nocturnal asthma attacks, which typically occurred around 4:00 A.M. Wheezing at night led to feelings of terror and fear of dying. The current treatment for her asthma was aminophylline 400 mg/day (a xanthine derivative, which relaxes the smooth muscle surrounding the bronchial tubes), plus two puffs on a beclomethasone inhaler (a steroid) twice daily. She also used an albuterol inhaler (a beta-agonist bronchodilator) irregularly, sometimes at bedtime. About once a year, an exacerbation of asthma would require a short course of systemic (oral) steroids.

Ms. Lazarus drank 5–8 cups of coffee daily. Alcoholic beverages precipitated wheezing and aggravated the delay in onset of sleep. Short-acting sedatives at bedtime caused a noticeable decrease in her ability to concentrate on work the following day. Evening relaxation exercises precipitated fears of being alone with a breathing problem and made her feel like "a skeleton with a pair of lungs."

During the consultation, Ms. Lazarus was articulate, smiling, and cheerful, and displayed a full range of emotions. She seemed to enjoy her own idiosyncrasies. She was quite talkative, organized, and informative, and easily able to discuss her feelings. She noted that it was ironic that she feared death so much yet loved to read about murders in fiction. "I guess it's been my way of feeling some sense of control."

Discussion of "Mystery Mastery"

Ms. Lazarus presents to the psychiatrist with a chief complaint of nightly insomnia (i.e., difficulty falling asleep) with consequent daytime sleepiness. Although some behavioral factors might be contributing to her difficulty falling asleep (i.e., nighttime anxiety, inconsistent bedtimes, engaging in engrossing stimulating activities at bedtime), her medication regimen for asthma appears to be the main culprit, because a number of the medications and substances she is using are likely to interfere with her ability to fall asleep. The aminophylline, the albuterol inhaler, the beclomethasone inhaler, and her 5–8 cups of coffee per day can exert long-lasting stimulation effects that are likely to interfere with good sleep quality. Thus, the DSM-5-TR diagnosis for Ms. Lazarus would be Caffeine/Aminophylline/Albuterol/Beclomethasone-Induced Sleep Disorder, Insomnia Type (DSM-5-TR, p. 468).

CHAPTER 13

Sexual Dysfunctions

DSM-5-TR describes Sexual Dysfunctions as a diverse group of disorders "characterized by a clinically significant disturbance in a person's ability to respond sexually or to experience sexual pleasure" (DSM-5-TR, p. 477). DSM-5-TR Sexual Dysfunctions are marked by a dysfunction in the processes that make up the sexual response cycle or by pain associated with sexual intercourse.

The sexual response cycle can be divided into four phases:

1. *Desire*: This phase consists of fantasies about sexual activity and the desire to have sexual activity.
2. *Excitement*: This phase consists of a subjective sense of sexual pleasure and excitement, accompanied by physiological changes. The major changes in men are penile tumescence and erection. In women, the physiological changes consist of vasocongestion in the pelvis, vaginal lubrication and expansion, and swelling of the external genitalia.
3. *Orgasm*: This phase consists of a peaking of sexual pleasure with release of sexual tension and rhythmic contraction of the perineal muscles and reproductive organs, along with ejaculation of semen in men.
4. *Resolution*: This phase consists of muscular relaxation and a general sense of well-being.

Table 13–1 lists DSM-5-TR Sexual Dysfunctions that can occur during the first three phases of the sexual response cycle (no dysfunction is associated with the resolution phase). Male Hypoactive Sexual Desire Disorder and Erectile Disorder involve dysfunctions in the desire and excitement phases, respectively, in men. Given that sexual desire and excitement are not as easily separable in women as they are in men, there is only a single disorder (Female Sexual Interest/Arousal Disorder) covering both of these phases in women. There are two types of dysfunctions in the orgasm phase in men, Premature (Early) Ejaculation and Delayed Ejaculation, as opposed to a single disorder in women, Female Orgasmic Disorder. Table 13–2 lists other DSM-5-TR Sexual Dysfunctions not related to the sexual response cycle: a disorder characterized by pain associated with intercourse (Genito-Pelvic Pain/Penetration Disorder) and a disturbance in sexual function caused by a substance or medication (Substance/

TABLE 13–1.   **Phases and disorders of the sexual response cycle**

Phase	Disorder	Affected sex	Key characteristics
Desire	Male Hypoactive Sexual Desire Disorder	Male	Lack of erotic thoughts, fantasies, and desire for sex
Desire/ Excitement	Female Sexual Interest/ Arousal Disorder	Female	Lack of sexual interest or erotic fantasies
			Lack of initiation of sex
			Lack of excitement/pleasure or genital sensations during sex
Excitement	Erectile Disorder	Male	Failure to obtain or maintain erections during sex
Orgasm	Premature (Early) Ejaculation	Male	Ejaculation within 1 minute of vaginal penetration and before wanted
	Delayed Ejaculation	Male	Delay in or inability to ejaculate despite stimulation
	Female Orgasmic Disorder	Female	Difficulty experiencing or reduced intensity of orgasm
Resolution	None		

Medication-Induced Sexual Dysfunction). An individual may have more than one DSM-5-TR Sexual Dysfunction at the same time—in such cases, each of the applicable Sexual Dysfunctions should be diagnosed.

A diagnosis of a DSM-5-TR Sexual Dysfunction is considered to be a "diagnosis of exclusion." That means that the clinician must first rule out specific explanations for the dysfunction before a diagnosis can be made. For example, the diagnosis should not be made if the person's inability to experience excitement or orgasm is the result of inadequate sexual stimulation. Similarly, diagnosis of a DSM-5-TR Sexual Dysfunction is not made if the dysfunction can be understood as being a symptom of another mental disorder, such as having low sexual desire during a Major Depressive Episode; erectile dysfunction caused by a nonpsychiatric medical condition such as pelvic nerve damage; or anorgasmia as a consequence of severe relationship distress or partner violence. In the case of a sexual dysfunction due to drugs or medications, the diagnosis should be Substance/Medication-Induced Sexual Dysfunction (see Section 13.8). Other factors that need to be considered when determining whether a person's presentation qualifies for diagnosis of a DSM-5-TR Sexual Dysfunction include cultural and religious factors that may influence the individual's expectations about or engender prohibitions about the experience of sexual pleasure, and the person's age, because aging may be associated with a normal decrease in sexual response.

Moreover, because transient sexual dysfunctions are often normal, such as those that occur in response to a life stressor, a diagnosis of a DSM-5-TR Sexual Dysfunction should not be made unless the symptoms are persistent. DSM-5-TR specifically requires a minimum duration of at least 6 months for a Sexual Dysfunction diagnosis (with the exception of Substance/Medication-Induced Sexual Dysfunction, which

TABLE 13–2. **Sexual Dysfunctions independent of the sexual response cycle**

Disorder	Key characteristics
Genito-Pelvic Pain/ Penetration Disorder	Difficulties with vaginal penetration during intercourse, vulvovaginal or pelvic pain during intercourse or penetration attempts, fear of pelvic pain related to vaginal penetration, tensing of pelvic floor muscles during attempted penetration
Substance/Medication-Induced Sexual Dysfunction	Disturbance in sexual function due to the direct effects of a substance or medication on the central nervous system

has no minimum duration but requires that the symptoms develop "soon after" exposure to the substance/medication). Finally, to qualify for a diagnosis, the dysfunction must be sufficiently problematic to cause the person distress. The person might be distressed by the dysfunction for a number of reasons. For example, Delayed Ejaculation, Premature Ejaculation, Erectile Disorder, and Genito-Pelvic Pain/Penetration Disorder might interfere with a couple's ability to conceive a child or may lead to avoidance of sexual encounters and interfere with the ability to develop intimate relationships. On the other hand, if the person is not particularly bothered by the dysfunction, a DSM-5-TR diagnosis should not be made. For example, there are individuals who identify themselves as asexual and view asexuality as an alternative sexual orientation, alongside heterosexuality, homosexuality, and bisexuality. These individuals, who may report a lifelong absence of sexual desire, would not qualify for a diagnosis of either Male Hypoactive Sexual Desire Disorder or Female Sexual Interest/ Arousal Disorder, because they lack the requisite distress.

DSM-5-TR provides subtypes that can be noted along with the diagnosis of a Sexual Dysfunction to indicate the course of the dysfunction and the context in which it occurs. The course of a particular DSM-5-TR Sexual Dysfunction can be *lifelong* (present from the time of the person's first sexual experiences) or *acquired* (developing after a period of relatively normal sexual functioning), and the context of occurrence can be *situational* (occurring only during certain sexual activities, such as intercourse, or with certain partners, such as the person's spouse) or *generalized* (occurring in all situations). Considering whether the Sexual Dysfunction is lifelong versus acquired and situational versus generalized can be helpful in determining its etiology and can also be helpful in conceptualizing the problem and recommending treatment. For example, sexual dysfunctions that are best understood as being a symptom of a nonpsychiatric medical condition generally have their start after the onset of the medical condition and tend to occur in all situations. On the other hand, dysfunctions that occur only during certain sexual activities or with certain partners (e.g., occurring only during intercourse but not during masturbation) suggest the presence of an interpersonal component that would need to be addressed in treatment.

13.1
Male Hypoactive
Sexual Desire Disorder

Male Hypoactive Sexual Desire Disorder involves a dysfunction in the first phase of the sexual response cycle, namely sexual desire. It is characterized by the reduction or absence of erotic thoughts or fantasies and desire for sexual activity. A man with this condition will neither initiate sexual activity nor respond to his partner's desire for sexual activity. A man with low sexual interest often is less troubled by the condition than is his partner, who may feel thwarted not only by the lack of physical affection and touch but also by the lack of opportunities for procreation. This problem may be particularly salient for a man who is involved in a relationship with a woman who wants to start a family; in such cases, the man's distress about having low sexual desire is more about its negative impact on their relationship than about not having an interest in sex itself. Male Hypoactive Sexual Desire Disorder may be specific to the partner or may not be limited to any potential partner.

Sexual desire problems are less common in younger men (ages 16–24 years; prevalence range 3%–14%) than in older men (ages 60–74 years; prevalence range 16%–28%). However, a persistent lack of interest in sex lasting 6 months or longer, as is required for the DSM-5-TR diagnosis of Male Hypoactive Sexual Desire Disorder, affects a smaller proportion of men (6%).

Perfect Gentleman

Jim Benson, a 34-year-old successful architect, consulted his family practitioner because of a lifelong history of minimal interest in sex. His scheduling an appointment is partially in response to pressure from his wife, who has been discussing divorce. He remembers wondering if he were somehow different in high school when his male friends appeared obsessed with sex, and he was not. He masturbated infrequently in high school, maybe two or three times a year. He does not recall any masturbatory fantasies and did not find pornography shared by his friends to be interesting. He pretended to be interested in pornography only in order to "fit in with them."

Mr. Benson recalls his first sexual experience as not being remarkable. After winning a baseball game, he and some of his teammates drank a case of beer and visited a local house of prostitution. He had sex with the prostitute mainly because of group pressure. He remembers the prostitute saying that of the team members, he was the only one who was a gentleman: "You weren't grabbing and squeezing me all over like the others." He dated very little in college, focusing on his studies, and finished in the top 5% of his class. His only dates during college were to fraternity events where he was required as a pledge to have a date. Mr. Benson does not remember having sex during college. His next sexual experience was after he married at age 28. His wife at first was impressed with how he was a perfect gentleman and did not pressure her to have sex like the other men she had dated. After marriage, she found that she was the one who had to initiate sex. Mr. Benson found sex pleasurable but would have been happy to have sex only once a year. In response to her pressure, they usually had sex every 3–4 months. He denies masturbation since marriage and also denies having sexual fantasies. He says that he notices other women who have good figures, but he denies wanting to have sex with them. He uses the following analogy: "I drive a Mercedes diesel. I notice the lines of a Porsche Carrera, but I don't lust after one."

A full endocrinological workup was done to check Mr. Benson's luteinizing hormone (stimulates production of testosterone), follicle-stimulating hormone (critical for the initiation of spermatogenesis), prolactin (when elevated, causes low libido in males), free testosterone (when low, can cause low libido, erectile dysfunction, and infertility in males), and thyroid indices. All results were within normal limits. There was no evidence of an atypical focus of sexual interest, such as being sexually attracted to children, and no evidence of his having had a homosexual orientation. Mr. Benson also did not have evidence of a mood disturbance (e.g., depression), did not abuse substances, and did not use any medications on a regular basis.

Discussion of "Perfect Gentleman"

As is typical for men with Male Hypoactive Sexual Desire Disorder, Mr. Benson went for help largely because of distress related to his wife's frustration with his low sexual desire, which is threatening his marriage. Before the diagnosis can be made, other causes for his low sexual desire with his wife need to be considered and ruled out. Many nonpsychiatric medical conditions (e.g., low testosterone), as well as the side effects of certain medications (e.g., selective serotonin reuptake inhibitor [SSRI] antidepressants), can cause low sexual desire. These causes are ruled out because Mr. Benson has normal hormone levels and does not use any medications or drugs of abuse. Other mental disorders, especially depression, can also cause low sex drive, but there is no evidence that Mr. Benson has any mood disturbance. Finally, another consideration is whether his preferred focus of sexual interest may not include his wife, either because his primary interests are paraphilic (see Chapter 19, "Paraphilic Disorders") or because he has a homosexual sexual orientation. However, the lifelong nature of his low sexual desire, which includes lack of interest in pornography of any type, plus the lack of his admission to having other sexual preferences, suggests that these potential explanations also do not explain his low desire. Thus, Mr. Benson's DSM-5-TR diagnosis is Male Hypoactive Sexual Desire Disorder (DSM-5-TR, p. 498). Because he has always experienced low sexual desire, the Lifelong subtype applies. Moreover, because his low sexual desire occurs in all situations and with all partners, the Generalized subtype also applies.

13.2
Female Sexual Interest/
Arousal Disorder

Although DSM-5-TR differentiates dysfunctions involving the desire phase of the sexual response cycle in men (Male Hypoactive Sexual Desire Disorder) from dysfunctions occurring in the excitement phase (Erectile Disorder), in women there is only a single diagnostic category in DSM-5-TR covering dysfunctions in both phases: Female Sexual Interest/Arousal Disorder. The use of a single diagnosis is because in women the relationship between desire and subjective arousal (excitement) is both complex and variable across women and not easily separable. Women tend to find it difficult to differentiate desire from arousal when sexually excited. Also, sexual desire precedes sexual arousal for some women but follows sexual arousal for other women.

Thus, the DSM-5-TR diagnosis of Female Sexual Interest/Arousal Disorder is defined in terms of both desire and arousal problems. The diagnosis can be made if at least three of the following six indicators of dysfunction are present: 1) reduced or absent interest in sexual activity; 2) reduced or absent erotic thoughts or fantasies; 3) lack of initiation of sexual activity and often being unreceptive to a partner's attempts to initiate sexual activity; 4) reduced or absent sexual excitement or pleasure during sexual activity; 5) reduced or absent sexual interest or arousal in response to written, verbal, or visual erotic cues; and 6) reduced or absent genital or nongenital sensations during sexual activity.

There may be different symptom profiles across women, as well as variability in how sexual interest and arousal are expressed. For example, Sexual Interest/Arousal Disorder may be expressed in one woman as a lack of interest in sexual activity, an absence of erotic or sexual thoughts, and reluctance to initiate sexual activity and respond to a partner's sexual invitations. In another woman, an inability to become sexually excited, an inability to respond to sexual stimuli with sexual desire, and a corresponding lack of signs of physical sexual arousal may be the primary features.

Before the diagnosis can be made, specific nonpsychiatric medical and substance/medication-induced causes must be ruled out. Low estrogen levels, especially after menopause, can cause desire and arousal difficulties. Although testosterone is often thought of as the "male" sex hormone, testosterone is also important in female sexual functioning, and low levels are associated with low sexual desire. Other nonpsychiatric medical problems that can cause desire or arousal problems in women include diabetes, thyroid disease, and cancer. A reduction in desire and arousal is a particularly common side effect of certain medications, especially antidepressant medications, antihypertensive medications, and anticancer drugs.

Approximately 30% of women experience chronic low desire, with approximately half of these reporting partner distress about the dysfunction and a quarter experiencing personal distress. The co-occurrence of sexual interest/arousal problems and other sexual difficulties is extremely common. Distressing low desire is associated with depression, thyroid problems, anxiety, urinary incontinence, and other nonpsychiatric medical factors.

No Sparkle

Martina Diaz is a 45-year-old woman referred to a sex therapist by her primary care physician for further evaluation and treatment, after she was nonresponsive to a 3-month course of treatment with flibanserin (a medication prescribed to treat low sexual desire in women). Her medical record indicates that she is experiencing perimenopause (with hot flashes, menstrual irregularity, and vaginal dryness) and is in good health, with hormone levels within the typical range.

Mrs. Diaz reports that she has been married for 20 years and has three adolescent children, ages 12, 15, and 17. She indicates an emotionally close, loving, and supportive relationship with her husband, with considerable nonsexual physical intimacy, including touching and hugging. She said that in the first decade of their relationship, she was much more sexually active, frequently initiating sex, and most of the time responsive sexually when her husband initiated. Over time, her interest in sex gradually decreased, and for the past 2 years, she has rarely initiated sexual activity and finds that she has little interest and has difficulty becoming aroused when her husband initiates. She sometimes experiences mild discomfort during penile-vaginal intercourse, associated with insufficient lubrication. Although she can still achieve orgasm on those infrequent occasions when her husband performs oral sex on her, she does not achieve orgasm as easily as in the past.

Mrs. Diaz trained as a lawyer and left practice after the birth of her first child. Five years ago, she returned to full-time employment in law and since then has been struggling with heavy time commitments with her career, as well as with driving her children to extracurricular activities. She hopes her oldest child will soon get a driver's license, and then Mrs. Diaz might have more time to herself. Her husband helps with household tasks but is also very busy in a sales position; most of the housework falls to Mrs. Diaz and part-time help the family hires to assist with cleaning.

Mrs. Diaz identifies as a practicing Catholic. She uses hormonal oral contraceptives and reports that she looks forward to menopause and being able to discontinue birth control, because neither she nor her husband wants additional children. She has a generally positive attitude toward sex, although she feels uncomfortable discussing her lack of sexual interest or her need for lubricant with her husband, fearing that he will think she does not find him attractive any more or she loves him less than she once did. She has never used vibrators and said she has not masturbated since she married, never having had much interest in or satisfaction from masturbation.

Recently, she has been assigned a younger male coworker who has been working on a complex case with her for extended periods of time. She reports occasionally noticing a "sparkle" of desire when she is near him, and she sometimes thinks of the coworker when her husband initiates sex, but then she immediately experiences guilt about these thoughts, which "shuts down" her desire for sex. She has not shared these thoughts with her spouse, and she states that the feelings are particularly confusing for her because she still loves her husband, and for both of them, it would be "immoral" and "unacceptable" to consider opening the relationship to nonmonogamy. She did not notice any improvement in her sexual desire or arousal while taking flibanserin and found the restrictions on moderate alcohol use inconvenient.

Mrs. Diaz shows no signs of depression or anxiety. Now that she has discontinued flibanserin, she has resumed drinking alcohol occasionally, a glass or two of wine a few times a week. She reports no tobacco or other psychoactive drug use and is not taking any medication except contraceptives. She is in generally good health, although her primary care physician has suggested she lose some weight and exercise more. She rarely has time or energy to cook or exercise, and the family regularly eats out together. She does not feel as if she has time to change these routines at the moment and is fearful that if she works less at her job, she might lose opportunities for advancement because she is considerably older than most junior associates in her law firm. She and her husband take an evening for a date night at least twice a month. Although she feels close to her husband during these dates and greatly enjoys them, they do little for her sexual interest.

The course of treatment on flibanserin was initiated and discontinued at her request, and she requested the referral for other types of treatment. Mrs. Diaz says she would like to enjoy sex as she once used to, and she is also concerned that long-term lack of interest in sex may adversely affect her relationship with her husband. Many of her college friends, who also married in their mid- to late 20s, have recently divorced after they or their partners had affairs, and she does not want this to happen to her. Stating that her marital relationship is otherwise good, Mrs. Diaz does not particularly want couples counseling and prefers to "solve this issue myself," adding that she has read online news articles on a multimodal approach to sexual issues but is not sure how couples counseling can help her, as she feels she already has a good relationship with her husband.

Mrs. Diaz's treatment proceeded with cognitive-behavioral sex therapy involving sensate focus, a therapeutic technique in which the person is encouraged to pay increased attention to their own senses and what feels good sexually. She was encouraged to explore fantasy as a way of increasing her interest in sex. After initial sessions, she invited her husband to join the therapy sessions so that they could work together on sensate focus and on introducing variations into their sexual routine (such as use of a vibrator and lubricants), focused on enhancing her pleasure. A gynecological consult was offered for vaginal estrogen, but Mrs. Diaz did not proceed with this consultation because she felt she had experienced sufficient improvement from psychotherapy alone. Although she still rarely wants to initiate sex, she reports that treatment has led to a significant increase in sexual response and pleasure when her husband initiates sex.

Discussion of "No Sparkle"

Mrs. Diaz presents for help for both low sexual interest and difficulty with sexual arousal. She reports virtually no interest in sexual activity, rarely initiating sex with her husband and failing to become aroused when her husband initiates intercourse, with concomitant insufficient lubrication. With the exception of the occasional "sparkle" of desire she experiences when near a younger male coworker, she rarely has any erotic thoughts.

Of the six possible symptoms included in the DSM-5-TR diagnostic criteria for Female Sexual Interest/Arousal Disorder, Mrs. Diaz has four of them: reduced interest in sexual activity, reduced erotic thoughts, rare initiation of sexual activity along with lack of response to her husband's attempts to initiate sex, and reduced sexual pleasure during most instances of sexual activity with her husband. Even though Mrs. Diaz is still capable of responding physiologically to orgasm as the recipient of oral sex, the reduction in physiological response and excitement/pleasure during most sexual encounters satisfies the fourth listed criterion. The evaluation by her primary care physician does not reveal any medical conditions that could account for her low desire and arousal. Although her vaginal dryness secondary to going through perimenopause might be a contributing factor, it could not account for the clinical picture, and she was not interested in a gynecological consult to address that problem. She does not have another mental disorder that might be associated with low desire (e.g., Major Depressive Disorder), and she has no nonpsychiatric medical problems and is taking no medication that could cause these symptoms. Finally, the symptoms are not a consequence of severe relationship distress. Given that this problem is not transient but has persisted for longer than 6 months and that it causes her significant distress, the DSM-5-TR diagnosis of Female Sexual Interest/Arousal Disorder (DSM-5-TR, p. 489) applies. Moreover, because Mrs. Diaz has had a history of normal sexual desire earlier in her life, the Acquired subtype applies. Finally, because the low desire does not appear to be limited to any particular situation or partner, the Generalized subtype applies as well.

13.3
Erectile Disorder

Erectile Disorder is characterized by a marked difficulty in obtaining an erection during sexual activity, marked difficulty in maintaining an erection until the completion of sexual activity, or a marked decrease in erectile rigidity that has persisted for at least 6 months and causes clinically significant distress in the individual. For the DSM-5-TR diagnosis to apply, the dysfunction must be experienced on all or almost all occasions of sexual activity, either in specific situational contexts (such as with certain types of stimulation or partners, in which case it is considered to be Situational) or in all contexts (in which case it is considered to be Generalized).

Specific causes of erectile dysfunction should be considered and ruled out before a diagnosis of Erectile Disorder is made. Nonpsychiatric medical causes include heart disease, clogged blood vessels (atherosclerosis), high cholesterol, diabetes, Parkinson's disease, multiple sclerosis, Peyronie's disease (development of scar tissue inside the penis associated with trauma), treatments for prostate cancer or enlarged prostate, and surgeries or injuries that affect the pelvic area or spinal cord. Erectile dysfunction can also be a side effect of certain medications, including diuretics and drugs to control high blood pressure, antidepressants, antianxiety drugs, antiepileptic drugs, antihistamines, gastric reflux medications, and muscle relaxants. Heavy alcohol use, tobacco use, and use of other drugs of abuse, such as cocaine, marijuana, and opiates, can also cause erectile dysfunction, as can anxiety and severe relationship stress. Mental disorders associated with erectile dysfunction include Major Depressive Disorder and Posttraumatic Stress Disorder. In all such cases, a DSM-5-TR diagnosis of Erectile Disorder is not made.

Many men are reluctant to discuss erectile dysfunction with their doctors because of embarrassment, and therefore the condition is underdiagnosed. The prevalence of Erectile Disorder in the general population is approximately 13%–21% among men ages 40–80 years. Rates appear to be lower than 10% among men younger than 40 years, about 20%–40% among men in their 60s, and 50%–75% among men older than 70 years. Erectile failure on first sexual attempt has been found to be related to having sex with a previously unknown partner, concomitant use of drugs or alcohol, not wanting to have sex, and peer pressure. Erectile Disorder can be comorbid with other DSM-5-TR Sexual Dysfunctions, such as Premature Ejaculation and Male Hypoactive Sexual Desire Disorder, as well as with Anxiety and Depressive Disorders.

(Un)Committed

Paul Petersen and his girlfriend Annie have been living together for the last 10 months and are contemplating marriage. Annie describes the problem that has brought them to the sex therapy clinic: "For about the last 6 months, he hasn't been able to keep his erection after he enters me." The psychologist turns to Paul and asks him how he sees the problem. Paul, embarrassed, agrees with Annie and adds, "I just don't know why."

The psychologist learns that Paul is 25 years old and a recently graduated lawyer, and that Annie is 24 and a successful buyer for a large department store. They both grew up in educated, middle-class, suburban families. They met through mutual friends and started to have sexual intercourse a few months after they met and recall no real problems at that time.

Two months later, Paul moved from his family home into Annie's apartment. The move was her idea, and Paul was unsure that he was ready for such an important step. Within a few weeks, Paul noticed that although he continued to be sexually aroused and wanted intercourse, as soon as he entered Annie, he began to lose his erection and could not stay inside. They would try again, but by then his desire had waned, and he was unable to achieve another erection. After the first few times this happened, Annie became so angry that she began punching him in the chest and screaming at him. Paul, who weighs 200 pounds, would simply walk away from his 98-pound lover, which would infuriate her even more.

The psychologist learned that sex was not the only area of contention in the relationship. Annie complained that Paul did not spend enough time with her and preferred to go to baseball games with his male friends. Even when he was home, he would watch all the sports events that were available on TV, and he was not interested in going to foreign films, museums, or the theater with her. Despite these differences, Annie was eager to marry Paul and was pressuring him to set a date.

Physical examination of the couple revealed no abnormalities, and there was no evidence that either partner was persistently depressed. Paul recently saw his internist for a regular medical examination with routine blood tests and urinalysis, and no medical problems were reported to be present. He was not taking any medication. Although he had an occasional glass of wine with dinner, he reported no problems with alcohol or drug abuse.

Neither partner was willing to discuss nonsexual problems. They were treated with Masters and Johnson–type sensate focus exercises over the next several months. In these exercises, the couple explored nongenital ways of giving physical pleasure to each other without the psychological demands of demonstrating sexual competence. Annie continually pressured Paul to translate the therapy into action. She saw herself as therapist and teacher, and Paul as patient and pupil. Although Paul passively avoided doing the exercises on many occasions, Paul's problem with maintaining an erection gradually resolved over a period of 8 months. They were married within 3 months after treatment ended.

Discussion of "(Un)Committed"

At the time of presentation to the sex therapy clinic, Paul reported the onset of an erectile problem—namely, the persistent inability to maintain his erection through the completion of sexual activity—that had lasted about 6 months and that was causing him distress. In considering a DSM-5-TR diagnosis of Erectile Disorder, the clinician must first determine whether the erectile dysfunction is persistent, is causing distress, and is not attributable to nonpsychiatric medical, substance, or other causes, such as severe relationship distress or partner violence, or to the presence of another mental disorder. Paul has had the erectile dysfunction for a sufficient time to meet the DSM-5-TR minimum requirement of a 6-month duration, and it is clearly causing him and his partner significant distress. Furthermore, there is no evidence suggesting that Paul has a nonpsychiatric medical problem or another mental disorder (e.g., Major Depressive Disorder), and he is not taking any medication or abusing alcohol or other drugs.

The timing of the onset of Paul's erectile dysfunction strongly suggests that there is likely a connection between his ambivalence about committing himself to a relationship with Annie and his sexual dysfunction. Although a diagnosis of a Sexual Dysfunction is not given if the clinician judges that the dysfunction is a result of severe relationship stress or partner violence, Paul's ambivalence about commitment is not deemed to meet the level of "severe relationship distress" that would preclude the diagnosis. Thus, the diagnosis is Erectile Disorder (DSM-5-TR, p. 481). Furthermore, because his erectile dysfunction began after a period of normal erectile functioning, the Acquired subtype applies.

13.4
Premature (Early) Ejaculation

DSM-5-TR includes two disorders involving orgasmic functioning in men, one for scenarios in which ejaculation occurs sooner during sexual intercourse than the man or his partner would like (i.e., Premature Ejaculation) and the other for situations in which ejaculation takes too long to happen or does not happen at all (i.e., Delayed Ejaculation; see Section 13.5). In DSM-5-TR, ejaculation is considered to be "premature" if it occurs during partnered sexual activity within approximately 1 minute following vaginal penetration and before the individual wishes it" (DSM-5-TR, p. 501). Despite the fact that the DSM-5-TR diagnosis of Premature Ejaculation is described in the context of sexual activity involving vaginal penetration, the diagnosis may also apply to individuals engaged in nonvaginal sexual activities, although specific duration guidelines have not been established for these activities. Biological causes of premature ejaculation include excess thyroid hormone, inflammation and infection of the prostate or urethra, and nerve damage from surgery or trauma.

Many men with Premature Ejaculation complain of a sense of lack of control over ejaculation and report apprehension about their anticipated inability to delay ejaculation in future sexual encounters. Premature Ejaculation may be associated with decreased self-esteem, a sense of lack of control, and adverse consequences for partner relationships. It may also cause personal distress and decreased sexual satisfaction in the sexual partner.

Ejaculation that occurs sooner than desired is one of the most common forms of male sexual dysfunction and has probably been experienced by most men at some point in their lives without sufficient distress to be considered a mental disorder. Estimates of the prevalence of the disorder vary widely, depending on the definition used, with a prevalence range of 8%–30% being reported across men of all ages. When the disorder is defined as ejaculation occurring within approximately 1 minute of vaginal penetration (as in DSM-5-TR), only 1%–3% of males would have symptoms that meet criteria for the diagnosis.

No Control

Liam and Melissa Crane are an attractive, gregarious couple, married for 15 years, who present to the therapist in the midst of a crisis over their sexual problems. Mr. Crane, age 38, is a successful restaurateur. Ms. Crane, age 35, has devoted herself to child rearing and managing the home since the couple married. She reports that throughout their marriage she has been extremely frustrated because sex has "always been hopeless for us." She is now seriously considering leaving her husband.

The difficulty is the husband's rapid ejaculation. Whenever any lovemaking is attempted, Mr. Crane becomes anxious, moves quickly toward intercourse, and reaches orgasm either immediately on entering his wife's vagina or within one or two strokes. He then feels humiliated and recognizes his wife's dissatisfaction, and they both lapse into silent suffering. He has severe feelings of inadequacy and guilt, and she experiences a mixture of frustration and resentment toward his "ineptness and lack of concern." Recently, they have developed a pattern of avoiding sex, which leaves them both frustrated but keeps overt hostility to a minimum.

Mr. Crane has always been a perfectionist, priding himself on his ability to succeed at anything he sets his mind to. As a child, he had always been a "good boy," in a vain effort to please his demanding father. His inability to control his ejaculation is a source of intense shame, and he finds himself unable to talk to his wife about his sexual "failures." Ms. Crane is highly sexual and easily aroused by foreplay, but she has always felt that intercourse is the only "acceptable" way to reach orgasm. Intercourse with her husband has always been unsatisfying, and she holds him completely responsible for her sexual frustration. As a result, they have developed other sexual techniques for pleasing each other. Because she cannot discuss the subject with Mr. Crane without feeling rage, she usually avoids talking about it.

In other areas of their marriage, including rearing of their two children, managing the family restaurant, and socializing with friends, the Cranes are highly compatible. Despite these strong points, however, they are near separation because of the tension produced by their mutual sexual disappointment.

Discussion of "No Control"

This couple presents with a sexual problem that is threatening their marriage. Mr. Crane's sexual difficulty is that he lacks a reasonable degree of voluntary control over ejaculation, so that he invariably ejaculates almost immediately on penetration during intercourse. As a result, Ms. Crane is never sexually satisfied, and Mr. Crane feels extremely inadequate. Because the problem has persisted throughout their marriage, is causing distress, does not appear to have a nonpsychiatric medical or substance-induced cause, and is not caused by another mental disorder or severe relationship distress such as partner violence, the diagnosis is Premature Ejaculation (DSM-5-TR, p. 501).

13.5
Delayed Ejaculation

In DSM-5-TR, Delayed Ejaculation is characterized by a marked delay in or inability to achieve ejaculation despite adequate sexual stimulation. Usually, the presenting complaint involves partnered sexual activity. DSM-5-TR does not offer a precise definition of the term *delayed*, because there is no consensus as to what constitutes an abnormally long time to reach orgasm. Instead, a man is probably experiencing Delayed Ejaculation if the delay is causing him distress or frustration, or if he has to stop sexual activity because of fatigue, physical irritation, loss of erection, or a request from his partner. Often, a man with Delayed Ejaculation might have difficulty reaching orgasm during sexual intercourse or other sexual activities with a partner, but will ejaculate without difficulty when masturbating.

Numerous nonpsychiatric medical conditions may lead to a delay in ejaculation, including spinal cord injury, stroke, multiple sclerosis, and diabetes. Alcohol abuse and cannabis use, as well as medications such as antihypertensive agents, antidepressants from the SSRI or serotonin-norepinephrine reuptake inhibitors (SNRI) class, and antipsychotic drugs, may be associated with delayed ejaculation. The prevalence of DSM-5-TR Delayed Ejaculation in the United States is estimated at 1%–5%, but rates as high as 11% have been reported in international studies because of differences in the definition.

In Jeopardy

Dennis Collins, a 33-year-old college professor, presented with the complaint that he has never been able to ejaculate while making love. He has had no trouble in attaining and maintaining an erection and no difficulties in stimulating his partner to her orgasm, but he could never be stimulated to ejaculation and would finally give up in boredom. He has always been able to reach ejaculation by masturbation, which he does about twice a week, but he has never been willing to allow a partner to masturbate him to orgasm. Previously, he resisted all of his girlfriend's attempts to persuade him to seek medical or psychological help, because he feels that intravaginal ejaculation is unimportant unless a person wants children.

Mr. Collins' current relationship is in jeopardy because his girlfriend is eager to marry and have children. He has never wanted to have children and is reluctant to become a father, but the pressures from his girlfriend have forced him to seek therapy. Throughout the interview, his attitude toward the problem is one of distance and disdain. He describes the problem as though he were a neutral observer, with little apparent feeling.

Discussion of "In Jeopardy"

Mr. Collins is able to have an erection without any difficulty and has no problem in sustaining the erection during intercourse, but he is unable to ejaculate during intercourse. Significantly, he has no trouble ejaculating when he masturbates, which excludes the possibility that a nonpsychiatric medical condition accounts for the problem, because in such a case the delay in ejaculation would be present in all circumstances. Moreover, the problem has persisted (it has been lifelong), is not due to substance use, is not a side effect of a medication, and is not attributable to another mental disorder. Although Mr. Collins does not appear to be particularly upset about his inability to ejaculate during intercourse, the facts that he is presenting for therapy and that his relationship with his girlfriend is "in jeopardy" suggest that the DSM-5-TR requirement that the dysfunction be causing distress is met, justifying a diagnosis of Delayed Ejaculation (DSM-5-TR, p. 478). The Situational and Lifelong subtypes also apply, because Mr. Collins is able to have orgasms during masturbation and he has never been able to have an orgasm with a partner.

13.6
Female Orgasmic Disorder

Female Orgasmic Disorder is characterized by either difficulty experiencing orgasm or significantly reduced intensity of orgasmic sensations, despite adequate sexual stimulation. There is wide variability in the type or intensity of stimulation that women need for orgasm. Similarly, women's subjective descriptions of orgasm are extremely varied, suggesting that it is experienced in very different ways, both among different women and on different occasions by the same woman. Because such variability is normal, a diagnosis of Female Orgasmic Disorder should be considered only if the orgasmic problems are experienced on almost all occasions of sexual activity.

Many women require clitoral stimulation to reach orgasm, and a relatively small proportion of women report that they always experience orgasm during penile-vaginal intercourse. Thus, a woman's experiencing orgasm through clitoral stimulation, but not during intercourse, would never justify a diagnosis of Female Orgasmic Disorder.

Many physiological factors, including nonpsychiatric medical conditions and medications, may influence a woman's experience of orgasm. Conditions such as multiple sclerosis, pelvic nerve damage from radical hysterectomy, and spinal cord injury can all influence orgasmic functioning in women. A wide variety of medica-tions, especially antidepressants that are SSRIs or SNRIs, can have a negative impact on a woman's ability to experience orgasm. If the orgasmic problems are clearly a side effect of a medication or substance, a diagnosis of Substance/Medication-Induced Sexual Dysfunction (see Section 13.8) should be considered.

The reported prevalence of orgasm problems in premenopausal women varies widely, from 8% to 72%, depending on multiple factors (e.g., age, cultural back-ground and context, duration, severity of symptoms). However, these estimates do not take into account the presence of distress, as required in the DSM-5-TR diagnosis. Internationally, approximately 10% of women do not experience orgasm throughout their lifetime.

Staying in Control

Lola Alvarez, a 25-year-old laboratory technician, has been married to a 32-year-old cabdriver for 5 years. The couple has a 2-year-old son, and the mar-riage appears harmonious.

The presenting complaint is Ms. Alvarez's lifelong inability to experience orgasm. She has never achieved orgasm, although during sexual activity she believes she has received what should have been sufficient stimulation. She has tried to masturbate, and on many occasions her husband has manually stimulated her patiently for lengthy periods of time. Although she does not reach climax, she is strongly attached to her husband, feels erotic pleasure during lovemaking, and lubricates copiously. According to both of them, her husband has no sexual difficulty.

Exploration of her thoughts as she nears orgasm reveals a vague sense of dread of some undefined disaster. More generally, she is anxious about losing control of her emotions, which she normally keeps closely in check. She is particularly uncomfortable about expressing any anger or hostility.

Physical examination reveals no abnormality.

Discussion of "Staying in Control"

Ms. Alvarez's sexual difficulties are limited to the orgasm phase of the sexual response cycle (she has no difficulty in desiring sex or in becoming aroused). During lovemaking there is what would ordinarily be an adequate amount of stimulation. Her report of a "vague sense of dread of some undefined disaster" as she approaches orgasm and her anxiety about losing control suggest that her inability to have orgasms represents a psychological inhibition. There is no suggestion of any other mental disorder, a nonpsychiatric medical condition, substance abuse, or medication use that could account for the orgasmic dys-function. Moreover, the problem has been persistent (i.e., she has never expe-rienced an orgasm) and it is causing her distress as evidenced by the fact that she is asking for help for this problem. Thus, the DSM-5-TR diagnosis is Fe-male Orgasmic Disorder, Lifelong, Generalized (DSM-5-TR, p. 485).

13.7
Genito-Pelvic Pain/
Penetration Disorder

Genito-Pelvic Pain/Penetration Disorder is a DSM-5-TR diagnosis that covers various aspects of sexual pain that occur in women. Presenting symptoms may include any of the following: 1) difficulty having vaginal intercourse; 2) marked vulvo-vaginal or pelvic pain during vaginal intercourse or other penetration attempts (e.g., gynecological examinations, tampon insertion); 3) marked fear or anxiety about vulvo-vaginal or pelvic pain in anticipation of, during, or as a result of vaginal penetration; and 4) marked involuntary tensing or tightening of the pelvic floor muscles around the vagina during attempted vaginal penetration, a phenomenon known as *vaginismus*.

As with the other Sexual Dysfunctions, Genito-Pelvic Pain/Penetration Disorder is not diagnosed if the problem can be explained by another mental disorder; is a consequence of severe relationship distress, such as partner violence; is attributable to a nonpsychiatric medical condition, such as endometriosis (a disease in which tissue that normally grows inside the uterus grows outside it), pelvic inflammatory disease (an infection of the upper part of the uterus, fallopian tubes, and ovaries, and inside the pelvis), or vulvovaginal atrophy (thinning, drying, and inflammation of the vaginal walls); or is a side effect of a medication.

Women with Genito-Pelvic Pain/Penetration Disorder often avoid sexual situations and opportunities and avoid gynecological examinations despite medical recommendations to the contrary. Commonly, women who have not succeeded in having sexual intercourse seek treatment only when they wish to conceive. Many women with this condition experience associated relationship or marital problems and also report that the symptoms significantly diminish their feelings of femininity.

Although 10%–28% of women of reproductive age in the United States report recurrent pain during intercourse, the actual prevalence of DSM-5-TR Genito-Pelvic Pain/Penetration Disorder, including the required 6-month minimum duration and the associated distress, is unknown. By definition, the diagnosis of Genito-Pelvic Pain/Penetration Disorder is given only to women. There is relatively new research concerning urological chronic pelvic pain syndrome in men, suggesting that men may experience some similar problems. The prevalence of genito-pelvic pain in men is estimated to be 2.2%–9.7% worldwide.

Sex Is a Nasty Business

Claire Whitaker, a 33-year-old secretary, was referred by her gynecologist to a sex therapist in a clinic specializing in sexual problems. The immediate reason for the referral was that the gynecologist had been unable to conduct a pelvic examination because of extreme contractions of Ms. Whitaker's perivaginal muscles (i.e., muscles around the vagina).

At the first visit to the therapist, Ms. Whitaker was visibly uncomfortable as she discussed her sexual problems. Since the birth of her son 2 years ago, she has been unable to have sexual intercourse because of vaginal spasms that are so extreme that neither her husband's nor her own little finger can be inserted into her vagina. She never looks forward to sexual contact with her husband and actively discourages his advances. Recently, her husband has been pressuring her to become pregnant again. She would like to become pregnant both to please him and because she herself wants another child.

The onset of the perivaginal muscle spasms, however, had been at an earlier time. Virginal at the time of her marriage 8 years previously, Ms. Whitaker had not been able to allow vaginal penetration for the first year. After a year of an "unconsummated marriage," she and her husband had seen a marriage counselor, who had helped them considerably so that they were able to have intercourse, at least episodically, over the next 5 years. Ms. Whitaker had always had some anxiety about and did not really like vaginal penetration, although she could be orgasmic, albeit rarely, with clitoral sexual stimulation.

Ms. Whitaker was unable to get pregnant during the first 5 years of her marriage, apparently because of chronic endometriosis, a common condition in which tissue that normally grows inside the uterus (endometrium) grows in other parts of the body, causing painful menstruation and sometimes infertility. When she finally gave birth, the baby was about 11 weeks premature and weighed only 3 pounds. Ms. Whitaker felt guilty about having caused the premature birth by taking estrogen for the endometriosis. Since the birth, she has been extremely fearful of becoming pregnant again and possibly delivering another premature child.

Ms. Whitaker recalled the difficulty that her mother had in talking to her about menstruation and sex. Her religious upbringing precluded any discussion of premarital sex, birth control, and abortion, which were all considered sinful. She knew nothing about the use of a condom as a birth-control device. She acknowledged not knowing where her clitoris was and was unable to identify it on a model. She had never masturbated, and indeed had learned about masturbation only recently. She expressed an aversion toward her husband's licking or sucking parts of her body, describing this as "yucky." She reported a lifelong fear of bathtub water getting into her vagina and "infecting" her. She recalled dreams in which large and frightening objects penetrated her body.

Treatment involved several sessions of couples therapy to deal with her husband's frustration, anger, and impatience and to secure his cooperation in exercises that were designed to focus on sensual pleasure without intercourse (sensate focus exercises). Ms. Whitaker also had individual sessions and was prescribed an antianxiety agent (alprazolam 0.5 mg, taken two or three times a day).

However, the main focus of Ms. Whitaker's treatment was on vaginal dilation using her fingers, while in a tub of warm water. Ms. Whitaker's progress with vaginal dilation was slow; she went through a series of gradual steps in which she introduced first the tip of one finger and then, gradually, two or three fingers. When the sensate focus exercises were added to the dilation, she disliked her husband's sucking, licking, and kissing; she had to spend a great deal of time trying to achieve some comfort with her own body. She later began attending group therapy for nonorgasmic women.

Seen at first weekly and then monthly, Ms. Whitaker slowly made progress, ultimately allowing penetration during intercourse. She was still frightened of pregnancy, even when her husband used a condom, expressing marked fear that the condom would break or slip off. After several more months of therapy, her fear of pregnancy diminished so that intercourse could take place without birth control.

Discussion of "Sex Is a Nasty Business"

Ms. Whitaker has a number of sexual dysfunctions, including low sexual interest and orgasmic difficulties, but her major problem at the present time and the one that brought her into treatment is contraction of her perivaginal muscles—demonstrated, as it often is, during a pelvic examination—that results in difficulties with intercourse. She also experiences marked anxiety related to the prospect of vaginal penetration. Her recurrent and persistent difficulties with vaginal penetration, which are a source of distress and are not due to the effects of a medication or attributable to a nonpsychiatric medical condition, justify the diagnosis of Genito-Pelvic Pain/Penetration Disorder (DSM-5-TR, p. 493).

13.8
Substance/Medication-Induced Sexual Dysfunction

A wide variety of medications as well as substances of abuse can cause problems in sexual functioning. Most (but not all) antidepressants have the potential to cause sexual dysfunction. Although the most commonly encountered problems involve difficulty with orgasm or ejaculation, problems with desire and erection can occur as well. Between 25% and 80% of individuals taking antidepressants report sexual side effects. Antipsychotic medications cause sexual side effects in approximately 50% of individuals who take them. Many nonpsychiatric medications, such as cardiovascular, cytotoxic (used to treat cancer, rheumatoid arthritis, and multiple sclerosis), gastrointestinal, and hormonal agents, are associated with disturbances in sexual function. Use of illicit substances is associated with decreased sexual desire, erectile dysfunction, and difficulty reaching orgasm. Chronic nicotine and chronic alcohol abuse are particularly strongly associated with erectile problems. Premature ejaculation can sometimes occur after cessation of opioid use and might justify a diagnosis of Opioid-Induced Sexual Dysfunction if the individual is significantly distressed by this.

Substance/Medication-Induced Sexual Dysfunctions can usually be reversed by lowering the dosage or stopping the medication.

Bad Side Effect

Amy Harris, a 36-year-old bank officer, is concerned about her extreme difficulty reaching orgasm. She remembers masturbating to orgasm in her early teens. Her first sexual partner was her high school boyfriend, the captain of the football team. After several months of sexual activity, she became orgasmic with him. She had only a few sexual partners in college but was usually orgasmic. She was an excellent student and was elected to the honor council at her college and was president of her sorority. After graduation, she accepted a beginning executive position at a local bank. She married at age 26 and was usually orgasmic with her husband. Initially, they were sexually active four to five times a week, but this frequency decreased to one to two times a week as the marriage progressed. She commented, "When I wanted to, I could reach orgasm. Sometimes, I just enjoyed the intimacy and did not make the effort." Sexual interest waxed and waned during attempts to become pregnant.

Approximately 6 months ago, Ms. Harris discovered that her husband had been sexually intimate with one of his female work associates. Shortly after that, Ms. Harris did not receive an expected promotion at work. She began experiencing self-doubt, questioning her competence both as a wife and as a businesswoman. She sought counseling, but her self-doubt increased, and she began wondering if she would be a bad mother even if she could become pregnant. Slowly, insomnia, anhedonia, fatigue, poor appetite, loss of sexual interest, and transient thoughts of suicide entered her life. Her work suffered, and she received a negative review, which increased her self-doubt.

Ms. Harris's primary care physician prescribed an antidepressant, paroxetine 20 mg/day, and Ms. Harris continued counseling with her therapist. After her depressive symptoms started to improve, she became receptive to her husband's sexual advances in spite of her anger about his affair and lingering doubts about her attractiveness. She had difficulty reaching orgasm but attributed this to her anger about her husband's affair. She still continued to have some depressive symptoms and returned to her primary care physician, who diagnosed an incomplete response to pharmacotherapy and increased her dosage of paroxetine to 40 mg/day. When she had coitus several weeks later, she was totally incapable of reaching orgasm. She also attempted masturbation and realized that she could not reach orgasm with masturbation. She read about SSRI-associated Sexual Dysfunction on the internet and contacted her primary care physician again. Her primary care physician gradually reduced her dosage of paroxetine to 20 mg/day, and her ability to reach orgasm with difficulty returned after several weeks.

Discussion of "Bad Side Effect"

This vignette starts out as a potential case of Female Orgasmic Disorder, given Ms. Harris's chief complaint of extreme difficulty reaching orgasm. The history indicates that this is a case of acquired orgasmic difficulty, because she had good orgasmic capacity during her teenage years and early 20s. The first signs of a sexual problem (i.e., loss of sexual interest) emerged in the context of a Major Depressive Episode that occurred after Ms. Harris's discovery that her husband had been sexually intimate with one of his female work associates. Given that low sexual desire is a common feature of Major Depressive Disorder, an additional diagnosis of Female Sexual Interest/Arousal Disorder would not have been appropriate.

After Ms. Harris's depression was successfully treated with an antidepressant, her sexual desire returned, but she discovered that she had a new problem: difficulty reaching orgasm, which she initially attributed to her anger about her husband's affair. After her primary care physician increased her antidepressant medication to deal with persistent depressive symptoms, Ms. Harris's orgasmic problems worsened to the point at which she was unable to achieve orgasm at all. Although it is possible that her orgasmic difficulties were psychologically mediated (e.g., arising from doubts about her attractiveness in the wake of her husband's affair), there are two reasons why her antidepressant medication is the most likely culprit. First, she was taking paroxetine, which is from a class of antidepressants, the SSRIs, that are especially likely to lead to orgasmic difficulties. Second, the fact that her orgasmic difficulties worsened when the dosage was increased from 20 mg/day to 40 mg/day, and improved when the dosage was lowered again to 20 mg/day, is completely consistent with a cause-and-effect relationship between her medication and her sexual dysfunction. Thus, Ms. Harris's diagnosis would be Paroxetine-Induced Sexual Dysfunction (DSM-5-TR, p. 504).

CHAPTER 14

Gender Dysphoria

Gender denotes the public and usually legally recognized lived role of a person as boy or girl, man or woman. In contrast, *sex* refers to the biological indicators of male and female, including reproductive capacity (e.g., sex chromosomes, gonads, sex hormones, external genitalia). Some individuals develop a social identity, or gender, as male or female that does not correspond to their biological sex. The term *gender dysphoria* refers to an individual's emotional and cognitive discomfort with their assigned gender—that is, the distress that may accompany incongruence between a person's experienced or expressed gender and their assigned gender based on biological characteristics. Not all people will experience distress as a result of this incongruence, but when they do, along with impairment in psychosocial functioning, they may qualify for a diagnosis of Gender Dysphoria. The DSM-IV diagnostic term for this disorder, *Gender Identity Disorder*, was replaced in DSM-5 (and continued in DSM-5-TR) by *Gender Dysphoria*, a more descriptive term that focuses on *distress* as the clinical problem rather than the person's gender identity itself.

DSM-5-TR presents two lists of diagnostic criteria for Gender Dysphoria: one for prepubescent children and one for adolescents and adults (see Table 14–1 for characteristic features). The criteria for children are age appropriate and inferential, and are somewhat more concrete and specific than the adult criteria, because children are usually less able to verbalize their desires and distress and have yet to develop sexually. When there is an actual physical disorder of sex development, such as congenital adrenal hyperplasia (a condition in which the child is born with an excess of male sex hormones, which in females can result in ambiguous genitalia such that it can initially be difficult to identify external genitalia as "male" or "female"), its presence can be noted with the specifier With a Disorder/Difference of Sex Development.

TABLE 14–1.   **Characteristic features of Gender Dysphoria**

Disorder	Key characteristics
Gender Dysphoria in Children	Desire to be of the other gender; strong preference for gender-affirming clothing, role-playing, toys and games, and playmates
	Rejection of toys, games, and activities of assigned gender; dislike of one's sexual anatomy; desire for sex characteristics of one's experienced gender
Gender Dysphoria in Adolescents and Adults	Incongruence between experienced gender and one's primary/secondary sex characteristics; desire to be rid of one's sex characteristics and to have sex characteristics of other gender
	Desire to be of the other gender and to be treated as such; conviction that one has feelings and reactions of other gender

14.1
Gender Dysphoria in Children

Gender Dysphoria in Children is defined as "a marked incongruence between one's experienced/expressed gender and assigned gender" (DSM-5-TR, p. 512) that persists for at least 6 months. There must be a strong desire to be the other gender or some alternative gender (i.e., neither stereotypically male nor female) that is different from the gender assigned at birth on the basis of biological characteristics. Among children with Gender Dysphoria, boys (assigned gender) have a strong preference for cross-dressing as a girl, and girls (assigned gender) have a strong preference for very boyish attire and a resistance to dressing in feminine clothing. There are also strong preferences for gender-affirming roles in play and fantasy life; for toys, games, and activities usually associated with the other gender; and for playmates of the other gender. Boys will reject typically masculine toys, games, and activities, such as competitive sports or toy cars and trucks, and will eschew rough-and-tumble play; girls will reject feminine toys, games, and activities, such as playing with dolls or feminine dress-up or role-play. These children will occasionally express a dislike of their own sexual anatomy and a desire to instead have sexual characteristics that are in concert with their experienced gender, although these verbal expressions of gender dysphoria are far less common in young children than they are in preadolescents or adolescents. When these strong desires and preferences are associated with significant distress and impairment in social, school, or other important areas of functioning, the diagnosis of Gender Dysphoria applies.

It is important to distinguish Gender Dysphoria from simple nonconformity to stereotypical gender role behavior (e.g., "tomboyism" in girls, "girly boy" behavior in boys). The DSM-5-TR diagnosis of Gender Dysphoria should be considered only for children who express a strong desire to be of another gender than the assigned one and who experience distress or impairment as a result of their desire to be another gender.

When Gender Dysphoria is diagnosed in a female, the desire to be male because of a profound discontent with being a female needs to be distinguished from the desire merely to have the perceived cultural advantages associated with being a male.

Gender Dysphoria is rare, although there are no large-scale population studies. Children assigned male at birth are more often affected than children assigned female at birth. Among adults seeking gender-affirming treatment in the United States and Europe, individuals assigned male at birth are also more common than individuals assigned female at birth.

In children who come to clinical attention, the onset of gender-affirming behaviors is usually between ages 2 and 4 years. There is a wide range in the rates of persistence of Gender Dysphoria in Children into adolescence and adulthood, with gender discomfort/discontent persisting in 2%–39% of individuals assigned male at birth and 12%–50% of individuals assigned female at birth. Among children whose Gender Dysphoria does not persist, the majority of those assigned male at birth will go on to be sexually attracted to males and self-identify as gay, whereas a somewhat smaller proportion of those assigned female at birth will go on to be sexually attracted to females and self-identify as lesbian.

Gender Dysphoria can interfere significantly with the development of peer relationships and can lead to social isolation. Some children may refuse to attend school because they are afraid of being teased or harassed. Suicidal ideation and suicide attempts are highly prevalent, and are estimated to affect up to 80% of individuals with the disorder. Comorbid Anxiety, Depression, Disruptive, Impulse-Control, and Autism Spectrum Disorders are common.

Dolls

Rocky is an 8-year-old boy for whom his parents seek treatment because "he wants to be a girl." The patient's major playmate is his younger sister, and although his parents are trying to foster friendships with other boys, Rocky prefers to play with girls or to be with his mother or a female babysitter. He refuses to participate in rough play with boys or physical fighting, although he is well-built, above average in height for his age, and well-coordinated. At home, he engages in much make-believe play, invariably assuming female roles. When playing house with his younger sister, he plays the "mother" or "big sister" role and leaves the male role to her. He likes to imitate female movie and TV figures, such as Anna from the movie *Frozen* or Bart Simpson's sister Lisa. Similarly, he likes to playact female characters from various children's books.

Rocky has never been interested in toy cars, trucks, or trains, but he is an avid player with dolls (baby, Barbie, and family dolls) and enjoys playing with kitchen toys. He also likes to play wedding, pregnancy, a female teacher, or a lady doctor. He is good at drawing and is very interested in drawing female figures. Although his parents try to restrict the activity, he engages in a lot of cross-dressing. He sometimes uses a quilt or a towel around his middle for skirts, or a T-shirt or nightgown for a dress. He does not use any female underwear or bathing suits. He likes bows in his hair and sometimes uses a slip or a veil on his head to imitate long hair. He loves dancing, preferably in dresses. He is very interested in jewelry, has plastic necklaces, and pretends at times to wear earrings. Also, he pretends to apply lipstick (using lip balm) and would use real lipstick and perfume if his mother would let him. He states, "I want to be a girl," often when he is unhappy, such as when he started kindergarten, or when he has felt in competition with his younger sister.

On physical examination, Rocky has normal male genitalia. His intellectual development is apparently normal. Although somewhat reluctantly, he is able to describe much of what his parents have related about his toy and game preferences. He says that he does not want to be a boy because he is afraid that he will have to play with soldiers or play army with other boys when he grows bigger. He wishes a fairy could change him into a girl. What he likes about being a girl is wearing dresses, long hair, and jewelry.

The family history, his mother's pregnancy, and Rocky's birth and early development are all normal. The parents do not show any overt psychopathology. Rocky's problems seem to have started with the birth of his younger sister, when he was 2 years old. For the first 4 months of her life, his sister had severe digestive problems and required a great deal of parental attention and care. Rocky then began to display definite signs of regression: he played the baby role again, wanting to drink from a bottle and to be held and carried. His mother gave in to some extent. Both parents and babysitters think that his cross-dressing and wanting to be a girl date back to that time, although before the birth of his sister, there were already some instances of the patient's imitating long hair by wearing a towel on his head. When Rocky was 4 years old, his sister got a baby doll, which he took from her. Around this same time, he spent a vacation with his sister at their grandparents' house and complained that his sister got more attention than he did, ending with the familiar, "Why can't I be a girl? Why didn't God make me a girl? Girls get to dress up, get to wear pretty things."

At age 3, Rocky was enrolled in nursery school, where he initially displayed much separation anxiety. He appeared more sensitive than the other children, always seemed to feel threatened by them, and did not stand up for himself. His teacher noted from the beginning that Rocky dressed up as a girl very frequently, announced that he wanted to be a mother when he grew up, and refused to engage in rough-and-tumble activities. In the second grade, he was so good at imitating a girl (e.g., voice inflection, walking) that the teacher wondered if he were an "intersex" (i.e., an individual with both male and female sexual characteristics).

Discussion of "Dolls"

Rocky has a strong and persistent identification of himself as a female. He frequently states his desire to be a girl. He is preoccupied with female stereotypical activity; he prefers to play with girls; he pretends that he is a girl; and he frequently cross-dresses. He plays exclusively with stereotypically female toys such as dolls. When imitating characters from books, movies, and TV, he always chooses female characters. There is also evidence of a persistent discomfort with being a boy. He rejects stereotypical male toys and activities and shows an aversion toward rough-and-tumble play. These are the characteristic features of Gender Dysphoria in Children, as seen in an individual assigned male at birth (DSM-5-TR, p. 512).

14.2
Gender Dysphoria
in Adolescents and Adults

Gender Dysphoria in Adolescents and Adults is characterized by a "marked incongruence between one's experienced/expressed gender and primary and/or secondary sex characteristics" (DSM-5-TR, p. 512). Primary sex characteristics include any structures of the body directly involved in reproduction, such as the penis, testes, ovaries, or vagina. Secondary sex characteristics are physical manifestations specific to each sex that are not essential to reproduction, such as breasts, fatty tissue distribution, muscle mass, facial hair, change in pitch of voice, and so on. In adolescents, the discomfort may be in anticipation of secondary sex characteristics. The affected person has a strong desire to be rid of primary or secondary sex characteristics or to prevent their development. The person expresses a strong desire to have the sex characteristics of the other gender, to be an individual of the other gender (or some alternative gender that is neither stereotypically male nor female), and to be treated as the other gender. The person believes very strongly that they have the typical feelings and reactions of the other gender. When this gender incongruence in a postpubertal individual is associated with significant distress and impairment in social, school, or other important areas of functioning, the diagnosis of Gender Dysphoria in Adolescents and Adults applies.

Some adults with Gender Dysphoria will dress and act like a person of their experienced gender and attempt to live as a different gender without seeking medical treatments to alter their sex characteristics. By living as their experienced gender, they resolve the felt incongruence. Some may adopt a gender role that is neither conventionally male nor female. Young adolescents may attempt to hide their secondary sex characteristics. Boys will bind their genitals to make them less obvious; girls may bind their breasts or wear loose clothing so that their breasts are less evident. Both older adolescents and adults may obtain (with or without a prescription) drugs to suppress gonadal hormones to delay or reverse the development of secondary sex characteristics and hormonal drugs to induce the development of the desired secondary sex characteristics. Some might also seek gender-affirming surgery.

Among individuals assigned male at birth, the onset of Gender Dysphoria can be either early (i.e., in childhood) or late (i.e., around puberty or even much later in life). Adolescents and adult individuals assigned male at birth with an early onset are almost always sexually attracted to men. Those with a later onset of Gender Dysphoria may engage in transvestic behavior for sexual excitement and are most often attracted to women or to other posttransitional (to women) individuals assigned male at birth who had a later-onset disorder. Among individuals assigned female at birth, by far the most common onset is early. Despite a period of time in which they may identify as lesbian, these individuals may later seek hormones and gender-affirming surgery.

It is important to distinguish Gender Dysphoria in males from Transvestic Disorder (see Section 19.8), because both conditions may involve cross-dressing behavior. In Gender Dysphoria, such cross-dressing behavior is a component of an overall pattern of engaging in activities stereotypically associated with the person's experienced gender. In Transvestic Disorder, a condition that occurs in heterosexual (or bisexual) adolescent and adult males (but rarely in females), the cross-dressing behavior is a source of intense sexual arousal. Notably, some individuals assigned male at birth who develop Gender Dysphoria during late adolescence or adulthood had Transvestic Disorder as a precursor (i.e., what started out as a sexual interest in cross-dressing shifted over time into a strong sense of gender incongruence).

Adolescents and adults with Gender Dysphoria often experience significant interpersonal problems, including sexual relationship problems. Because Gender Dysphoria is associated with high levels of stigmatization, discrimination, and victimization, these individuals may have low self-esteem, may develop other mental disorders such as Major Depressive Disorder, may drop out of school, and may be economically challenged as a result of work problems. It is often difficult for them to find accepting and informed medical and psychological care.

She Wants to Be a Boy

Kelly, a 16-year-old Canadian girl from British Columbia, is referred to a gender identity clinic at the suggestion of her family physician and with her parents' agreement and participation. According to her mother, "Kelly wants a sex change. She wants to be a boy very desperately." Kelly echoes this statement, saying that she has wanted to be a boy "since I was 2." The current referral was precipitated by Kelly's relationship with another girl, Anna, who has been living with the family for the past few months. Kelly's mother became agitated about the girls' relationship, feeling that it was sexual: "They always have their legs crossed, arms around each other, and once were lying naked with their breasts exposed reading dirty books."

Since reaching puberty, Kelly has continued to show a number of signs suggesting that she is very uncomfortable with being a female. She finds her menstrual periods "horrible" and dislikes having to wear a bra. Kelly has continued to say that she wants to be a boy, including having a penis. Last year, she learned of the possibility of gender-affirming surgery. She knows that it would include a mastectomy, removal of her internal reproductive organs, and hormone injections. She is not sure whether she could have a penis surgically constructed.

Kelly's physical appearance is ambiguous with regard to her biological sex. Her hair is short, she is dressed casually in blue jeans, and she wears no makeup. Kelly says that she does not care if others perceive her as a male or as a female, preferring to be seen as a "human being." As she speaks, it becomes clear that she prefers that people not ask her if she is a male or a female.

Kelly quit school after the seventh grade. She reports that she is now in a youth group, training to be in the military. She very much enjoys this because even though she is known to be a female, "They treat you like a buddy—the same as the other guys." She takes great delight in ordering around her cadet peers, relishing "being mean; they all hate me" when she demands that they do 100 push-ups. Kelly spoke in great detail about using an AK-47 assault rifle and said she had been practicing weapon use for several years. She is attracted by "gory things, blood, and living dangerously." Kelly says that the thought of war appeals to her because "they push you so hard and you are down on your knees, begging them to stop."

Kelly's mother tried to find out about her daughter's sexuality by having Kelly read a "pornographic" book and underline those passages that excited her or, as Kelly put it, gave her a "twingy" feeling, during which she felt "weird inside." The passages that elicited such a feeling involved lovemaking between women. Kelly says that she is not sure if boys or girls turn her on. She jogs whenever she begins to have "twingy feelings" and denies that she has ever masturbated. "I think it's sick."

She denies ever experiencing sexual images either in dreams or fantasy. She says she has never had any sexual experiences with another person and has no desire to marry. When asked about lesbianism, she claims not to want to know very much about the gay subculture: "It's their life."

When she appeared for the physical examination, she apologized for not having shaved her legs. An endocrine evaluation was performed and indicated that the sex chromosomes were XX (i.e., she was genetically female), there was no abnormally elevated level of testosterone (the male sex hormone), and there were no signs of physical hermaphroditism (an intersex condition in which an individual is born with both ovarian and testicular tissue).

At a 4-year follow-up, Kelly remained preoccupied with changing her gender, yet she continued to live in an ambivalent gender role; for example, she was employed in a typically "masculine" occupation (as a plumber's assistant) but claimed that no one asked, or cared, if she was male or female. In the past year, Kelly made an application to an adult gender identity clinic with the hope that she would eventually be able to have gender-affirming surgery. She failed to keep her appointment.

Discussion of "She Wants to Be a Boy"

Kelly has a strong and persistent desire to be a male, which goes beyond any perceived cultural advantages of being male. She has a stated desire to become a male, including the possibility of having gender-affirming surgery. She is comfortable passing as a male, has hidden her secondary sex characteristics, believes that she has the feelings and reactions of a male, and has a stated desire to live and be treated as a male. In addition, she indicates a persistent discomfort with being female. All of these features are characteristic of Gender Dysphoria in Adolescents and Adults (DSM-5-TR, p. 512).

There are a few notable aspects of this case that deserve clarification. It is important to keep in mind the differences between a person's gender identity (whether a person identifies as male, female, or a third gender) and that person's sexual orientation (whether a person is sexually attracted to men, women, to both [bisexual], or to neither [asexual]). Kelly's mother's attempt to determine her daughter's "sexuality" by having her read a pornographic book and underline the passages that "excited" her (they involved lovemaking between women), coupled with the behaviors she exhibited with her best friend ("they always have their legs crossed, arms around each other"), suggest that she is most likely attracted to women. Thus, Kelly's sexual orientation is gynephilic (attracted to women)—as opposed to androphilic (attracted to men). Also notable for its atypicality is Kelly not caring whether others perceive her as a male or as a female; most individuals with Gender Dysphoria prefer that others treat them as their experienced gender.

Living as a Man

A 25-year-old patient who was assigned female at birth and now calls himself Charles Northrup requested a "sex change operation." He had for 3 years lived socially and been employed as a man. For the last 2 of these years, he had been the housemate of, economic provider for, and husband-equivalent for a bisexual woman who had fled from a bad marriage. Her two young children regarded Mr. Northrup as their stepfather, and there was a strong, affectionate bond between them.

In appearance, the patient passed as a somewhat androgynous male whose sexual development in puberty might be conjectured to have been extremely delayed or hormonally deficient. His voice was pitched low but not baritone. His shirt and jacket were bulky and successfully camouflaged tightly bound, flattened breasts. A strap-on penis produced a masculine-looking bulge in the pants; it was so constructed that in case of social necessity, it could be used as a urinary conduit in the standing position. The patient had tried without success to obtain a mastectomy, so that in summer he could wear only a T-shirt while working at his job on a textile factory assembly line. He had also been unsuccessful in obtaining a prescription for testosterone to produce male secondary sex characteristics and suppress menses. The patient wanted a hysterectomy (surgical removal of the uterus) and oophorectomy (surgical removal of the ovaries), and as a long-term goal looked forward to obtaining a successful phalloplasty (surgical construction of a penis).

The patient was straightforward in his account of progressive recognition in adolescence of being able to fall in love only with a woman, following a tomboyish childhood that had finally consolidated into the transgender role and identity.

Physical examination revealed normal female anatomy, which the patient found personally repulsive and incongruous, and which was a source of continual distress. The endocrine laboratory results were within normal limits for a female.

Discussion of "Living as a Man"

The diagnosis of Gender Dysphoria in Adolescents and Adults (DSM-5-TR, p. 512) is certainly indicated in this case. Mr. Northrup desperately wants to get rid of his primary female sex characteristics and acquire male sex characteristics because of a persistent discomfort with those characteristics and a strong sense of incongruence between his experienced gender and his birth-assigned gender. This case also demonstrates another characteristic feature of Gender Dysphoria when present in an adult: a strong and persistent identification as being of the other gender, manifested by dressing, living socially, and being employed as a person of the experienced/expressed gender. As is almost always the case, there is no evidence of physical intersex or genetic abnormality.

Adults who develop the desire to physically change their gender (previously referred to as transsexualism) almost invariably report having struggled with gender-related dysphoria since in childhood. The onset of the full syndrome, however (as in Mr. Northrup's case), most often occurs in late adolescence or early adulthood.

CHAPTER 15

Disruptive, Impulse-Control, and Conduct Disorders

The DSM-5-TR Disruptive, Impulse-Control, and Conduct Disorders are characterized by problems in the self-control of behavior and emotions. Many disorders in other DSM-5-TR diagnostic classes, such as Bipolar and Related Disorders, also involve problems in emotional and/or behavioral regulation, but the disorders in this chapter are unique in that these problems are manifested in behaviors that invariably violate the rights of others (e.g., aggression, property destruction) or that bring the individual into conflict with social norms or authority figures. All of the disorders are related to an underlying personality dimension of "externalizing," whereby individuals are more prone to act antagonistically toward people or things in their environment to express their problems outwardly, in contrast to "internalizing," in which individuals inwardly experience distress.

The disorders in this group vary in age at onset (usually beginning during childhood or adolescence, but sometimes in adulthood), but importantly also vary in the degree to which they involve lack of control over behavior versus lack of control over emotions. Conduct Disorder is characterized predominantly by poor behavioral regulation, whereas Intermittent Explosive Disorder is characterized predominantly by uncontrolled emotions, such as anger. Oppositional Defiant Disorder has an age at onset in childhood and is characterized by poor control of both behavior and emotions. Pyromania is a disorder of poor behavioral impulse control that involves fire setting, Kleptomania involves stealing. Both Pyromania and Kleptomania are associated with a buildup of internal tension before the person engages in the act and thus appear to have a tension-relieving function.

Antisocial Personality Disorder is a pervasive pattern of disregard for and violation of the rights of others; the disorder shares many features of other disorders on the externalizing spectrum, but because it has features in common with other Personality Disorders (e.g., problems in self- and interpersonal functioning), it is classified within that DSM-5-TR diagnostic class (see Section 18.5). Finally, Substance Use Dis-

TABLE 15–1.　Characteristic features of Disruptive, Impulse-Control, and Conduct Disorders

Disorder	Key characteristics
Oppositional Defiant Disorder	Pattern of angry/irritable mood, argumentative/defiant behavior, or vindictiveness lasting at least 6 months
Intermittent Explosive Disorder	Recurrent behavioral outbursts representing failure to control aggressive impulses out of proportion to provocation or psychosocial stressor
	Outbursts not premeditated or committed to achieve tangible objective
	Chronological age at least 6 years
Conduct Disorder	Repetitive and persistent pattern of behavior in which basic rights of others or societal norms or rules are violated
	Pattern manifested by aggression toward people and animals, destruction of property, deceitfulness or theft, and/or serious violations of rules
Pyromania	Deliberate and purposeful fire setting more than once
	Tension or affective arousal before the act
	Fascination with, interest in, curiosity about, or attraction to fire
	Pleasure, gratification, or relief when setting fires
Kleptomania	Recurrent failure to resist impulse to steal objects that are not needed
	Increasing tension before committing theft
	Pleasure, gratification, or relief at time of theft

orders and Gambling Disorder also involve behavioral loss of control (i.e., over the use of psychoactive substances or over problematic gambling, respectively) and thus also lie on the externalizing spectrum. They, too, are classified elsewhere in DSM-5-TR, under Substance-Related and Addictive Disorders (see Chapter 16). Table 15–1 lists characteristic features of the Disruptive, Impulse-Control, and Conduct Disorders that are discussed in this chapter.

15.1
Oppositional Defiant Disorder

Oppositional Defiant Disorder is defined as "a pattern of angry/irritable mood, argumentative/defiant behavior, or vindictiveness" (DSM-5-TR, p. 522) that persists for at least 6 months and that causes distress either in the affected individual or in those around them, or that negatively impacts psychosocial functioning. The angry or irritable mood that is characteristic of individuals with Oppositional Defiant Disorder is manifested by frequent loss of temper, being "touchy" or easily annoyed, or being often angry or resentful. Argumentative or defiant behavior is exhibited by frequent arguments with adults or other authority figures, defying or refusing to go along with requests made by authority figures, deliberately annoying others, or blaming others for the individual's own mistakes. Vindictiveness or spitefulness is often also present.

Given that many of these behaviors are normal during childhood, the clinician should take several caveats into account before making this diagnosis. First, the symptoms cannot be entirely explained as a consequence of sibling rivalry; that is, the behaviors must occur during interactions with individuals apart from the child's siblings. Second, the DSM-5-TR requirement that four or more symptoms be present within the preceding 6 months must be met and must result in significant impairment in functioning. Finally, the persistence and frequency of the symptoms should go beyond what is normative given the child's age, developmental level, gender, and culture. For example, it is not unusual for preschool children to have temper tantrums on a weekly basis. For a preschool child's temper outbursts to be considered indicative of Oppositional Defiant Disorder, they must occur much more often than normal (e.g., on most days); the outbursts must occur along with at least three other Oppositional Defiant Disorder symptoms; and, together with the other symptoms, they must cause significant impairment in functioning (e.g., the child's being asked to leave school because of destruction of property that was the result of the temper outbursts). The severity of the disorder is noted as Mild if the antagonistic emotions and behaviors occur in only one social setting (i.e., at home, at school, at work, with peers); as Moderate if symptoms are present in at least two settings; and as Severe if symptoms occur in three or more settings.

The earliest symptoms of Oppositional Defiant Disorder usually appear in the preschool years and rarely later than early adolescence. Some children with Oppositional Defiant Disorder may go on to develop Conduct Disorder. The defiant, argumentative types of Oppositional Defiant Disorder may elevate the risk for the later development of Conduct Disorder, whereas the angry, irritable types may predispose to the later development of Anxiety or Depressive Disorders. The average estimated prevalence of Oppositional Defiant Disorder is 3.3%. The disorder appears to be somewhat more prevalent in boys than in girls before adolescence, but this male predominance is not consistently found in samples of adolescents or adults (DSM-5-TR, p. 524). Oppositional Defiant Disorder occurs at high rates in children, adolescents, and adults with Attention-Deficit/Hyperactivity Disorder (ADHD). It also co-occurs with Substance Use Disorders in adolescents and adults.

No Brakes

Jeremy, age 9 years and in the 4th grade, was brought by his mother to a mental health care clinic because he had become increasingly disobedient and difficult to manage at school. Several events during the previous month had convinced his mother that she had to do something about her son's behavior. Several weeks ago, he swore at his teacher and was suspended from school for 3 days. Last week he was reprimanded by the police for riding his three-wheeler in the street, something his mother had repeatedly cautioned him about. The next day he failed to use his pedal brakes and rode his bike through a store window, shattering it. He has not engaged in any offenses of higher severity, although he once broke a window when he was riding his bike with a friend.

Jeremy has been difficult to manage since nursery school. The problems have slowly escalated. Whenever he is without close supervision, he gets into trouble. He has been reprimanded at school for teasing and kicking other children, tripping them, and calling them names. He is described as bad-tempered and irritable, even though at times he seems to enjoy school. He often appears to be deliberately trying to annoy other children, although he always claims that others have started the arguments. He has not become involved in serious fights.

Jeremy sometimes refuses to do what his two teachers tell him to do, and this year he has been particularly difficult with the teacher who has him in the afternoon for arithmetic, art, and science lessons. He gives many reasons why he should not have to do his work, and he argues when told to do it. Many of the same problems were experienced last year, when he had only one teacher. Despite these problems, his grades are good and have been getting better over the course of the year, particularly in arithmetic and art, which are subjects taught by the teacher with whom he has the most difficulty.

At home Jeremy's behavior is quite variable. On some days he is defiant and rude to his mother, needing to be told to do everything several times before he will do it; however, eventually he usually complies. On other days he is charming and volunteers to help. His mother says that his unhelpful days predominate. "The least little thing upsets him, and then he shouts and screams." Jeremy is described as spiteful and mean toward his younger brother; even when Jeremy is in a good mood, he is unkind to his brother.

Jeremy's concentration is generally good, and he does not leave his work unfinished. His mother describes him as "on the go all the time" but not restless. His teachers have expressed concern about his attitude, not about restlessness. His mother also comments that he tells many minor lies, although when pressed, he is truthful about important things.

Discussion of "No Brakes"

Jeremy's defiant and reckless behavior suggests the possibility of both Conduct Disorder (see Section 15.3) and ADHD (see "Into Everything" in Section 1.7). Although Jeremy has annoyed other children and adults, he has not violated their basic rights or displayed any of the more serious forms of behavior, such as cruelty, stealing, truancy, running away from home, or destroying property, that would justify a diagnosis of Conduct Disorder. His encounter with the police was over a petty violation, and the damage he caused to a shop window was not done with any destructive intent. Although Jeremy does quite well academically, he has problems with teachers and peers. He has a high energy level but is not aimlessly hyperactive and does not appear to have the other characteristics of ADHD.

The persistent argumentative, irritable, defiant, annoying, and resentful behaviors that Jeremy displays are characteristic symptoms of Oppositional Defiant Disorder (DSM-5-TR, p. 522). The severity in Jeremy's case is noted as Severe, because his emotional outbursts and defiant behavior occur at home, in school, and with peers.

Some clinicians consider Oppositional Defiant Disorder to be merely a mild form of Conduct Disorder, but many children with the disorder never develop any higher-severity behavioral problems and grow out of those they have.

Special Dinners

At their wits' end, the parents of Caleb, a 6-year-old boy, brought him to a child psychologist for evaluation. Their already shaky marriage was being severely tested by conflict over their son's behavior at home. The mother complained bitterly that the father, who was frequently away from home on business, "over-indulged" their son during the times he was at home. In point of fact, the son would argue and throw temper tantrums and insist on continuing games, books, or other activities whenever his father tried to put him to bed, so that the 7:30 P.M. bedtime was often delayed until 10:30, 11:00, or even 11:30 P.M. Similarly, the father had been known to cook four or five different meals for his son's dinner if the son stubbornly insisted that he would not eat what had been prepared. Increasingly, Caleb had become easily annoyed and "touchy" when interacting with his parents.

On questioning by the psychologist, the parents denied that their son had ever been destructive of property, lied excessively, or stolen anything. When interviewed, the child was observed to be cheerful and able to sit quietly in his chair, listening attentively to the questions that were asked of him. His answers, however, were brief, and he tended to minimize the extent of the problems he was having with his parents.

Discussion of "Special Dinners"

In contrast to the previous case ("No Brakes"), all of Caleb's oppositional defiant behavior is confined to the home setting. He has frequent temper tantrums, is easily annoyed, often argues with both parents, and refuses to comply with rules about bedtime or to eat the food that has been prepared for him. There is no evidence that his problematic behavior extends into school. Because Caleb's behavior does not involve the violation of the basic rights of others or of major age-appropriate societal norms or rules (e.g., physical aggression or truancy from school), this is not a case of Conduct Disorder (see "Shoelaces" in Section 15.3).

Because there is no evidence that Caleb has a more serious disorder, such as Schizophrenia (see Section 2.1) or Autism Spectrum Disorder (see Section 1.6), the diagnosis of Oppositional Defiant Disorder (DSM-5-TR, p. 522) is made. Given that Caleb's problematic behaviors are confined to the home setting and are not apparent in his interactions with his teachers or friends, the severity of the Oppositional Defiant Disorder would be considered Mild. As with many cases of Oppositional Defiant Disorder, there is a relational component to the clinical picture in that Caleb's oppositional defiant behavior is being perpetuated by his father's inability to set appropriate limits on his son's unreasonable behavior, suggesting that family therapy should be a crucial part of the treatment plan.

15.2
Intermittent Explosive Disorder

The hallmark features of Intermittent Explosive Disorder are recurrent emotional and behavioral outbursts that reflect a failure to control aggressive impulses. The outbursts can be verbal (e.g., temper tantrums, verbal arguments) or physical. DSM-5-TR sets two different thresholds for the minimum number of behavioral outbursts, depending on their severity (in terms of impact on others and on property). If the behavioral outbursts are confined to verbal assaults or physical assaults that do not hurt other people or damage property, a minimum frequency of twice weekly on average for a period of at least 3 months is required. For physical assaults that result in hurting animals or other people or that result in damage or destruction of property, only three such episodes in a 1-year period are required. Moreover, to warrant a diagnosis of Intermittent Explosive Disorder, the aggressive outbursts should be 1) out of proportion to any provocation or psychosocial stressor; 2) impulsive and not premeditated or designed for personal gain; and 3) a cause of distress or of impairment in psychosocial functioning or associated with financial or legal consequences.

Many other mental disorders may be associated with aggressive outbursts, such as Bipolar Disorder (see Chapter 3, "Bipolar and Related Disorders"), Disruptive Mood Dysregulation Disorder (see Section 4.1), a Psychotic Disorder (see Chapter 2, "Schizophrenia Spectrum and Other Psychotic Disorders"), or a Personality Disorder, such as Antisocial or Borderline Personality Disorder (see Section 18.5 and Section 18.1, respectively). In general, if the aggressive outbursts are better explained by another mental disorder, a nonpsychiatric medical disorder (e.g., head trauma, Alzheimer's disease), or the physiological effects of a substance or a medication, Intermittent Explosive Disorder would not be diagnosed. However, the diagnosis can be made in addition to other mental disorder diagnoses, such as ADHD, Conduct Disorder, Oppositional Defiant Disorder, or Autism Spectrum Disorder, if the outbursts are more severe than those usually seen in these disorders and require additional clinical attention.

The 1-year prevalence of Intermittent Explosive Disorder is estimated at 2.6% in the United States. This disorder is more commonly found in younger adults than in older ones. It rarely begins after age 40 years. It may affect men slightly more often than women, and it has an episodic but recurrent course. It can have devastating social, occupational, financial, and legal consequences, because affected individuals alienate and drive away friends and partners, lose jobs, destroy property, and are charged in civil and criminal proceedings. Intermittent Explosive Disorder often co-occurs with other Disruptive Behavior Disorders, Depressive Disorders, Anxiety Disorders, Eating Disorders, Substance Use Disorders, Posttraumatic Stress Disorder, and Antisocial and Borderline Personality Disorders.

Hothead Harry, Gnome Assassin

Harry Axelrod, a 35-year-old marketing director, contacted an anger and aggression treatment clinic after having a heated argument with his fiancée. As Mr. Axelrod later explained, after being "nagged to death" by his fiancée to mow the lawn, he took a baseball bat and destroyed the couple's lawn gnome (his initial target was the lawn mower, but he thought better of it). After this outburst, Mr. Axelrod's fiancée gave him the ultimatum to "get help or get lost."

Mr. Axelrod stated that throughout his adulthood, he has engaged in frequent aggressive outbursts, including "heated arguments" and acts of property destruction ("too many to count"). He described several episodes in which he kicked in his TV screen, smashed in a stranger's car window, and threw his cell phone at the wall—all in response to relatively minor provocations. Over the past few years, Mr. Axelrod estimated that he had engaged in approximately three arguments and one act of property destruction per week. In addition to jeopardizing his current relationship with his fiancée, his aggression had "ruined" past relationships, alienated his coworkers, and almost cost him his job. The patient explained that he became angry "at the drop of a hat…over anything…over nothing," and that the urge to be aggressive often felt overwhelming. His eyes began to tear up as he described the shame and remorse he felt following his aggressive acts, although he also reported feeling a huge sense of relief at the same time.

Difficulties with anger were not new for Mr. Axelrod or his family. He grew up in a middle-class family living in the suburbs. His father, an accountant, although not physically abusive, "definitely had a hair-trigger temper" and would often berate Mr. Axelrod in front of his friends for minor transgressions, such as arriving home a few minutes late. Mr. Axelrod's sister and three brothers also had problems with verbal and physical aggression, so that family functions often turned into "war zones." Mr. Axelrod did quite well academically while growing up, although he mentioned having difficulties getting along with classmates, which he attributed to having low self-esteem. He reported that his first aggressive acts emerged during childhood, when he would occasionally break small toys or school supplies when he was angry or frustrated. Mr. Axelrod's impulsive aggression became more prominent in adolescence, when he found himself becoming involved in frequent arguments (one to four a week) with friends, classmates, and family members.

After graduating from high school, Mr. Axelrod left home to attend college, where he obtained a bachelor's degree in marketing. He was able to develop friendships and a few romantic relationships in college; however, his aggression difficulties continued unabated. His friend gave him the nickname "Hothead Harry" after an incident in which Mr. Axelrod responded to receiving a poor test score by kicking his chair and "accidentally" breaking it.

Mr. Axelrod began working for a marketing firm right out of college but left the firm after 6 months because he "couldn't stand" how the company was run. He also admitted to not getting along with his coworkers, whom he considered "unprofessional idiots." In his 20s, he dated a woman for 3 years until they broke up over his irritability and outbursts. He was clinically depressed for approximately 1 month afterward. During this time, he considered seeking help but decided that "there is no pill to stop you from being an asshole." He reported that there were several times in his life when he "drank too much," but he had never felt that his drinking was "out of control," and he went for long periods without drinking alcohol at all.

Throughout his late 20s and early 30s, Mr. Axelrod worked at the same company. His dedication to his work helped offset his interpersonal problems; however, his verbal outbursts alienated his coworkers. This situation came to a head when Mr. Axelrod grabbed and pushed a coworker (his only reported act of physical assault) after an altercation in which he yelled at the coworker for not completing a task. The coworker told him to "chill out and start drinking decaf." After the incident, Mr. Axelrod was mandated to see an employee assistance program counselor for five sessions. He did not find these sessions useful, explaining that "We really didn't do anything."

Mr. Axelrod was introduced to his fiancée 2 years ago. Their relationship was tumultuous, and his fiancée warned Mr. Axelrod on several occasions to control his anger after incidents in which he would yell or break objects. He described a pattern of his feeling guilty and angry with himself after an outburst, after which he would attempt to apologize, only to become defensive and verbally aggressive again when his fiancée expressed her anger at his overreaction. Mr. Axelrod was quick to add that he never threatened his fiancée or put his hands on her in anger, stating, "I am not that bad a guy, really. It is just my goddamned temper."

Discussion of "Hothead Harry, Gnome Assassin"

Mr. Axelrod's history of aggression is consistent with a diagnosis of Intermittent Explosive Disorder (DSM-5-TR, p. 527). He has a pattern of generalized reactive aggression that has resulted in numerous acts of verbal aggression and numerous acts of serious property destruction. These acts were not instrumental (i.e., they were not used as a means to intimidate others or to gain a tangible reward such as money); rather, the aggressive acts were a consequence of his feelings of intense anger. Although Mr. Axelrod had a history of possible alcohol abuse and a previous episode of Major Depressive Disorder, the aggressive behavior was not confined to those periods where he was using alcohol or was depressed.

Calisthenics

Camille Fortunato, a 31-year-old stay-at-home mother, sought help because of a 2- to 3-year history of temper outbursts associated with increasing marital discord. During the past few years, she had had increasing difficulty with her husband, whom she suspected of having an affair with his secretary. She ruminated angrily about his possible deception whenever he claimed to be working late. During such ruminative episodes, Ms. Fortunato felt her tension "building up," and she would often attempt to "discharge it" through calisthenics, but she still found herself "exploding" when her husband eventually came home. On one occasion, she threw a glass at him; on another, she banged on the walls of her house with her high-heeled shoe, causing the plaster to crumble; and on yet another she put her hand through a window when her husband left abruptly after one of her outbursts. Before each outburst she tried to remain calm, but she often experienced a headache and a feeling of "strangeness" when she saw her husband coming home. At this point she would usually lose control and become violent. Following the outburst Ms. Fortunato felt depressed and remorseful, recognizing that her outbursts were "crazy," even if her suspicions were justified. She also admitted that when the children cried or were impatient when she was in one of her ruminative periods, she was overzealous in her discipline and often found herself slapping them or punishing them more harshly than she ordinarily would. At one point, she had lost her temper when one of her children would not go to sleep and had slapped him hard enough to cause a bruise on his face.

The episodes of loss of control occurred one to two times a month but had seemed to be increasing over the past year. In between these episodes, Ms. Fortunato was generally calm and displayed no signs of aggressiveness.

Past history revealed that at age 8, Ms. Fortunato had been knocked unconscious for a short period of time in a roller-skating accident but had not had medical intervention for this injury. Apparently, she had sustained repeated accidental, minor head injuries, to the point that the family urged her to "wear a football helmet" because she was so clumsy. An electroencephalogram (EEG) done after Ms. Fortunato entered therapy revealed a nonspecific abnormality, a 6- to 14-second dysrhythmia (a disturbance or irregularity in the rhythm of brain waves).

During the course of her treatment, Ms. Fortunato confronted her husband, who finally acknowledged that he was having an affair with his secretary.

Discussion of "Calisthenics"

Ms. Fortunato entered therapy because she realized that even if her suspicions about her husband were warranted, her angry outbursts were inappropriate and markedly at variance with her normally unaggressive behavior. The patient has experienced intermittent temper outbursts that have resulted in property damage and in physical harm to one of her children, whom she had slapped. These emotional and behavioral outbursts suggest a Disruptive, Impulse-Control, or Conduct Disorder, most likely Intermittent Explosive Disorder (DSM-5-TR, p. 527).

The diagnosis in this case hinges on two issues: 1) whether the outbursts result in serious assault or destruction of property and 2) whether the behavior is grossly out of proportion to any provocation or precipitating psychosocial stressor. Ms. Fortunato had on one occasion broken a window with her fist, and on another had damaged a wall with her shoe. She also hit one of her children and bruised the child's face. The acts of destruction of property just make it past the threshold of three attacks in a 1-year period that cause damage to property or physical harm to others. Some could argue that no degree of rage is "out of proportion" to the provocation of a lying, unfaithful husband. However, her loss of control with her child when he refused to go to sleep is grossly out of proportion to the provocation. Therefore, the clinician in this case made a provisional diagnosis of Intermittent Explosive Disorder, because of uncertainty about the boundary between this disorder and the "normal" temper outbursts to which relations between spouses and between parents and children may give rise. In this case, particularly because of the potential for child abuse, the clinician felt that the preferred action was to err on the side of making a diagnosis that justified treatment directed at Ms. Fortunato's loss of impulse control.

Ms. Fortunato's EEG dysrhythmia suggests an underlying abnormality of the central nervous system, as is often found in patients with this disorder. Aggressive and violent behaviors have been associated with epilepsy, especially temporal or frontal lobe seizures. However, the abnormality is not specific to any diagnosable neurological disorder that could cause Ms. Fortunato's aggressive outbursts. The student reader might wonder about a diagnosis of traumatic brain injury (TBI), an acquired brain injury resulting from sudden, violent trauma to the brain, or chronic traumatic encephalopathy (CTE), a progressive degenerative disease of the brain found in athletes and others who have had repeated concussions or even subconcussive hits to the head. There is no history in this case suggesting the severe head trauma usually associated with TBI. CTE is associated with memory loss, confusion, impaired judgment, problems with impulse control, aggression, depression, and eventually dementia (dementia is discussed in Chapter 17, "Neurocognitive Disorders"). Besides her problems controlling her anger and feeling depressed and remorseful after an outburst, Ms. Fortunato does not appear to have any of these symptoms, although she did not undergo neuropsychological testing. CTE is a neuropathological diagnosis made on autopsy of the brain after death.

15.3
Conduct Disorder

Conduct Disorder is defined as "a repetitive and persistent pattern of behavior in which the basic rights of others or major age-appropriate societal norms or rules are violated" (DSM-5-TR, p. 530). DSM-5-TR divides the 15 behaviors that make up the criteria for Conduct Disorder into four groups:

1. *Aggression to people and animals*: often bullying, threatening, or intimidating others; often initiating physical fights; using a weapon that can cause harm to others; being physically cruel to people or animals; stealing while confronting the victim (e.g., mugging, purse snatching, extortion, armed robbery); forcing someone to have sex
2. *Destruction of property*: deliberate setting of fire with the goal of damaging property; deliberately destroying others' property in some other way
3. *Deceitfulness or theft*: breaking into someone's house, building, or car; lying or "conning" others to obtain goods or favors or to avoid obligations; stealing items of nontrivial value without confronting a victim (shoplifting, forgery)
4. *Serious violations of rules*: repeatedly staying out beyond parental curfew; running away from home; being truant from school

When at least three of these behaviors occur within a 12-month period, and they cause impairment in social, academic, or occupational functioning, the diagnosis of Conduct Disorder applies.

The Conduct Disorder diagnosis is further delineated according to subtypes defined by the age at onset of symptoms:

• If some sign of Conduct Disorder appeared before age 10 years, it is called Childhood-Onset Type. Individuals with this form of Conduct Disorder are generally considered to have a worse prognosis. Childhood-Onset Type is more common in boys, is more often associated with physical aggression toward others, and is characterized by poor peer relationships. These children may have received a diagnosis of Oppositional Defiant Disorder (see Section 15.1) when they were younger and may have concurrent ADHD (see Section 1.7) or other neurodevelopmental problems. Their problems are much more likely to persist into adulthood and may presage the development of Antisocial Personality Disorder (see Section 18.5).
• If no characteristic sign occurred before age 10 in a child or adolescent with Conduct Disorder, it is called Adolescent-Onset Type. Individuals with this type are as likely to be girls as boys, are less likely to engage in aggressive behavior, tend to have normal relationships with peers, and are less likely to have conduct problems that persist into adulthood.

In addition, there are certain antagonistic personality traits that qualify a child with Conduct Disorder for the specifier With Limited Prosocial Emotions. These traits also portend more aggression toward others and a poorer prognosis. Children or adolescents with limited prosocial emotions do not show remorse or guilt about doing something wrong; are callous and lack empathy for the feelings of others that they harm; are unconcerned about their performance in school or work; and express very shallow, insincere, and superficial emotions.

Finally, Conduct Disorder varies in severity, based on the number of signs present and their effects on other people. *Mild* indicates that the individual has few conduct problems (beyond what are required for the diagnosis), and the problems cause relatively minor harm to others (e.g., lying, truancy). *Moderate* indicates that the individual has more problems that have somewhat more of a harmful effect on others. *Severe* indicates that the individual has many conduct problems, including problems that cause considerable harm to others (e.g., forced sex, physical cruelty, use of a weapon, stealing with confrontation of a victim).

In the United States and other largely high-income countries, the estimated 1-year prevalence of Conduct Disorder in children and adolescents is 2%–10%, with a median of 4%. Prevalence rates increase from childhood to adolescence and are higher among men than among women. Prevalence of Adolescent-Onset Conduct Disorder is associated with psychosocial stressors, such as being a member of a socially oppressed ethnic group facing discrimination.

The onset of Conduct Disorder can be in the preschool years but is most commonly between middle childhood and middle adolescence. Physically aggressive signs are more common in childhood, and nonaggressive signs are more common in adolescence. The course is variable, with Childhood-Onset Type predicting a worse prognosis in adulthood, including an increased risk of criminal behavior and Substance-Related Disorders. The Adolescent-Onset Type is more likely to remit by adulthood, with affected individuals achieving adequate social and occupational adjustment.

Conduct Disorder has serious implications for the functioning of the person with the disorder and for society in general. The individual may be suspended or expelled from school, have trouble at work, have legal difficulties, contract and propagate sexually transmitted diseases, become pregnant as a young teenager, or be injured in physical fights or accidents. The individual may abuse substances and engage in reckless or risky behavior. These psychosocial impairments are generally more severe and long-lasting than those associated with other mental disorders of childhood or adolescence. Conduct Disorder is associated with higher-than-expected rates of suicidal thoughts, suicide attempts, and deaths by suicide. Co-occurrence of other mental disorders—both externalizing and internalizing (see Chapter 18, "Personality Disorders")—is common.

Killer

Alfred, a 10-year-old boy, was brought before juvenile authorities on charges that he had pushed a 6-year-old girl from a rooftop to her death. Although initially the girl's death was thought to be an accident, Alfred was later overheard bragging about the incident. Another neighborhood child, who cared very little for Alfred, told his parents, who encouraged the girl's mother to go to the police.

Alfred is known to be a peculiarly solitary and destructive child, who roams his neighborhood at all hours of the night. He has frequently been absent from school and never does his assignments or appears to care about his failing grades. On many of the days when he attends school, he has numerous arguments and physical fights with other boys he tries to intimidate. Since age 8, he has been caught several times in his neighborhood setting fires and breaking windows. When questioned by police, he readily admitted to pushing the girl, stating that she refused to give him money. When arrested, he expressed no emotion, concern, or remorse about what he had done. He appeared not to care what effect his action had on the young victim's family. The judge remanded the boy to the hospital for psychiatric consultation.

Discussion of "Killer"

Alfred's pattern of antisocial behavior began with his staying out late at night, being truant from school, and engaging in intimidation and physical aggression with his peers. In addition, he set fires and destroyed property (breaking windows), and his antisocial behavior culminated in his horrific killing of a young girl. Such a pattern of antisocial behavior involving serious violations of social rules and physical aggression against people and property, with an onset before age 10, indicates Severe Conduct Disorder, Childhood-Onset Type (DSM-5-TR, p. 530). Alfred's lack of remorse, callous lack of empathy, lack of concern about school performance, and unemotional reaction to what he had done are all characteristic of the symptom cluster captured by the specifier With Limited Prosocial Emotions for Conduct Disorder, which is commonly observed in individuals with Severe Conduct Disorder, Childhood-Onset Type, and suggests a grave prognosis.

Shoelaces

Javier is a 16-year-old boy who was admitted to the hospital from a juvenile detention center following a serious suicide attempt. He had wrapped shoelaces and tape around his neck, causing respiratory impairment. When found, he had cyanosis (a bluish discoloration of the skin due to deficient oxygen in the blood) and was semiconscious. He had been admitted earlier that day to the detention center, where it had been noted that he was quite withdrawn.

On admission, Javier was reluctant to speak except to say that he would kill himself and nobody could stop him. He did, however, admit to a 2-week history of depressed mood, difficulty sleeping, decreased appetite, decreased interest, guilt feelings, and suicidal ideation.

According to his parents, Javier had had no emotional difficulties until age 13, when he became involved in drugs, primarily LSD, marijuana, and nonopioid sedatives. His grades dropped drastically, he ran away from home on several occasions after arguments with his parents, he began to skip going to school, and he made a suicide gesture by overdosing on aspirin. A year later, Javier was expelled from school after threatening the principal during an argument about whether Javier was bringing drugs into the school. Because he was unable to control his behavior at home or at school, his parents had him evaluated in a mental health care clinic, and a recommendation was made for placement in a group home. He apparently did well in the group home, and his relationship with his parents improved immensely with family counseling. He was quite responsible in holding a job and attending school and was involved in no illegal activities, including use of drugs.

Six months before admission to the hospital, however, he became reinvolved with drugs, and over a 2-week period engaged in 10 instances of breaking and entering, all of which he did alone. He remembers being depressed at this time but cannot recall whether the mood change was before or after reinvolvement with drugs. He was then sent to the juvenile detention center, where he did so well that he had been discharged to his parents' care 3 weeks previously. One day after returning home, he impulsively left with his buddies in a stolen car for a trip to Texas. He said that his depression began shortly thereafter and that his guilt about what he had done to his parents led to his suicide attempt.

Discussion of "Shoelaces"

Since age 13, Javier has displayed a repeated and persistent pattern of conduct in which he has violated the basic rights of others and major age-appropriate societal norms or rules. This behavior has included being truant from school; threatening the principal, leading to expulsion from school; purchasing illegal drugs; running away from home; and incidents of breaking and entering and car theft. This pattern of antisocial behavior, with an onset after age 10, justifies the diagnosis of Conduct Disorder, Adolescent-Onset Type (DSM-5-TR, p. 530). This type generally has a better prognosis than Childhood-Onset Type. The severity is noted as Severe, because of the repeated episodes of breaking and entering, which cause considerable harm to others. He expresses guilt about the problems he has caused for his parents, does not appear to be cold and uncaring, shows that he can be responsible in holding a job and attending school, and is not shallow or insincere, so the specifier With Limited Prosocial Emotions would not apply in Javier's case.

Javier's serious suicide attempt that occasioned admission to the hospital is clearly a symptom of a Major Depressive Episode. There is a 2-week history of depressed mood with many of the characteristic symptoms of the depressive syndrome. Although there is mention of the patient's being depressed 6 months previously, it is not clear whether at that time he had the full depressive syndrome. There is also a reference to his having made a suicide gesture by overdosing on aspirin at age 13, but it is unclear whether that was in the context of a Major Depressive Episode. Thus, an additional diagnosis would be Major Depressive Disorder, Single Episode, Severe (DSM-5-TR, p. 183).

Javier has had many episodes of maladaptive use of substances, including LSD, marijuana, and sedatives. Even with the little information available, it seems likely that the patient has had one or more Substance Use Disorders—Cannabis Use Disorder (DSM-5-TR, p. 575), Other Hallucinogen Use Disorder (LSD) (DSM-5-TR, p. 590), and/or Sedative, Hypnotic, or Anxiolytic Use Disorder (DSM-5-TR, p. 620)—given that his drug use has resulted in his failure to fulfill his obligations at school (his "grades dropped drastically" and he was expelled) and has caused him persistent interpersonal problems with his parents and his school principal. These two manifestations alone within a 12-month period indicate at least a Mild Substance Use Disorder.

This case illustrates the common clinical finding that Conduct Disorder can be complicated by other co-occurring mental disorders, which might require treatment in their own right.

Seizure

Rene, a 16-year-old girl who is a junior in high school, was hospitalized on the psychiatric service for behavior problems. She had been in trouble with school authorities since age 12 for truancy and petty thefts. More recently, she had been expelled from school for smoking marijuana in the locker room. Finally, a series of thefts from neighborhood stores and an incident in which she and a companion set a fire in a vacant lot brought her into court and prompted a judge to remand her to a psychiatric ward for evaluation. Her parents said they were unable to control her.

On the ward, Rene befriended other adolescent kids. The staff found her to be demanding and emotionally volatile. She frequently stormed out of community meetings when decisions were made that did not go her way. She tried to have the ward recreational activities revolve around her and would be very enthusiastic about them at first but later would appear angry and pouty when she was not permitted to monopolize the activity. Despite Rene's superficial bravado, however, the nursing staff found her to be insecure and dependent.

One evening about a week into her hospitalization, after being refused a pass to go out of the hospital, Rene stormed down the hall to her room. Minutes later, a scream was heard. When the first nurse reached her, Rene was writhing on the floor on her back, making jerking movements of her pelvis, arms, and legs and rolling her eyes upward. When the staff and patients had congregated near her room, her violent shaking stopped. She laid nearly still, eyes closed, with a slight trembling visible over her body. She had not bitten her tongue or voided urine or feces. When a nurse held Rene's hand above her face and dropped it, the hand repeatedly fell to the side of Rene's head each time, rather than on her face. Finally, the nurse, noting her to be fully alert, asked her some questions, which Rene answered appropriately, although she stated that she could not yet move. Fifteen minutes later, she walked to the examining room to be evaluated by the doctor on call.

Discussion of "Seizure"

The doctor on call would have no difficulty in making a diagnosis of the behavioral problems that led to Rene's hospitalization. For at least 4 years, Rene has been getting into trouble. She has repeatedly violated important age-appropriate societal rules (truancy, smoking marijuana at school) and the basic rights of others (stealing). This repetitive and pervasive pattern indicates a diagnosis of Conduct Disorder (DSM-5-TR, p. 530). Because her violation of rules and the rights of others has involved primarily nonaggressive acts that have caused little harm to others, the Conduct Disorder is noted as Mild in severity. Because the onset was after age 10 years, this would be an example of a better-prognosis Adolescent-Onset Type. Although Conduct Disorder more commonly occurs in boys, Adolescent-Onset Type has a more equal gender distribution.

The immediate diagnostic problem for the doctor on call is how to characterize Rene's "fit." Several features suggest that it was not a genuine epileptic seizure. During a genuine tonic-clonic (grand mal) seizure, the clinician would expect urinary and possibly fecal incontinence. The clinician would also expect a period of postictal (postseizure) confusion during which the patient would not be fully alert and able to protect herself from hitting herself in the face when her hand was dropped.

There are three diagnostic possibilities for Rene's fit: Functional Neurological Symptom Disorder (Conversion Disorder) (see Section 9.3), Factitious Disorder (see Section 9.5), and the non–mental disorder Malingering (see DSM-5-TR, p. 835). Both Malingering and Factitious Disorder assume that the symptom is consciously faked. In this case, there is no evidence to support the notion that the patient had voluntary control over and thus falsified the fit. Without additional evidence of her conscious production of the fit, it seems preferable to give her the benefit of the doubt, assume that the symptom was not falsified, and diagnose it as Functional Neurological Symptom Disorder, With Attacks or Seizures (DSM-5-TR, p. 360). Two additional specifiers for Functional Neurological Symptom Disorder capture the heterogeneity of this case: Acute Episode (symptoms lasting for less than 6 months) and With Psychological Stressor (Rene was "refused a pass to go out of the hospital").

A degree of diagnostic uncertainty can be indicated by qualifying the Functional Neurological Symptom Disorder diagnosis as "provisional." If Rene were later to acknowledge that because she was angry with the staff, she decided to give them a hard time by faking the fit, the clinician could diagnose Malingering (see DSM-5-TR, p. 835), because Rene would then be considered to be deliberately trying to manipulate the staff to get more attention or privileges. Malingering is not a DSM-5-TR mental disorder per se but rather is a codable behavior or condition that could be a focus of clinical attention—these entities sometimes are referred to as "Z codes" (formerly known as "V codes") because of the ICD-10-CM code assigned to them. In the unlikely event that

Rene goes on to develop a pattern of exhibiting fake fits for no purpose other than to appear ill or impaired, the diagnosis would be changed to Factitious Disorder Imposed on Self (see Section 9.5).

15.4
Pyromania

Pyromania is defined as "deliberate and purposeful fire setting on more than one occasion" (DSM-5-TR, p. 537). As is often the case in disorders of impulse control, the act of fire setting is preceded by tension or emotional arousal and pleasure, gratification, or relief on setting the fire. Individuals with Pyromania typically have a fascination with, interest in, curiosity about, or attraction to fire and its situational contexts (e.g., paraphernalia, uses, consequences). Such individuals are often regular "watchers" at fires in their neighborhoods, may set off false alarms, and may spend time at the local fire department, set fires in order to be affiliated with the fire department, or even become firefighters. Fire setting in Pyromania is not done for financial, political, or criminal purposes. It is also not an act of anger or vengeance, a response to a delusion or hallucination, or a result of impaired judgment (e.g., as in Major Neurocognitive Disorder [see Section 17.2] or Intellectual Developmental Disorder [see Section 1.1]).

Pyromania is a very rare mental disorder—most cases of fire setting are not attributable to Pyromania. Fire-setting behavior occurs most often in men. Fire setting in adults is usually not related to another mental disorder and is done for a variety of reasons: for monetary gain, to improve the individual's living circumstances, to express anger or vengeance, to conceal criminal activity, or to attract attention or recognition (e.g., setting a fire in order to be the one to discover it and save the day). When fire setting is related to a mental disorder, it is most often associated with the impaired judgment characteristic of Substance Intoxication, with a Major Neurocognitive Disorder, or in response to a delusion or hallucination. Pyromania may have a typical age at onset in late adolescence. Children and adolescents who often set fires rarely meet the full criteria for Pyromania. Instead, the behavior more likely represents developmental experimentation in childhood (e.g., playing with matches) or is related to another mental disorder, such as Conduct Disorder (see Section 15.3) or Intellectual Developmental Disorder (see Section 1.1).

Brrr

Kelvin is a 6-year-old boy whose single mother brought him to the emergency room because she was frightened that she could not prevent the child from setting fires, which he had done several times in the last year and a half. Although he had so far managed to put out all the fires he set himself, his mother was afraid that he would set the house afire while she and his sister were asleep. She complained that he was sneaky about setting the fires, making it impossible for her to control him or to know how many fires he had actually set.

Kelvin says that he has set fires because a "man in my head tells me to." This "man" stays in his room when he is awake and "goes away" when he is asleep. The man makes a noise ("brrr"), which Kelvin interprets as a command to "set fires." He is afraid to talk to anyone about the man or not to obey his commands, "because he might beat me up." His mother apparently does not take the voice seriously, stating that he has offered a variety of different reasons for setting fires, depending on to whom he was talking. Both Kelvin and his mother agree that he sets fires partly in retaliation against his mother when he is angry with her.

Kelvin has been fascinated with setting fires for the last 2 years. His mother remembers that he and a friend set their first fire by burning holes in the plastic sheets on his and his sister's beds. His mother found out about the incident later and reacted by hitting him on his hands and telling him how dangerous fires were. During the next fire-setting incident, Kelvin used a lighter to try to burn a doorframe that his mother had just painted. This time he was not hit but was forbidden to ride his bicycle for a week. His mother was sleeping during a third episode, in which he set the garbage on fire with a table lighter. He then took a broom and beat out the fire. His mother awoke to a funny smell and remembers that he was running all over the house in a peculiar manner. She related this incident with amusement at the child's antics.

The most recent fires had taken place 3 weeks previously, when Kelvin first tried to burn a dish towel on a gas flame. After he burned the fringe, he rolled up the towel and threw it in the garbage. His mother, who was just outside the house at the time, sent him to bed and later explained to him again about the dangers of fire setting. During the last incident, he took a plastic container that held a Super Mario action figure and burned holes with a lighter into the front of the container.

Apart from these incidents, his mother reports that Kelvin has often found matches or gone into the bathroom with a lighter and tried to smoke. His mother has talked to him at length about fires, describing that they get bigger with alcohol and can be put out with water. He becomes excited during these discussions, but then promises never again to play with fire.

At present, his mother reports, Kelvin is unhappy in school and misses his former friends from the neighborhood the family left 3 months before the current hospital admission. She says that he has made no new friends outside school, and that he and his sister complain frequently of boredom. Aside from the fire setting, there is no history of any other aggressive or antisocial behavior. His mother reports that Kelvin has been difficult to discipline, mainly because he ignores her. Kelvin's schoolteacher was surprised to hear of his fire setting. When interviewed, she described him as a lovely, bright, obedient child who plays and works well with both the teacher and his peers. On further inquiry, she added that at times he became a "little wild" in play.

Kelvin lives with his 10-year-old sister and 26-year-old mother, who herself was hospitalized as an adolescent after she had been truant from school for 7 months in retaliation for her mother's remarriage. In an initial discussion with the interviewer, Kelvin's mother acknowledged that at times she becomes violently angry, to the point that she is unable to control herself.

The findings of Kelvin's physical examination were within normal limits except for a second-degree burn on his hand, which his mother initially said came from her attempts to "teach him that fire hurts" by insisting that he put his hand in a gas flame. (She later denied this action, but Kelvin insisted that she had done it.)

Kelvin and his mother were referred for further outpatient evaluation. When interviewed by the evaluating psychologist, Kelvin was somewhat guarded and distrustful at first. This behavior seemed to be a manifestation of shyness and fear of what his mother would say or do. Over the course of several evaluation sessions, Kelvin's play revolved around themes of fires getting bigger and out of control. He said that he knows that he can get burned and that a big fire could burn down his house and "I would die." When talking about fires, his affect was either inappropriate (laughter) or blunted (emotionless). When discussing the "man" and his "command hallucinations," Kelvin seemed to be nonchalant and unconcerned. He denied suicidal ideation, although his mother reported that he had recently said that he wished to die.

Discussion of "Brrr"

Recurrent setting of fires may be a symptom of Conduct Disorder (see "Killer" in Section 15.3); Kelvin, however, is described by his teacher as a "lovely, bright, obedient child who plays and works well with both the teacher and his peers," and he apparently engages in no antisocial activities other than fire setting.

It does appear that Kelvin has committed deliberate and purposeful fire setting on several occasions; that he derives pleasure from the fire setting; that he is very fascinated with fires, as evidenced by his excitement during his mother's discussions with him about the specifics of fires; and that there is no understandable goal, such as monetary gain from insurance. The diagnosis is therefore Pyromania (DSM-5-TR, p. 537).

Although the DSM-5-TR diagnostic criteria for this disorder technically require "tension or affective arousal before the act," this feature can only be inferred from the available information, as this subjective experience is often not easily documented in a person as young as Kelvin.

Kelvin's claim that he has set fires because a "man in my head tells me to" raises the question of whether the fire setting is a result of Kelvin's obeying a command hallucination, in which case the diagnosis of Pyromania would not apply. His mother's evaluation that the "man" in his head is one of a number of stories that he provides to explain his behavior, coupled with his nonchalant behavior during the interview when discussing the "man," suggests that Kelvin is likely making up this explanation to avoid taking responsibility for his behavior.

15.5
Kleptomania

Kleptomania is characterized by "recurrent failure to resist impulses to steal objects that are not needed for personal use or for their monetary value" (DSM-5-TR, p. 539). Individuals with Kleptomania experience an increasing sense of tension immediately before stealing, as well as pleasure, gratification, or relief from committing the act. The stealing is not an act of anger or vengeance, is not done in response to a delusion or hallucination, and is not better explained by another mental disorder, such as stealing for thrills during a Manic Episode in Bipolar I Disorder (see Section 3.1) or stealing as part of a pattern of antisocial behavior in Conduct Disorder (see Section 15.3) or Antisocial Personality Disorder (see Section 18.5). Individuals with Kleptomania typically attempt to resist the impulse to steal, and they are aware that the act is wrong and senseless. They frequently fear being apprehended and often feel depressed or guilty about the thefts.

Although shoplifting may be rather common, true Kleptomania is a very rare mental disorder, with a prevalence of 0.3%–0.6% in the U.S. general population. Women are three times as likely as men to have the disorder. Onset of Kleptomania most commonly occurs during adolescence, although the behavior can begin at any time from childhood through late adulthood. The course can be sporadic, with brief episodes separated by long periods of remission; episodic, with longer periods of both stealing and remission; or chronic, with some degree of fluctuation. The consequences of Kleptomania can be severe, because it can cause serious legal, family, and career problems. Kleptomania has been found to be associated with an increased risk of suicide attempts. Co-occurrence both with other externalizing disorders and with internalizing disorders has been observed (see Chapter 18, "Personality Disorders" for a discussion of externalizing and internalizing disorders).

Lobsterman

Mario Rossi was stopped as he was leaving a grocery store with three cans of lobster hidden in his pockets. He was charged with shoplifting, but the court asked for a psychological evaluation after determining that he had no prior criminal record and no particular need for the food he had stolen.

Mr. Rossi, age 42, is married, with two teenage sons. He has worked in insurance for 15 years and has never been arrested before. He admits to the psychologist that he has been shoplifting for years, following a pattern that only this time resulted in his arrest. He describes how he entered the store impulsively, without any specific purpose. While walking around in the store, he had an increasing sense of tension, which grew in intensity the longer he remained in the store. Then he had a desire to take the cans of lobster. He had no particular need for the food and actually does not like seafood. He had not been asked by anyone to buy canned lobster, and it is something that neither he nor his family members usually eat. He had more than enough money in his wallet to pay for the lobster had he wanted to. The tension increased until he could no longer resist it. He took the cans and stuffed them in his pockets, after which he experienced a sense of relief. He went on to explain that he knew nothing about this particular grocery store or its owners. The choice of the store was apparently random.

For the previous few years, Mr. Rossi had been having similar urges to steal, which he could not resist. The urges usually came on suddenly and for no apparent reason. Typically, he would be in a store and would have an increasing sense of tension and feel that he needed to pick up something and leave the store without paying for it. The items he shoplifted were never expensive and were usually nothing that he particularly needed or wanted. For reasons that he did not understand, he most commonly would steal canned seafood. A few moments after the shoplifting, he would have strong feelings of guilt and resolve never to do this again, but would be able to resist the urge for only 2 or 3 weeks before again succumbing to the impulse.

He and his wife both have excellent jobs and no financial problems. He can think of no particular stresses either in his family or at work that might be related to the impulse to steal. He does not know why he takes these "useless little things" and wishes he were able to control the urge to steal.

For the past 2 years, Mr. Rossi says he has had a growing sense of futility about his life. His children are approaching the point where they will be leaving home, and he has no interests or hobbies that do not revolve specifically around the children. Although he occasionally feels that "life is not worth living," he denies active suicidal thoughts, or other persistent symptoms of depression. His feelings of shame and guilt are limited to his shoplifting. Otherwise, he considers himself to be a hardworking, law-abiding person, who contributes to his community by coaching sports.

Mr. Rossi is the only child of an alcoholic father, who physically abused his wife. There were many periods during which Mr. Rossi and his mother lived away from his father, and he has always felt very close to her, and as an adult has been a dutiful and supportive son.

He describes himself as having been an irritable and quite aggressive adolescent. He was often in fights, usually with boys larger than himself who had made some kind of derogatory remark about his size. Usually, his response was grossly out of proportion to the remark.

Discussion of "Lobsterman"

Although superficially Mr. Rossi acts like an ordinary shoplifter, he is not motivated simply by the desire to have what he takes without paying for it. He has no particular need or desire for the things that he takes and does not even understand why he often takes seafood. He knows only that he has recurrent impulses to steal objects that he does not need and, with an increasing sense of tension, he inevitably gives in to the impulse and steals, after which he feels relief, guilt, and remorse. He does not plan to steal but succumbs to the impulse once he is in a store. These are the characteristic features of Kleptomania (DSM-5-TR, p. 539).

Kleptomania is more common in females than in males, so Mr. Rossi's case is somewhat unusual. Kleptomania is a rare condition, and even among arrested shoplifters, only a minority give a history that is consistent with the disorder. It is assumed that in some of these cases, the history is fabricated by the individuals to conform to the stereotype of the disorder and thereby avoid criminal prosecution. The onset is usually in adolescence, but the disorder may begin as early as childhood. In Mr. Rossi's case, the onset appears to have been in adulthood and the course episodic (i.e., with protracted periods of stealing and remission).

The Heiress

Martha Wellington is a wealthy and beautiful 34-year-old woman, who presented to a psychiatric social worker with a "marital problem." She was an heiress of a wealthy European family, and her husband was the president of a small importing company. She felt he was insensitive and demanding, and she claimed that he accused her of being self-centered, impulsive, and a "compulsive" liar. Over the course of their 10-year marriage, each had had numerous affairs, most of which eventually came into the open. Both would resolve to deal with their marital frustrations and to stop having affairs, and a brief period of reconciliation would follow, but soon one or the other would again surreptitiously begin an affair.

Ms. Wellington also described a special problem that worried her and that she had never disclosed to her husband. Periodically, she experienced the urge to walk into one of the more elegant department stores in the city and steal an article of clothing. Over the course of the previous 3 or 4 years, she had stolen several blouses, a couple of sweaters, and a skirt. Considering that her husband's income alone was more than $400,000 a year and her investments worth many times that, she recognized the "absurdity" of her acts. She also indicated that what she stole was rarely very expensive and sometimes not enough to her liking for her to wear. Ms. Wellington would become aware of the desire to steal something several days before she actually did it. The thoughts would increasingly occupy her mind until, on impulse, she walked into a store, plucked an item off the rack, and stuffed it under her coat or into a bag she happened to be carrying. Once out the door she felt a sense of relaxation and satisfaction, but at home she experienced anxiety and guilt when she realized what she had done. Ms. Wellington was caught on one occasion but gave a long, involved story about intending to pay after she had gone elsewhere in the store and then "forgot." She was released by the store security officers with a warning and suspiciously raised eyebrows.

Ms. Wellington spent considerable time describing her own accomplishments, talents, and abilities. Her affairs, she said, proved that she was indeed beautiful and of superior "stock." She thought that she and her husband, who was handsome, aggressive, and successful, should be a perfect match. According to her, the problems with her husband stemmed from the little attention he paid her and the expectations he seemed to have that she would be at his beck and call. The frequent arguments they had upset her greatly, and thus it was her idea that they each seek professional help. Regarding the charge that she was a compulsive liar, she admitted that she often found it easier to tell "white lies" than to face up to something "stupid" that she had done.

Discussion of "The Heiress"

Although not the reason for her seeking treatment, the stealing that Ms. Wellington describes has the classic features of Kleptomania (DSM-5-TR, p. 539). She gives in to recurrent impulses to steal objects she does not like and does not need. There is a mounting sense of tension that builds until she gives in to the impulse to steal; this is followed by a sense of release, and then remorse at what she has done. There is no evidence of other motivations or psychopathology that would better explain the stealing.

Ms. Wellington's marital problem, which is the reason for her seeking professional help, is apparently unrelated to the Kleptomania. It may be related to certain narcissistic personality traits, such as her exaggerated sense of her own importance (belief that she is of "superior stock"), her need for attention and admiration (her affairs), and her apparent lack of empathy (blaming her husband for their marital problems). Because there is no evidence of other characteristics of Narcissistic Personality Disorder (e.g., arrogant and haughty behavior, envy of others, being interpersonally exploitative; see "Unrecognized Genius" in Section 18.6), the Personality Disorder diagnosis is not made, but the presence of narcissistic personality traits could be noted.

CHAPTER 16

Substance-Related and Addictive Disorders

The Substance-Related Disorders in DSM-5-TR encompass 10 separate classes of drugs: alcohol; caffeine; cannabis; hallucinogens (with separate categories for phencyclidine (PCP) [or similarly acting arylcyclohexylamines] and other hallucinogens); inhalants; opioids; sedatives, hypnotics, or anxiolytics; stimulants (amphetamine-type substances, cocaine, and other stimulants); tobacco; and other (or unknown) substances, a category that in DSM-5-TR includes anabolic steroids, corticosteroids, antiparkinsonian medications, antihistamines, nitrous oxide, and amyl, butyl, or isobutyl nitrites. It should be noted that the term *substance* in DSM-5-TR refers to any exogenous substance and includes alcohol, tobacco, and other drugs of abuse, as well as medications (a number of which can be abused by individuals for their psychoactive effects).

Gambling Disorder is a behavioral addiction covered in this chapter, reflecting evidence that gambling behavior activates reward systems similar to those activated by drugs of abuse and are associated with symptoms that appear comparable to many of the symptoms associated with Substance Use Disorders. For this reason, the name of this chapter was changed from "Substance-Related Disorders" in DSM-IV to "Substance-Related and Addictive Disorders" in DSM-5 to accommodate the addition of behavioral addictions. DSM-5-TR includes two such behavioral addictions: Gambling Disorder, which appears in the "Substance-Related and Addictive Disorders" chapter, and Internet Gaming Disorder, which is not an official category in DSM-5-TR but rather is located in the "Conditions for Further Study" chapter in Section III ("Emerging Measures and Models"). Internet Gaming Disorder is also included in the "Disorders Due to Addictive Behaviors" section in the World Health Organization's International Classification of Diseases, 11th Revision (ICD-11).

DSM-5-TR divides the Substance-Related Disorders into Substance Use Disorders and Substance-Induced Disorders, defined as follows:

- A diagnosis of a Substance Use Disorder is given when an individual has a problematic pattern of substance use that leads to clinically significant impairment or distress.

- A diagnosis of a Substance-Induced Disorder is given when an individual experiences psychological or behavioral symptoms that are caused by the direct physiological effects of the substance on the central nervous system. Substance-Induced Disorders include Substance Intoxication, Substance Withdrawal, and the Substance/Medication-Induced Mental Disorders.

Although a Substance Use Disorder and a Substance-Induced Disorder involving the same substance commonly co-occur because individuals who have a pattern of excess substance use are also likely to experience psychological or behavioral symptoms caused by that substance, they are distinct conditions warranting separate DSM-5-TR diagnoses. For example, consider an individual whose life is in a shambles because they are unable to control their cocaine use, who are brought into an emergency room because of severe agitation and paranoid delusions caused by heavy cocaine use. Such an individual would qualify for both Cocaine Use Disorder and Cocaine-Induced Psychotic Disorder. These two diagnoses have different treatment implications.

Not every substance class is known to be associated with Substance Use Disorder, Substance Intoxication, Substance Withdrawal, or Substance/Medication-Induced Mental Disorders. For example, inhalants are not known to cause a clinically significant withdrawal syndrome, and cannabis is not known to cause a bipolar-like presentation. Table 16–1 shows the classes of substances that are associated with diagnoses of Substance Use Disorder, Substance Intoxication, and Substance Withdrawal. Table 16–2 summarizes the recognized combinations of classes of substances and Substance/Medication-Induced Mental Disorders.

TABLE 16–1.   **Substance classes corresponding to Substance Use Disorder, Substance Intoxication, and Substance Withdrawal**

Substance class	Use Disorder	Intoxication	Withdrawal
Alcohol	X	X	X
Sedatives, Hypnotics, or Anxiolytics	X	X	X
Stimulants (amphetamines and cocaine)	X	X	X
Caffeine		X	X
Tobacco	X		X
Cannabis	X	X	X
Hallucinogens/Phencyclidine	X	X	
Opioids	X	X	X
Inhalants	X	X	
Other (or Unknown) Substances	X	X	X

TABLE 16–2. Substance classes with corresponding Substance/Medication-Induced Mental Disorders

Substance class	Psychotic Disorders	Bipolar Disorders	Depressive Disorders	Anxiety Disorders	Obsessive-Compulsive and Related Disorders	Sleep Disorders	Sexual Dysfunctions	Delirium	Neurocognitive Disorders
Alcohol	X	X	X	X		X	X	X	X
Sedatives, Hypnotics, or Anxiolytics	X	X	X	X		X	X	X	X
Stimulants (amphetamines and cocaine)	X	X	X	X	X	X	X	X	X
Caffeine				X		X			
Tobacco						X			
Cannabis	X			X		X		X	
Hallucinogens/ Phencyclidine	X[a]	X	X	X				X	
Opioids			X	X		X	X	X	
Inhalants	X	X	X	X				X	X
Other (or Unknown) Substances	X	X	X	X	X	X	X	X	X

[a]Also includes Hallucinogen Persisting Perception Disorder.

Source. Adapted from American Psychiatric Association: "Substance-Related and Addictive Disorders," in *Diagnostic and Statistical Manual of Mental Disorders*, 5th Edition, Text Revision. Washington, DC, American Psychiatric Association, 2022, p. 545. Copyright © 2022 American Psychiatric Association. Used with permission.

Substance Use Disorders

Substance Use Disorders are characterized by a cluster of cognitive, behavioral, and physiological symptoms indicating that the individual continues using a substance despite significant substance-related problems. Individuals with Substance Use Disorders experience an underlying change in brain circuits that may persist beyond abstinence, such that many are prone to repeated relapses and intense drug craving when exposed to drug-related stimuli, such as drug paraphernalia. DSM-5-TR lists 11 symptom criteria to define a Substance Use Disorder, at least two of which must occur within a period of 12 months to qualify for the diagnosis.

The first four criteria (A1–4) involve different manifestations of impaired control over substance use. Individuals who recognize that their substance use is problematic may set limits on the amount of the substance they intend to use or the amount of time they intend to spend taking the substance, only to regularly exceed their own preset limits. Similarly, they may express a persistent desire to cut down or regulate their substance use, and often report multiple unsuccessful efforts to do so. Depending on the ease of availability of the substance in question, individuals may spend an inordinate amount of time and effort obtaining the substance. They may spend a great deal of time using the substance or recovering from its effects. For individuals with severe forms of Substance Use Disorder, virtually all of the individual's daily activities revolve around the substance. Many individuals develop craving for the substance, manifested as an intense desire or urge to use the drug, that may occur at any time but is more likely to occur when an individual finds themself in an environment where they have previously obtained or used the drug.

The next three criteria (A5–7) reflect social and occupational impairment related to the inability to control substance use. Recurrent substance use may result in the person's being unable to fulfill major role obligations at work, school, or home, as manifested, for instance, by repeated absences from work or poor work performance; absences, suspensions, or expulsions from school; or neglect of children or household responsibilities. Moreover, the individual may continue to use the substance despite having persistent or recurrent social or interpersonal problems that are caused or exacerbated by the effects of taking the substance, such as marital strain caused by spousal arguments about substance use or physical fights that occur during periods of intoxication. Important social, occupational, or recreational activities may be reduced or completely given up because of substance use. Examples would include an amateur athlete who has stopped participating in sports activities because of substance use or a person who has stopped seeing all their good friends so they can stay home and get high.

The next two criteria (A8 and A9) focus on risky use of the substance. Risky use may take the form of repeatedly using the substance in situations in which it is physically hazardous to do so, such as becoming intoxicated before driving a car or operating potentially dangerous machinery. The individual may continue substance use despite having a persistent or recurrent physical or psychological problem that they know has been caused or exacerbated by the substance. Examples of physical problems caused by substance use include serious damage to nasal mucosa from sniffing cocaine and esophageal bleeding due to excessive drinking. Examples of psychological problems include cocaine-induced paranoia or panic attacks and alcohol-related "blackouts" (memory loss for events that occurred while intoxicated with alcohol).

The final two criteria (A10 and A11) describe consequences of the person's having become physiologically dependent on the substance, as manifested by evidence of tolerance or the development of withdrawal symptoms when the person cuts down or stops using the substance. Tolerance is indicated when the person either requires a markedly increased amount of the substance in order to get high or experiences a markedly reduced effect from the substance over time when the usual dose is consumed. Withdrawal symptoms occur when blood or tissue concentrations of a substance decline in someone who has had prolonged heavy use of the substance. Withdrawal symptoms vary greatly across the different classes of substances and are most obvious during withdrawal from the depressant and opioid drug classes, which involve the development of withdrawal symptoms such as hand tremor, sweating, nausea, vomiting, diarrhea, agitation, and fever. Symptoms of withdrawal from either the stimulant class or cannabis tend to be less obvious, involving dysphoric mood and fatigue. Significant withdrawal symptoms from PCP and other hallucinogens and from inhalants have not been documented in humans. It should be noted that the development of physiological dependence (as manifested by the development of tolerance and withdrawal) often occurs during appropriate medical treatment with certain prescribed medications, such as opioid analgesics, sedatives, and stimulants. If tolerance and withdrawal develop in the context of the individual's taking medication as prescribed, those symptoms should not count toward a diagnosis of a Substance Use Disorder. However, given the high prevalence of prescription drug abuse, if tolerance and withdrawal occur in the context of an individual's taking a medication at higher dosages or more often than prescribed, it would be appropriate to count these symptoms toward the diagnosis of a Substance Use Disorder.

The severity of Substance Use Disorders can vary from mild to severe, with severity based on the number of DSM-5-TR symptom criteria that are present from criteria A1–A11: *Mild* Substance Use Disorder is indicated by the presence of two to three symptoms, *Moderate* by four to five symptoms, and *Severe* by six or more symptoms. DSM-5-TR also offers course specifiers for indicating whether the Substance Use Disorder is current or in remission: In Early Remission applies if no criteria have been met for at least 3 months but less than 12 months, and In Sustained Remission applies if no criteria have been met for 12 months or longer. An individual is not considered to be in remission if they have been free of symptoms for less than 3 months, given the particularly high propensity for relapse during such a short period.

Substance-Induced Disorders

The DSM-5-TR Substance-Induced Disorders include Substance Intoxication, Substance Withdrawal, and the various Substance/Medication-Induced Mental Disorders (e.g., Substance-Induced Psychotic Disorder, Substance-Induced

Anxiety Disorder). Substance Intoxication and Substance Withdrawal are considered to be Substance-Induced Disorders because they involve the development of symptoms attributable to the effects of the substance on the brain.

Substance Intoxication

Substance Intoxication is diagnosed when problematic behavioral or psychological changes, such as belligerence, mood lability, or impaired judgment, occur during use of a substance and are attributable to the physiological effects of the substance on the person's central nervous system. The most common changes involve disturbances of perception, wakefulness, attention, thinking, judgment, psychomotor behavior, and interpersonal behavior. The specific set of symptoms that occur in the context of intoxication depends on the specific substance. For example, intoxication with a depressant drug or medication (e.g., respectively, either alcohol or a sedative, hypnotic, or anxiolytic medication) may be characterized by inappropriate sexual or aggressive behavior, mood lability, impaired judgment, slurred speech, incoordination, and/or impairment in attention and memory, whereas Caffeine Intoxication is characterized primarily by symptoms such as restlessness, nervousness, excitement, insomnia, flushed face, sweating, muscle twitching, increased heart rate, and rambling flow of thought and speech. Substance Intoxication is common among individuals with a Substance Use Disorder, but it also occurs frequently in individuals without a Substance Use Disorder.

Substance Withdrawal

Substance Withdrawal is characterized by the development of substance-specific behavioral changes accompanied by certain physiological and cognitive disturbances that are due to the cessation of, or reduction in, heavy and prolonged substance use and that cause clinically significant distress or impairment in social, occupational, or other important areas of functioning. Withdrawal is usually, but not always, associated with a Substance Use Disorder, because it generally develops only after prolonged use of the substance. The symptoms characteristic of the substance-specific withdrawal syndromes are often the opposite of the symptoms occurring during intoxication. For example, whereas Stimulant Intoxication is typically characterized by euphoria, increased sociability, and loss of appetite, Stimulant Withdrawal involves dysphoric mood, fatigue, and increased appetite.

Substance/Medication-Induced Mental Disorders

The Substance/Medication-Induced Mental Disorders are potentially severe and usually temporary, but sometimes persisting, psychiatric syndromes that develop in the context of the effects of substances of abuse, medications, or several toxins. Nine specific types of Substance/Medication-Induced Mental Disorders are included in DSM-5-TR that differ based on the nature of the psychiatric symptoms caused by a substance. These include Substance/Medication-Induced Psychotic Disorder, Substance/Medication-Induced Bipolar and Related Disorder, Substance/Medication-Induced Depressive Disorder, Substance/Medication-Induced Anxiety Disorder,

Substance/Medication-Induced Obsessive-Compulsive and Related Disorder, Substance/Medication-Induced Sleep Disorder, Substance/Medication-Induced Sexual Dysfunction, Delirium (i.e., Substance-Induced Delirium, Substance Withdrawal Delirium, and Medication-Induced Delirium), and Substance/Medication-Induced Neurocognitive Disorder. As noted earlier in this chapter, given that only certain substances have the potential to cause particular psychiatric symptoms, not every substance or medication causes a Substance/Medication-Induced Mental Disorder (see Table 16–2).

Substance-Related Disorders in Case Examples

This chapter includes cases representing various Substance Use Disorders and Substance-Induced Disorders. Specifically, cases are presented to illustrate the following diagnoses:

- In Alcohol-Related Disorders (Section 16.1): Alcohol Use Disorder ("Vodka"), Alcohol Intoxication ("Joe College"), and Alcohol Withdrawal ("The Reporter")
- In Sedative-, Hypnotic-, or Anxiolytic-Related Disorders (Section 16.2): Diazepam Use Disorder and Diazepam Withdrawal ("August Days")
- In Stimulant-Related Disorders (Section 16.3): Cocaine Use Disorder ("Cocaine Problem")
- In Caffeine-Related Disorders (Section 16.4): Caffeine Withdrawal ("Coffee Machine")
- In Tobacco-Related Disorders (Section 16.5): Tobacco Use Disorder ("Junkie")
- In Cannabis-Related Disorders (Section 16.6): Cannabis Intoxication ("Freaking Out") and Cannabis Withdrawal ("Fidgety and Grumpy")
- In Phencyclidine-Related Disorders (Section 16.7): Phencyclidine Use Disorder and Phencyclidine Intoxication ("Peaceable Man")
- In Hallucinogen-Related Disorders (Section 16.8): Hallucinogen Persisting Perception Disorder ("A Man Who Saw the Air")
- In Opioid-Related Disorders (Section 16.9): Opioid Use Disorder ("Cough Medicine")
- In Inhalant-Related Disorders (Section 16.10; also includes discussion of Other [or Unknown] Substance–Related Disorders): Inhalant Intoxication ("Better Living Through Chemistry")

The chapter concludes with a case of Gambling Disorder ("Loan Sharks") (Section 16.11).

Other Substance/Medication-Induced Mental Disorder cases are included in other chapters in this book, reflecting their placement in DSM-5-TR in the chapters with which they share symptoms:

- In Chapter 2 ("Schizophrenia Spectrum and Other Psychotic Disorders"): Substance/Medication-Induced Psychotic Disorder ("Agitated Businessman" and "Threatening Voices" in Section 2.7)
- In Chapter 3 ("Bipolar and Related Disorders"): Substance/Medication-Induced Bipolar and Related Disorder ("Sleepless Mother" in Section 3.4)
- In Chapter 12 ("Sleep-Wake Disorders"): Substance/Medication-Induced Sleep Disorder ("Mystery Mastery" in Section 12.10)
- In Chapter 13 ("Sexual Dysfunctions"): Substance/Medication-Induced Sexual Dysfunction ("Bad Side Effect" in Section 13.8)
- In Chapter 17 ("Neurocognitive Disorders"):
  - Substance/Medication-Induced Delirium ("Traction" and "Thunderbird" in Section 17.1)
  - Substance/Medication-Induced Major Neurocognitive Disorder ("Chief Petty Officer" in Section 17.2; "Disabled Vet" in Section 4.3)

16.1
Alcohol-Related Disorders

Alcohol and the class of drugs known as sedatives, hypnotics, or anxiolytics (covered in the next section) are considered to be "depressants"—they lower neurotransmission levels, an effect that serves to depress or reduce arousal or stimulation in various areas of the brain. Depressants exert their effects through a number of different pharmacological mechanisms, the most prominent being activation of γ-aminobutyric acid, a major inhibitory neurotransmitter, and inhibition of excitatory glutamatergic and monoaminergic neurotransmitters. For this reason, alcohol and drugs from the sedative, hypnotic, or anxiolytic class are considered to be "cross-tolerant"—i.e., someone who has developed tolerance to the effects of alcohol will also be tolerant to the effects of sedative, hypnotic, or anxiolytic medications, and vice versa. Moreover, the DSM-5-TR diagnostic criteria for Alcohol Intoxication and for Sedative, Hypnotic, or Anxiolytic Intoxication are nearly identical, as are the DSM-5-TR diagnostic criteria for Alcohol Withdrawal and for Sedative, Hypnotic, or Anxiolytic Withdrawal.

In most cultures, alcohol is the most frequently used intoxicating substance and is a cause of considerable morbidity and mortality. Repeated intake of large amounts of alcohol can affect nearly every organ system in the body, especially the gastrointestinal tract, the cardiovascular system, and the central and peripheral nervous systems. Alcohol Use Disorder is an important contributor to suicide risk during severe intoxication, and there is an increased risk of suicidal behavior, as well as of completed suicide, among individuals with Alcohol Use Disorder.

Alcohol Use Disorder is common. Among adults in the United States, lifetime prevalence rates of Alcohol Use Disorder are estimated to be 29.1% overall, with 8.6% of cases being of mild severity, 6.6% of moderate severity, and 13.9% severe. Rates vary widely by age. Men have higher rates of drinking and Alcohol Use Disorder (36.0% lifetime prevalence) than women (22.7% lifetime prevalence). However, because women generally weigh less than men and have more fat and less water in their bodies, they are likely to develop higher blood alcohol levels per drink than men do. Among individuals who drink heavily, women may also be more vulnerable than men to some of the physical consequences associated with alcohol, including liver disease.

For most people, the first episode of Alcohol Intoxication is likely to occur during the mid-teens. Most individuals who develop Alcohol-Related Disorders do so before reaching their late 30s. The initial signs of withdrawal typically manifest after other aspects of an Alcohol Use Disorder have already emerged. Adolescents who have preexisting conduct problems and those who start drinking at an earlier age are more likely to experience an earlier onset of Alcohol Use Disorder.

Alcohol Use Disorder tends to be characterized by periods of remission and relapse. A decision to stop drinking, often in response to a crisis, is likely to be followed by a period of weeks or more of abstinence, which is often followed by limited periods of controlled or nonproblematic drinking. However, once alcohol intake resumes, it is highly likely that consumption will rapidly escalate and that severe problems will once again develop.

Alcohol Use Disorder is frequently misunderstood as an insurmountable condition, possibly because it is well-known that individuals seeking alcohol treatment often have a long history of severe alcohol-related issues. However, it is important to note that these severe cases represent only a small proportion of individuals with this disorder, and the average person with Alcohol Use Disorder has a significantly more positive outlook for recovery.

Both Alcohol Intoxication and chronic heavy alcohol use are associated with suicide. Compared with nondrinking individuals, individuals under the acute influence of alcohol have a nearly sevenfold increase in the risk of a suicide attempt. Moreover, the acute co-use of alcohol and sedatives has an even stronger association with a suicide attempt compared with the acute use of alcohol alone.

Vodka

Violet Gottfried, a 45-year-old, twice-married woman, has been drinking a pint of vodka daily for 13 years. Before that, she had been a light drinker. During the period of her divorce from her first husband, she became depressed and found that alcohol made her feel better. While drinking in a bar, she met her second husband, also a heavy drinker. They continued to drink at home in the evenings. She increasingly found reasons not to go to work and was eventually dismissed from her job. She began drinking throughout the day, allowing herself an ounce of vodka per hour, interspersed with occasional beers. She hid bottles and beer cans so her husband would not know she was drinking so much. Her husband, finding her intoxicated on his return home, began complaining and threatened to leave her. Ms. Gottfried vowed to drink only beer. She kept this up for a month, drinking two or three six-packs a day. Then she became worried about her weight and decided not to drink at all except for "two drinks before dinner." The two drinks became three, and soon she was drinking a pint of vodka again. She began having memory lapses. Once she burned a hole in the sofa and did not remember doing it. Her husband moved out after a violent argument. Drinking alone, she cried a good deal and thought about suicide. She finally contacted Alcoholics Anonymous for help.

Discussion of "Vodka"

This case illustrates a number of the characteristic features of Alcohol Use Disorder (DSM-5-TR, p. 553), including Ms. Gottfried's impaired control over her use of alcohol combined with negative social and occupational consequences. Her inability to control her alcohol use is indicated by her setting drinking limits that she repeatedly exceeds (i.e., after setting a limit of two drinks, she ended up drinking an entire pint), unsuccessful efforts to cut back or stop drinking, spending a great deal of time drinking (i.e., throughout the day), continuing to drink even though her drinking led to arguments with her husband that culminated in his moving out, and her continuing to drink despite having potentially dangerous memory lapses caused by her drinking. Another negative consequence was her being dismissed from her job because of her drinking. Finally, the fact that Ms. Gottfried is drinking a pint of vodka a day is indicative of her having developed tolerance. Although she did not develop withdrawal symptoms when she switched from a pint of vodka to two or three six-packs of beer a day, that change in the amount of alcohol consumed daily may not have been enough to trigger withdrawal, so her propensity to develop withdrawal is not currently known. The presence of at least eight definitive symptoms indicates Severe Alcohol Use Disorder.

Joe College

Joseph Schiavone, a 19-year-old college freshman, spends an afternoon drinking beer with his fraternity brothers. After 8–10 glasses, he becomes argumentative with one of his larger frat brothers and suggests that they step outside and fight. Normally a quiet, unaggressive person, Joseph now speaks in a loud voice and challenges the larger man to fight with him, apparently for no good reason. When the fight does not develop, he becomes morose and spends long periods looking into his beer glass. He seems about to cry. After more beers, he begins telling long, indiscreet stories about former girlfriends. His attention drifts when others talk. He tips over a beer glass, which he finds humorous, laughing loudly until the bartender gives him a warning look. He starts to get up and say something to the bartender but trips and falls to the floor. His friends help him to the car. Back at the fraternity house, he falls into a deep sleep, awaking with a headache and a bad taste in his mouth. He is again the quiet, shy person his friends know him to be.

This is the first time that Joseph has ever become drunk. He grew up with parents who were very strict about alcohol and drug use, and he hung out with high school friends who rarely drank.

Discussion of "Joe College"

Although intoxication in the physiological sense occurs in social drinking, maladaptive behavior is required for the DSM-5-TR diagnosis of Substance Intoxication. In Joseph's case there is evidence of disinhibition of aggressive impulses (picking a fight), impaired judgment (telling indiscreet stories), mood lability (argumentative, then crying and morose), and physiological signs (incoordination and unsteady gait) of intoxication. Alcohol is obviously the offending substance, so this is clearly a case of Alcohol Intoxication (DSM-5-TR, p. 561).

Because it does not appear that Joseph has demonstrated this kind of behavior before this incident, an additional diagnosis of an Alcohol Use Disorder would not be warranted. If, however, this pattern continues, Joseph may be headed for a future diagnosis of Alcohol Use Disorder.

The Reporter

Mitchell Dodge, a 29-year-old newspaper reporter, had been a heavy drinker for 10 years. One evening after work, having finished a feature article, he started drinking with friends and continued to drink throughout the evening. He fell asleep in the early morning hours. On awakening he had a strong desire to drink again and decided not to go to work. Food did not appeal to him, and instead he had several Bloody Marys. He later went to a local tavern and drank beer throughout the afternoon. He met some friends and continued drinking into the evening.

Mr. Dodge's pattern of drinking throughout the day persisted for the next 7 days. On the eighth morning, Mr. Dodge tried to drink a cup of coffee and found that his hands were shaking so violently he could not get the cup to his mouth. He managed to pour some whiskey into a glass and drank as much as he could. His hands became less shaky, but at this point he was nauseated and began having "dry heaves." He tried repeatedly to drink but could not keep alcohol down. He felt ill and intensely anxious and decided to call a doctor friend. The doctor recommended hospitalization.

When evaluated on admission, Mr. Dodge is alert; he has a marked tremor of the hands, and his tongue and eyelids are tremulous. He has feelings of "internal" tremulousness. Lying in the hospital bed, he finds the noises outside his window unbearably loud and begins seeing "visions" of animals and, on one occasion, a dead relative. He is terrified and calls a nurse, who gives him a tranquilizer. He becomes quieter, and his tremor is less pronounced. At all times he realizes that the visual phenomena are "imaginary." He always knows where he is and is otherwise oriented. He has no memory impairment. After a few days, the tremor disappears, and Mr. Dodge no longer hallucinates. He still has trouble sleeping but otherwise feels normal. He vows never to drink again.

When questioned further about his history of drinking, Mr. Dodge claims that although during the last 10 years he has developed the habit of drinking several glasses of scotch each day, his drinking has never interfered with his work or relations with colleagues or friends. He denies having aftereffects of drinking other than occasional mild hangovers, claims never to have gone on binges before this one, and denies needing to drink every day in order to function adequately. He admits, however, that he has never tried to reduce or stop his drinking.

Discussion of "The Reporter"

Mr. Dodge markedly increases his amount of drinking for a week and then stops drinking as he becomes sick with nausea and vomiting. He then develops visual hallucinations; tremor of the hands, tongue, and eyelids; and anxiety. Significantly, he has intact reality testing in that he realizes that the hallucinations are imaginary, and he remains alert, fully oriented, and without memory impairment. These symptoms, associated with the reduction in heavy alcohol use, indicate Alcohol Withdrawal (DSM-5-TR, p. 564). Furthermore, the specifier With Perceptual Disturbances would be noted to indicate the presence of hallucinations occurring with intact reality testing.

Some readers might wonder whether the most appropriate diagnosis for Mr. Dodge would be Alcohol Withdrawal Delirium (commonly called delirium tremens ["the DTs"]) (see "Thunderbird" in Section 17.1) because of the visual hallucinations. Delirium, however, requires reduced ability to maintain attention to external stimuli accompanied by reduced awareness of the environment, both of which are absent in Mr. Dodge's case. The visual hallucinations with intact reality testing that Mr. Dodge experienced are rather common in Alcohol Withdrawal.

Although Mr. Dodge denies impaired control of his drinking and claims that his drinking does not interfere with his work or social relations, his pattern of drinking would still meet the criteria for a Mild Alcohol Use Disorder. He has evidence of tolerance (drinking several scotches every day), and he developed a full-blown withdrawal syndrome when he cut down on drinking, thus fulfilling the minimum requirement of at least two Alcohol Use Disorder symptoms. Given that it is common for individuals with Alcohol Use Disorder to overestimate their ability to control their drinking and to minimize the impact of their drinking on their lives, the clinician would want to be watchful about Mr. Dodge's ongoing drinking pattern to see if it continues to cause him problems, as it did in this instance.

16.2
Sedative-, Hypnotic-,
or Anxiolytic-Related Disorders

As indicated by its name, the sedative, hypnotic, and anxiolytic drug class includes a wide variety of medications that are prescribed to calm people down (the "sedative" part of the name), to help people sleep ("hypnotic"), and to reduce anxiety ("anxiolytic"). The class includes the benzodiazepines—medications that are generally indicated for the treatment of anxiety (e.g., diazepam, lorazepam, clonazepam, alprazolam)—and benzodiazepine-like medications that are used as sleep aids (e.g., zolpidem, zaleplon). Most other medications in the sedative, hypnotic, and anxiolytic drug class, such as carbamates (e.g., meprobamate), barbiturates (e.g., secobarbital), and barbiturate-like sleep aids (e.g., methaqualone), were much more popular in the 1950s–1970s but are now rarely used in medical contexts because of their higher risk of causing addiction or leading to death from overdose in comparison with benzodiazepines and benzodiazepine-like medications.

Sedative, hypnotic, and anxiolytic substances are available both by prescription and illegally. Sedative, Hypnotic, or Anxiolytic Use Disorder often is associated with other Substance Use Disorders (e.g., Alcohol, Cannabis, Opioid, Stimulant Use Disorders) when sedatives are used to alleviate the unwanted effects of these other substances.

The usual course of Sedative, Hypnotic, or Anxiolytic Use Disorder involves onset when individuals are in their teens or 20s, followed by escalation in occasional use of sedative, hypnotic, or anxiolytic medication to the point at which problems develop that meet criteria for a diagnosis. An initial pattern of intermittent social use (e.g., at parties) can evolve into a pattern of daily use and the development of high levels of tolerance. A less frequently observed clinical course begins with medication originally obtained by prescription from a physician, usually for the treatment of anxiety, insomnia, or somatic complaints. As the patient develops tolerance (i.e., a need for higher doses of the medication), they gradually increase the dose and frequency of self-administration. The individual is likely to justify their continued use of the antianxiety or sleep medication on the basis of the original symptoms of anxiety or insomnia, but substance-seeking behavior becomes more prominent, and the person may end up seeking out multiple physicians to obtain sufficient supplies of the medication. Tolerance can reach high levels, and withdrawal (including seizures and withdrawal delirium) may occur.

The 12-month prevalence of Sedative, Hypnotic, or Anxiolytic Use Disorder in the United States is highest among individuals ages 18–29 years (0.5%) and lowest among individuals ages 65 years and older (0.04%). Rates have not been consistently shown to vary by sex.

U.S. epidemiological studies show that hypnotics are associated with suicide, but it is unclear to what degree this association is attributable to underlying psychiatric conditions such as depression or insomnia, which are themselves risk factors for suicide.

August Days

PSYCHIATRIST (DR): "Hello?"
PATIENT (PT): "Hello, is this Dr. Sharkey?"
DR: "Yes."
PT: "This is Ms. Dudek. I am a patient of Dr. Black's. He said you were covering for him while he was on vacation."
DR: "Yes. What can I do for you?"

So began a telephone consultation with a 55-year-old divorced schoolteacher and a young psychiatrist one August morning. The teacher had recently, against medical advice, signed herself out of a psychiatric unit of a general hospital where she had gone to be evaluated for anxiety and to be "detoxified" from a benzodiazepine drug (i.e., to have the antianxiety drug discontinued under medical supervision).

Ms. Dudek had a 5-year history of mouth pain, which had been alternately diagnosed as trigeminal neuralgia (a chronic pain disorder characterized by episodes of intense pain in the face) and as temporomandibular joint (TMJ) dysfunction (pain and dysfunction in the jaw joint and the muscles that move the jaw). For this pain, she had taken an acetaminophen-oxycodone combination medication (a narcotic pain medication) and diazepam (an antianxiety medication that also has muscle-relaxant properties). The drugs relieved the symptoms somewhat, but the beneficial effects would gradually wear off, necessitating an increase in the dosage. She had seen numerous internists, neurologists, and psychiatrists, some of whom were reluctant to prescribe medications indefinitely because of their addictive potential. Attempts to treat the pain with carbamazepine (a nonaddictive anticonvulsant medication used in treating pain) and amitriptyline (a nonaddictive antidepressant medication often used in treating pain) had been short-lived because of side effects she said were "horrendous."

Nine months earlier, Ms. Dudek's ex-husband had died suddenly of a heart attack. During the ensuing months, the pain in her mouth became worse and anxiety developed. She increased her diazepam dosage to 90 mg/day (the maximum daily dosage recommended by the U.S. Food and Drug Administration is 8–40 mg/day), but she still complained of feeling shaky and weak, having difficulty falling asleep, and awakening at 3 A.M. with inability to fall back to sleep without taking at least 15–20 mg of diazepam. She was increasingly absent from work, feeling either "hungover" or "exhausted" in the morning. Depressed mood and vegetative signs of depression (i.e., physical symptoms such as changes in appetite, sleep) were not prominent. Ms. Dudek described one acute attack of anxiety that sounded like a panic attack, for which she had seen a cardiologist, who said that her heart was normal.

She had signed out of the hospital because she could not stand the anxiety and pain that developed as the diazepam was being reduced. She had obtained Dr. Black's name from a friend; he had seen the patient once. She had pleaded with him to allow her to try being detoxified from diazepam as an outpatient. He had suggested that she might profit from a trial of venlafaxine (an antidepressant medication) or lithium (a mood-stabilizing medication).

At the time she called Dr. Sharkey, Ms. Dudek had exhausted the supply of diazepam she had been given to use while reducing her dosage and had taken no diazepam within the past 24 hours. She reported rapid heartbeat, sweating, weakness in her knees, shaking hands, nausea, anxiety, and insomnia.

Discussion of "August Days"

Ms. Dudek has both problems with her pattern of use of diazepam and symptoms indicative of diazepam withdrawal. She shows evidence of tolerance ("She increased her diazepam dosage to 90 mg/day… but she still complained of feeling shaky and weak, having difficulty falling asleep"), her diazepam use results in a failure to fulfill major role obligations at work ("she was increasingly absent from work, feeling either 'hungover' or 'exhausted' in the morning"), and she has withdrawal symptoms when she cuts down on her use of diazepam ("rapid heartbeat, sweating, weakness in her knees, shaking hands, nausea, anxiety, and insomnia"), justifying a diagnosis of Diazepam Use Disorder (DSM-5-TR, p. 620). It should be noted that DSM-5-TR has an instruction advising against counting the tolerance and withdrawal criteria toward the diagnosis in "individuals taking sedatives, hypnotics, or anxiolytics under medical supervision" (DSM-5-TR, p. 621); this note is intended to prevent giving the diagnosis to individuals who develop physiological dependence (i.e., tolerance and withdrawal) in the course of taking sedative, hypnotic, or anxiolytic medication as prescribed. Ms. Dudek's pattern of diazepam use would *not* be considered to be under medical supervision because she has increased the dosage on her own and is attempting to obtain more diazepam than prescribed by going to multiple physicians. Moreover, because her current presentation is characterized by the development of symptoms characteristic of the diazepam withdrawal syndrome, an additional current diagnosis of Diazepam Withdrawal would also apply (DSM-5-TR, p. 628).

As is common, especially for adults, Ms. Dudek's use of a benzodiazepine (diazepam) started after it had been legitimately prescribed for TMJ. Unfortunately, her use of diazepam has escalated to the point that it is out of control: she wants to stop but is unable to, she has developed tolerance and withdrawal, and it has interfered with her life. She has resorted to desperate techniques, such as trying to convince a doctor who is completely unfamiliar with her case to prescribe more of the drug for her. In fact, given her need to procure the medication, it is possible that she may have fabricated part of her medical history to provide the covering doctor with a legitimate enough story to convince him to prescribe the diazepam. Assuming that she was in actuality beginning to exhibit symptoms of benzodiazepine withdrawal at the time of the telephone call, it might be justified for the covering doctor to prescribe at least 1 or 2 days' worth of diazepam to prevent her from developing a full-blown withdrawal syndrome, given that sedative withdrawal can evolve into a potentially life-threatening Sedative-Induced Withdrawal Delirium (for the alcohol-induced version of this condition, see "Thunderbird" in Section 17.1).

Whether Ms. Dudek also has an independent Anxiety Disorder is a bit unclear, given that one of the main symptoms of sedative withdrawal is the development of symptoms of anxiety and even panic attacks like she has experienced before. In Ms. Dudek's case, the only way to know whether she also has an underlying independent Anxiety Disorder is to evaluate her again several months after discontinuing the diazepam. If she is free of anxiety symptoms, the clinician can assume that all of her recent anxiety symptoms were a manifestation of her diazepam use. If the anxiety symptoms continue to persist, an additional Anxiety Disorder diagnosis might be warranted.

16.3
Stimulant-Related Disorders

The stimulants discussed in this section include both amphetamine and amphetamine-type stimulants such as dextroamphetamine and methamphetamine, as well as other stimulants with similar effects, such as methylphenidate and cocaine. (Although caffeine and nicotine are technically stimulants, these legal substances are covered in the next two sections [16.4 and 16.5, respectively].) Amphetamines and other stimulants (excluding cocaine) may be obtained by prescription for the treatment of obesity, Attention-Deficit/Hyperactivity Disorder, and Narcolepsy and are sometimes diverted into the illegal market. Cocaine comes in various forms (i.e., cocaine hydrochloride powder, which may be inhaled through the nostrils or dissolved in water and injected intravenously, and cocaine alkaloids such as freebase and crack) that differ in potency because of varying levels of purity and rapidity of onset.

When injected or smoked, stimulants typically produce an instant feeling of well-being, confidence, and euphoria. Dramatic behavioral changes can rapidly develop with Stimulant Use Disorder. Chaotic behavior, social isolation, aggressive behavior, and sexual dysfunction can result from long-term Stimulant Use Disorder.

Individuals exposed to amphetamine-type stimulants or cocaine can develop Stimulant Use Disorder in as short a time as 1 week, although the onset is not always this rapid. Regardless of the route of administration, tolerance almost invariably occurs with repeated use. Withdrawal symptoms, particularly excessive sleepiness, increased appetite, and dysphoria, can occur and can enhance craving.

Stimulant use may be chronic or episodic, with binges punctuated by brief periods of abstinence. Aggressive or violent behavior is common when high doses are smoked, ingested, or administered intravenously. Intense temporary anxiety resembling Panic Disorder (see Section 5.5) or Generalized Anxiety Disorder (see Section 5.7), as well as paranoid ideation and psychotic episodes that resemble Schizophrenia, can occur with high-dose use. Withdrawal states are associated with temporary but intense depressive symptoms that can resemble a Major Depressive Episode (DSM-5-TR, p. 183), although the depressive symptoms usually resolve within a week of stopping use.

Some individuals with Stimulant Use Disorder begin using stimulants to control their weight or to improve their performance in school, work, or athletics. Examples include obtaining medications such as methylphenidate or amphetamine salts that were prescribed for others for the treatment of Attention-Deficit/Hyperactivity Disorder.

The 12-month prevalence of amphetamine-type Stimulant Use Disorder in the United States is 0.1% among individuals ages 12–17 years, 0.5% among those ages 18–25 years, and 0.4% among those age 26 years and older. Rates for Cocaine Use Disorder are similar: 0.1% among individuals ages 12–17 years, 0.7% among those ages 18–25 years, and 0.3% among those age 26 years and older.

Cocaine Problem

Al Santini, a 39-year-old restaurant owner, is referred by a marriage counselor to a private outpatient substance abuse treatment program for evaluation and treatment of a possible "cocaine problem." According to the counselor, attempts to deal with the couple's marital problems have failed to produce any signs of progress over the past 6 or 7 months. The couple continues to have frequent, explosive arguments, some of which have led to physical violence. Fortunately, neither spouse has been seriously injured, but the continuing chaos in their relationship has led to a great deal of tension at home and appears to be contributing to the acting-out behavior and school problems of their two children, ages 9 and 13.

Several days ago, Mr. Santini admitted to the counselor and to his wife that he has been using cocaine "occasionally" for at least the past year. His wife became angry and tearful, stating that if her husband failed to obtain treatment for his drug problem, she would separate from him and inform his parents of the problem. He reluctantly agreed to seek professional help, insisting that his cocaine use was "not a problem," and that he felt capable of stopping his drug use without entering a treatment program.

During the initial evaluation interview, Mr. Santini reports that he is currently using cocaine intranasally 3–5 days a week, and that this pattern has been ongoing for at least the past 2 years. On average, he consumes a total of 1–2 grams of cocaine weekly, for which he pays $200 per gram. Most of his cocaine use occurs at work, in his private office or in the bathroom. He usually begins thinking about "coke" while driving to work in the morning. When he arrives at work, he finds it nearly impossible to avoid thinking of the cocaine vial in his desk drawer. Although he tries to distract himself and postpone using it as long as possible, he usually snorts his first "line" within an hour of arriving at work. On some days he may snort another two or three lines over the course of the day. On other days, especially if he feels stressed or frustrated at work, he may snort a line or two every hour from morning through late afternoon. His cocaine use is sometimes fueled by offers of the drug from his business partner, whom the patient describes as a more controlled, infrequent user of the drug.

Mr. Santini rarely uses cocaine at home, and never in the presence of his wife or children. Occasionally, he snorts a line or two on weekday evenings or during weekends at home when everyone else is out of the house. He denies current use of any other illicit drug but reports taking 10–20 mg of the antianxiety drug diazepam (prescribed by a physician friend) at bedtime on days when cocaine leaves him feeling restless, irritable, and unable to fall asleep. When diazepam is unavailable, he drinks two or three beers instead.

He first tried cocaine 5 years ago at a friend's party. He enjoyed the energetic, euphoric feeling and the absence of any unpleasant side effects, except for a slightly uncomfortable "racing" feeling in his chest. For nearly 3 years thereafter, he used cocaine only when it was offered by others, and never purchased his own supplies or found himself thinking about the drug between episodes of use. He rarely snorted more than four or five lines on any single occasion of use. During the past 2 years, his cocaine use escalated to its current level, coincident with a number of significant changes in his life: his restaurant business became financially successful, he bought a large home in the suburbs, he had access to large sums of cash, and the pressures of a growing business made him feel entitled to the relief and pleasures offered by cocaine.

He denies any history of other alcohol or drug abuse problems. The only other drug he has ever used is marijuana, which he smoked infrequently in college but never really liked. He also denies any history of other emotional problems and, except for marriage counseling, reports that he has never needed help from a mental health care professional.

During the interview Mr. Santini remarks several times that although he thinks his cocaine use "might be a problem," he does not consider himself to be "addicted" and is still not sure that he really requires treatment. In support of this view, he lists the following evidence: 1) his current level of cocaine use is not causing him any financial problems or affecting his standard of living; 2) he is experiencing no significant drug-related health problems that he is aware of, with the possible exception of feeling lethargic the next day following a day of heavy use; 3) on many occasions he has been able to stop using cocaine on his own, for several days at a time; and 4) when he stops using the drug, he experiences no withdrawal syndrome and no continuous drug craving. On the other hand, he also admits the following: 1) he often uses much more cocaine than intended on certain days; 2) the drug use is impairing his functioning at work because of negative effects on his memory, attention span, and attitude toward employees and customers; 3) even when he is not actively intoxicated with cocaine, the aftereffects of the drug cause him to be short-tempered, irritable, and argumentative with his wife and children, leading to numerous family problems, including a possible breakup of his marriage; 4) although he seems able to stop using cocaine for a few days at a time, somehow he always goes back to it; and 5) as soon as he starts to use cocaine again, the craving and the preoccupation with the drug are immediately as intense as before he stopped using it.

At the end of the interview, Mr. Santini agrees that although he came for the evaluation largely under pressure from his wife, he can see the potential benefits of trying to stop using cocaine on a more permanent basis. With a saddened expression, he explains how troubled and frightened he feels about the problems with his wife and children. He says that although marital problems existed before he started snorting cocaine, his continuing drug use has made them worse, and he now fears that his wife might leave him. He also feels extremely guilty about not being a "good father." He spends very little time with his children, and often is distracted and irritable with them because of his cocaine use.

Mr. Santini entered the outpatient treatment program. His treatment included individual, group, and marital counseling combined with supervised urine screening and participation in a self-help group (Cocaine Anonymous). He initially had difficulty in fully acknowledging and accepting the seriousness of his drug dependency problem. He harbored fantasies about returning to "controlled" cocaine use and disputed the program's requirement of total abstinence from all mood-altering substances, arguing that because he had never experienced problems with alcohol, he saw no reason to deny himself an occasional drink with dinner or at social gatherings. During the first 3 months of treatment, he had two short "slips" back to taking cocaine, one of which was precipitated by drinking a glass of wine, which led to intense craving for cocaine.

Subsequently, Mr. Santini remained completely abstinent for the duration of the program (12 months) and became increasingly committed to maintaining a drug-free lifestyle. His relationship with his wife and children improved considerably. The violent arguments stopped immediately with the cessation of cocaine use, and spending more time with his children became much easier without the negative influence of cocaine on his mood and mental state.

Discussion of "Cocaine Problem"

Mr. Santini, like many people with a serious drug problem, does not like to think of himself as "addicted." However, his use of cocaine illustrates the core concept of a Substance Use Disorder: a cluster of cognitive, behavioral, and physiological symptoms indicating that the person has impaired control over their substance use and continues use of the substance despite adverse consequences. Mr. Santini craves cocaine and cannot stop himself from the first hit of cocaine in the morning; he uses it more often than he plans to; he keeps returning to it after stopping for a few days; he experiences withdrawal symptoms (lethargy); he has gradually reduced his participation in important social activities with his family because of his cocaine-related mood changes; and he continues to use cocaine despite the psychological problems resulting from his use (i.e., negative effects on his memory, attention span, and attitude). Therefore, because six of the criteria have been met, his diagnosis is Severe Cocaine Use Disorder (DSM-5-TR, p. 632).

16.4
Caffeine-Related Disorders

Caffeine is the most widely consumed psychoactive substance in the world. It is available in a wide variety of sources, including coffee, tea, caffeinated soda, "energy" drinks, over-the-counter analgesics and cold remedies, weight-loss aids, and chocolate. More than 85% of adults and children in the United States regularly consume caffeine, with adult caffeine consumers ingesting about 280 mg/day on average. Some caffeine users do display symptoms consistent with problematic use, including tolerance and withdrawal; however, given that data are not available at this time to determine the clinical significance and prevalence of a diagnosis of Caffeine Use Disorder, the diagnosis is not included in the main part of DSM-5-TR (although it is included in the DSM-5-TR Section III chapter "Conditions for Further Study"). DSM-5-TR does include diagnostic criteria for Caffeine Intoxication and Caffeine Withdrawal, because there is evidence that these conditions are clinically significant and sufficiently prevalent.

In particularly vulnerable individuals such as children, the elderly, and individuals who have not been previously exposed to caffeine, symptoms such as restlessness, nervousness, excitement, insomnia, flushed face, sweating, and gastrointestinal complaints can occur with doses as low as 200 mg (the amount in a single strong cup of coffee). At higher levels of caffeine (e.g., more than 1 g/day), symptoms such as muscle twitching, rambling flow of thought and speech, increased or irregular heartbeat, periods of inexhaustibility, and physical restlessness may occur. Because caffeine-related symptoms are relatively common in the general population, the diagnosis of Caffeine Intoxication should be made only if the symptoms cause clinically significant distress or impairment in social, occupational, or other important areas of functioning. Impairment from Caffeine Intoxication may have serious consequences, including social indiscretions or dysfunction at work or school. Moreover, extremely high doses of caffeine (5–10 g) ingested in a short period of time can be fatal.

In individuals with prolonged heavy daily ingestion, Caffeine Withdrawal can develop after abruptly stopping or substantially reducing caffeine use. Headache is the hallmark feature of Caffeine Withdrawal. In the United States, headache may occur in approximately 50% of cases of caffeine abstinence. Other symptoms include marked fatigue or drowsiness, depressed or irritable mood, difficulty concentrating, and flu-like symptoms (e.g., nausea, vomiting, muscle pain and stiffness). Because caffeine ingestion is often integrated into social customs and daily rituals (e.g., coffee break, teatime), some caffeine consumers may be unaware of their physical dependence on caffeine. Thus, Caffeine Withdrawal symptoms could be unexpected and misattributed to other causes (e.g., the flu, migraine). Furthermore, Caffeine Withdrawal symptoms may occur when individuals are required to abstain from foods and beverages before medical procedures; during religious rituals, such as fasting; or when a usual caffeine dose is missed because of a change in routine (e.g., during travel, on weekends). This relatively common phenomenon should be considered worthy of a DSM-5-TR diagnosis only if the withdrawal syndrome causes clinically significant distress or impairment in social, occupational, or other important areas of functioning. Examples of functional impairment include being unable to work, exercise, or care for children; staying in bed all day; and ending a vacation early.

Coffee Machine

Eliot Evans is a 41-year-old attorney whose internist has referred him for a psychiatric consultation. He has been complaining of fatigue, loss of motivation, sleepiness, headaches, nausea, feeling unsociable, and having difficulty concentrating. His symptoms occur mostly on weekends, and as a result he often begs off weekend social activities, causing his wife to be very annoyed with him. She complains that he is fine during the week but never feels like going out with friends or playing with the children on weekends. He is in good health, with no recent history of any medical conditions.

Mr. Evans works a 60-hour week in a busy law practice and barely sees his family during the week. At work he is often anxious, restless, and constantly busy. He often has trouble sleeping on weeknights because he worries about his job. He denies marital or family problems, other than those caused by his not wanting to do anything on the weekends.

He has a history of alcohol problems but has not had a drink for 5 years. He used to smoke 20 cigarettes a day but stopped 2 months ago, hoping that quitting would improve his condition. (It did not.) At work he drinks four cups of coffee a day. He has stopped using coffee on the weekends because he suspected it might be contributing to his anxiety and sleeplessness.

The psychiatrist was impressed with the relationship between Mr. Evans's cessation of coffee drinking on weekends and the onset of the symptoms of headache, fatigue, difficulty concentrating, sleepiness, and loss of motivation. Mr. Evans was advised to decrease his coffee drinking during the week, but he found that he could not function well without his usual dose of coffee. Instead, Mr. Evans decided to resume drinking coffee on the weekends, because there was no medical contraindication to his regular use of caffeine. He decided to live with the anxiety and difficulty sleeping that had originally prompted his giving up his weekend coffee.

Discussion of "Coffee Machine"

Many people recognize that they need a cup of coffee to get going in the morning. They likely do not recognize, however, that by taking a cup or more of coffee, they are avoiding the development of Caffeine Withdrawal symptoms. Typically, withdrawal symptoms begin approximately 12 hours after the last cup of coffee. Often, a heavy coffee drinker who has coffee with dinner starts to develop withdrawal symptoms the next morning if they, for some reason, do not have coffee at breakfast.

Mr. Evans's presenting symptoms of fatigue, loss of motivation, sleepiness, feeling unsocial, and having difficulty concentrating are certainly suggestive of a Depressive Disorder (see Chapter 4), and some people with depression may report that they feel worse on the weekends when removed from the structure of a typical workday. The astute clinician, noticing the connection between Mr. Evans's reduction in coffee consumption and the development of symptoms (especially the headache), diagnosed Caffeine Withdrawal (DSM-5-TR, p. 571). This diagnosis can be confirmed by demonstrating a resolution of symptoms if Mr. Evans drinks coffee at home over the weekend at the same level he drinks while in the office.

16.5
Tobacco-Related Disorders

Nicotine is the primary psychoactive substance contained in tobacco products. Although cigarettes are the most commonly used tobacco product, use of other tobacco products (especially e-cigarettes) has become more common. In the United States, 19% of adults used a tobacco product in the last year. One-fourth (24%) of current U.S. smokers are nondaily smokers. In the United States, among people age 12 years or older in 2020, 8.5% reported experiencing symptoms of nicotine dependence within the past 30 days.[1]

Tobacco Use Disorder can develop with use of all forms of tobacco (e.g., cigarettes, chewing tobacco, snuff, pipes, cigars, electronic nicotine delivery devices such as electronic cigarettes [e-cigarettes]) and with prescription nicotine-containing medications (nicotine gum and patch). The relative ability of these products to produce Tobacco Use Disorder or to induce withdrawal is associated with the rapidity of the route of administration (smoked over oral over transdermal) and the nicotine content of the product. Tobacco Use Disorder is common among individuals who use cigarettes and smokeless tobacco daily and is uncommon among individuals who do not use tobacco daily or who use nicotine medications. Smoking within 30 minutes of waking, smoking daily, smoking a larger number of cigarettes per day, and waking at night to smoke are indications of Tobacco Use Disorder. Cessation of tobacco use can produce a well-defined withdrawal syndrome that can impair a person's ability to stop tobacco use. The symptoms that occur after abstinence from tobacco are in large part attributable to nicotine deprivation and are much more intense among individuals

---

[1]National Institute on Drug Abuse: Tobacco, Nicotine, and E-Cigarettes Research Report: "What is the scope of tobacco, nicotine, and e-cigarette use in the United States?" December 14, 2023. Available at: https://nida.nih.gov/publications/research-reports/tobacco-nicotine-e-cigarettes/what-scope-tobacco-use-its-cost-to-society. Accessed June 25, 2024.

who smoke cigarettes or use smokeless tobacco than among those who use nicotine medications. Tobacco Withdrawal is common among daily tobacco users who stop or reduce use, but it can also occur among nondaily users.

More than 80% of individuals who use tobacco attempt to quit at some time, but 60% relapse within 1 week. However, most individuals who use tobacco make multiple attempts to quit, and 50% of tobacco users eventually become abstinent. National U.S. survey data show that past-year cigarette use is associated with a two- to threefold increased risk of suicidal thoughts and behavior, with earlier age at first tobacco use further increasing this risk.

Junkie

Stuart Havel, a 54-year-old administrator at a Midwestern university, was asked to tell the story of his struggle to give up cigarettes. He has not smoked at all for 2 years, following a 6-week treatment with a nicotine patch that was prescribed by a colleague who runs a smoking cessation research program.

Mr. Havel began smoking when he was 18 years old, usually smoking one or two packs a day. Beginning in his late 30s, he vowed to stop every morning, but by 9:30 A.M., "It was over, and I was lighting my first cigarette of the day." When he was age 45 and under a lot of pressure from family, friends, and his cardiologist, he asked his colleague to prescribe clonidine, a medication used to treat high blood pressure that has also been used to help smokers stop smoking by reducing nicotine withdrawal symptoms. Over 4 days, the clonidine dosage was gradually increased, and Mr. Havel did not smoke. On the fourth day, he began to feel "like I was on an LSD trip." He reported that his surroundings seemed unreal; "people opened and closed their mouths, but no words came out"; and, frightened about what was happening to him, he stopped the drug abruptly. For the next few weeks, he still felt drugged but did not smoke. Back to normal, he fell into smoking again and was soon up to a pack or two a day.

Over the next 5 years, there was more social pressure for him to stop. Smoking was outlawed in his office building, and his wife and doctor were relentless in their badgering. He also began to notice that he was short of breath when he walked up a few flights of steps. He again asked his colleague for help and was given a nicotine patch. "I had always thought that I smoked because it was a part of my life, but then I got the patch and didn't need to smoke, and in that moment, I realized I was a junkie."

Discussion of "Junkie"

Mr. Havel referred to himself as a "junkie" because he recognized that he was as dependent on nicotine as any heroin user might be on heroin. He was repeatedly unable to cut down or control his smoking, he smoked all day, and he smoked despite the knowledge that it was causing him physical problems (shortness of breath when walking upstairs). Therefore, for many years, Mr. Havel had To-bacco Use Disorder (DSM-5-TR, p. 645).

Periodically, as Mr. Havel sought to cut down on his smoking, he tried to avoid withdrawal symptoms by using drugs such as clonidine or by using a nicotine patch, which slowly administers a low dose of nicotine into the bloodstream.

16.6
Cannabis-Related Disorders

DSM-5-TR uses the term *cannabis* to refer to all forms of cannabis-like sub-stances, including synthetic cannabinoid compounds. Synthetic oral formulations (pills, capsules) of Δ^9-tetrahydrocannabinol (THC) are available by prescription for a number of approved medical indications (e.g., chronic pain, chemotherapy-induced nausea and vomiting, anorexia and weight loss associated with HIV/AIDS). Other synthetic cannabinoid compounds have been manufactured and distributed for non-medical use in the form of plant material that has been sprayed with a cannabinoid formulation (e.g., K2, Spice). Although such synthetic cannabinoids are designed to mimic cannabis effects, their chemical composition, potency, effects, and duration of action are unpredictable, and they may cause more severe adverse effects than canna-bis plant products, including seizures, cardiac conditions, psychosis, and even death. Among the generally available formulations of cannabis, potency (THC concentra-tion) varies greatly, averaging 10%–15% in typical cannabis plant material, 30%–40% in hashish, and 50%–55% in hash oil (concentrated extraction of the cannabis plant).

Cannabis Use Disorder and the Cannabis-Induced Disorders include problems that are associated with substances derived from the cannabis plant and chemically similar synthetic compounds. Cannabis is most commonly smoked but is sometimes ingested orally, typically by mixing it into food. More recently, devices have been developed in which cannabis is "vaporized," which involves heating the plant material to release psychoactive cannabinoids for inhalation. As with other psychoactive substances, smoking and vaporization typically produce more rapid onset and more intense expe-riences of the desired effects. Intoxication develops within minutes if the cannabis is smoked but may take a few hours to develop if the cannabis is ingested orally.

Some individuals with Cannabis Use Disorder use cannabis throughout the day over a period of months or years, and thus spend many hours a day under the influ-ence. Some other individuals use less frequently, but their use causes recurrent prob-lems related to family, school, work, or other important activities (e.g., repeated absences at work). Still others may smoke occasionally without any ill effects.

Regular cannabis users become tolerant to many of the acute effects of cannabis, and stopping regular cannabis use generally leads to a Cannabis Withdrawal syn-drome, which can contribute to difficulty quitting or relapse among individuals try-ing to quit. Cannabis Withdrawal symptoms include irritability, anger or aggression, anxiety, depressed mood, restlessness, difficulty sleeping, and decreased appetite or weight loss. Moreover, because of the growing perception that cannabis use is harmless, individuals may fail to realize that the symptoms they experience, including withdrawal symptoms, are related to a Cannabis Use Disorder.

Individuals who regularly use cannabis often report that they use it to cope with mood, sleep, pain, or other problems, and those diagnosed with Cannabis Use Disorder frequently have other concurrent mental disorders.

Among youth in the United States (ages 12–17 years), the past-year prevalence of Cannabis Use Disorder ranges from 2.7% to 3.1%, and among adults, it ranges from 1.5% to 2.9%. Among individuals reporting any past-year use of cannabis, the prevalence of Cannabis Use Disorder is 20.4% among youth and 30.6% among adults. Cannabis has commonly been considered as a "gateway" drug because individuals who use cannabis have a substantially greater lifetime probability than nonusers of subsequently using other, more risky substances (e.g., opioids, cocaine).

Freaking Out

In the middle of a rainy October night in 1970, a family doctor living in a Chicago suburb was awakened by an old friend who begged him to get out of bed and come quickly to a neighbor's house, where he and his wife had been visiting. The caller, Lou Wolff, was very upset because his wife, Sybil, had smoked some marijuana and was "freaking out."

The doctor, extremely annoyed, arrived at the neighbor's house to find Mrs. Wolff lying on the couch looking quite frantic and unable to get up. She said she was too weak to stand, was dizzy, was having palpitations, and could feel her blood "rushing through [her] veins." She kept asking for water, because her mouth was so dry that she could not swallow. She was sure there was some poison in the marijuana. Mrs. Wolff was relieved to see the doctor because she had believed the neighbors would not let her husband call him for fear of being arrested for possession of marijuana, and she was sure that without medical help, she would die.

Mrs. Wolff, age 42, worked as a librarian at a university, and she and her husband had three teenage sons. She was a very controlled, well-organized woman who prided herself on her rationality. She had smoked a small amount of marijuana only once before, and the only reaction she detected was that it made her feel "slightly mellow." It was she who asked the neighbors to share some of their high-quality homegrown marijuana with her, because she "wanted to see what all the fuss was about."

Her husband said that she took four or five puffs of a joint and then wailed, "There's something wrong with me. I can't stand up." Her husband and the neighbors tried to calm her, telling her she should just lie down, and she would soon feel better; but the more they reassured her, the more convinced she became that something was really wrong with her, and that her husband and neighbors were just trying to cover it up.

The doctor examined her. The only notable findings were that her heart rate was increased, and her pupils were dilated. Adopting his best bedside manner, the doctor said to her, "For Christ's sake, Sybil, you're just a little stoned. Go to bed and stop making such a fuss." Mrs. Wolff seemed reassured. The doctor then walked into another room and told her husband, "If that doesn't work, we'll have to take her to the emergency room."

Mrs. Wolff was helped up to her bed by her husband (she still could not stand up). She stayed in bed for 2 days, feeling "spacey" and weak, but no longer terribly anxious. She realized that because the marijuana was home-grown, there was no reason to think that it contained any poison. However, she still believed that her neighbors did not want to call the doctor because they were afraid of the police. She vowed never to smoke marijuana again.

Discussion of "Freaking Out"

Mrs. Wolff's bad experience with marijuana (cannabis) resulted in characteristic physical symptoms such as dry mouth and increased heart rate. It was the psychological symptoms, however, that caused her husband to seek help. Mrs. Wolff became extremely anxious and had paranoid ideation (that the marijuana was poisoned and that her neighbors would not let her husband call the doctor). This maladaptive reaction to the recent use of cannabis, combined with her extreme distress, indicates that a DSM-5-TR diagnosis of Cannabis Intoxication is appropriate (DSM-5-TR, p. 582).

An additional consideration in this case is whether Mrs. Wolff's paranoid thinking could justify a diagnosis of Cannabis-Induced Psychotic Disorder (DSM-5-TR, p. 126) instead of Cannabis Intoxication, which would be the case if her paranoid thinking crossed the line into full-blown delusions (see Chapter 2, "Schizophrenia Spectrum and Other Psychotic Disorders," for a more detailed discussion of this differentiation) and if these symptoms predominated in the clinical picture and were sufficiently severe to warrant clinical attention. The clinician decided that the diagnosis of Cannabis-Induced Psychotic Disorder did not apply, because Mrs. Wolff's paranoid thinking did not reach the level of being delusional for a couple of reasons: First, the fact that her neighbors would not let her husband call the doctor may have been realistic (and not evidence of a delusion), because they would have had to admit that they were smoking an illegal substance, which at the time this case occurred (i.e., 1970) would likely have been a more serious concern than it is now, with the current climate of legalization of cannabis in a number of states. Second, Mrs. Wolff was reassured by the doctor that the marijuana did not contain poison, whereas, by definition, a delusion is a false belief that is firmly held despite evidence to the contrary.

Fidgety and Grumpy

Dorothy Calkins is a 24-year-old waitress who comes in to see her doctor be-cause her long-standing anxiety problems, which she has been self-treating with cannabis, have reappeared along with new symptoms of depression. She reports generalized anxiety, crying spells, poor sleep, a 10-pound weight loss, mild abdominal pain, and headaches. She has smoked cannabis one or two times daily for the last 6 years and has not been able to go without cannabis for more than 2–3 days because her anxiety symptoms get worse when she stops. Ten days ago, however, Ms. Calkins decided to stop because she is be-ginning a new, challenging job that will require her to focus carefully for extend-ed periods of time and to multitask. Moreover, the job also requires urine testing for drugs. Over the last week or so, she has been "grumpy" and has had fights with her boyfriend, plus she has been "fidgety." These symptoms have im-proved somewhat in the last week, but she still has had to leave work early on 2 days, mostly because of poor sleep and "wild" dreams the night before. On reflection, Ms. Calkins states that the symptoms began a couple of days after she stopped using cannabis and worries that she might need cannabis to cope. She has not changed her moderate use of alcohol and caffeine, or her occasional tobacco use. She has not used any other drugs in the past month.

Discussion of "Fidgety and Grumpy"

Ms. Calkins presents for treatment because of what she perceives to be a re-emergence of her long-standing anxiety symptoms, but this time accompanied by depression. The typical waxing and waning nature of many Anxiety and Depressive Disorders suggests that her presentation may simply represent a worsening of her underlying Anxiety Disorder. However, the timing of the on-set of her symptoms, occurring soon after she stopped her daily cannabis use, plus the presence of additional symptoms not typical of anxiety and depres-sion (e.g., disturbing dreams and abdominal pain), indicate that these symp-toms are in fact attributable to Cannabis Withdrawal (DSM-5-TR, p. 584), which developed after she stopped using marijuana because of her new job. Her lack of awareness of the connection between her symptoms and her can-nabis use was likely related to two factors. First, the fact that cessation of daily cannabis use can lead to clinically significant withdrawal symptoms is not generally well known by the public, given that Cannabis Withdrawal was in-troduced as a DSM diagnosis only fairly recently (2013, in DSM-5). Second, be-cause Ms. Calkins perceived her marijuana use to be successfully treating her anxiety, the return of her anxiety symptoms after she stopped smoking mari-juana most likely appeared to be a result of her cessation of "treatment" rather than part of a withdrawal syndrome.

16.7
Phencyclidine-Related Disorders

The diagnosis of substance-related disorders attributed to PCP (also known as "angel dust") includes related substances that are less potent but similarly acting compounds, such as ketamine (the "S" form [esketamine] of which is FDA-approved for treatment-resistant depression), methoxetamine, and dizocilpine. These substances were first developed as dissociative anesthetics in the 1950s and became street drugs in the 1960s. At low doses, they produce feelings of separation from mind and body (hence "dissociative"), and at high doses, stupor and coma can result. Although the primary psychoactive effects of PCP last only a few hours, the drug typically takes 8 days or longer to be totally eliminated from the body. In vulnerable individuals, however, the hallucinogenic effects may last for weeks and may precipitate a persistent psychotic episode resembling Schizophrenia. Phencyclidine Intoxication is characterized by disorientation, confusion, hallucinations or delusions, a catatonic-like syndrome, and coma. Violent behavior can also occur with PCP use, as intoxicated individuals may believe that they are being attacked.

Data on the prevalence of Phencyclidine Use Disorder are not available, but rates appear to be low (less than 0.1%). Furthermore, among U.S. substance use treatment facility admissions, only 0.3% of the admitted individuals identified PCP as their primary drug.

Peaceable Man

Leo Boyer is a 20-year-old man who was brought to the hospital, trussed in ropes, by his four brothers. This is his seventh hospitalization in the last 2 years, each for similar behavior. One of his brothers reports that he "came home crazy" late one night, threw a chair through a window, tore a gas heater off the wall, and ran into the street. The family called the police, who apprehended him shortly thereafter as he stood naked, directing traffic at a busy intersection. He assaulted the arresting officers, escaped from them, and ran home screaming threats at his family. Once home, his brothers were able to subdue him.

On admission, Leo was observed to be agitated, his mood fluctuating between anger and fear. He had slurred speech and staggered when he walked. He remained extremely violent and disorganized for the first several days of his hospitalization; then he began having longer and longer lucid intervals, still interspersed with sudden, unpredictable periods in which he displayed great suspiciousness, a fierce expression, slurred speech, and clenched fists.

After calming down, Leo denied ever having been violent or acting in an unusual way ("I'm a peaceable man," he said) and stated that he could not remember how he got to the hospital. He admitted using alcohol and marijuana socially, but denied PCP use except once, experimentally, 3 years previously. Nevertheless, blood and urine tests were positive for PCP, and his brother believes "he gets dusted every day."

According to his family, Leo was perfectly normal until about 3 years before. He made above-average grades in school, had a part-time job and a girlfriend, and was of a sunny and outgoing disposition. Then, at age 17, he had his first episode of emotional disturbance. This episode was of very sudden onset, with symptoms similar to those of the current episode. Leo quickly recovered entirely from that first episode, went back to school, and graduated from high school. With subsequent episodes, however, his improvement was less and less encouraging.

After 3 weeks of the current hospitalization, the patient is sullen and watchful, and is quick to remark sarcastically on the smallest infringement of the respect due him. He is mostly quiet and isolated from others, but is easily provoked to fury. His family reports that "this is as good as he gets," and that he has returned to his baseline functioning.

Discussion of "Peaceable Man"

Leo's hospitalization was occasioned by the acute effects of PCP on the central nervous system: violence, bizarre and disorganized behavior, psychomotor agitation, emotional lability, slurred speech, and ataxia. This presentation is typical of Phencyclidine Intoxication (DSM-5-TR, p. 594).

In addition, Leo has a history of regular use of PCP, resulting in many similar episodes of disturbed behavior. This patient is frequently intoxicated when he would be expected to be working (his brother reports that "Leo gets dusted every day"); spends a great deal of time recovering from the effects of PCP use; continues to use PCP despite knowledge that it causes him to get into trouble over and over again; and has given up important social and occupational activities (i.e., he lies around the house, does no work) because of PCP use. These behaviors point to an additional diagnosis of Phencyclidine Use Disorder (DSM-5-TR, p. 587).

16.8
Hallucinogen-Related Disorders

Hallucinogens comprise a diverse group of substances that despite having different chemical structures and possibly involving different molecular mechanisms, produce similar alterations of perception, mood, and cognition in users. Hallucinogens encompass the phenylalkylamines, such as mescaline, DOM (2,5-

dimethoxy-4-methylamphetamine), and MDMA (3,4-methylenedioxymethamphet-amine; also called "ecstasy" or "molly"); the indoleamines, including dimethyltrypt-amine (DMT) and psilocybin (and its metabolite psilocin, the compound primarily responsible for the psychedelic effects of hallucinogenic mushrooms); and the ergo-lines, such as LSD (lysergic acid diethylamide) and morning glory seeds. Even though PCP can be considered to be a hallucinogen because one of its main effects is to cause hallucinations, it was placed in its own drug lass because of the more significant and problematic behavioral changes associated with PCP intoxication (e.g., belligerence, assaultiveness, impulsiveness, unpredictability, psychomotor agitation, impaired judg-ment) in comparison with intoxication with other hallucinogens. Although cannabis (and its psychoactive compound, THC) can cause perceptual disturbances, it is not con-sidered to be part of the hallucinogen drug class because of significant differences in its associated psychological and behavioral effects.

The duration of effects varies across types of hallucinogens. Some hallucinogens (i.e., LSD, MDMA) have an extended duration of action such that users may spend hours to days using and/or recovering from their effects, whereas other hallucino-genic drugs (e.g., DMT, salvia) are short acting. MDMA/ecstasy as a hallucinogen may have distinctive effects attributable to both its hallucinogenic and its stimulant properties. In comparison with users of other hallucinogens, users of MDMA/ecstasy have a higher risk of developing a Hallucinogen Use Disorder.

In U.S. population surveys, past-year use of hallucinogens is reported by 0.62%, and any lifetime use is reported by 9.32%.[2] Hallucinogen Use Disorder, on the other hand, is relatively uncommon, with a low risk of development following exposure to hallucinogens.

Hallucinogen Intoxication may involve development of anxiety or depression, ideas of reference, fear of "losing one's mind," paranoid ideation, and impaired judg-ment. Hallucinogen Intoxication may lead to increased suicidal thoughts or behavior, although suicide is rare among individuals who use hallucinogens.

Hallucinogen Persisting Perception Disorder is a condition in which an individual reexperiences, while sober, the types of perceptual disturbances that were previously experienced when under the influence of hallucinogens. This persistence of effects is in contrast to the effects of almost all of the Substance/Medication-Induced Mental Disorders, which eventually resolve once the substance is no longer in the body. In most cases, the perceptual disturbances are visual and are characterized by phenom-ena such as geometric hallucinations, false perceptions of movement in the peripheral visual fields, flashes of color, intensified colors, or halos around objects. In some peo-ple, these visual disturbances are episodic, and in others, they are nearly continuous and may last for weeks, months, or years. In any case, the diagnosis is made only if the visual disturbances cause distress or impairment in functioning. This condition occurs primarily (but not exclusively) after LSD use, and there does not appear to be a strong correlation between developing this disorder and the number of occasions of

---

[2]Shalit N, Rehm J, Lev-Ran S: Epidemiology of hallucinogen use in the U.S. results from the Na-tional epidemiologic survey on alcohol and related conditions III. *Addictive Behaviors* 89:35-43, 2019 30245407.

LSD use, given that there are reports of the disorder occurring with only minimal exposure to hallucinogens. It has been estimated that the prevalence of Hallucinogen Persisting Perception Disorder among individuals who use hallucinogens is approximately 4%.

A Man Who Saw the Air

James Van Dorf, a 21-year-old undergraduate, presented with a chief complaint of "seeing the air." The visual disturbance consisted of perception of white pinpoint specks in both the central and peripheral visual fields too numerous to count. They were constantly present and were accompanied by the perception of trails of moving objects left behind as they passed through the patient's visual field. Attending a hockey game was difficult, because the brightly dressed players left streaks of their own images against the white of the ice for seconds at a time. James also described the false perception of movement in stable objects, usually in his peripheral visual fields; halos around objects; and positive and negative afterimages.

Other symptoms included mild depression, daily bitemporal headache, and a loss of concentration in the last year.

The visual syndrome had gradually emerged following experimentation with LSD on three separate occasions in the prior 3 months. He feared he had suffered some kind of "brain damage" from the drug experiences. He denied use of any other agents, including amphetamines, PCP, or opioids, and denied drinking alcohol to excess. He had smoked marijuana twice a week for a period of 7 months at age 17.

James had consulted two ophthalmologists, both of whom confirmed that the white pinpoint specks were not vitreous floaters (diagnostically insignificant particulate matter floating in the vitreous humor—that is, the clear gel between the lens and the retina of the eye—that can cause the perception of "specks"). A neurologist's examination also proved negative.

Discussion of "A Man Who Saw the Air"

James is experiencing a variety of visual disturbances that are presumably similar to those that he experienced when he was intoxicated with the hallucinogen LSD. Mild and transient perceptual disturbances that occur long after cessation of use of a hallucinogen may be common. When the perceptual disturbance is severe enough to cause marked distress, as in this patient, it is called Hallucinogen Persisting Perception Disorder (DSM-5-TR, p. 598). Usually, such perceptual disturbances last for just a few seconds. More rarely, as in this patient, they are experienced throughout the day for long periods of time. The symptoms are often triggered by emergence from a dark environment or use of cannabis.

16.9
Opioid-Related Disorders

Opioids are prescribed as analgesics to treat pain, as anesthetics, as antidiarrheal agents, or as cough suppressants. The opioids include natural opioids (e.g., morphine), semisynthetics (e.g., heroin), and synthetics with morphine-like action (e.g., codeine, hydromorphone, methadone, oxycodone, meperidine, fentanyl). Medications such as pentazocine and buprenorphine, which have both opioid agonist effects (i.e., they activate a receptor to produce euphoria) and antagonist effects (i.e., they block the action of an agonist and thus are useful in treatment), are also included in this class because—especially at lower dosages—their agonist properties produce effects (e.g., euphoria) similar to the effects produced by other medications in this class.

Opioid Use Disorder includes signs and symptoms that reflect compulsive, prolonged self-administration of opioid substances that either are used entirely for recreational purposes (i.e., for no legitimate medical purpose) or, if a medical condition is present that requires opioid treatment, are used at dosages greatly exceeding the amount actually needed for the medical condition (e.g., a person prescribed analgesic opioids for pain relief uses significantly more than prescribed in order to get high rather than to alleviate persistent pain). Opioids are usually purchased on the illegal market, but they may also be obtained from physicians by falsifying or exaggerating medical problems or by going to multiple physicians to receive multiple simultaneous prescriptions.

Most individuals with Opioid Use Disorder have significant levels of tolerance and will experience withdrawal on abrupt discontinuation. Opioid Intoxication is accompanied by pupillary constriction and drowsiness (described as being "on the nod"), which may progress to slurred speech, impairment in attention or memory, and coma. Opioid Withdrawal is characterized by symptoms that are the opposite of intoxication, including pupillary dilation, anxiety, restlessness, irritability, and increased sensitivity to pain.

Attempts to achieve Opioid Intoxication may result in a fatal or nonfatal opioid overdose. Opioid overdose is characterized by unconsciousness, respiratory depression, and pinpoint pupils. Opioid overdoses have increased exponentially in the United States since 1999. Up to 2009, opioid overdoses mainly involved prescribed opioids, but since 2010, overdoses involving heroin began a sharp rise, and additionally, since 2015, fatal overdoses involving synthetic opioids other than methadone (generally fentanyl) have outnumbered overdoses with prescribed opioids.

Among U.S. adults, the prevalence of nonmedical prescription opioid use (i.e., taking an opioid in a manner or at a dose other than prescribed, taking someone else's prescription opioid, or taking a prescription opioid for the feelings that it produces) is 4.1%–4.7%, with rates of use higher in adults ages 18–25 than in those age 26 and older (5.5% vs. 3.4%, respectively). The prevalence of heroin use in the United States is 0.3%–0.4% and is higher among adults ages 18–25 (0.5%–0.7%) than in other age groups. In contrast, the prevalence of prescription Opioid Use Disorder among U.S. adults is 0.6%–0.9%, and the prevalence of Heroin Use Disorder is 0.1%–0.3%. Once Opioid Use Disorder develops, it usually continues over a period of many years, with brief periods of abstinence in some individuals, but long-term abstinence only in a minority. Opioid Use Disorder is associated with a heightened risk for suicide attempts and suicide.

Cough Medicine

Scott LaGrange, a 42-year-old executive in a public relations firm, was referred for psychiatric consultation by his surgeon, who discovered that Mr. LaGrange had sneaked large quantities of a codeine-containing cough medicine into the hospital via a visitor. The patient had been a heavy cigarette smoker for 20 years and had a chronic, hacking cough. He had come into the hospital for a hernia repair and found the pain from the incision unbearable when he coughed.

An operation on his back 5 years before had led Mr. LaGrange's doctor to prescribe codeine to help relieve the incisional pain at that time. Over the intervening 5 years, however, Mr. LaGrange had continued to use the tablets, which contained 5 mg of codeine, and had increased his intake to 60–90 tablets daily. He stated that he often "just took them by the handful—not to feel good, you understand, but just to get by." He had spent considerable time and effort developing a circle of physicians and pharmacists to whom he would "make the rounds" at least three times a week to obtain new supplies of pills. He had tried several times to stop using codeine but had failed. During this period, he lost two jobs because of lax work habits and was divorced by his wife of 11 years.

Discussion of "Cough Medicine"

Although Mr. LaGrange's opioid use was initiated in the context of postsurgical pain relief, over the years it escalated into a problematic pattern of use. Spending a great deal of time obtaining a supply of a substance, repeated unsuccessful efforts to cut down use, tolerance (markedly increased amounts are needed to achieve the desired effect: his taking 60–90 tablets a day), and use of the substance to avoid withdrawal symptoms all point to Opioid Use Disorder (DSM-5-TR, p. 608).

16.10
Inhalant-Related Disorders and Other (or Unknown) Substance–Related Disorders

Two DSM-5-TR drug classes are included in this section: Inhalant-Related Disorders and Other (or Unknown) Substance–Related Disorders. The Inhalant-Related Disorders involve use of volatile hydrocarbons from glues, fuels, paints, and other volatile compounds. Disorders arising from inhalation of nitrous oxide or of amyl, butyl, or isobutyl nitrites ("poppers") are considered Other Substance–Related Disorders. The Other Substance–Related Disorders involve use of anabolic steroids; nonsteroidal anti-inflammatory drugs; cortisol; antiparkinsonian medications; antihistamines; betel nut, which is chewed in many cultures to produce mild euphoria and a floating sensation; kava (from a South Pacific pepper plant), which produces sedation, incoordination, weight loss, mild hepatitis, and lung abnormalities; and cathinones (including khât plant agents and synthetic chemical derivatives), which produce stimulant effects. In some cases, the person may have developed symptoms after ingesting a substance of which the identity is unknown (e.g., a new black market drug not yet identified). In such situations, the category Unknown Substance-Related Disorder would be applicable.

Individuals who use inhalants to get high do so by inhaling the aliphatic and aromatic hydrocarbons found in substances such as gasoline, glue, paint thinners, and spray paints. The active ingredients include toluene, benzene, acetone, tetrachloroethylene, and methanol. Volatile hydrocarbon use impairs neurobehavioral function and can cause various neurological, gastrointestinal, cardiovascular, and pulmonary problems. Because of inherent toxicity, use of inhalants can be fatal. Death can occur from anoxia, cardiac dysfunction, extreme allergic reaction, severe injury to the lungs, vomiting, accidents or injury, or central nervous system depression. Moreover, inhalation of any agent in this class may produce "sudden sniffing death" from cardiac arrhythmia. Fatalities may occur even on the first inhalant exposure and are not thought to be dose related.

Inhalant Intoxication develops during, or immediately after, intended or unintended inhalation of a volatile hydrocarbon substance. Typically, the intoxication clears within a few minutes to a few hours after the exposure ends. Thus, Inhalant Intoxication usually occurs in brief episodes that may recur.

Among American youth ages 12–17 years, about 2.3% have used inhalants in the past 12 months, with 0.1% having symptoms that meet criteria for an Inhalant Use Disorder. Among U.S. adults, past 12-month prevalence of inhalant use is about 0.21%, with 0.04% having symptoms that meet criteria for an Inhalant Use Disorder. Among U.S. adolescents and adults, inhalant use and Inhalant Use Disorder are associated with suicidal thoughts and behavior, especially in individuals reporting symptoms of anxiety and depression and a history of trauma.

Youth ages 12–17 years who progress to Inhalant Use Disorder tend to exhibit multiple other problems, such as Conduct Disorder and other Substance Use Disorders.

Better Living Through Chemistry

Danny Bridges, age 17 years, is brought by his older brother Roy to the emergency room at 3:00 A.M. on a Sunday morning. On returning home from a date, Roy found Danny stumbling around their parents' basement den crying and mumbling, "Everything is blurry and double." Roy says that his brother "cussed him out" on the way to the hospital. He says that Danny drinks alcohol and smokes both tobacco and marijuana, but Roy does not know if Danny uses any other drugs.

The examining physician notes that Danny is wearing an earring and a T-shirt that bears the inscription "Better Living Through Chemistry." Around his neck on a chain is a coke spoon hanging outside his shirt. His breath has an odor suggestive of an organic solvent. There is a symmetrical red rash about his mouth and nose. His pupils are symmetrical and responsive to light, although the whites of his eyes are markedly inflamed. Close inspection reveals transparent viscous material just inside both nostrils.

While questioning Danny, the doctor notes that the patient has an extremely short attention span. His manner at one moment is apathetic and disinterested, and at the next, belligerent and abusive. Neurological examination reveals no signs of localized neurological impairment. Danny appears intoxicated, with slurred speech and unsteady, staggering gait. His reflexes are bilaterally depressed, his muscular strength is generally diminished, and he manifests an intentional tremor (a tremor of the hand that appears only when it is extended) and horizontal and vertical nystagmus (involuntary rapid movements of the eyeballs). Examination of the oral and pharyngeal mucosa (tissue in the mouth and back of the throat) reveals diffuse irritation. Several times during the examination, Danny attempts to leave, and at one point takes the reflex hammer and starts testing the doctor. The physical examination is otherwise unremarkable.

Over the 45-minute course of the examination, Danny comments that the blurring of his vision and the double vision have disappeared. Over the same period, the doctor observes that the patient's reflexes have become more vigorous. Despite these changes, Danny's affect continues to vacillate between apathy and hostility.

A urine specimen is collected for a drug toxicology screening, and Danny is placed in a holding area while a psychiatric consultant is called. Danny waits a short while and then, against medical advice, leaves the hospital. All attempts to reach his parents are unsuccessful. Subsequently, the urine drug toxicology screen revealed aromatic inhalants.

Discussion of "Better Living Through Chemistry"

Roy says that his brother uses only marijuana and alcohol, but the doctor smells an organic solvent on Danny's breath, notices a rash around his nose and mouth, and therefore wonders whether he may be intoxicated from inhaling a volatile substance such as gasoline, glue, paint, or paint thinner. The doctor's suspicion that Danny was under the influence of a volatile inhalant is confirmed by the urine drug test.

Individuals who inhale aromatic substances sometimes soak a rag with the substance, apply the rag to the mouth and nose, and breathe in the vapors. Alternatively, they might inhale the substance directly from containers or from aerosols. The inhalants quickly reach the lungs and bloodstream and cause an acute intoxication state. Danny's visual symptoms, slurred speech, unsteady gait, lethargy, depressed reflexes, tremor, and muscle weakness are characteristic of intoxication with a volatile inhalant. The DSM-5-TR diagnosis of Inhalant Intoxication (DSM-5-TR, p. 605) is made when these symptoms are accompanied by maladaptive behavioral changes, such as belligerence alternating with apathy, as in this case.

The most serious complication of recurrent Inhalant Intoxication is brain damage, which, when severe, takes the form of a Substance-Induced Major Neurocognitive Disorder (see Chapter 17). Because Danny's current symptoms of cognitive impairment (i.e., extremely short attention span) are due to the acute effects of the drug (intoxication), it is not possible to determine whether some of these symptoms might represent an incipient Inhalant-Induced Mild Neurocognitive Disorder.

16.11
Gambling Disorder

Gambling involves risking something of value in the hopes of obtaining something of greater value. In many cultures, individuals gamble on games and events, and most do so without experiencing problems. However, some individuals lose control over their gambling behavior so that it disrupts personal, family, academic, or occupational pursuits.

Some individuals who develop Gambling Disorder become preoccupied with gambling, for example, by reliving past gambling experiences or spending a lot of time planning the next gambling venture. Most of these individuals report that they gamble more for the excitement than for the money, and thus may develop a tolerance-like effect in which they need to gamble with increasingly larger bets to continue to get the same thrill. They often continue to gamble despite their repeated efforts to control, cut back on, or stop gambling. Analogous to withdrawal phenomena in Substance Use Disorders, the attempts to cut down on or stop gambling may cause individuals with Gambling Disorder to become restless or irritable. Many individuals gamble when they feel distressed, as a way of escaping from problems or to relieve a dysphoric mood. Commonly, a pattern of "chasing one's losses" develops, wherein the individual experiences an urgent need to gamble in order to recoup money lost during previous gambling experiences. Individuals may lie to family members, therapists, or others to conceal how much time or money they have spent gambling or to cover up illegal behaviors such as forgery, theft, or embezzlement, which were done to obtain money with which to gamble. Often, such individuals have jeopardized or lost a significant relationship, job, or educational opportunity because of their gambling. Individuals may also engage in "bailout" behavior, turning to family or others for help with a desperate financial situation that was caused by gambling. Some individuals with Gambling Disorder are impulsive, competitive, energetic, restless, and easily bored; they may be overly concerned with the approval of others and may be generous to the point of extravagance when winning. Other individuals with Gambling Disorder are depressed and lonely, and they may gamble when feeling helpless, guilty, or depressed.

In the U.S. general population, the past-year prevalence rate of Gambling Disorder is about 0.2%–0.3%, and the lifetime prevalence rate is about 0.4%–1.0%. For women, the lifetime prevalence rate of Gambling Disorder is about 0.2%, and for men, it is about 0.6%. Generally, Gambling Disorder develops over the course of years, although its progression appears to be more rapid in women than in men.

Loan Sharks

Steven Dawson, a 48-year-old attorney, was interviewed while he was being detained awaiting his sentencing. He had been arrested for taking funds from his firm, which he stated he had fully intended to return after he had a "big win" at gambling. He appeared deeply humiliated and remorseful about his behavior, although he had a previous history of near-arrests for defrauding his company of funds. His father had provided funds to extricate him from previous financial difficulties but refused to assist him this time. Mr. Dawson had to resign from his job under pressure from his firm. This outcome distressed him greatly, because he had worked diligently and effectively at his job, although he had been spending more and more time away from work in order to pursue gambling.

Mr. Dawson had gambled on horse racing for many years. He spent several hours each day studying the results of the previous day's races in the newspaper. He had been losing heavily recently and had resorted to illegal borrowing to increase his bets and win back his losses. He was now being pressured by loan sharks for payment. He stated that he embezzled the money to pay off these illegal debts because the threats of the loan sharks were so frightening to him that he could not concentrate or sleep. He admitted to having problems with his friends and wife since he had borrowed from them. His friends were now alienated and gave him little emotional support because they no longer had any faith in his repeated promises to limit his gambling. His wife had decided to leave him and live with her parents.

During the interview, Mr. Dawson was tense and restless, at times having to stand up and pace. He said he was having a flare-up of a duodenal ulcer. He was somewhat tearful throughout the interview. He said that although he realized his problems stemmed from his gambling, he still had a strong urge to gamble.

Discussion of "Loan Sharks"

Mr. Dawson is preoccupied with gambling, which has led to his being arrested for embezzlement and defaulting on debts, and the disruption of his marriage. After losing money gambling, he borrows more to gamble again. He has destroyed relationships and lost his job because of his gambling. He relies on others to support his gambling habit. All of these features are clearly beyond the bounds of recreational gambling and indicate a behavioral addiction, Gambling Disorder (DSM-5-TR, p. 661).

Although Mr. Dawson has engaged in antisocial behavior, a diagnosis of Antisocial Personality Disorder (see Section 18.5) is not appropriate because the antisocial behavior is limited to attempts to obtain money to pay off gambling debts, and there is neither a childhood history of antisocial behavior nor evidence of impaired occupational and interpersonal functioning other than that associated with his gambling.

CHAPTER 17

Neurocognitive Disorders

Neurocognitive Disorders are characterized by acquired deficits in cognitive functioning that represent a decline from a previously attained level of functioning. This acquired decline is in contrast to the cognitive deficits in Neurodevelopmental Disorders such as Intellectual Developmental Disorder (see Section 1.1), which have been present since birth or early life. Although cognitive deficits are present in many mental disorders (e.g., Schizophrenia, Bipolar and Related Disorders, Major Depressive Disorder), only disorders whose identifying features involve cognitive impairments are included in the DSM-5-TR Neurocognitive Disorders diagnostic class.

Cognitive domains that are affected in the DSM-5-TR Neurocognitive Disorders include the following:

1. *Complex attention*: Deficits involve problems with sustaining attention for a particular task, dividing attention between two or more tasks, or selectively paying attention to a task while filtering out extraneous stimuli and distractions. Individuals with deficits in complex attention have difficulty functioning in environments with multiple stimuli (e.g., TV, radio, conversations); have difficulty holding new information in mind, such as recalling phone numbers or addresses just given or reporting what was just said; or may be unable to perform mental calculations. Because of these attentional problems, all mental functions take longer than usual to perform, so cognition is generally slowed.

2. *Executive function*: Deficits involve difficulties in planning or decision-making, problems with working memory (inability to hold and manipulate information in memory), difficulties with feedback/error utilization (inability to benefit from feedback to improve the ability to solve a problem), and problems with mental flexibility (inability to shift between concepts). Individuals with executive function deficits lose their ability to plan and sequence a task because they can no longer prioritize each segment of an activity. Therefore, such individuals need to rely on others to plan instrumental activities of daily living (i.e., activities that are not necessary for fundamental functioning, but that allow an individual to live independently, such as performing housework or preparing meals) or help them make decisions.

3. *Learning and memory*: Deficits can involve 1) immediate memory (e.g., being unable to immediately repeat lists of numbers or words); 2) recent memory (e.g., free recall—being unable to freely recall a list of words or the elements of a story after a few minutes—or cued recall—being unable to recall a list of words or elements of a story even after being given cues, such as "tell me all of the food items on that list of words"); and 3) very-long-term memory, including semantic memory (i.e., memory for facts), autobiographical memory (i.e., memory for personal events or people), or memory for procedural learning (i.e., how to perform tasks). Individuals with deficits in memory and learning might repeat themselves in conversation, be unable to keep track of a short list of items while shopping, and require frequent reminders as to the task at hand.

4. *Language*: Deficits involve expressive language (including problems naming objects and word finding, fluency in speech, and problems with grammar and syntax) or receptive language (including trouble following verbal directions, understanding a story, or understanding figurative language).

5. *Perceptual-motor*: Deficits include problems in visual perception (e.g., inability to recognize faces), visuoconstructional problems (e.g., problems with drawing or copying figures or with block assembly), agnosia (e.g., problems recognizing what a familiar object is used for), and apraxia (e.g., problems with the ability to carry out a previously learned movement). Individuals with perceptual-motor deficits may have significant difficulties with previously familiar activities, such as using tools or driving a motor vehicle.

6. *Social cognition*: Deficits include problems with recognizing emotions in others and an inability to take into consideration other people's thoughts, desires, and intentions. For example, there may be insensitivity to social standards of modesty in dress or of political, religious, or sexual topics of conversation, or the person might focus excessively on a topic despite a group's disinterest or direct feedback.

There are three cognitive syndromes (i.e., collections of symptoms that occur together) that make up the Neurocognitive Disorders in DSM-5-TR: Delirium, Major Neurocognitive Disorder, and Mild Neurocognitive Disorder (see Table 17–1 for characteristic features). The first step in making a diagnosis of a DSM-5-TR Neurocognitive Disorder is to determine which of the three cognitive syndromes is present. Delirium is a distinct syndrome characterized by the acute onset of a fluctuating disturbance in attention to and awareness of the environment. It is independent of the Major or Mild Neurocognitive Disorder distinction because symptom severity in Delirium by definition fluctuates over the course of a day. Major and Mild Neurocognitive Disorders represent more and less severe categories, respectively, on a continuum of neurocognitive dysfunction. Major Neurocognitive Disorder is defined by a decline in one or more cognitive domains that is severe enough to significantly interfere with a person's everyday independence. Mild Neurocognitive Disorder involves a more modest decline that is not severe enough to significantly interfere with the person's capacity for independence in everyday activities.

Once the diagnosis of the appropriate neurocognitive syndrome is made on the basis of the symptom pattern and course (for Delirium) or severity (for Major and Mild Neurocognitive Disorders), the etiology of the neurocognitive syndrome must then

TABLE 17–1. **Characteristic features of Neurocognitive Syndromes**

Disorder	Key characteristics
Delirium	Disturbance in attention to and reduced awareness of the environment
	Develops over a short period of time and tends to fluctuate in severity over the course of a day
	Additional disturbance in cognition is required (e.g., memory deficits, disorientation, language, visuospatial ability, or perception)
Major Neurocognitive Disorder	Significant cognitive decline from a previous level of performance
	Deficits interfere with independence in everyday activities
Mild Neurocognitive Disorder	Modest cognitive decline from a previous level of performance on cognitive testing
	Deficits do not interfere with capacity for independence

be determined. These neurocognitive syndromes can be caused by any one of various nonpsychiatric medical conditions (e.g., Alzheimer's disease, head trauma, HIV infection, metabolic disturbances) or by the direct effects of a substance or medication. The appropriate DSM-5-TR diagnosis is constructed by combining the name of the syndrome with its etiology. For example, if an individual presents with a syndrome of Delirium that is caused by the metabolic effects of liver failure, the DSM-5-TR diagnosis would be Delirium Due to Hepatic Encephalopathy.

17.1
Delirium

The syndrome of Delirium is characterized by a disturbance of attention to and awareness of the environment (sometimes referred to as "clouding of consciousness") that develops over a short period of time (usually hours to a few days) and represents a change from the person's baseline levels of attention and awareness. A hallmark of Delirium is its tendency to fluctuate in severity over the course of a day, often worsening in the evening and night when external orienting stimuli are usually decreased. The attentional disturbance is manifested by a "reduced ability to direct, focus, sustain, and shift attention" (DSM-5-TR, p. 672). Questions must be repeated because the person's attention wanders, or the person may perseverate with an answer to a previous question rather than appropriately shifting attention to the next question. The disturbance in awareness is manifested by affected individuals being disoriented to where they are, to the time of day or day of the week, and at times even to themselves or other people such as family members.

The problems with attention and awareness are accompanied by other disturbances in cognition that may include impairments in memory and learning (particularly recent memory), alteration in the ability to speak or understand language, and perceptual disturbances (usually visual) that can include misinterpretations of stimuli (illusions) or frank hallucinations.

The syndrome of Delirium may result from an underlying nonpsychiatric medical condition, from medication or substance use, or from a combination of these factors. The most common causes are medication use, particularly anticholinergic medications; intoxication with or withdrawal from alcohol or psychoactive drugs; dehydration; and infections, such as pneumonia and septicemia (infection in the blood). Many other nonpsychiatric medical conditions can also cause Delirium, including strokes; head trauma; endocrine disorders, such as Cushing's syndrome and hyperthyroidism; and metabolic abnormalities, such as fluid and electrolyte abnormalities and those caused by liver or kidney failure.

The DSM-5-TR diagnosis of Delirium requires a determination of the presumed cause, given that treatment of Delirium requires that the underlying condition or exposure be addressed. The cause of the Delirium must be specified as one of the following etiological subtypes: Substance Intoxication Delirium, Substance Withdrawal Delirium, Medication-Induced Delirium, Delirium Due to Another Medical Condition, and Delirium Due to Multiple Etiologies.

Delirium may occur at any age but is more common among elderly persons. The prevalence of Delirium among individuals admitted to the hospital ranges from 18% to 35%, and estimates of the occurrence of Delirium arising during hospitalization range from 29% to 64% in general hospital populations. The prevalence of Delirium among individuals in nursing homes or post-acute care settings is 20%–22%, and the prevalence among individuals with terminal illness may be as high as 88%. When Delirium occurs in younger people, it is usually due to drug use or a life-threatening systemic (i.e., affecting the whole body) nonpsychiatric medical condition. The majority of individuals with Delirium make a full recovery with or without treatment, especially in individuals who are not elderly. However, Delirium may progress to stupor, coma, seizures, or death, particularly if it is undetected and the underlying cause(s) remains untreated.

Traction

Diego Hernandez is a previously healthy 32-year-old carpenter from Nevada who was involved in a motor vehicle accident as he was returning from a 3-month trip to Mexico. He was found by the state police and taken to the hospital. On admission, he was found to have multiple fractures involving his pelvis, toes on his right foot, and several ribs on his left side. He also sustained two small cuts on his head that required stitches. Mr. Hernandez reported that he had lost consciousness during the accident and had had a period of amnesia of about 15 minutes following it, but these were not witnessed. He was alert and complained of severe back pain; he was not disoriented. He was treated with a narcotic pain killer (meperidine, 125 mg intramuscularly every 3 hours) and a sleeping pill (zolpidem, 10 mg by mouth at bedtime). The following day, his back pain was unimproved, and his pain medication was changed to morphine.

Four days after admission, Mr. Hernandez developed a fever and was sweaty and tremulous. Because a history of drinking five to six beers a day had been elicited, the diagnosis of Alcohol Withdrawal was considered, and a benzodiazepine (diazepam, 5 mg by mouth every 6 hours) was added to his daily medication regimen, which at this time included a combination preparation of oxycodone 10 mg (narcotic) and acetaminophen 325 mg (analgesic), 1 or 2 capsules by mouth every 3–4 hours, and zolpidem (sleep medication), 10 mg at bedtime. The next day he was described as anxious, agitated, and constantly scratching. Two days later he was still febrile (had fever). Blood cultures (a blood test looking for bacteria in the blood), urinalysis, and chest X-ray were negative. An antihistamine (hydroxyzine, 25 mg by mouth 4 times a day) was given to relieve itching.

Eight days after admission, Mr. Hernandez was noted to be disoriented. He complained that it took him some time to realize where he was on awakening. His temperature was still elevated. He was receiving morphine (3–10 mg every 3 hours for pain), a muscle relaxant (diazepam, 5 mg by mouth every 6 hours), and a hypnotic (zolpidem, 10 mg by mouth at bedtime). The next day, his pain medication was again changed, this time to a combination preparation of the narcotic oxycodone (10 mg) and acetaminophen (325 mg, 1 or 2 tablets every 3 hours) and the narcotic pain killer meperidine (75 mg intramuscularly every 4 hours).

One day later, Mr. Hernandez underwent an open reduction (surgery to realign a bone fracture) for a fractured left acetabulum (the socket of the hip bone). The surgery, conducted under general anesthesia, was tolerated well; however, immediately following the procedure, the patient was disoriented to time and place and was noted to be picking at things in the air. His temperature was still elevated, although there was no documented source of infection. At this time the patient was receiving meperidine (75–100 mg intramuscularly every 4 hours), hydroxyzine (75 mg every 3 hours), and acetaminophen every 4 hours.

Over the next few days, Mr. Hernandez's mental status improved, although he was still disoriented at times and confessed, "You know, sometimes I can't pay attention to what you're saying." His temperature was still moderately elevated. Medication consisted of a synthetic opioid, hydromorphone (2–4 mg every 3–4 hours). The continuing periods of disorientation disturbed his doctors, and a psychiatric consultation was requested.

At the initial interview with the psychiatrist, now 17 days after the accident, Mr. Hernandez was alert, fully oriented, and in good spirits. Results of mental status testing were normal. The patient admitted having had difficulties in thinking and "hallucinations" at times during the previous couple of weeks. He described them as "opiate dreams," caused by his pain medication.

Over the next few days, Mr. Hernandez's condition was generally improved during the daytime hours, but at night, he was frequently found to be taking his traction apparatus apart. When discovered, he would sometimes talk incoherently about the "traction thingamajig." If questioned the next day, he always denied having dismantled the equipment. At this time, he was taking an acetaminophen-oxycodone combination (2 capsules every 6 hours) for pain. He often complained of severe pain, many times arguing with his doctors in an attempt to persuade them to give him his pain medication more often. The psychiatrist was called in again to help, and the pain medication was given more frequently. It was felt that the patient's addiction potential was not very high at that time.

Several days later, Mr. Hernandez was observed to be playing with fecal matter in his bed and once again dismantling his traction apparatus. When discovered, he admitted to these acts, was so upset that he could not sleep that night, and asked to see a psychiatrist. When interviewed, he appeared anxious and angry. He stated that he did not understand what was happening to him and was very upset about his behavior. He said he had not been sleeping more than 2–3 hours a night for at least 2 weeks. He was very frightened by the thought that his mind was doing things he was not aware of and could not control. He asked for a "game plan" to stop this behavior and even suggested stopping all pain medication if necessary. Over the next few days, the pain medication was reduced. The patient now appeared alert and oriented, and there were no further episodes of disturbed behavior at night.

Discussion of "Traction"

Mr. Hernandez's presentation has all of the hallmarks of a Delirium. Beginning 8 days after admission to the hospital and continuing for several weeks, Mr. Hernandez intermittently showed reduced awareness of and decreased ability to maintain attention to external stimuli ("I can't pay attention to what you're saying"). He had additional symptoms, such as disorientation to place and time and visual hallucinations (he picked at things in the air and had "opiate dreams"). The symptoms came on suddenly and fluctuated throughout the day, but were often worse during the nighttime.

There is no difficulty in identifying several physical factors that could have contributed to the development of Delirium: infection, fever, and the large number of analgesics and sedatives that the patient received. (It is not clear from the case record why Mr. Hernandez's medications were changed so often.) The diagnosis is therefore Delirium Due to Multiple Etiologies (DSM-5-TR, p. 674). Once the causes of the Delirium were corrected (i.e., resolution of his medical problems and a reduction in his medication), the Delirium completely resolved.

Thunderbird

Tremaine Graves, a 43-year-old divorced construction worker, is examined in the hospital emergency room because for the last few days he has been confused and unable to take care of himself. The patient's sister is available to provide some information. The sister reports that the patient has consumed large quantities of cheap wine daily for more than 5 years. He had a reasonably stable home life and job record until his wife left him for another man 5 years previously. The sister indicates that Mr. Graves drinks more than a bottle of wine a day and that this has been an unvarying pattern since the divorce. He often has had blackouts from drinking and has missed work; consequently, he has been fired from several jobs. Fortunately for him, with the recent building boom, construction workers have been in great demand, so he has been able to provide marginally for himself during these years. However, 3 days ago, he ran out of money and wine and had to beg on the street to buy a meal. The patient has been poorly nourished, eating perhaps one meal a day and evidently relying on the wine as his primary source of nourishment.

The morning after his last day of drinking (3 days earlier), Mr. Graves felt increasingly tremulous—his hands were shaking so grossly that it was difficult for him to light a cigarette. Accompanying these physical sensations was an increasing sense of inner panic, which had made him unable to sleep. A neighbor became concerned about the patient when he seemed not to be making sense and was clearly unable to take care of himself. The neighbor contacted the sister, who took Mr. Graves to the hospital.

On examination, Mr. Graves alternates between apprehension and chatty, superficial warmth. He is quite keyed up and talks almost constantly in a rambling and unfocused manner. At times he recognizes the doctor, but at other times he gets confused and thinks the doctor is his older brother. Twice during the examination, he calls the doctor by his older brother's name and asks when he arrived, evidently having entirely lost track of the interview up to that point. He has a gross hand tremor at rest, and there are periods when he picks at "bugs" he sees on the bedsheets. He is disoriented to time and place (he thinks that he is in a supermarket parking lot rather than in a hospital). He indicates that he feels he is fighting against a terrifying sense that the world is ending in a holocaust. He is startled every few minutes by sounds and scenes of fiery car crashes (evidently evoked by the sound of rolling carts in the hall). Efforts at testing his memory and calculation fail because his attention shifts too rapidly.

Discussion of "Thunderbird"

Mr. Graves, who has a long history of heavy alcohol use, has developed severe withdrawal symptoms after he stopped drinking. He has the characteristic symptoms of a Delirium: a disturbance in attention (his attention shifts too rapidly to test his memory and ability to do calculations) and awareness (he thinks that he is in a supermarket parking lot rather than in a hospital), accompanied by other cognitive deficits, including disorganized thinking (rambling), perceptual disturbances (he sees scenes of car crashes evoked by the sound of rolling carts in the hall), and confusion (he mistakes the doctor for his brother). The appearance of a Delirium, with marked autonomic hyperactivity (hand tremors), shortly after cessation or reduction of heavy alcohol ingestion indicates Alcohol Withdrawal Delirium (DSM-5-TR, p. 673). Alcohol Withdrawal Delirium, commonly known as delirium tremens (DTs), is potentially life-threatening because of the possibility of respiratory failure and cardiac arrhythmias and requires hospital admission and administration of intravenous sedatives. It typically occurs only in people with a high intake of alcohol for more than 1 month and occurs 3–10 days following the last drink. About half of people with Alcohol Use Disorder will develop withdrawal symptoms after reducing alcohol use. Of these, 3%–5% develop DTs or have seizures.

Although Mr. Graves' treatment will initially be directed at the Alcohol Withdrawal Delirium, the additional diagnosis of Alcohol Use Disorder (DSM-5-TR, p. 553) can be assumed from the information that he has been a heavy daily user of alcohol for more than 5 years, has lost jobs because of his alcohol use, and has been poorly nourished.

17.2
Major Neurocognitive Disorder

The syndrome of Major Neurocognitive Disorder, historically referred to as "dementia," is characterized by an acquired cognitive decline in one or more of the domains discussed in the introductory section to this chapter (i.e., complex attention, executive function, learning and memory, language, perceptual-motor, and social cognition). DSM-5 introduced the term *major neurocognitive disorder* as a replacement for the term *dementia* to help reduce the stigma associated with both the earlier word (which comes from the Latin word *demens*, which means "out of one's mind") and the condition to which it refers.

The evidence for cognitive decline can come from any of a number of possible sources: from the individual, who might complain, for example, of difficulties remembering a short grocery list or planning a holiday meal; from a friend or family member who might observe the person having difficulties performing certain tasks, such as driving a car; or from a clinician, who might observe the presence of cognitive deficits during a mental status examination (see "Backstage With Rosie" in Section 17.3). In addition, however, there must also be evidence of substantial impairment in performance on cognitive testing, preferably documented by neuropsychological testing, in which the person's performance is compared with standardized norms appropriate to the person's age, educational attainment, and cultural background. A diagnosis of Major Neurocognitive Disorder typically requires performance on testing that is two or more standard deviations below the norms (i.e., 3rd percentile or below). Finally, for the diagnosis of Major Neurocognitive Disorder to apply, the cognitive deficits must be severe enough to interfere with the person's ability to function independently. At a minimum, a person with Major Neurocognitive Disorder would require assistance with complex instrumental activities of daily living, such as paying bills or managing medications.

A number of additional cognitive, perceptual, emotional, and behavioral features are commonly part of the presentation of a Major Neurocognitive Disorder. These include psychotic features such as paranoia, other delusions, or hallucinations, which may occur in any modality; mood disturbances, including depression, anxiety, and elation; agitation, which may arise as combative behaviors particularly in the context of resisting caregiving duties such as bathing and dressing; sleep disturbances, which may include symptoms of insomnia, sleeping excessively, and circadian rhythm disturbances; apathy, which may include diminished motivation, reduced goal-directed behavior, and decreased emotional responsiveness; and other behavioral symptoms, including wandering, disinhibition, hyperphagia (overeating), and hoarding. When such features are severe enough to be clinically significant, the appropriate specifier—With Agitation; With Anxiety; With Mood Symptoms (e.g., dysphoria, irritability, euphoria); With Psychotic Disturbance (i.e., delusions and/or hallucinations); and either With or Without Other Behavioral or Psychological Disturbance (e.g., apathy, aggression, disinhibition, disruptive behaviors or vocalizations, sleep or appetite/eating disturbance)—can be assigned, along with the diagnosis of Major Neurocognitive Disorder.

After it is determined that the syndrome of Major Neurocognitive Disorder is present, the specific DSM-5-TR diagnosis depends on the etiology of the cognitive deficits. Major Neurocognitive Disorder can be caused by a variety of nonpsychiatric medical conditions. The most common form (60%–70% of cases) is due to Alzheimer's disease, a chronic neurodegenerative disease associated with the development of plaques (abnormal clusters of chemically "sticky" proteins called β-amyloid that build up between nerve cells) and tangles (twisted strands of a protein called tau, which can be seen on microscopic examination) in the brain. Other nonpsychiatric medical conditions that can cause Major Neurocognitive Disorder include frontotemporal lobar degeneration (a neurodegenerative disease preferentially affecting the frontal and temporal lobes of the brain), Lewy body disease (a neurodegenerative disease in which protein deposits called Lewy bodies develop in nerve cells in the brain), vascular disease (which can cause a series of large or small strokes), traumatic brain injury (from an impact to the head or to rapid movement or displacement of the bran within the skull), Parkinson's disease (a neurodegenerative disorder that affects predominately the dopamine-producing neurons in a specific area of the brain called substantia nigra), Huntington's disease (an inherited disease that causes the progressive breakdown [degeneration] of nerve cells in the brain), prion disease (caused by microscopic infectious agents made of protein), and HIV infection (now uncommon due to availability of combination antiretroviral therapy). Substance use (particularly inhalant abuse and chronic heavy alcohol or sedative use) can also cause severe cognitive deficits (especially memory impairment) that persist long after the person has stopped using the substance. Certain medications (e.g., those with anticholinergic properties such as scopolamine for motion sickness and diphenhydramine for allergies) can cause neurocognitive impairment, especially in the elderly.

Finally, Major Neurocognitive Disorder can be caused by multiple co-occurring etiologies (e.g., both vascular disease and Alzheimer's disease).

Among individuals older than 60 years, the prevalence of Neurocognitive Disorders increases steeply with age. Overall prevalence estimates for Major Neurocognitive Disorder are approximately 1%–2% at age 65 years and as high as 30% by age 85 years. Female gender is associated with a higher prevalence of dementia overall, and especially of Alzheimer's disease, but this difference is largely, if not wholly, attributable to the greater longevity of women. Large-scale studies indicate that rates of suicidal behavior are elevated in individuals with a Neurocognitive Disorder (due to a variety of etiologies) compared with those without a Neurocognitive Disorder.

The Hiker

At age 61, Samuel Walling, a science department head at a small rural high school and an experienced and enthusiastic camper and hiker, became extremely fearful while on a trek in the mountains. Gradually, over the next few months, he lost interest in his usual hobbies. Formerly a voracious reader, he stopped reading. He had difficulty doing computations and made gross errors in home financial management. On several occasions he became lost while driving in areas that were formerly familiar to him. He began to write notes to himself so that he would not forget to do errands. Very abruptly, and in uncharacteristic fashion, he decided to retire from work, without discussing his plans with his wife. Intellectual deterioration gradually progressed. He spent most of the day piling miscellaneous objects in one place and then transporting them to another spot in the house. He became stubborn and querulous. Eventually, he required assistance in shaving and dressing.

When examined during a follow-up evaluation at age 67, 6 years after the first symptoms had developed, Mr. Walling was alert and cooperative. He was disoriented with respect to place (he did not know where he was) and time (he did not know the year, month, or day of the week). He could not recall the names of five objects after a 5-minute interval of distraction. He could not remember the names of his college and graduate school or the subject in which he had majored. He could describe his job by title only. In 2023, he thought that Barack Obama was president of the United States. His speech was fluent and well-articulated, but he had considerable difficulty finding words and used many long, essentially meaningless phrases. He called a cup a "vase," and identified the rims of eyeglasses as "the holders." His performance of simple calculations was poor. He could not copy a cube or draw a house. He had no insight into the nature of his problems. When asked about what the proverb "people who live in glass houses shouldn't throw stones" means, Mr. Walling replied, "you have to be careful of falling stones if you have too many windows in your house."

An elementary neurological examination revealed nothing abnormal, and routine laboratory tests were also negative. A computed tomography (CT) scan of the brain, however, showed marked cortical (i.e., white matter) atrophy (a decrease in amount). Other, more sophisticated (and more expensive) laboratory testing that is more specific for diagnosing Alzheimer's disease, like a positron emission tomography scan, was not available in his small community.

Discussion of "The Hiker"

Mr. Walling has memory impairment (both short term, in that he was unable to remember five objects after 5 minutes, and long term, in that he was unable to remember where he attended college or what subject was his major); impairment in abstract thinking (concrete interpretation of proverbs); and other disturbances in higher cortical functioning (severe language problems). These signs of global cognitive impairment, severe enough to interfere significantly with work and social activities, and not occurring exclusively during the course of Delirium, indicate a Major Neurocognitive Disorder. Furthermore, although not a required feature, Mr. Walling's change in personality (becoming stubborn and querulous) is a common associated feature that can contribute to difficulties in managing the condition.

Up until relatively recently, the only way to make a definitive diagonals of Alzheimer's disease was by microscopically examining the person's brain after their death. While there is no single laboratory test that can determine if a person is living with Alzheimer's disease, the diagnosis can be made with a high degree of confidence if characteristic clinical features are present, combined with laboratory testing. These clinical features include the presence of a characteristic course (steadily progressive, gradual decline in cognition, without extended plateaus) and a characteristic pattern of symptoms (clear evidence of decline in memory and learning, and impairment involving at least one other cognitive domain). Laboratory tests that are specifically useful for making a diagnosis of Alzheimer's disease include brain positron emission tomography scans showing deposition of amyloid beta 42 (protein fragments deposited in the brain in plaques, which are increased in Alzheimer's disease) and increased tau protein in the cerebrospinal fluid. In Mr. Walling's case, he has impairment in short- and long-term memory, as well as in several other domains. Moreover, the onset of his decline was insidious, and the course of his deterioration has been gradual and steady over the past 6 years. Finally, the normal findings on the neurological examination and on routine laboratory testing and the lack of evidence of vascular disease on the CT scan suggest that other potential causes of the Major Neurocognitive Disorder can be ruled out. Thus, the diagnosis is Major Neurocognitive Disorder Due to Alzheimer's Disease (DSM-5-TR, p. 690). Although the CT finding of marked cortical atrophy is certainly consistent with a diagnosis of Alzheimer's disease, it is too nonspecific to be of diagnostic value.

Certified Public Accountant

Maurice Rosen was age 69 when he made an appointment for a neurological evaluation. He had recently noticed that his memory was slipping and he had problems with concentration that were beginning to interfere with his work as a self-employed tax accountant. He complained of slowness and losing his train of thought. Recent changes in the tax laws were hard for him to learn, and his wife said he was becoming more withdrawn and reluctant to initiate activities. However, he was still able to take care of his personal finances and to accompany his wife on visits with friends. Although mildly depressed about the decline in his cognitive abilities, he denied other symptoms of depression, such as disturbed sleep or appetite, feelings of guilt, or suicidal ideation.

Mr. Rosen has a long history of treatment for episodes of depression, beginning in his 20s. He has taken a number of different antidepressant medications, and once was treated with a course of electroconvulsive therapy (a procedure done under general anesthesia, in which small electrical currents are passed through the brain, intentionally triggering a brief seizure). As recently as 6 months before the current evaluation, he had been taking the antidepressant drug fluoxetine. Two years earlier, he had developed an intermittent resting tremor in his left hand and a shuffling gait. Although the diagnosis of Parkinson's disease was considered by his psychiatrist at that time, it was not confirmed by a neurologist, and therefore no additional treatment was given.

The neurologist who was now evaluating Mr. Rosen found that his spontaneous speech was hesitant and unclear (dysarthric). Findings from the cranial nerve examination (an examination of the nerves that emanate directly from the brain) were normal. Motor tone was increased slightly in his neck and in all limbs. Rapid alternating movements of his hands were performed slowly. His left arm had a slight intermittent tremor at rest. His reflexes were symmetrical (the same strength on both sides). A diagnosis of idiopathic Parkinson's disease was made, and Mr. Rosen was placed on a low dosage of carbidopa-levodopa, a medication that alleviates the symptoms of Parkinson's disease.

A neuropsychological examination performed 3 weeks later revealed average performance on the Wechsler Adult Intelligence Scale; Mr. Rosen had a full-scale IQ of 104, a verbal IQ of 118, and a performance IQ of 84. Memory was poor, as assessed by a 12-item, 10-trial selective reminding task, with no more than seven items recalled on any trial, and only three words recalled after a 15-minute delay, although Mr. Rosen could recognize the remaining words. He showed marked difficulty in drawings of overlapping figures and parallel lines. He was unable to draw three-dimensional figures. He demonstrated impaired naming in language testing. In summary, he had evidence of impairment in memory, naming, and constructional abilities. His deficits were believed to be due to Parkinson's disease. Additional evaluation included magnetic resonance imaging, which revealed only generalized atrophy, and an electroencephalogram, which was significant for background generalized slowing.

Mr. Rosen's motor function improved as he continued taking Parkinson's medication, but his memory worsened, and he described occasional difficulty telling time and writing checks. His wife said he would immediately forget conversations or movie plots. He was again treated with the antidepressant medication fluoxetine, but without improvement in his cognitive status. He then had a small stroke that temporarily affected his motor function. With all of these new difficulties, he decided to retire. The following year, he reported increasing difficulty in decision-making, memory impairment, and more word-finding problems. His Parkinson's disease had also worsened. In the second year after his evaluation, his speech became more difficult to understand, and he had "freezing" episodes (his foot "sticking" to the floor because he could not lift it), resulting in falls. He frequently used the wrong words in conversation. His memory continued to worsen, and he was unable to care for himself without a great deal of assistance from his wife.

Discussion of "Certified Public Accountant"

Although the first neurologist who saw Mr. Rosen did not make a diagnosis of Parkinson's disease, the subsequent development of an intermittent resting tremor and abnormalities in speech and other motor functions confirmed the diagnosis. The second neurological evaluation was prompted primarily by the patient's cognitive symptoms, which included failing memory, problems with concentration, and difficulty in the initiation of goal-directed activities. On neuropsychological examination, Mr. Rosen showed impairment in memory, naming, and constructional abilities. All of these symptoms, when they are sufficiently severe to cause significant impairment in functioning, indicate the presence of a Major Neurocognitive Disorder. Because the onset of Parkinson's disease clearly preceded the onset of the Major Neurocognitive Disorder, the impairments had insidious onset and gradual progression, and there was no evidence of a mixed etiology, the diagnosis indicated in Mr. Rosen's case is Major Neurocognitive Disorder Due to Parkinson's Disease (DSM-5-TR, p. 723).

The prevalence of Parkinson's disease in the United States steadily increases with age, from approximately 0.4% of individuals between ages 60 and 69 years to 1.4% of those between ages 80 and 89 years. Parkinson's disease is more common in men than in women. Among individuals with Parkinson's disease, as many as 80% will develop a Major Neurocognitive Disorder sometime in the course of their disease.

Chief Petty Officer

A medical student on rotation at a chronic-disease hospital was assigned to present at rounds a 56-year-old retired chief petty officer. Will Genardo was a long-time heavy consumer of alcoholic beverages. Following his divorce many years previously, his drinking had become exceptionally heavy, and he underwent a change in personality. He was often belligerent, even when sober, and on several occasions had assaulted members of his family. This disturbing behavior had necessitated two brief admissions to mental hospitals. Mr. Genardo persisted in his heavy drinking, and on several other occasions had been admitted to hospitals for tremulousness and hallucinations associated with Alcohol Withdrawal. As far as was known, he had never had major head trauma or a stroke. Finally, because of his inability to care for himself properly, he had been sent to live in a nursing home, but because of his belligerent and disruptive behavior, admission to this hospital had been found necessary 7 years earlier.

When examined by the student, Mr. Genardo was somewhat peevish and inattentive. His consciousness was not clouded, however, and he was not hallucinating. He knew the name of the hospital but not the correct date. He could not retain the names of five objects after a brief interval of distraction. He remembered events of his youth and young manhood but not those of more recent years. He remembered the events of 9/11 but had no recollection of the 2021 U.S. withdrawal from Afghanistan. His language was normal, but he could not copy the drawing of a two- or three-dimensional figure. He could not do even simple calculations, and he interpreted proverbs very concretely. Neurological examinations revealed somewhat diminished ankle jerk reflexes, and he had mild unsteadiness of gait. Laboratory tests failed to reveal any positive evidence for the etiology of the disturbance.

Discussion of "Chief Petty Officer"

Mr. Genardo's short-term and recent memory disturbances, combined with his marked loss of intellectual abilities, poor judgment, and other disturbances of higher cortical functioning (e.g., inability to copy drawings and do calculations, concrete responses to proverbs) that significantly interfere with his ability to take care of himself, all indicate the presence of a Major Neurocognitive Disorder. The differential diagnosis of a Major Neurocognitive Disorder involves a search for specific causes, such as head trauma (particularly important in someone with a history of Alcohol Use Disorder, given the increased risk of accidents and physical altercations during intoxication) or a brain tumor. In Mr. Genardo's case, the absence of a history of trauma and the failure of the laboratory tests to reveal the etiology of the Neurocognitive Disorder make prolonged heavy drinking the most likely etiological agent; thus, the diagnosis is Alcohol-Induced Major Neurocognitive Disorder (DSM-5-TR, p. 712). Because of his history of clinically significant belligerence and disruptive behavior, the specifier With Other Behavioral or Psychological Disturbance would apply (DSM-5-TR, p. 713). A diagnosis of Major Neurocognitive Disorder Due to Alzheimer's Disease is ruled out because the course has remained relatively stable over many years.

17.3
Mild Neurocognitive Disorder

Most healthy people experience a gradual decline in mental abilities as part of aging. In someone with Mild Neurocognitive Disorder, however, the decline in mental abilities is greater than would be seen in normal aging. For example, it's common for anyone to find themselves in their kitchen without remembering why they are there or to run into an acquaintance in the grocery store and forget their name. But when these types of occurrences happen repetitively and on a daily basis, the symptoms are often beyond features of normal aging.

It is also important to distinguish the syndrome of Mild Neurocognitive Disorder from its more severe counterpart, Major Neurocognitive Disorder. In contrast to Major Neurocognitive Disorder, in which there is a significant decline in cognitive functioning, the level of cognitive decline in Mild Neurocognitive Disorder is only "modest." Moreover, whereas performance on neuropsychological testing is in the 3rd percentile or lower for Major Neurocognitive Disorder, in Mild Neurocognitive Disorder, tested performance typically lies one to two standard deviations below average range (between the 3rd and 16th percentiles). Finally, whereas the cognitive impairments in Major Neurocognitive Disorder are severe enough to interfere with independence in everyday activities, the decline in cognitive functioning that is characteristic of Mild Neurocognitive Disorder, by definition, does not interfere with the person's capacity for independence in everyday activities, such as paying bills or managing medications, although greater effort or extra time, the use of compensatory strategies, or other accommodations may be required. Mild Neurocognitive Disorder was added to DSM-5 with the intention of providing an opportunity for early detection and treatment of cognitive decline before patients' deficits become more pronounced and progress to Major Neurocognitive Disorder or other debilitating conditions.

As with the diagnosis of Major Neurocognitive Disorder, the actual DSM-5-TR diagnosis for Mild Neurocognitive Disorder depends on the etiology of the cognitive deficits (see DSM-5-TR, p. 681, for a list of conditions and substances that can cause Mild Neurocognitive Disorder).

Estimates of the prevalence of Mild Neurocognitive Disorder among older individuals are quite variable and are sensitive to how it has been defined in different studies. Prevalence estimates range from 2% to 10% at age 65 and from 5% to 25% by age 85.

Backstage With Rosie[1]

Rosie Shapiro, a 70-year-old lifelong New Yorker, was brought by her niece to an evaluation and treatment center specializing in problems in the elderly. The niece, who lives in a rural community 70 miles away, had become concerned after a regular monthly visit to her aunt's apartment in the city. On the visit, the niece noticed that her aunt's supply of food was unusually low. The few fruits and vegetables in the refrigerator were rotten, and unopened mail was piling up. When she asked her aunt about these, the elderly woman looked surprised and said, "Well, I guess I didn't get around to my chores this week!" Otherwise, she seemed her normal self.

---

[1]Adapted from Skodol AE: *Problems in Differential Diagnosis: From DSM-III to DSM-III-R in Clinical Practice.* Washington, DC, American Psychiatric Press, 1989, pp. 93–94. Copyright © 1989 American Psychiatric Press. Used with permission.

In fact, Mrs. Shapiro's niece had become increasingly uneasy about her aunt's living situation over the past year. Her aunt had no children of her own and, since her husband's death 5 years before, had been living alone in an apartment that she had inhabited for 35 years. The niece, as the closest living family member, had assumed the responsibility for a monthly drive to the city to visit and check on Mrs. Shapiro's well-being.

In earlier years, Mrs. Shapiro had had a weekly routine that she always followed: going on Mondays to the grocery store, doing her laundry on Tuesdays, and so forth. But for a year, her schedule seemed to have become disrupted. She seemed also to be constantly misplacing things in her apartment and repeating stories and details of her daily life that she had told her niece on previous visits.

When the psychiatrist interviewed Mrs. Shapiro, he found that she was a woman with a rich and exciting past. Both she and her husband had been in the theater, her husband a manager and Mrs. Shapiro a wardrobe designer. Her eyes lit up as she spoke of shows like *Cabaret* and *A Chorus Line* and shared some ancient gossip about romantic liaisons between actors and actresses who starred in movies and who were on the covers of magazines when the psychiatrist was a child.

When asked to name the current president of the United States, she replied, "you know, what's his name." But no matter how hard she tried, Mrs. Shapiro could not remember the president's name. In addition, many other current common facts and events eluded Mrs. Shapiro's recall. She would look up at the ceiling and then at the psychiatrist, shaking her head and saying, "I knew that, you know. I just can't seem to think of it right now." As for her reason for coming to the hospital, she said, "Well, I was due for a checkup. A friend of the family is an internist and he insisted that I come over."

Mrs. Shapiro was unable to remember any of three objects a few minutes after she had repeated them. She struggled but performed the serial 7s task (i.e., a test of cognitive functioning in which a person is asked to count backward from 100 by 7s) with only two mistakes. She was able to repeat six numbers and find similarities between objects and, except for some difficulty with word and name finding, showed no marked aphasia (language impairment), apraxia (impairment in ability to perform purposeful movements), or agnosia (impairment in the ability to interpret sensations and hence to recognize things). She had difficulty correctly copying the figure of intersecting pentagons, which is part of the MMSE (Mini-Mental State Examination), which surprised her, as she reported always having been good at copying things. She admitted that her forgetfulness was "getting to be a problem" and agreed to let the psychiatrist and her niece arrange for some home assistance.

A workup for the presence of a nonpsychiatric medical problem that might be responsible for Mrs. Shapiro's memory decline was negative except for the beginning signs of cortical atrophy (shrinkage of her cerebral cortex) on a CT scan.

Discussion of "Backstage With Rosie"

Mrs. Shapiro has clearly experienced a decline in cognitive functioning, primarily in the domain of memory, that has gradually developed over the past several years. As is commonly the case with individuals with Neurocognitive Disorders, the patient came to clinical attention because of concerns raised by a family member (in this case her niece) rather than by the patient herself. In addition to her niece noticing that her aunt's food supply had gotten low and that mail was piling up unopened, the niece noticed that her aunt seemed to be constantly misplacing things and that she was repeating stories and details of her daily life that she had told her niece on previous visits. There was also accompanying objective evidence of memory impairment, as evidenced by her inability during the mental status examination to remember any of the three objects that the psychiatrist asked her to remember and her inability to remember the name of the current U.S. president. Given that her memory problems are not yet sufficiently severe to interfere with her capacity for independence in everyday activities (i.e., she is still able to live independently, albeit with some home assistance for complex tasks like grocery shopping), Mrs. Shapiro would be diagnosed as having the syndrome of Mild Neurocognitive Disorder rather than Major Neurocognitive Disorder.

As is required for a diagnosis of Major Neurocognitive Disorder, the DSM-5-TR diagnosis of Mild Neurocognitive Disorder requires specification of a presumed etiology. Given that 1) there is clear evidence of decline in memory and learning and impairment in at least one other cognitive domain (impaired visual motor ability, as evidenced by the patient's inability to correctly copy the intersecting pentagons portion of the MMSE), and 2) the course of the development of the cognitive deficits is consistent with the typical course of Alzheimer's disease (i.e., a steadily progressive, gradual decline in cognition, with insidious onset, and without extended plateaus), the DSM-5-TR diagnosis in Mrs. Shapiro's case would be Mild Neurocognitive Disorder Due to Possible Alzheimer's Disease (DSM-5-TR, p. 690).

The most likely pressing issue for Mrs. Shapiro and her niece is what the future is likely to hold for Mrs. Shapiro in terms of the likelihood of continued cognitive decline that would justify a change in diagnosis from Mild Neurocognitive Disorder to Major Neurocognitive Disorder Due to Alzheimer's Disease. Longitudinal studies of patients with Mild Neurocognitive Disorder suggest that most individuals do eventually progress to Major Neurocognitive Disorder Due to Alzheimer's Disease (with an estimated 10%–15% "converting" each year in clinical samples).

CHAPTER 18

Personality Disorders

Personality Disorders are among the most impairing of mental disorders, are difficult to diagnose, and are challenging to treat. Personality Disorders are typified by significant problems in self-appraisal and self-regulation and by impaired interpersonal relationships. Up to 50% of all patients evaluated in clinical settings have a Personality Disorder, often in combination with other mental disorders, making Personality Disorders among the most common disorders seen by mental health care professionals. Personality Disorders are associated with high rates of social and occupational impairments, and the presence of a comorbid Personality Disorder predicts a slower recovery, a higher risk of relapse, and a more chronic course for a host of other mental disorders.

DSM's exclusively categorical approach to the diagnosis of Personality Disorders, however, has been criticized ever since the publication of DSM-III in 1980. Well-documented problems with the categorical approach include the extensive co-occurrence of Personality Disorders, such that most patients receiving a Personality Disorder diagnosis have personality features that meet criteria for more than one Personality Disorder; the extreme heterogeneity among patients with the same Personality Disorder diagnosis, meaning that two patients with a particular Personality Disorder may have very few features in common; the instability of Personality Disorders over time, occurring at rates that are incompatible with the basic definition of a Personality Disorder; the arbitrary diagnostic thresholds, set with little or no empirical basis, resulting in the reification of disorders as present or absent, with variable levels of underlying pathology and limited validity and clinical utility; the poor coverage of personality pathology; and the poor convergent validity of Personality Disorder criterion sets, such that patient groups diagnosed by different methods may be only weakly related to one another.

Although these problems were well recognized during the development of DSM-5 and a new model of personality psychopathology designed to rectify them was developed, it was decided that there were not enough empirical data to support the new model, or clear evidence of its clinical utility, at the time of DSM-5's publication in 2013. Therefore, two models of Personality Disorders were provided in DSM-5 and were continued unchanged in DSM-5-TR:

- In the main section of DSM-5-TR (i.e., Section II, "Diagnostic Criteria and Codes"), a Personality Disorder is defined as "an enduring pattern of inner experience and behavior that deviates markedly from the norms and expectations of the individual's culture, is pervasive and inflexible, has an onset in adolescence or early adulthood, is stable over time, and leads to distress or impairment" (DSM-5-TR, p. 733). The pattern is manifested in two or more of the following areas: cognition, affectivity, interpersonal functioning, and impulse control.

- In Section III, "Emerging Measures and Models," an Alternative DSM-5 Model for Personality Disorders is provided, because the Personality Disorder features described in DSM-5-TR Section II are not sufficiently specific to Personality Disorders and may characterize other chronic mental disorders. According to this alternative empirically derived model, Personality Disorders are characterized by impairments in personality functioning, including the areas of identity, self-direction, empathy, and intimacy, and by the presence of pathological personality traits (DSM-5-TR, p. 881). *Impairments in personality functioning* have been demonstrated to be core features of personality psychopathology and to accurately identify Personality Disorders, thus aiding in the discrimination of Personality Disorders from other types of mental disorders. *Pathological personality traits* describe the myriad manifestations in the presentations of personality pathology.

The manifestations of personality pathology, according to either of the DSM-5-TR models described above, are relatively pervasive, meaning that they are exhibited in a wide range of contexts and situations, not only in a particular situation or with a given person. The Alternative Model describes Personality Disorders as "relatively stable" (Section III, Criterion D, p. 881) rather than simply "stable" (Section II, Criterion D, p. 735) because longitudinal research has shown that Personality Disorders change over time and have a clinical course that tends toward improvement or remission.

Co-occurrence of mental disorders is very common in clinical populations and in the community because certain types of signs and symptoms tend to vary together. This covariation has led to attempts to understand the organization of psychopathology by identifying dimensions that might underlie groups of disorders by factor analyses of disorder manifestations. Two broad dimensions, or "spectra," referred to as "internalizing" and "externalizing" (DSM-5-TR, p. 12), have been identified that encompass a large number of nonpsychotic mental disorders. Simply put, *internalizing* involves the individual expressing problems via negative feelings and behaviors directed at themself and includes, for example, symptoms of depression and anxiety. In contrast, *externalizing* involves the individual expressing problems via negative feelings and behaviors directed at other people or things in the environment and includes, for example, symptoms of aggression, violence, and defiance. A third identified spectrum—referred to as the "thought disorder spectrum" (not discussed specifically in DSM-5-TR)—includes Psychotic Disorders and Bipolar I Disorder. Even though disorders within these three broad domains are assigned to different diagnostic classes in DSM-5-TR, they have been shown to share genetic, environmental, and temperamental risk factors; exhibit common cognitive and emotional processing abnormalities; and respond to similar treatments. A classification of mental problems based on empirical methods may include both symptoms—relatively transient forms of psychopathology—and maladaptive personality traits that are thought to form the stable core of many mental disorders.

The Alternative DSM-5 Model for Personality Disorders describes personality pathology in terms of five broad trait domains, within the internalizing, externalizing, and thought disorder spectra. The domains and their definitions are as follows (DSM-5-TR, pp. 899–901):

1. *Negative Affectivity*: Frequent and intense experiences of high levels of a wide range of negative emotions (e.g., anxiety, depression, guilt/shame, worry, anger) and their behavioral (e.g., self-harm) and interpersonal (e.g., dependency) manifestations.
2. *Detachment*: Avoidance of socioemotional experience, including both withdrawal from interpersonal interactions (ranging from casual, daily interactions to friendships to intimate relationships) and restricted affective experience and expression, particularly limited hedonic capacity.
3. *Antagonism*: Behaviors that put the individual at odds with other people, including an exaggerated sense of self-importance and a concomitant expectation of special treatment, as well as a callous antipathy toward others, encompassing both unawareness of others' needs and feelings and a readiness to use others in the service of self-enhancement.
4. *Disinhibition*: Orientation toward immediate gratification, leading to impulsive behavior driven by current thoughts, feelings, and external stimuli, without regard for past learning or consideration of future consequences.
5. *Psychoticism*: Exhibiting a wide range of culturally incongruent odd, eccentric, or unusual behaviors and cognitions, including both process (e.g., perception, dissociation) and content (e.g., beliefs).

Each of the five broad trait domains includes more specific, component trait facets. The trait facets and their definitions can be found in Table 18–1.

Whether considered from the main or Alternative Model presented in DSM-5-TR, Personality Disorders vary in their manifestations and complexity. Some Personality Disorders are related to other internalizing mental disorders, such as Depressive Disorders (see Chapter 4) or Anxiety Disorders (see Chapter 5), because they are characterized primarily by traits of Negative Affectivity (e.g., depressivity, anxiousness). Dependent Personality Disorder is an example of a Personality Disorder within the internalizing spectrum of psychopathology. Some Personality Disorders are related to other externalizing disorders, such as Disruptive, Impulse-Control, and Conduct Disorders (see Chapter 15) or Substance Use Disorders (see Chapter 16), because they are characterized by traits of Disinhibition (e.g., impulsivity, risk taking) and of Antagonism (e.g., callousness, deceitfulness, grandiosity). Antisocial Personality Disorder is an example of a Personality Disorder within the externalizing spectrum of psychopathology. Some Personality Disorders have characteristics of both internalizing and externalizing disorders. Borderline Personality Disorder is the classic example. Finally, some Personality Disorders are related to Psychotic Disorders (see Chapter 2). These are characterized by traits of Psychoticism (e.g., cognitive and perceptual dysregulation, unusual beliefs and experiences) and of Detachment (e.g., suspiciousness, with-

TABLE 18–1.　**Definitions of DSM-5 Personality Disorder (Alternative Model) trait facets**

Domains and facets	Definition
Negative Affectivity	
Emotional lability	Instability of emotional experiences and mood; emotions that are easily aroused, intense, and/or out of proportion to events and circumstances.
Anxiousness	Feelings of nervousness, tenseness, or panic in reaction to diverse situations; frequent worry about the negative effects of past unpleasant experiences and future negative possibilities; feeling fearful and apprehensive about uncertainty; expecting the worst to happen.
Separation insecurity	Fears of being alone due to rejection by—and/or separation from— significant others, based in a lack of confidence in one's ability to care for oneself, both physically and emotionally.
Submissiveness	Adaptation of one's behavior to the actual or perceived interests and desires of others even when doing so is antithetical to one's own interests, needs, or desires.
Hostility	Persistent or frequent angry feelings; anger or irritability in response to minor slights and insults; mean, nasty, or vengeful behavior. See also Antagonism.
Perseveration	Persistence at tasks or in a particular way of doing things long after the behavior has ceased to be functional or effective; continuance of the same behavior despite repeated failures or clear reasons for stopping.
Depressivity	See Detachment.
Suspiciousness	See Detachment.
Restricted affectivity (lack of)	The lack of this facet characterizes low levels of Negative Affectivity. See Detachment for definition of this facet.
Detachment	
Withdrawal	Preference for being alone to being with others; reticence in social situations; avoidance of social contacts and activity; lack of initiation of social contact.
Intimacy avoidance	Avoidance of close or romantic relationships, interpersonal attachments, and intimate sexual relationships.
Anhedonia	Lack of enjoyment from, engagement in, or energy for life's experiences; deficits in the capacity to feel pleasure and take interest in things.
Depressivity	Feelings of being down, miserable, and/or hopeless; difficulty recovering from such moods; pessimism about the future; pervasive shame and/or guilt; feelings of inferior self-worth; thoughts of suicide and suicidal behavior.
Restricted affectivity	Little reaction to emotionally arousing situations; constricted emotional experience and expression; indifference and aloofness in normatively engaging situations.
Suspiciousness	Expectations of—and sensitivity to—signs of interpersonal ill intent or harm; doubts about loyalty and fidelity of others; feelings of being mistreated, used, and/or persecuted by others.

TABLE 18–1. **Definitions of DSM-5 Personality Disorder (Alternative Model) trait facets *(continued)***

Domains and facets	Definition
Antagonism	
Manipulativeness	Use of subterfuge to influence or control others; use of seduction, charm, glibness, or ingratiation to achieve one's ends.
Deceitfulness	Dishonesty and fraudulence; misrepresentation of self; embellishment or fabrication when relating events.
Grandiosity	Believing that one is superior to others and deserves special treatment; self-centeredness; feelings of entitlement; condescension toward others.
Attention seeking	Engaging in behavior designed to attract notice and to make oneself the focus of others' attention and admiration.
Callousness	Lack of concern for the feelings or problems of others; lack of guilt or remorse about the negative or harmful effects of one's actions on others.
Hostility	See Negative Affectivity.
Disinhibition	
Irresponsibility	Disregard for—and failure to honor—financial and other obligations or commitments; lack of respect for—and lack of follow-through on—agreements and promises; carelessness with others' property.
Impulsivity	Acting on the spur of the moment in response to immediate stimuli; acting on a momentary basis without a plan or consideration of outcomes; difficulty establishing and following plans; a sense of urgency and self-harming behavior under emotional distress.
Distractibility	Difficulty concentrating and focusing on tasks; attention is easily diverted by extraneous stimuli; difficulty maintaining goal-focused behavior, including both planning and completing tasks.
Risk taking	Engagement in dangerous, risky, and potentially self-damaging activities, unnecessarily and without regard to consequences; lack of concern for one's limitations and denial of the reality of personal danger; reckless pursuit of goals regardless of the level of risk involved.
Rigid perfectionism (lack of)	Rigid insistence on everything being flawless, perfect, and without errors or faults, including one's own and others' performance; sacrificing of timeliness to ensure correctness in every detail; believing that there is only one right way to do things; difficulty changing ideas and/or viewpoint; preoccupation with details, organization, and order. The lack of this facet characterizes low levels of Disinhibition.
Psychoticism	
Unusual beliefs and experiences	Belief that one has unusual abilities, such as mind reading, telekinesis, thought-action fusion; unusual experiences of reality, including hallucination-like experiences.
Eccentricity	Odd, unusual, or bizarre behavior, appearance, and/or speech; having strange and unpredictable thoughts; saying unusual or inappropriate things.

TABLE 18–1.   **Definitions of DSM-5 Personality Disorder (Alternative Model) trait facets (continued)**

Domains and facets	Definition
Cognitive and perceptual dysregulation	Odd or unusual thought processes and experiences, including depersonalization, derealization, and dissociative experiences; mixed sleep-wake state experiences; thought-control experiences.

Source.   Adapted from American Psychiatric Association: *Diagnostic and Statistical Manual of Mental Disorders,* Fifth Edition, Text Revision. Washington, DC, American Psychiatric Association, 2022, pp. 899–901. Copyright © 2022 American Psychiatric Association. Used with permission.

drawal). Schizotypal Personality Disorder is an example of this type of Personality Disorder. Detachment also characterizes some Personality Disorders in the internalizing spectrum, such as Avoidant Personality Disorder.

All of the Personality Disorders in Section II of DSM-5-TR can be characterized by pathological personality traits in one or more of the Alternative Model's trait domains of Negative Affectivity, Detachment, Antagonism, Disinhibition, and Psychoticism. Some of the Personality Disorders have traits in only one domain (e.g., Narcissistic Personality Disorder has traits only in the Antagonism domain; Dependent Personality Disorder has traits limited to the Negative Affectivity domain). Some of the more complex Personality Disorders have traits in more than one domain (e.g., Antisocial Personality Disorder has traits in both the Antagonism and Disinhibition domains; Schizotypal Personality Disorder has traits in both the Detachment and Psychoticism domains). Complexity in clinical presentation is also reflected by the common co-occurrence of Personality Disorders with each other and with other mental disorders. Co-occurring disorders frequently (but not always) reflect the same psychopathological spectrum or trait domain.

The discussion of each specific Personality Disorder in this chapter first addresses aspects of the disorder in the main model of DSM-5-TR, followed by a synopsis of the Alternative DSM-5 Model for that particular disorder. Some specific elements of the Alternative DSM-5 Model that are included in the specific disorder discussions are described as follows:

- The Alternative DSM-5 Model covers six specific Personality Disorders—Antisocial, Avoidant, Borderline, Narcissistic, Obsessive-Compulsive, and Schizotypal—selected for inclusion because of their empirical bases or their utility for clinicians. The other four Personality Disorders in the main section of DSM-5-TR (i.e., Dependent, Histrionic, Paranoid, and Schizoid), as well as any other Personality Disorder presentations that would be diagnosed as Other Specified Personality Disorder in DSM-5-TR (see Section 18.12), are diagnosed in the Alternative Model as Personality Disorder—Trait Specified.
- Included with the Alternative DSM-5 Model is the Level of Personality Functioning Scale (DSM-5-TR, pp. 891–892, 895–898), a construct of the severity of impairment in personality functioning across the areas of identity, self-direction, empathy, and intimacy. This scale has utility for a broad range of theoretical and treatment ap-

proaches, including the interpersonal, cognitive, psychodynamic, attachment, and social cognitive approaches. The scale provides ratings for the specific level of impairment in areas of personality functioning as follows: "0—little or no impairment," "1—some impairment," "2—moderate impairment," "3—severe impairment," or "4—extreme impairment."

- In the Alternative Model, both the specific level of impairment (listed above) and the specific pathological personality traits (see Table 18–1) that describe the person would be noted for patients diagnosed with Personality Disorder—Trait Specified. In the Alternative DSM-5 Model, a Personality Disorder diagnosis requires at least moderate impairment in personality functioning, because a moderate level of impairment has been empirically shown to identify Personality Disorders with maximal combined sensitivity ("true positive rate"—i.e., the proportion of affected people correctly identified as having a Personality Disorder) and specificity ("true negative rate"—i.e., the proportion of nonaffected people who are correctly identified as not having a Personality Disorder).

This chapter integrates both Personality Disorder models presented in DSM-5-TR in Section II and Section III. All 10 of the Personality Disorders organized by clusters of descriptive similarity in Section II of DSM-5 (i.e., Cluster A, Cluster B, Cluster C) are presented; however, the organization of disorders by cluster has instead been replaced with an order that reflects the dimensions of personality (e.g., internalizing and externalizing). Thus, the presentation of disorders and cases in this chapter begins with Borderline Personality Disorder. Borderline Personality Disorder is the central and most clinically important Personality Disorder on the basis of growing evidence that it is related to a general personality disorder factor (DSM-5-TR, pp. 734–735, 881) that is common to all Personality Disorders and thus reflects the severity of personality psychopathology. The DSM-5-TR Personality Disorders are then presented according to those with prominent internalizing features, those with prominent externalizing features, and those with prominent features of psychoticism, respectively. The chapter concludes with 1) cases of Personality Change Due to Another Medical Condition and 2) cases that do not fit into the existing 10 DSM-5-TR officially recognized categories and that would be diagnosed as Other Specified Personality Disorder in DSM-5-TR. Table 18–2 lists the characteristic features of Personality Disorders in the order in which they are discussed in this chapter.

18.1
Borderline Personality Disorder

Borderline Personality Disorder is defined by "a pervasive pattern of instability in interpersonal relationships, self-image, and affects, and marked impulsivity" (DSM-5-TR, p. 752). Central to the psychopathology of this disorder are an impaired capacity for attachment to others and maladaptive behavior related to separation from others on whom the individual depends. People with this disorder have

TABLE 18–2.   **Characteristic features of Personality Disorders**

Disorder	Key characteristics[a]
Borderline Personality Disorder	Pervasive pattern of instability of interpersonal relationships, self-image, and affects and marked impulsivity
Dependent Personality Disorder	Pervasive and excessive need to be taken care of that leads to submissive and clinging behavior and fears of separation
Avoidant Personality Disorder	Pervasive pattern of social inhibition, feelings of inadequacy, and hypersensitivity to negative evaluation
Obsessive-Compulsive Personality Disorder	Pervasive pattern of preoccupation with orderliness, perfectionism, and mental and interpersonal control at the expense of flexibility, openness, and efficiency
Antisocial Personality Disorder	Pervasive pattern of disregard for and violation of the rights of others since age 15 years
	History of Conduct Disorder before age 15 years
	Current age of at least 18 years
Narcissistic Personality Disorder	Pervasive pattern of grandiosity (in fantasy or behavior), need for admiration, and lack of empathy
Histrionic Personality Disorder	Pervasive pattern of excessive emotionality and attention seeking
Schizotypal Personality Disorder	Pervasive pattern of social and interpersonal deficits marked by acute discomfort with, and reduced capacity for, close relationships, as well as by cognitive or perceptual distortions and eccentricities of behavior
Schizoid Personality Disorder	Pervasive pattern of detachment from social relationships and restricted range of emotional expression
Paranoid Personality Disorder	Pervasive distrust and suspiciousness of others such that their motives are interpreted as malevolent
Personality Change Due to Another Medical Condition[b]	Persistent personality disturbance that represents a change from a previous characteristic personality pattern
	Disturbance is the direct pathophysiological consequence of a nonpsychiatric medical condition
Other Specified Personality Disorder	Symptoms characteristic of a Personality Disorder that do not meet full criteria for any of the disorders in the Personality Disorders diagnostic class

[a]Descriptions are based on DSM-5-TR diagnostic criteria presented in DSM-5-TR Section II, "Personality Disorders."
[b]In DSM-5-TR, this Personality Disorder is discussed only in Section II, "Personality Disorders." Disorders without this note are presented in both Section II (see "Personality Disorders") and Section III (see "Alternative DSM-5 Model for Personality Disorders").

a significant identity disturbance characterized by a markedly unstable self-image or sense of self. They chronically feel "empty" inside. Individuals with Borderline Personality Disorder make frantic efforts to avoid real or imagined abandonment. They have a pattern of unstable and intense interpersonal relationships, characterized by alternating between idealization (another person can do no wrong), when they feel cared for and supported by another person, and devaluation (another person can do no right), when they feel rejected or abandoned. People with Borderline Personality Disorder are subject to intense affective instability or lability, in which they experience mood swings characterized by intense episodes of dysphoria (a state of feeling unwell or unhappy), irritability, or anxiety for hours or a few days at a time, often in reaction to disappointing interpersonal events or encounters. They may also experience intense anger and have problems controlling anger. People with Borderline Personality Disorder are subject to transient dissociative or paranoid reactions when under stress. They may engage in recurrent suicidal behavior, gestures, or threats, and in self-mutilating behavior. They may also have other problems with impulsivity and engage in other potentially self-damaging acts, such as having indiscriminate sex, abusing substances, driving recklessly, binge eating, or overspending.

Borderline Personality Disorder is included as a specific Personality Disorder in the Alternative DSM-5 Model for Personality Disorders (DSM-5-TR, p. 886). The proposed diagnostic criteria describe disorder-specific impairments in personality functioning (e.g., poorly developed and unstable self-image, instability in goals and values, compromised ability to recognize the needs and feelings of others associated with interpersonal hypersensitivity, and intense and unstable close relationships) and pathological traits in the domains of Negative Affectivity (the traits of emotional lability, anxiousness, separation insecurity, and depressivity), Disinhibition (the traits of impulsivity and risk taking), and Antagonism (the trait of hostility).

Borderline Personality Disorder is a relatively common Personality Disorder and is particularly prevalent in clinical populations. The estimated median population prevalence of Borderline Personality Disorder, based on seven epidemiological studies, is 2.7%. In clinical samples, Borderline Personality Disorder is more common among women than men, but in community samples, there is no sex difference. This is believed to be the case because women are more likely than men to seek help for problems. The prevalence of Borderline Personality Disorder is about 6% among patients in primary care settings, about 10% among individuals seen in outpatient mental health care clinics, and about 20% among psychiatric inpatients.

The onset of Borderline Personality Disorder is usually in late adolescence or early adulthood, although in some adolescent treatment settings, individuals as young as 12 or 13 years have been found to have personality pathology that meets criteria for the disorder. The course of Borderline Personality Disorder is waxing and waning. Over time, many patients experience sustained symptomatic improvement, especially with appropriate treatment. Impulsive symptoms remit most rapidly, while affective symptoms are more persistent. It is one of the most impairing of the Personality Disorders, however, with significant negative impacts on social relationships and work functioning. Attaining and maintaining symptomatic remission and good psychosocial functioning (i.e., "recovery") is more difficult than achieving symptomatic remission alone.

Borderline Personality Disorder commonly co-occurs with other DSM-5-TR mental disorders, including Depressive Disorders, Bipolar and Related Disorders, Substance Use Disorders, Anxiety Disorders (e.g., Panic Disorder, Social Anxiety Disorder), Eating Disorders (e.g., Bulimia Nervosa, Binge-Eating Disorder), Posttraumatic Stress Disorder, Attention-Deficit/Hyperactivity Disorder, and Other Personality Disorders.

Empty Shell

Zoe Barnes is a 23-year-old veterinary assistant admitted for her first psychiatric hospitalization. She arrived late at night, referred by a local psychiatrist. She stated, "I don't really need to be here."

Three months before admission, Ms. Barnes learned that her mother had become pregnant. She began drinking heavily, ostensibly to help her sleep at night. While drinking, she became involved in a series of "one-night stands." Two weeks before admission, she began feeling panicky and experiencing episodes in which she felt as if she were removed from her body and in a trance. During one of these episodes, she was stopped by the police while wandering on a bridge late at night. While she was at work the next day, in response to hearing a voice repeatedly telling her to jump off a bridge, Ms. Barnes sought out her supervisor and asked for help. Her supervisor, seeing Ms. Barnes's distress and also noting scars from a recent wrist-slashing, referred her to a psychiatrist, who arranged for her immediate hospitalization.

At the time of the hospital admission, Ms. Barnes appeared as a disheveled and frail waif. She was cooperative, coherent, and frightened. Although she did not feel hospitalization was needed, she welcomed the prospect of relief from her anxiety and depersonalization. She acknowledged that she had had feelings of loneliness and inadequacy and frequent brief periods of depressed mood and anxiety since adolescence. Recently, she had been having fantasies that she was stabbing herself or a little baby with a knife. She confided that she felt like "just an empty shell that is transparent to everyone."

Ms. Barnes's parents had divorced when she was age 3, and for the next 5 years she lived with her maternal grandmother and her mother, who had a severe drinking problem. Ms. Barnes had night terrors during which she would frequently end up sleeping with her mother. At age 6, she went to a special boarding school for a year and a half, after which she was withdrawn by her mother, against the advice of the school. When she was age 8, her maternal grandmother died; Ms. Barnes recalls trying to conceal her grief over this death from her mother. She spent most of the next 2 years living with various relatives, including a period with her father, whom she had not seen since the divorce. When she was age 9, her mother was hospitalized with a diagnosis of Schizophrenia. From age 10 through college, Ms. Barnes lived with an aunt and uncle, but had ongoing and frequent contacts with her mother. Her school record was consistently good.

Since adolescence, Ms. Barnes has dated regularly and has had an active but rarely pleasurable sex life. Her relationships with men usually end abruptly after she becomes angry with them when they disappoint her in some apparently minor way. She then concludes that they were "no good to begin with." She has had several roommates but has had trouble establishing a stable living situation because of her jealousy of sharing her roommates with others and her manipulative efforts to keep them from seeing other people.

Since college, Ms. Barnes has worked steadily and successfully as a veterinary assistant. At the time of admission, she was working the night shift in a veterinary hospital and living alone.

When she left the hospital, Ms. Barnes resumed work and saw a woman therapist on a twice-weekly schedule. Her therapist felt that they had a tenuous relationship in which the patient sometimes seemed to seek nurturance or special favors and at other times was belligerent and viewed therapy as useless. After 3 months, Ms. Barnes became involved with a new boyfriend and soon thereafter quit therapy, with the complaint that her therapist "didn't really care or understand her."

Discussion of "Empty Shell"

Ms. Barnes demonstrates the characteristic features of Borderline Personality Disorder (DSM-5-TR, p. 752). She clearly has a pattern of unstable interpersonal relationships, self-image, affects, and control over impulses. Her relationships with men have been intense and unstable, and the relationships end when she becomes angry and devalues them. She reports that she feels like an "empty shell," evidence of her chronic feelings of emptiness and distorted self-image. Affective instability is suggested by her having experienced frequent brief periods of depressed mood and anxiety since adolescence. In addition, at least during the most recent episode, she demonstrates impulsivity (drinking and sex) and suicidal gestures or self-mutilating acts (slashing her wrists). It is quite likely that these characteristics have also been present during periods of stress in the past.

Ms. Barnes's recent symptoms present reasons to consider other DSM-5-TR disorders. In the last 3 months, since hearing of her mother's pregnancy, Ms. Barnes has begun drinking heavily, has had several episodes of what appears to be depersonalization, and has been anxious, depressed, and suicidal. These symptoms might suggest a co-occurring Anxiety or Depressive Disorder, but the symptoms are too transient for either of these disorders to be diagnosed and more likely are reflections of the characteristic affective instability of Borderline Personality Disorder. In addition, the patient briefly had auditory hallucinations telling her to kill herself. The diagnosis of a Psychotic Disorder, such as Other Specified Schizophrenia Spectrum and Other Psychotic Disorder (see Section 2.8), for the current episode is not warranted because the brief hallucination and the patient's reaction to it (i.e., knowing that it was not real) is an example of the transient stress-related psychotic experiences that are often a feature of Borderline Personality Disorder. For the same reason, a diagnosis of Depersonalization/Derealization Disorder (see "Foggy Student" in Section 8.3) to account for Ms. Barnes's recent symptoms of depersonalization would be superfluous. DSM-5-TR also includes a symptom code for noting the presence or history of Nonsuicidal Self-Injury (DSM-5-TR, p. 822) to alert clinicians to problems such as self-mutilating behavior and to the need to address them in treatment. The criteria for a Nonsuicidal Self-Injury Disorder (see DSM-5-TR,

Section III, chapter "Conditions for Further Study") indicate, however, that the behavior should not be "better explained by another mental disorder," such as Borderline Personality Disorder.

Disco Di

Diana Miller, age 25, entered a long-term treatment unit of a psychiatric hospital after a serious suicide attempt. Alone in her enormous suburban house, with her parents away on vacation, depressed and desperately lonely, she made herself a diazepam and scotch cocktail, drank it, and then called her psychiatrist.

Ms. Miller had been a tractable child, with a mediocre school record, until she was age 12. Her disposition, which had been cheerful and outgoing, changed drastically: she became demanding, sullen, and rebellious, shifting precipitously from a giddy euphoria to tearfulness and depression. She took up with a "fast" crowd, became sexually promiscuous, abused marijuana and hallucinogens, and ran away from home at age 15 with a 17-year-old boy. Two weeks later, having eluded the private investigators her parents had hired, they both returned. She reentered school but dropped out for good in her junior year of high school. Her relationships with men were stormy, full of passion, unbearable longing, and violent arguments. She craved excitement. She would get drunk and dance wildly on tabletops in discos and then leave with strange men and have sex in their cars. If she refused, she was sometimes put out on the street. After one such incident, at age 17, she made her first suicide attempt, cutting her wrist severely, leading to her first hospitalization.

After her first hospitalization, Ms. Miller was referred to a therapist for intensive, twice-weekly psychodynamic psychotherapy, for which she had little aptitude. She filled up most of her sessions with a litany of complaints against her family, from whom she expected "100% attention." She called her therapist several times a day about one "crisis" or another.

During her long period of unsuccessful outpatient treatment, punctuated by several brief hospitalizations, Ms. Miller had many symptoms. She was afraid to travel even to her doctor's office without one of her parents. She was depressed, with suicidal preoccupations and feelings of hopelessness. She drank excessively and used up to 40 mg/day of diazepam. She had eating binges, followed by crash diets to get back to her normal weight. She was obsessed with calories and with the need to have her foods cut into particular shapes and arranged on her plate in a particular manner. If her mother failed to comply with these rules, Ms. Miller had tantrums, sometimes so extreme that she broke dishes and had to be physically restrained by her father.

Ms. Miller had never worked except for a few months as a receptionist in her father's company. She never had an idea of what she wanted to do with her life, apart from being with a "romantic man." She had never had female friends, and her only source of solace was her dog. She was often "eaten alive" with boredom. Efforts by her therapist to set limits had little effect. She refused to join Alcoholics Anonymous or to attend a day program or vocational rehabilitation center, regarding these as "beneath" her. Instead, she languished at home, grew more depressed and agoraphobic, and escalated her diazepam use to 80 mg/day. It was a serious suicide attempt that led to her current (seventh) psychiatric hospitalization.

In the hospital Ms. Miller complained that the nurses were "cruel" to her and that other patients "hated" her. Her parents attended many of their own therapy sessions, where they were counseled to resist their daughter's pleas to return home. She was exquisitely sensitive to the slightest decrement in her diazepam dosage, such that the medication could be reduced by only 1 mg/day. At this rate, it took 3 months for her to be "off" the drug. Afterward, her progress was unexpectedly good. Her disposition became cheerful. She grew cooperative toward the staff and friendly toward other patients. She learned secretarial skills in a hospital rehabilitation program, and she became less fearful of going outside and less fussy about food. By the end of her 10-month stay, she developed a friendship with another convalescing patient, and the two arranged to share an apartment. Both found part-time work, and Ms. Miller continued therapy once a week as an outpatient.

Ms. Miller responded primarily to a supportive mode of psychotherapy, one that emphasized education, exhortation, encouragement, and limit setting. She was too anxious and too action prone to benefit from a psychodynamic approach that required introspection and reflection. Brief hospitalizations could not stem the tide of her multiple and intense symptoms, of which her substance abuse was the most threatening. For Ms. Miller, what seemed to work best was a long-term hospitalization, where the substance abuse could be properly dealt with, and where vocational rehabilitation could take hold. The enforced separation from her parents helped her and her mother realize that each could survive without the other. During 7 years of follow-up, Ms. Miller has held her ground, continues to work, lives with the same roommate, and is able to visit her parents with regularity, and without falling back into the old pattern of mother-daughter interdependence. Sensation seeking remains a noticeable part of her adaptation—she likes flashy clothes, clubs, and rock concerts—but she is less impulsive, abstains from alcohol and other drugs, and no longer places herself in jeopardy with strange men.

Discussion of "Disco Di"

Ms. Miller's history of many different symptoms over many years suggests several different mental disorders. The depression and suicide attempt that prompted her last hospitalization suggest the diagnosis of Major Depressive Disorder (see "Worthless Wife" in Section 4.2) or Persistent Depressive Disorder (see "Junior Executive" in Section 4.3). Because this case was presented several years after the hospitalization, insufficient information is available to make these diagnoses.

Ms. Miller's escalating dosage of diazepam (with the resulting development of tolerance) and her continued use despite its negative effect on her life suggest a diagnosis of Benzodiazepine (Sedative, Hypnotic, or Anxiolytic) Use

Disorder (DSM-5-TR, p. 620). Her binge eating may also have been frequent enough to warrant the additional diagnosis of Binge-Eating Disorder (DSM-5-TR, p. 392).

Most striking, however, are Ms. Miller's chronically chaotic life and her pervasive pattern of instability in mood, interpersonal relationships, and impulse control. These suggest that the primary disturbance is a Personality Disorder, specifically Borderline Personality Disorder (DSM-5-TR, p. 752). Ms. Miller demonstrates at least five of the characteristic symptoms of the disorder. She has unstable and intense interpersonal relationships, and the "violent arguments" she has had with men suggest an alternation between extremes of idealization and devaluation of them. She has an identity disturbance (no goals in life), impulsive behavior in many areas (sex, substance abuse, eating), recurrent suicidal behavior, affective instability (sudden shifts of mood), and inappropriate and intense anger. Additionally, her feeling of being "eaten alive" with boredom is likely evidence of chronic feelings of emptiness.

DSM-5-TR provides a symptom code for Suicidal Behavior (DSM-5-TR, p. 822) that can be added to any DSM-5-TR diagnosis to alert clinicians to this problem. Located in the chapter "Other Conditions That May Be a Focus of Clinical Attention," the code requires that the person has "engaged in potentially self-injurious behavior with at least some intent to die" (DSM-5-TR, p. 822).

As is common in individuals with severe Personality Disorders, Ms. Miller has features of several other Personality Disorders: Narcissistic (e.g., Alcoholics Anonymous was "beneath" her), Histrionic (craving excitement), Obsessive-Compulsive (rigidity about food), and Dependent (inability to manage without her parents). As is illustrated in Ms. Miller's case, patients with Borderline Personality Disorder commonly have other emotional problems that fall into both the internalizing and the externalizing spectra of psychopathology.

18.2
Dependent Personality Disorder

Dependent Personality Disorder is characterized by "a pervasive and excessive need to be taken care of that leads to submissive and clinging behavior and fears of separation" (DSM-5-TR, p. 768). People with Dependent Personality Disorder are able to take care of themselves, but they grossly underestimate their abilities and judgment. They view others as more capable and stronger than they are and therefore look to others to help them with even everyday decisions, to tell them what they should do and think, and to be responsible for them. They have problems disagreeing with others for fear they will lose support or approval and will even offer to do unpleasant, self-sacrificing things to obtain nurturance and support. They feel very uncomfortable and helpless when alone because they feel unable to care for themselves, and they feel the need to find someone new to depend on when a close relationship ends.

According to the Alternative Model, Dependent Personality Disorder is not a specific Personality Disorder but rather is diagnosed as Personality Disorder—Trait Specified (DSM-5-TR, p. 890). The level of impairment in personality functioning is typically moderate, and the relevant personality traits are submissiveness, separation insecurity, and anxiousness, all of which are traits from the Negative Affectivity trait domain.

The estimated median population prevalence of Dependent Personality Disorder, based on six epidemiological studies, is 0.4%, making it one of the least common Personality Disorders. The disorder is more common among women than among men. Dependent behavior (e.g., on parents) is developmentally appropriate in children and adolescents to an extent, but people ordinarily become more self-sufficient and independent as they move through the developmental milestones of leaving home, forming close relationships outside of the nuclear family, and achieving financial independence from their families. Periods of economic recession and unemployment may affect the timelines for achieving these goals. Some cultures and societies may be more accepting of passivity, politeness, and deferential behavior, and cultural and subcultural norms should be considered in making a diagnosis. Dependent Personality Disorder is associated with moderate impairment in quality of life and psychosocial dysfunction. Individuals with the disorder are at increased risk of Depressive Disorders, Anxiety Disorders, Adjustment Disorders, and other Personality Disorders (e.g., Borderline, Avoidant, Histrionic).

Blood Is Thicker Than Water

Morgan Stewart is a 34-year-old single man who lives with his mother and works as an accountant. He seeks treatment because he is very unhappy after having just broken up with his girlfriend. His mother had disapproved of his marriage plans, ostensibly because their family was Presbyterian and Deborah, the woman he wanted to marry, was Jewish. Mr. Stewart felt trapped and forced to choose between his mother and his girlfriend, and because "blood is thicker than water," he had decided not to go against his mother's wishes. Nonetheless, he is angry at himself and at her; he believes that she will never let him marry and is possessively hanging on to him. He says that his mother "wears the pants" in the family and is a very domineering woman who is used to getting her way. Mr. Stewart is afraid of disagreeing with his mother for fear that she will not be supportive of him, and then he will have to fend for himself. He criticizes himself for being weak, but also admires his mother and respects her judgment; he says, "Maybe Deborah wasn't right for me after all." He alternates between resentment and a "Mother knows best" attitude. He feels that his own judgment is poor.

Mr. Stewart works at a job several grades below what his education and talent would permit. On several occasions he has turned down promotions because he did not want the responsibility of having to supervise other people or make independent decisions. He has worked for the same boss for

10 years, gets on well with him, and is, in turn, highly regarded as a dependable and unobtrusive worker. He has two very close friends whom he has known since early childhood. He has lunch with one of them every single workday and feels lost if his friend is sick and misses a day.

Mr. Stewart is the youngest of four children and the only boy. He was "babied and spoiled" by his mother and elder sisters. He had considerable separation anxiety as a child—difficulty falling asleep unless his mother stayed in the room, mild school refusal, and unbearable homesickness when he occasionally tried "sleepovers." As a child he was teased by other boys because of his lack of assertiveness and was often called a baby. He has lived at home his whole life except for 1 year of college, from which he returned because of homesickness. He started dating girls in high school and has had several medium-term relationships with women since then, a couple of which were sexual, but he has been unable to leave his mother to live with another woman.

Mr. Stewart's therapist treated him with a combination of behavior therapy and psychodynamic psychotherapy for several years. He has also been in group therapy. After a year of therapy, he moved out of his mother's house and married his girlfriend. When the therapist last heard from him, he said he was fairly happy in his marriage.

Discussion of "Blood Is Thicker Than Water"

Mr. Stewart allowed his mother to make the important decision as to whether he should marry a girlfriend, and this seems to be merely one instance of a pattern of subordinating his own needs and wishes to those of his domineering mother. At work, he demonstrates lack of initiative and reluctance to rely on his own judgment and abilities by avoiding promotions and working below his potential. He apparently feels uncomfortable when he is alone and has always worried about being left to take care of himself. Mr. Stewart is afraid of disagreeing with his mother. This dependent and submissive behavior is severe enough to interfere significantly with his social and occupational functioning and therefore justifies the diagnosis of Dependent Personality Disorder (DSM-5-TR, p. 768). Although Dependent Personality Disorder is more common among women than men, this case illustrates that men can have the disorder.

18.3
Avoidant Personality Disorder

The hallmark of Avoidant Personality Disorder is "a pervasive pattern of social inhibition, feelings of inadequacy, and hypersensitivity to negative evaluation" (DSM-5-TR, p. 764). People with Avoidant Personality Disorder have a very poor self-image. They feel inadequate and believe that they are socially inept, personally unappealing, and generally inferior. Consequently, individuals with Avoidant Personality Disorder avoid occupational activities that involve significant interpersonal interaction because they fear criticism and disapproval. They are very reticent in their social lives because they want guarantees that they will be liked and are afraid that they will be rejected, shamed, or ridiculed. They tend to avoid new activities because they worry that they will embarrass themselves. They are generally risk averse.

Avoidant Personality Disorder is included as a specific Personality Disorder in the Alternative DSM-5 Model for Personality Disorders (DSM-5-TR, p. 885). It is characterized by moderate impairments in personality functioning (e.g., self-appraisal as socially inept, reluctance to pursue goals or take personal risks, preoccupation with and sensitivity to criticism or rejection, reluctance to get involved with others unless being certain of being liked); the trait of anxiousness (required) from the Negative Affectivity trait domain; and the traits of (social) withdrawal, anhedonia, and intimacy avoidance from the Detachment domain.

The estimated median population prevalence of Avoidant Personality Disorder is 2.1%, based on six epidemiological studies. In population-based samples, the disorder is slightly more common in women than in men. Avoidant behavior often begins in infancy or childhood, with excessive shyness and fear of strangers or novel situations. Whereas most children outgrow childhood shyness, those who go on to develop Avoidant Personality Disorder may get increasingly withdrawn in adolescence or early adulthood, when expanding their social network outside of the family becomes important for development. Avoidant Personality Disorder is associated with impairment in both social and occupational spheres. Other disorders that commonly co-occur with Avoidant Personality Disorder include Depressive Disorders, Anxiety Disorders (especially Social Anxiety Disorder), and Substance Use Disorders.

Sad Sister

Barbara Nowak is a 26-year-old teacher's aide who seeks counseling. For several years she has been feeling increasingly lonely and "lost," particularly since her 28-year-old sister married and moved out of town 3 months ago. This sister and one close friend from high school have been the patient's only real social contacts; otherwise, Ms. Nowak has no other girlfriends, and she is extremely afraid of men. As far back as she can remember, Ms. Nowak has felt that she has very little to offer others. She has always anticipated that men, even if attracted to her, would quickly find fault with her and "drop" her. Although she would like to be married, she characteristically cuts off potential relationships with men after two or three dates because of her fear of eventual rejection. Her relationships with others are superficial and usually structured through work, civic groups, or her church club. Ms. Nowak is rarely critical of others or able to get angry at them, except in regard to social or political issues. She champions the causes of minorities, ecology, and liberalism against the rich and powerful, but she is more likely to volunteer to spend a Saturday stuffing leaflets in envelopes than canvassing door to door to collect money.

Discussion of "Sad Sister"

Throughout most of her life, Ms. Nowak has had significant difficulty establishing relationships with other people. Because she has significant impairments in her self-concept and in her capacity to develop close interpersonal relationships with others, she likely has a Personality Disorder. Social isolation is commonly seen in Schizotypal Personality Disorder (see Section 18.8), but the absence of oddities of behavior and thinking rules out that diagnosis in Ms. Nowak's case. In Schizoid Personality Disorder (see Section 18.9), the isolation is apparently the result of a basic emotional coldness and indifference to others. In this case, however, Ms. Nowak obviously has a strong desire for affection and acceptance, which is inhibited by anticipation of disapproval and rejection—a characteristic feature of Avoidant Personality Disorder (DSM-5-TR, p. 764). Ms. Nowak also displays poor self-esteem (she feels she has little to offer others), another characteristic feature of this disorder. It is because of the patient's Personality Disorder that she was particularly vulnerable to the stressor of her sister's moving. Although the exacerbation of Ms. Nowak's long-standing problems since her sister moved away has caused her to seek treatment at this time, this reaction does not represent a new illness (e.g., an Adjustment Disorder [see Section 7.6]), but instead is an expression of her Avoidant Personality Disorder.

The Jerk

Leon Mitchell is a single 45-year-old postal employee who was evaluated at a clinic specializing in the treatment of depression. He claims to have felt constantly depressed since first grade, without a period of "normal" mood for more than a few days at a time. His depression has been accompanied by lethargy, little or no interest or pleasure in anything, trouble concentrating, and feelings of inadequacy, pessimism, and resentment. His only periods of normal mood occur when he is home alone, listening to music or watching TV.

On further questioning, Mr. Mitchell reveals that he cannot ever remember feeling comfortable socially. Even before kindergarten, if he was asked to speak in front of a group of his parents' friends, his mind would "go blank." He felt overwhelming anxiety at children's social functions, such as birthday parties, which he either avoided or attended in total silence. He could answer questions in class only if he wrote down the answers in advance; even then, he frequently mumbled and could not get the answer out. He met new children with his eyes lowered, fearing their scrutiny, expecting to feel humiliated and embarrassed. He was convinced that everyone around him thought he was "dumb" or "a jerk."

As he grew up, Mr. Mitchell had a couple of neighborhood playmates, but he never had a "best friend." His school grades were good but suffered when oral classroom participation was expected. As a teenager, he was terrified of girls, and to this day has never gone on a date or even asked a girl for a date. This bothers him, although he is so often depressed that he feels he has little energy or interest in dating.

Mr. Mitchell attended college and did well for a while, then dropped out as his grades slipped. He remained very self-conscious and "terrified" of meeting strangers. He had trouble finding a job because he was unable to answer questions in interviews. He worked at a few jobs for which only a written test was required. He passed a civil service examination at age 24 and was offered a job in the post office on the evening shift. He enjoyed this job because it involved little contact with others. He was offered, but refused, several promotions because he feared the social pressures. Although by now he supervises a number of employees, he still finds it difficult to give instructions, even to people he has known for years. He has no friends and avoids all invitations to socialize with coworkers. During the past several years, he has tried several therapies to help him get over his "shyness" and depression.

Mr. Mitchell has never experienced sudden anxiety or a panic attack in social situations or at other times. Rather, his anxiety gradually builds to a constant high level in anticipation of social situations. He has never experienced any psychotic symptoms.

Discussion of "The Jerk"

Mr. Mitchell comes to the clinic complaining of lifelong depression. Indeed, he has been depressed and has experienced only limited interest and enjoyment ever since he was a child. Although his depressed mood has been associated with pessimism, low energy, and difficulty concentrating, other symptoms of a Major Depressive Episode, such as appetite and sleep disturbances, have not been present. This chronic mild depression is diagnosed as Persistent Depressive Disorder (DSM-5-TR, p. 193), which is further qualified as Early Onset (before age 21).

In addition, Mr. Mitchell has lifelong social anxiety that makes it difficult for him to maintain even the most minimal social contact. His fear is that he will have nothing to say and will be thought of as "a jerk." This fear seems to be independent of his Persistent Depressive Disorder and therefore justifies the additional diagnosis of Social Anxiety Disorder (DSM-5-TR, p. 229).

This patient illustrates a frequent problem in diagnosing Social Anxiety Disorder, in that the symptoms overlap considerably with those of Avoidant Personality Disorder. Mr. Mitchell has certainly displayed a pervasive pattern of social inhibition, feelings of inadequacy, and hypersensitivity to negative evaluation throughout his life. He believes he is socially inept, avoids occupational activities that involve significant interpersonal contact, and is inhibited in new interpersonal situations because of feelings of inadequacy. He undoubtedly is also preoccupied with being rejected in social situations and is probably unwilling to become involved with people unless he is certain of being liked. Therefore, we also make the diagnosis of Avoidant Personality Disorder (DSM-5-TR, p. 764). Future research is needed to clarify whether

Avoidant Personality Disorder and Social Anxiety Disorder merely reflect different perspectives on the same disorder or whether they are different. At the present time, it appears that the impairments in personality functioning that characterize Avoidant Personality Disorder are more pervasive and severe than the social anxiety experienced by patients with Social Anxiety Disorder in the absence of Avoidant Personality Disorder.

18.4
Obsessive-Compulsive Personality Disorder

The characteristic personality pattern of Obsessive-Compulsive Personality Disorder is one of "preoccupation with orderliness, perfectionism, and mental and interpersonal control, at the expense of flexibility, openness, and efficiency" (DSM-5-TR, p. 771). For people with Obsessive-Compulsive Personality Disorder, potentially virtuous traits such as neatness, punctuality, organization, and conscientiousness become so extreme that they end up causing either distress (mostly in others) or some amount of functional impairment. For example, while preparing lists and organizing things, the person might forget the point of the activity. The individual might be such a perfectionist that they never get tasks done. The person may also be so devoted to work and productivity that they never have time for leisure activities or even friendships or relationships. These individuals not only are interested in controlling the details in their own lives but often exert their control over others. At work, they will be reluctant to delegate tasks unless things are done in exactly their way. In relationships, they will also try to control others, attempting to get others to think and act as they themselves would. Individuals with Obsessive-Compulsive Personality Disorder tend to be unemotional and have great difficulty expressing warm and caring feelings toward others. They tend to be somewhat miserly and are often "hoarders" of worthless objects.

Obsessive-Compulsive Personality Disorder is included as a specific Personality Disorder in the Alternative DSM-5 Model for Personality Disorders (DSM-5-TR, p. 888). It is characterized by specific impairments in personality functioning at the moderate level (sense of self derived from work or productivity, difficulty completing tasks and realizing goals, difficulty understanding ideas and feelings of others, rigidity and stubbornness that negatively affect relationships) and by the traits of rigid perfectionism (required), perseveration (Negative Affectivity), and intimacy avoidance and restricted affectivity (both Detachment).

Obsessive-Compulsive Personality Disorder is one of the most common Personality Disorders, with an estimated median population prevalence (based on five epidemiological studies) of 4.7%. It is equally common in men and women.

Because of the extreme control that people with Obsessive-Compulsive Personality Disorder need to exert over others and their restricted range of emotionality and inability to let others get emotionally close to them, they will often have significant impairment in interpersonal functioning, characterized by few intimate relationships or by a history of breakups, separations, and divorces. In cultures where work and productivity are especially emphasized and rewarded, individuals with Obsessive-Compulsive Personality Disorder can be quite occupationally successful (as long as they are willing to work as long as it takes them to satisfy their need for perfection), to the extent that some mental health care professionals question whether it is a disorder at all. Individuals with Obsessive-Compulsive Personality Disorder are at increased risk for an Anxiety Disorder (e.g., Generalized Anxiety Disorder, Social Anxiety Disorder), a Depressive Disorder, an Obsessive-Compulsive and Related Disorder, or an Eating Disorder.

The Workaholic

Jacob Nielsen is a 45-year-old lawyer who seeks treatment at his wife's insistence. She is fed up with their marriage: she can no longer tolerate his emotional coldness, rigid demands, bullying behavior, sexual disinterest, long work hours, and frequent business trips. Mr. Nielsen feels no particular distress in his marriage and has agreed to the consultation only to humor his wife.

It soon becomes clear, however, that Mr. Nielsen is troubled by problems at work. He is known as the hardest-driving member of a hard-driving law firm. He was the youngest full partner in the firm's history and is known for being able to handle many cases at the same time. Lately, he finds himself increasingly unable to keep up. He is too proud to turn down a new case and too much of a perfectionist to be satisfied with the quality of work performed by his assistants. Displeased by their writing style and sentence structure, he finds himself constantly correcting their briefs, and therefore unable to stay abreast of his schedule. People at work complain that his extreme attention to detail and inability to delegate responsibility are reducing his efficiency. Mr. Nielsen has had two or three secretaries a year for 15 years. No one can tolerate working for him for very long because he is so critical of any mistakes made by others. When assignments get backed up, he cannot decide which to address first. He starts making schedules for himself and his staff, but then is unable to meet the demand of those schedules and works 15-hour days to keep up. He finds it difficult to be decisive now that his work has expanded beyond his own direct control.

Mr. Nielsen discusses his children as if they were mechanical dolls, but also with a clear underlying affection. He describes his wife as a "suitable mate" and has trouble understanding why she is dissatisfied. He is punctilious in his manners and dress, slow and ponderous in his speech, dry and humorless, with a stubborn determination to get his point across.

Mr. Nielsen is the product of two upwardly mobile, extremely hardworking parents. He grew up feeling that he was never working hard enough, that he had much to achieve and very little time. He was a superior student, a "book-worm," who was awkward and unpopular in adolescent social pursuits. He has always been competitive and a high achiever. He has trouble relaxing on vacations, develops elaborate activity schedules for every family member, and becomes impatient and furious if they refuse to follow his plans. He likes sports but has little time for them and refuses to play if he cannot be at the top of his form. He is a ferocious competitor on the tennis courts and a poor loser.

Discussion of "The Workaholic"

Although the marital problem is the entry ticket, it is clear that Mr. Nielsen has many personality traits that are quite maladaptive. He is cold, rigid, excessively perfectionistic, and preoccupied with details. He is indecisive but insists that others do things his way. His interpersonal relationships suffer because of his excessive devotion to work. These are the characteristic features of Obsessive-Compulsive Personality Disorder (DSM-5-TR, p. 771).

18.5
Antisocial Personality Disorder

The core feature of Antisocial Personality Disorder is a pattern of socially irresponsible behaviors that show a "disregard for and violation of the rights of others" (DSM-5-TR, p. 748). People with Antisocial Personality Disorder frequently engage in unlawful acts. Their personalities are characterized by the traits of deceitfulness (e.g., lying, using aliases, conning others for pleasure or profit), impulsivity (e.g., failure to plan ahead), irritability and aggressiveness (e.g., engaging in physical fights or assaults), recklessness (e.g., disregard for the safety of self or others), irresponsibility (e.g., failure to consistently hold a job or honor financial obligations), and callousness or lack of remorse (e.g., indifference to or rationalizing having hurt, mistreated, or stolen from another person). Antisocial Personality Disorder is the only Personality Disorder in DSM-5-TR to have a minimum age limit; it can only be diagnosed in individuals age 18 years and older. To qualify for the diagnosis, the individual must also have evidence of Conduct Disorder (see Section 15.3) with an onset before age 15 years.

Antisocial Personality Disorder is included as a specific Personality Disorder in the Alternative DSM-5 Model for Personality Disorders (DSM-5-TR, p. 884). There are disorder-specific impairments in personality functioning at a moderate level (e.g., egocentrism, absence of prosocial internal standards for behavior, lack of concern for feelings or needs of others, exploitation and intimidation as means of relating to others) and pathological personality traits from two trait domains: Antagonism (the traits of manipulativeness, callousness, deceitfulness, and hostility) and Disinhibition (the traits of risk taking, impulsivity, and irresponsibility).

Antisocial Personality Disorder is one of the most common Personality Disorders. The estimated median population prevalence (based on seven epidemiological studies) is 3.6%. The highest prevalence of Antisocial Personality Disorder (>70%) is among samples of males with Alcohol Use Disorder and samples from substance abuse clinics, prisons, and other forensic settings. Antisocial Personality Disorder is three times more common in men than in women. The course of Antisocial Personality Disorder is chronic, beginning with evidence of Conduct Disorder before age 15 years (required), and often with oppositional behavior and Attention-Deficit/ Hyperactivity Disorder (very common). Later in life (i.e., by the mid-40s), criminal behavior and other manifestations may decrease. Antisocial Personality Disorder frequently co-occurs with Anxiety Disorders, Depressive Disorders, Somatic Symptom Disorder, Substance Use Disorders, and Gambling Disorder. Other Personality Disorders, particularly Borderline, Narcissistic, and Histrionic Personality Disorders, also commonly co-occur with Antisocial Personality Disorder.

Belligerent Boy

While being detained in jail awaiting trial for attempted robbery, a 21-year-old man named Myles Sugarman was interviewed by a psychiatrist. Myles had a history of multiple arrests for drug charges, robbery, and assault and battery.

Past history revealed that Myles had been expelled from junior high school for truancy, fighting, and generally poor performance in school. Following a car theft when he was 14 years old, he was placed in a juvenile detention center. Subsequently, he spent brief periods in a variety of institutions, from which he usually ran away. At times his parents attempted to let him live at home, but he would get angry, disruptive, and threaten them with physical harm. After one such incident during which he "exploded" and threatened them with a knife, Myles was admitted to a psychiatric hospital. He signed himself out against medical advice, 1 day later. Without a place to go, he went back to living "on the street."

Myles has never formed close personal relationships with his parents, his two older brothers, or friends of either sex. He is a loner and a drifter and has not worked for more than 2 months at any one job. He expresses neither remorse for any of his past behaviors nor any feelings about the people he obviously had harmed. Recently, after 3 weeks of enrollment in a vocational training program, he was expelled because of poor attendance and picking fights.

Myles tried to get the psychiatrist to say that he was "mental" and should be sent back to a hospital rather than to jail. He tried to say that the most recent charge, like others before, had been "trumped up" by the police who "had it in for him." When the psychiatrist said that he could not send him to a hospital, Myles got furious and kicked his chair across the room. He was taken, kicking and screaming, from the examining room by burly guards and put into a cell.

Discussion of "Belligerent Boy"

Myles's multiple arrests for criminal activity, and his hostility and aggressiveness, irresponsible failure to attend school or work consistently, impulsivity, callous lack of remorse, manipulativeness, and deceitfulness all suggest Antisocial Personality Disorder (DSM-5-TR, p. 748). A history of antisocial behavior before age 15 (truancy, expulsion from school, fighting, thefts) confirms the diagnosis.

18.6
Narcissistic Personality Disorder

A "pervasive pattern of grandiosity..., need for admiration, and lack of empathy" are the hallmark signs of Narcissistic Personality Disorder (DSM-5-TR, p. 760). In the traditional view, people with Narcissistic Personality Disorder have a grandiose sense of self and are preoccupied with fantasies of unlimited success, power, brilliance, and so forth, often without a commensurate level of achievement. They believe that they are "special," feel entitled to be treated as such by others, and require constant admiration. They will take advantage of others, have little regard for the feelings or needs of others, and are envious and arrogant.

A more modern and more valid clinical perspective on people with Narcissistic Personality Disorder recognizes that a grandiose self-image actually often shields the person from feelings of inferiority and is an attempt at compensating for inadequacies. Thus, the person with Narcissistic Personality Disorder will feel vulnerable and react with strong feelings of hurt or anger to even small slights, rejections, defeats, or criticisms. There are also less overt forms of pathological narcissism in which a conviction of superiority is hidden behind social withdrawal and a façade of self-sacrifice.

Narcissistic Personality Disorder is included as a specific Personality Disorder in the Alternative DSM-5 Model for Personality Disorders (DSM-5-TR, p. 887). The model recognizes that self-appraisal may be either inflated (i.e., the grandiose presentation) or deflated (i.e., the vulnerable presentation) and that entitlement may be either overt or covert. Typical impairments in personality functioning are at the moderate level (e.g., excessive reference to others for self-esteem regulation, goal setting based on gaining approval of others, inability to recognize the feelings and needs of others, superficial relationships existing to serve self-esteem regulation), and relevant traits include grandiosity and attention seeking (both in the Antagonism domain). The Alternative Model also allows for further description of the person with Narcissistic Personality Disorder by means of trait specifiers (DSM-5-TR, p. 888), such as the following:

- An individual with "vulnerable narcissism" might also exhibit the traits of anxiousness and depressivity from the Negative Affectivity trait domain, which are not part of the proposed diagnostic criteria for Narcissistic Personality Disorder but can be used as diagnostic modifiers.

- Narcissistic Personality Disorder in its most extreme form bears a strong resemblance to Antisocial Personality Disorder (see Section 18.5). Thus, additional traits from the Antagonism domain, such as manipulativeness, deceitfulness, or callousness, may also be used as trait specifiers. When a number of additional Antagonism traits apply, the condition has been called "malignant narcissism."

Narcissistic Personality Disorder is relatively uncommon (estimated median population prevalence of 1.6% based on five epidemiological studies) compared with other Personality Disorders, although pathological narcissism—the pathology of self-appraisal—is frequently present in Personality Disorders other than Narcissistic Personality Disorder. Most individuals with Narcissistic Personality Disorder are men. People with Narcissistic Personality Disorder often are successful in certain aspects of their lives (e.g., their careers) but not in others (e.g., close relationships). People with Narcissistic Personality Disorder also have particular difficulty in later life, when inherent physical and occupational limitations arise. In individuals with Narcissistic Personality Disorder, suicidal ideation may be evoked by exposure to their imperfections or failures. Suicide attempts are more likely to be planned rather than impulsive, and tend to be of higher lethality than attempts associated with other Personality Disorders.

Narcissistic Personality Disorder may co-occur with Depressive Disorders, Anorexia Nervosa, and Substance Use Disorders, especially Cocaine Use Disorder. Histrionic, Borderline, Antisocial, and Paranoid Personality Disorders also commonly co-occur with Narcissistic Personality Disorder.

Unrecognized Genius

Jonathan Wagner, a 25-year-old single graduate student, complains to his psychoanalyst of difficulty completing his doctorate in English literature and expresses concerns about his relationships with women. He believes that his thesis topic may profoundly increase the level of understanding in his discipline and make him famous, but so far, he has not been able to get past the third chapter. His mentor does not seem sufficiently impressed with his ideas, and Mr. Wagner is furious at him, but he is also self-doubting and ashamed. He blames his mentor for his lack of progress and believes that he deserves more help with his grand idea and that his mentor should help with some of the research. The patient brags about his creativity and complains that other people are "jealous" of his insight. He is very envious of students who are moving along faster than he, whom he regards as "dull drones and ass-kissers." He prides himself on the brilliance of his classroom participation and imagines someday becoming a great professor.

Mr. Wagner becomes rapidly infatuated with women and has powerful and persistent fantasies about each new woman he meets, but after several experiences of sexual intercourse he feels disappointed in them and finds them dumb, clinging, and physically repugnant. He has many "friends," but they turn over quickly, and no one relationship lasts very long. People get tired of his continual self-promotion and lack of consideration of them. For example, he was going to be alone this past Christmas and tried to insist that his best friend stay in town rather than visit his family. The friend refused, criticizing the patient's self-centeredness; the patient, enraged, decided never to see this friend again.

Discussion of "Unrecognized Genius"

Mr. Wagner's narcissistic personality traits are clear: grandiosity about the importance of his thesis, preoccupation with fantasies of great success in his career and in his relationships with women, beliefs that he is special and entitled to have his mentor do some of his work, need for excessive admiration, envy of others, and lack of empathy. Because these traits significantly interfere with both his academic achievement and his success in friendships and heterosexual relationships, a diagnosis of Narcissistic Personality Disorder (DSM-5-TR, p. 760) is appropriate. Interestingly, the patient also shows his vulnerable side: he feels anger, self-doubt, and shame when his mentor is not sufficiently impressed with his work. Patients with Narcissistic Personality Disorder often vacillate between grandiose and vulnerable presentations. Although it is not specifically stated that the traits of Narcissistic Personality Disorder in this case are of long duration, this is a reasonable assumption. (There is no description in the literature of episodic narcissism.)

False Rumors

Bob Bailey, a 21-year-old man, comes to the psychologist's office, accompanied by his parents, on the advice of his college counselor. Bob begins the interview by announcing that he has no problems. His parents are always overly concerned about him, and it is only to get them "off my back" that he has agreed to the evaluation. "I am dependent on them financially but not emotionally."

The psychologist was able to obtain the following story from Bob and his parents. Bob had apparently spread malicious and false rumors about several of the teachers who had given him poor grades, implying that they were having homosexual affairs with students. This, following the loss of a girlfriend, as well as increasingly erratic attendance at his classes over the past term, prompted the college counselor to suggest to Bob and his parents that help was urgently needed. Bob claimed that his academic problems were exaggerated, his success in theatrical productions was being overlooked, and he was in full control of the situation. He did not deny that he spread the false rumors, but he showed no remorse or apprehension about possible repercussions for himself.

Bob is a tall, stylishly dressed young man with a dramatic wave in his hair. His manner is distant but charming, and he obviously enjoys talking about a variety of intellectual subjects and current affairs. However, he assumes a condescending, cynical, and bemused manner toward the psychologist and the evaluation process. He conveys a sense of superiority and control over the evaluation.

Accounts of Bob's development were complicated by his bland dismissal of its importance and by the conflicting accounts about it by his parents. His mother was an extremely anxious, immaculately dressed, outspoken woman. She described Bob as having been a beautiful and joyful baby, who was always extremely gifted and brilliant. She recalled that after a miscarriage, when Bob was 1 year old, she and her husband had become even more devoted to his care, giving him "the love for two." The father was a rugged-looking, soft-spoken, successful man. He recalled a period in Bob's early life when they had been very close, and he had even confided in Bob about very personal matters and expressed deep feelings. He also noted that Bob had become progressively more resentful with the births of his two siblings. The father laughingly commented that Bob "would have liked to have been the only child." He recalled a series of conflicts between Bob and authority figures over rules, and remembered that Bob had expressed disdain both for his peers at school and for his siblings.

In his early school years, Bob seemed to play and interact less with other children than most others do. In fifth grade, after a change in teachers, he became arrogant and withdrawn and refused to participate in class. Nevertheless, he maintained excellent grades. In high school, he had been involved in an episode similar to the one that had led to the current evaluation. At that time, he had spread false rumors about a classmate with whom he was competing for a role in the school play.

In general, it became clear that Bob had never been "one of the boys." He liked dramatics and movies but had never shown an interest in athletics. He always appeared to be a loner but did not complain of loneliness. When asked, he claimed to take pride in "being different" from his peers. He also distanced himself from his parents and often responded with silence to their overtures for more communication. His parents felt that behind his guarded demeanor was a sad, alienated, lonely young man. Although he was well-known to classmates, the relationships he had with them were generally under circumstances in which he was looked up to for his intellectual or dramatic talents.

Bob conceded that others viewed him as cold or insensitive. He readily acknowledged these qualities, and the fact that he had no close friends, but he dismissed these characteristics as unimportant. They represented strength to him. He went on to note that when others complained about these qualities in him, it was largely because of their own weakness. In his view, they envied him and longed to have him care about them. He believed they sought to gain by having an association with him.

Bob had occasional dates but no steady girlfriends. Although the exact history remains unclear, he acknowledged that the girl whose loss seemed to have led to his escalating school problems had been someone whom he cared about. She was the first person with whom he had had a sexual relationship. The relationship had apparently dissolved after she had expressed an increasing desire to spend more time with her girlfriends and to go to school social events.

Discussion of "False Rumors"

This case is an example of Narcissistic Personality Disorder (DSM-5-TR, p. 760), and the reader will certainly be struck by Bob's grandiosity and insensitivity to others (lack of empathy). In addition, he is extremely jealous of his siblings, he spreads rumors about teachers who gave him poor grades and a student with whom he was competing, and he believes others envy him. Inference from the limited case material presented identifies behaviors that meet two additional criteria required for the diagnosis. Bob's trouble with authorities about conforming to school rules suggests that he does not believe the rules should apply to him, a behavior that is an indication of entitlement. His spreading rumors about teachers and peers can be considered evidence that he is interpersonally exploitative. Finally, his need for constant attention and admiration is suggested by his dramatic presentation.

Bob's case illustrates the clinical observation and research data that indicate that Narcissistic Personality Disorder might not always manifest with expressions of extremely overt grandiosity, but rather sometimes with more subtle and covert attitudes and behaviors. The case also reveals that grandiosity and entitlement often mask a vulnerable and insecure self-concept. Finally, some severe cases of Narcissistic Personality Disorder have features of Antisocial Personality Disorder (see Section 18.5). In Bob's case, in addition to being interpersonally exploitative and lacking empathy (two criteria for Narcissistic Personality Disorder), Bob shows signs of being deceitful and manipulative (spreading false rumors about teachers to get revenge and about other students to achieve his goals). Bob's case is an example of what has been referred to as "malignant narcissism."

18.7
Histrionic Personality Disorder

Histrionic Personality Disorder is characterized by "a pervasive pattern of excessive emotionality and attention seeking" (DSM-5-TR, p. 757). Patients with Histrionic Personality Disorder need to be the center of attention and will go to great lengths to use their physical appearance and inappropriate sexually seductive or provocative behavior to draw attention to themselves. Affected persons display exaggerated, effusive, but labile and shallow emotions; are very dramatic in their interpersonal styles; and have a very impressionistic style of speaking. They often believe that their relationships with others are considerably closer and more intimate than they actually are.

According to the Alternative DSM-5 Model for Personality Disorders, Histrionic Personality Disorder would be diagnosed as Personality Disorder—Trait Specified (DSM-5-TR, p. 890). The level of impairment in personality functioning is typically moderate, and the relevant domains and personality traits are as follows: emotional lability (Negative Affectivity domain) and attention seeking and manipulativeness (both in the Antagonism domain).

Histrionic Personality Disorder is one of the least common Personality Disorders, with an estimated median population prevalence of 0.9% (based on five epidemiological studies). Although more women than men receive this diagnosis in clinical settings, the actual ratio (i.e., in the general population) of women to men with the disorder is believed to be more equal. Romantic relationships end up being disappointing, leading to depression or somatic problems of unclear etiology. Disorders commonly co-occurring with Histrionic Personality Disorder include Borderline, Narcissistic, Paranoid, Dependent, and Antisocial Personality Disorders; Substance Use Disorders; Somatic Symptom Disorders (e.g., Functional Neurological Symptom Disorder [Conversion Disorder]); and Major Depressive Disorder. Individuals with this disorder may be prone to making suicidal gestures and threats.

Coquette

Carla Peters is a 30-year-old cocktail waitress who sought treatment with a clinical psychologist after breaking up with her 50-year-old boyfriend. Although initially she was tearful and expressed suicidal thoughts, she brightened up within the first session and became animated, dramatic, and coquettish with the male interviewer. During the intake evaluation interviews, she was always attractively and seductively dressed, wore carefully applied facial makeup, and crossed her legs in a revealing fashion. Ms. Peters related her story with dramatic inflections and seemed very concerned with the impression she was making on the interviewer. Although she often cried during sessions, her grief appeared to be without depth and mainly for effect. Several times she asked that the next appointment be changed to accommodate her plans; when this was not possible, she became anxious and depressed and expressed the feeling that her therapist must not like her.

Ms. Peters' history reveals that she is frequently the life of the party and has no problem making friends, although she seems to lose them just as easily and feels lonely most of the time. People apparently accuse her of being selfish, immature, and unreliable. She is often late for appointments; borrows money that she rarely returns; and breaks dates on impulse or if someone more attractive turns up. She is competitive with and jealous of other women, believes that they are catty and untrustworthy, and is known for being particularly seductive with her friends' boyfriends.

Discussion of "Coquette"

Ms. Peters' seductive behavior, both in the interview situation and with her friends' boyfriends, and her behavior at parties are evidence of consistent attention seeking. This, combined with her dramatic storytelling (self-dramatization) and her intense disappointment at not being able to reschedule her appointments to accommodate her plans, is presumably characteristic of her personality style. Her frequent crying for effect in the interviews is indicative of shallowness, and there is ample evidence of her self-indulgent lack of consideration for others, such as not returning borrowed money and often breaking dates. All of these personality traits, which clearly cause significant interpersonal problems for Ms. Peters (e.g., she loses friends easily, people "accuse her of being selfish, immature, and unreliable"), add up to a prototypical description of Histrionic Personality Disorder (DSM-5-TR, p. 757).

Although Ms. Peters has narcissistic traits (e.g., her constantly seeking attention and admiration, sense of entitlement, exploitative behavior in interpersonal relationships), the absence of grandiosity or a sense of uniqueness precludes the diagnosis of Narcissistic Personality Disorder (see Section 18.6). There are also borderline personality traits, such as emotional lability, but no evidence of most of the other characteristics of Borderline Personality Disorder, such as instability in self-image and impulsivity (see Section 18.1).

18.8
Schizotypal Personality Disorder

Persons with Schizotypal Personality Disorder experience "cognitive or perceptual distortions" and have "eccentricities of behavior," in addition to a "pattern of social and interpersonal deficits marked by acute discomfort with, and reduced capacity for, close relationships" (DSM-5-TR, p. 744). Common cognitive and perceptual distortions include ideas of reference (i.e., the belief that casual incidents and external events have particular and unusual meaning that is specific to them), bodily illusions (e.g., sensing that another person is present when no one else is there), and unusual beliefs (e.g., that they have unusual telepathic or clairvoyant powers) that are not held with delusional conviction. In part because of these experiences, persons with Schizotypal Personality Disorder exhibit odd and eccentric behavior. They may talk to themselves in public, gesture for no apparent reason, or dress in a strange or unkempt fashion. Their speech is often odd and idiosyncratic, perhaps unusually circumstantial (talking around a point without ever getting to it), metaphorical, or vague. Their emotional expression is constricted or inappropriate (e.g., they may laugh when discussing their problems). On top of these problems, individuals with Schizotypal Personality Disorder are suspicious of others and are socially anxious. Therefore, they have very few close friends or confidants.

Schizotypal Personality Disorder is included as a specific Personality Disorder in the Alternative DSM-5 Model for Personality Disorders (DSM-5-TR, p. 889). It is characterized by disorder-specific impairments in personality functioning (e.g., confused boundaries between self and others, unrealistic or incoherent life goals, misinterpretation of others' motivation and behavior, marked impairment in developing close relationships with others because of mistrust) at the extreme level and by traits in two personality trait domains: Psychoticism (the traits of cognitive and perceptual dysregulation, unusual beliefs and experiences, and eccentricity) and Detachment (the traits of restricted affectivity, withdrawal, and suspiciousness).

Schizotypal Personality Disorder is one of the least common Personality Disorders, with an estimated median population prevalence of 0.6% (based on five epidemiological studies). The disorder is slightly more common in men than in women. It may begin in childhood or adolescence as solitary behavior, poor peer relationships, social anxiety, underachievement in school, and hypersensitivity. In addition, the young person may express peculiar thoughts and bizarre fantasies and may appear odd or eccentric to others and attract teasing. Schizotypal Personality Disorder is one of the most impairing Personality Disorders with respect to psychosocial functioning. Despite its symptomatic similarity to the prodrome of Schizophrenia (see Section 2.1), Schizotypal Personality Disorder usually has a relatively stable course over time and rarely evolves into Schizophrenia or another Psychotic Disorder. It appears, however, that there may be a strong genetic relationship between Schizophrenia and Schizotypal Personality Disorder, given that some of the symptoms and abnormalities in brain chemistry, brain structure, and brain functioning found in people with Schizophrenia can also be found in people with Schizotypal Personality Disorder. Schizoid, Paranoid, Avoidant, and Borderline Personality Disorders may co-occur with Schizotypal Personality Disorder.

Clairvoyant

Destiny Carter is a 32-year-old single unemployed woman receiving public assistance, who complains that she feels "spacey." She reports that her feelings of detachment have gradually become stronger and more uncomfortable. For many hours each day, she feels as if she were watching herself move through life, and the world around her seems unreal. She feels especially strange when she looks in a mirror. For many years, she has felt able to read people's minds by a "kind of clairvoyance I don't understand." According to her, several people in her family apparently also have this ability. She is preoccupied by the thought that she has some special mission in life, but she is not sure what it is; she is not particularly religious. Ms. Carter is very self-conscious in public, often feels that people are paying special attention to her, and sometimes thinks that strangers cross the street to avoid her. She is lonely and isolated and spends much of each day lost in fantasies or watching TV soap operas. She speaks in a vague, abstract, digressive manner, generally just missing the point, but she is never incoherent. She seems shy, suspicious, and afraid she will be criticized. She has no gross loss of reality testing (i.e., psychosis), such as hallucinations or delusions. She has never had treatment for emotional problems. She has had occasional jobs but drifts away from them because of lack of interest.

Discussion of "Clairvoyant"

Although Ms. Carter's signs and symptoms have become more distressing to her recently, they are manifestations of a long-standing maladaptive pattern that suggests a Personality Disorder rather than the new development of another mental disorder. Her symptoms include depersonalization (feelings of detachment and feeling as if she were watching herself), derealization (feeling that "the world around her seems unreal"), magical thinking (clairvoyance), ideas of reference (strangers cross the street to avoid her), social isolation, odd speech (vague, abstract, digressive), and suspiciousness. These are the hallmarks of Schizotypal Personality Disorder (DSM-5-TR, p. 744). This Personality Disorder is more complex than either Paranoid Personality Disorder (see Section 18.10) or Schizoid Personality Disorder (see Section 18.9), because it is characterized by traits of both Psychoticism and Detachment (DSM-5-TR, p. 899).

It is reasonable to explore if Ms. Carter's belief in her ability to read people's minds is a delusion that would indicate a Psychotic Disorder (see Chapter 2, "Schizophrenia Spectrum and Other Psychotic Disorders") rather than merely an example of magical thinking. Her statement that she herself does not understand the process suggests that it is probably not a belief that is firmly held, as is characteristic of a delusion. The reader might be curious about the likelihood that Ms. Carter has had a previous psychotic episode, in which case the current symptoms would be indicative of the residual phase of Schizophrenia (see "The Witch" in Section 2.1). In the absence of such a history, however, a diagnosis of Schizotypal Personality Disorder is most appropriate.

Wash Before Wearing

Seymour Goldstein is a 41-year-old man who was referred to a community mental health care center's activities program for help in improving his social skills. He has a lifelong pattern of social isolation, with no real friends, and spends long hours worrying that his angry thoughts about his older brother would cause his brother harm. He previously worked as a civil service clerk but lost his job because of poor attendance and low productivity.

On interview by the intake social worker, Mr. Goldstein is distant and somewhat distrustful. He describes in elaborate and often irrelevant detail his rather uneventful and routine daily life. He tells the interviewer that he has often spent 1½ hours in a pet store deciding which of two brands of fish food to buy, and then he explains their relative merits. He describes how for 2 days he studied the washing instructions on a new pair of jeans, considering whether "Wash before wearing" means that the jeans are to be washed before wearing the first time or that, for some reason, they need to be washed each time before they are worn again. He does not regard concerns such as these as senseless, although he acknowledges that the amount of time spent thinking about them might be excessive. Mr. Goldstein describes how he often buys several different brands of the same item, such as different kinds of can openers, and then keeps them in their original bags in his closet, expecting that at some future time he will find them useful. He is usually very reluctant, however, to spend money on things that he actually needs, although he has a substantial bank account. He can recite from memory his most recent monthly bank statement, including the amount of every check and the running balance as each check was written. He knows his balance on any particular day but sometimes gets anxious if he considers whether a certain check or deposit has actually cleared.

Mr. Goldstein asked the interviewer whether, if he joined the program, he would be required to participate in groups. He said that groups made him very nervous because he feels that if he reveals too much personal information, such as the amount of money that he has in the bank, people will take advantage of him or manipulate him for their own benefit.

Discussion of "Wash Before Wearing"

Mr. Goldstein's long-standing maladaptive pattern of behavior indicates a Personality Disorder. Prominent symptoms include the absence of close friends or confidants, magical thinking (worrying that his angry thoughts would cause his brother harm), constricted affect (observed to be "distant" in the interview), odd speech (providing elaborate and often irrelevant details), and social anxiety associated with paranoid fears. These features are characteristic of Schizotypal Personality Disorder (DSM-5-TR, p. 744).

Although Autism Spectrum Disorder (see Section 1.6) is characterized by problems in social communication and social interaction, this disorder can be distinguished from Schizotypal Personality Disorder in that individuals with Autism Spectrum Disorder have a much more pronounced lack of social awareness and emotional reciprocity, as well as stereotyped behaviors and interests.

Although the absence of close friends or confidants is also characteristic of Schizoid Personality Disorder (see Section 18.9), Mr. Goldstein's eccentricities of thought and speech preclude that diagnosis. There are many similarities between Schizotypal Personality Disorder and the symptoms seen in the residual phase of Schizophrenia (see Section 2.1), but the absence of a history of overt psychotic symptoms rules out that diagnosis.

Mr. Goldstein's concerns with choosing the best brand of fish food and understanding the instructions for washing his jeans suggest obsessions, but because the concerns are not experienced by the patient as intrusive and unwanted and he does not try to suppress them or neutralize them with some other thought or action, they are not true obsessions, which would be indicative of Obsessive-Compulsive Disorder (see "Lady Macbeth" in Section 6.1), but rather examples of the personality trait of perfectionism. He is also preoccupied with organizing his financial affairs and is miserly with his money.

Despite having these traits of Obsessive-Compulsive Personality Disorder (DSM-5-TR, p. 771), Mr. Goldstein does not seem to meet the full criteria for the disorder. This case illustrates the common finding that individuals with Personality Disorders often have at least traits or features of other Personality Disorders, which make each case somewhat distinctive.

18.9
Schizoid Personality Disorder

Schizoid Personality Disorder is characterized by "a pervasive pattern of detachment from social relationships and a restricted range of expression of emotions in interpersonal settings" (DSM-5-TR, p. 741). Individuals with Schizoid Personality Disorder have little desire for social relationships and consequently are very socially isolated. They prefer solitary activities, take pleasure in few activities, and have little interest in having sexual experiences with another person. They have few or no close friends, seldom date or get married, and often work at jobs that have little interpersonal contact (e.g., night watchman). These individuals lack emotional expressivity and appear cold, detached, and aloof. They also seem indifferent to the praise or criticism of others.

According to the Alternative DSM-5 Model for Personality Disorders, Schizoid Personality Disorder would be diagnosed as Personality Disorder—Trait Specified (DSM-5-TR, p. 890). The level of impairment in personality functioning would typically be extreme, and the relevant pathological personality traits all come from the Detachment trait domain: withdrawal, intimacy avoidance, anhedonia, and restricted affectivity.

Schizoid Personality Disorder is a relatively rare Personality Disorder (median population prevalence of 1.3%, based on six epidemiological studies). The disorder is particularly uncommon in clinical settings. It appears to be more common in men than in women. Like Schizotypal Personality Disorder (see Section 18.8), Schizoid Personality Disorder may first become apparent in childhood and adolescence with solitariness, poor peer relationships, and underachievement in school. By definition, individuals with Schizoid Personality Disorder have very poor social relationships. The disorder most often co-occurs with Schizotypal, Paranoid, and Avoidant Personality Disorders.

Man's Best Friend

Kyle Murphy is a 50-year-old single man who seeks treatment a few weeks after his dog was run over and killed. Since that time, he has felt sad and tired, and has had trouble sleeping and concentrating.

Mr. Murphy lives alone and for many years has had virtually no conversational contacts with other human beings beyond a "Hello" or "How are you?" He prefers to be by himself, finds talk a waste of time, and feels awkward when other people try to initiate a relationship. He occasionally spends some time in a bar, but always off by himself and not trying to follow the general conversation. He reads newspapers avidly and is well informed in many areas, but he takes no particular interest in the people around him. He is employed as a security guard but is known by fellow workers as a "cold fish" and a "loner." They no longer even notice or tease him, especially because he never seemed to pay attention to or care about their teasing anyway.

Mr. Murphy has gone through most of his adult life without relationships except with his dog, which he dearly loved. At Christmas, he would buy his dog elaborate gifts and in return would receive a wrapped bottle of scotch that he bought for himself as a gift from the dog. He believes that dogs are more sensitive and loving than people, and he can in return express toward them a tenderness and emotion not possible in his relationships with people. The losses of his pets have been the only events in his life that have caused him sadness. He experienced the death of his parents without emotion and feels no regret whatever at being completely out of contact with the rest of his family. He considers himself different from other people and regards emotionality in others with bewilderment.

Discussion of "Man's Best Friend"

Mr. Murphy's long-standing pattern of social isolation, inability to express tenderness or emotion for people, and general indifference to others, coupled with an absence of oddities and eccentricities of behavior, speech, or thought, is indicative of Schizoid Personality Disorder (DSM-5-TR, p. 741). It is the presence of the Schizoid Personality Disorder that has made him particularly vulnerable to the stress of his pet's death. If there were evidence of unusual perceptions or thinking, such as recurrent illusions or ideas of reference, the diagnosis Schizotypal Personality Disorder (see Section 18.8) would need to be considered.

As is common in patients with Personality Disorders, it is often something distressing that is not necessarily symptomatic of the Personality Disorder (in this case, the Adjustment Disorder as a result of the dog's death) that leads the person to seek treatment.

18.10
Paranoid Personality Disorder

Individuals with Paranoid Personality Disorder have a "pervasive distrust and suspiciousness of others such that their motives are interpreted as malevolent" (DSM-5-TR, p. 737). Such individuals suspect that others may be out to exploit, harm, or deceive them and therefore may question, without justification, the loyalty or trustworthiness of friends or associates and often have unjustified suspicions about the fidelity of their spouses or sexual partners. They are reluctant to confide in others for fear that the information will be used against them. Persons with Paranoid Personality Disorder are likely to find "evidence" for their distrust by reading hidden or threatening meaning into benign remarks or events. These individuals are very sensitive to perceived "attacks" on their character or reputation and are likely to be unforgiving of insults, injuries, or slights. They will be quick to react angrily and to counterattack when they feel threatened. Persons with Paranoid Personality Disorder can be extremely litigious. Some individuals with Paranoid Personality Disorder appear quietly and tensely aloof and hostile, whereas others are openly angry and combative.

According to the Alternative DSM-5 Model for Personality Disorders, Paranoid Personality Disorder would be diagnosed as Personality Disorder—Trait Specified (DSM-5-TR, p. 890). It would be characterized by severe or extreme impairment in personality functioning, and relevant descriptive pathological personality traits would include suspiciousness and hostility from the Negative Affectivity domain.

Paranoid Personality Disorder is a fairly common Personality Disorder, with a median population prevalence of 3.2% based on six epidemiological studies. The disorder is more often found in men than in women. Paranoid Personality Disorder often first manifests in childhood or adolescence as a solitary persona, with poor peer relationships, social anxiety, school underachievement, and hypersensitivity to teasing. Because people with Paranoid Personality Disorder are so suspicious of others, they are typically socially isolated and have trouble with intimate relationships, with bosses, and with coworkers.

Commonly co-occurring other mental disorders include Agoraphobia, Obsessive-Compulsive Disorder, and Schizotypal, Schizoid, Narcissistic, Avoidant, and Borderline Personality Disorders.

Useful Work

An 85-year-old man named Peter Grace is seen by a social worker at a senior citizens center for evaluation of health care needs for Mr. Grace and his bedridden wife. He is apparently healthy, with no evidence of impairment in thinking or memory. He has been caring for his wife but has been reluctantly persuaded to seek help because her condition has deteriorated, and his strength and energy have decreased with age.

A history is obtained from the subject and his daughter. Mr. Grace has never been treated for mental illness, and in fact has always claimed to be "immune to psychological problems" and to act only on the basis of "rational" thought. He had a moderately successful career as a lawyer and businessman. He has been married for 60 years, and his wife is the only person for whom he has ever expressed tender feelings and is probably the only person he has ever trusted. He has always been extremely careful about revealing anything of himself to others, assuming that they are out to take something away from him. He refuses obviously sincere offers of help from acquaintances because he suspects they have underlying motives. Mr. Grace never reveals his identity to a caller without first questioning the person as to the nature of their business. Throughout his life there have been numerous occasions on which he has displayed exaggerated suspiciousness, sometimes of almost delusional proportions (e.g., storing letters from a client in a secret safe deposit box so that he could use them as evidence in the event that the client attempted to sue him for mismanagement of an estate).

Mr. Grace has always involved himself in "useful work" during his waking hours and claims never to have time for play, even during the 20 years since he has been retired. He spends many hours monitoring his stock market investments and has had altercations with his broker when he suspected that an error on a monthly statement was evidence of the broker's attempt to ruin his reputation.

Discussion of "Useful Work"

This gentleman demonstrates pervasive and unwarranted distrust and suspiciousness of others. Mr. Grace expects to be exploited or deceived by others (he assumes others are out to take something from him; he questions callers before revealing his identity). He perceives attacks on his character and is quick to react angrily and counterattack (he has had altercations with his broker when he suspects an attempt to ruin his reputation). He questions the loyalty or trustworthiness of others (his wife is the only person he has ever trusted). He is reluctant to confide in others (he is extremely careful about revealing anything about himself). These lifelong features, in the absence of any evidence of persistent persecutory delusions or any other psychotic symptoms, characterize Paranoid Personality Disorder (DSM-5-TR, p. 737).

This case illustrates the ego-syntonic nature of Paranoid Personality Disorder (i.e., Mr. Grace does not believe that there is anything wrong with him). For this reason, treatment is rarely sought by individuals with this disorder. A number of other Personality Disorders share this feature. It is often only the people with whom the individual has contact who recognize the person's attitude or behavior as problematic. This case also demonstrates the frequently associated features of the quiet and tense presentation of Paranoid Personality

Disorder: an inability to relax (e.g., never has time for recreation) and restricted affectivity or emotionality (e.g., pride in being "rational").

Mr. Grace has several schizoid and obsessive-compulsive features, but not enough to warrant the additional diagnosis of either Schizoid Personality Disorder (see Section 18.9) or Obsessive-Compulsive Personality Disorder (see Section 18.4).

18.11
Personality Change Due to Another Medical Condition

The diagnosis of Personality Change Due to Another Medical Condition is made when "a persistent personality disturbance that represents a change from the individual's previous characteristic personality pattern" (DSM-5-TR, p. 775) occurs as a result of a nonpsychiatric medical condition, such as a brain tumor or head trauma. The predominant features of the personality change are specified according to various subtypes: Labile Type (if the predominant feature is emotional lability), Disinhibited Type (poor impulse control), Aggressive Type (aggressive behavior), Apathetic Type (marked apathy and indifference), Paranoid Type (suspiciousness and paranoid ideation), Other Type, Combined Type, or Unspecified Type.

Using the Alternative Model, any of the 25 DSM-5-TR pathological personality traits can be used to describe the personality features of a Personality Change Due to Another Medical Condition, either alone or in combination.

The level of associated impairment and the clinical course of these disorders will depend on the nature and extent of the causative other medical disorder and its treatability and reversibility. When making this diagnosis, the name of the nonpsychiatric medical condition causing the personality change is noted.

Coma

Dominick Wozniak, a 34-year-old former schoolteacher, lives in a halfway house. For the last 2 years, he has been unemployed and separated from his wife and children, who avoid him. Two years ago, he was in a serious auto accident, which resulted in a coma from which he made a gradual recovery with only supportive medical treatment. He now has no significant neurological signs except a very minor loss in one visual field. His verbal and performance IQs are about 120.

According to the family, Mr. Wozniak has changed since the accident. He is frequently impulsive and argumentative, often misses buses and trains to familiar places, and gets lost. He displays poor social judgment and financial irresponsibility; for example, he makes long-distance phone calls (including one to the Pope at the Vatican) and then sends the bills to his family.

When seen by the clinician, Mr. Wozniak was disheveled and joked frequently but with an undercurrent of bitterness and hostility. A computed tomography (CT) scan demonstrated large areas of brain tissue destruction, principally in the frontal lobes.

Discussion of "Coma"

The abrupt change in Mr. Wozniak's personality and functioning after his recovery from coma secondary to head trauma suggests a Neurocognitive Disorder. However, while there is some evidence of memory impairment (he often misses buses and trains, gets lost), his high IQ is inconsistent with the generalized loss in intellectual functioning of a Major Neurocognitive Disorder (see "The Hiker" in Section 17.2). Instead, the most prominent features in this case are impulsivity, argumentativeness, poor judgment, and deterioration in self-care, all of which have led to severe occupational and social impairments. These changes in personality, associated with a specific medical factor known to be etiological to the disturbance (history of trauma and CT scan indicating frontal lobe brain damage), indicate a Personality Change Due to Traumatic Brain Injury (DSM-5-TR, p. 775).

18.12
Other Specified Personality Disorder

The diagnosis of Other Specified Personality Disorder is used to indicate clinical disturbances that have the general characteristics of a Personality Disorder and cause significant distress or impairment in psychosocial functioning but do not meet the criteria for any of the specific disorders in the DSM-5-TR Personality Disorders class. In prior DSM classifications, a similar residual Personality Disorder diagnosis—Personality Disorder Not Otherwise Specified—was actually found to be the most commonly used by clinicians. The frequent use of this category occurs because there are many forms in which personality psychopathology can be manifest, not simply the specified types. Some of these alternative Personality Disorders have appeared in previous DSM editions but were subsequently deleted for lack of validity (e.g., Passive-Aggressive Personality Disorder) or have been candidates for inclusion that did not become adopted (e.g., Depressive or Self-Defeating Personality Disorders). The Other Specified Personality Disorder category can also be used if a patient meets the general criteria for a Personality Disorder (DSM-5-TR, p. 734), has features of several types, and does not meet the criteria for any one specific Personality Disorder; such a case would receive the diagnosis Other Specified Personality Disorder, With Mixed Personality Features (DSM-5-TR, p. 778).

Using the Alternative DSM-5 Model for Personality Disorders, the diagnosis for all such cases would be Personality Disorder—Trait Specified (DSM-5-TR, p. 890), with the prominent personality traits listed. For example, Passive-Aggressive Personality Disorder would be Personality Disorder—Trait Specified with listed traits of submissiveness and hostility; and Depressive Personality Disorder would be Personality Disorder—Trait Specified with depressivity, anxiousness, and anhedonia. The Alternative Model provides considerable flexibility in describing the myriad presentations of personality pathology that do not fit one of the specific types.

Stubborn Psychiatrist

A 34-year-old psychiatrist named Derek Cooper is 15 minutes late for his first appointment. He had recently been asked to resign from his job in a mental health care center because, according to his supervisor, he had frequently been late for work and meetings, missed appointments, forgot about assignments, was late with his statistics, refused to follow instructions, and seemed unmotivated. The patient was surprised and resentful; he thought he had been doing a particularly good job under trying circumstances and experienced his supervisor as excessively obsessive and demanding. Nonetheless, he reported a long-standing pattern of difficulties with authority.

Dr. Cooper had a childhood history of severe and prolonged temper tantrums that were a legend in his family. He had been a bossy child who demanded that other kids "play his way" or else he would not play at all. With adults, particularly his mother and female teachers, he was sullen, insubordinate, oppositional, and often unmanageable. He had been sent to an all-boys preparatory school that had primarily male teachers, and he gradually became more subdued and disciplined. Dr. Cooper continued, however, to stubbornly want things his own way and to resent instruction or direction from teachers. He was a brilliant but erratic student, working only as hard as he wanted to, and he "punished" teachers he did not like by not doing their assignments. He was argumentative and self-righteous when criticized, and complained that he was not being treated fairly.

Dr. Cooper is unhappily married. He complains that his wife does not understand him and is a "nitpicker." She complains that he is unreliable and stubborn. He refuses to do anything around the house and often forgets to complete the few errands he has accepted as within his responsibility. Tax forms are submitted several months late, and bills are not paid. The patient is sociable and has considerable charm, but friends generally become annoyed at his unwillingness to go along with the wishes of the group; for example, if a restaurant is not his choice, he may sulk all night or forget to bring his wallet.

Discussion of "Stubborn Psychiatrist"

Whenever Dr. Cooper feels that demands are being made on him, either socially or occupationally, he passively resists through such characteristic maneuvers as procrastination (e.g., sending tax returns late, not paying bills), stubbornness (e.g., being unwilling to go along with the wishes of his friends), and forgetfulness (e.g., forgetting errands for his wife and assignments at work). His behavior has resulted in impaired work performance and marital difficulties. Such a long-standing pattern of resistance to demands for adequate performance in role functioning is a prototype of Passive-Aggressive Personality Disorder, included for further study in DSM-IV but not retained in DSM-5 (or DSM-5-TR). This is an example of a situation in which an Other Specified Personality Disorder (DSM-5-TR, p. 778) would be diagnosed, because the behavior pattern does not correspond to any of the 10 specific Personality Disorders included in DSM-5-TR Section II. Although passive-aggressive behavior is quite common in situations in which assertive behavior is not encouraged or is actually punished (e.g., in the military service), a Personality Disorder diagnosis is made only if the behavior occurs in situations in which more assertive behavior is possible.

This case demonstrates that neither a high IQ nor membership in a mental health care profession conveys immunity to a Personality Disorder.

Goody Two-Shoes

Maryann West is a single 35-year-old magazine editor who lives alone. She was referred for psychotherapy by her female family doctor, who suggested that Ms. West needed to work on problems in her relationships with men. Ms. West resisted following through on the referral for a year, saying, "I don't like getting help. I like giving it."

When she first met with the male therapist, Ms. West appeared to be highly intelligent; she was affable and articulate and spoke in a breathy voice. She had metal-black hair, was dressed all in black (leather skirt and jacket and black top), and wore "punkish" glasses. She said, at the beginning of the interview, that she did not want a male therapist because she was mistrustful of men, who in her experience wanted only to exploit women. However, with the exception of her family doctor, she had no close women friends.

Her story was that she had just extricated herself from a "destructive" relationship with a man, "my outlaw love," who was a heroin addict, and she was fighting her wish to return to him. Once, 4 years earlier, he had hit her and made her cry, but she told him that if he did that again, she would leave, and such an attack never recurred. She claimed she was not frightened of him and actually blamed herself for his attacking her. "I often tell him things he should know about himself, and he gets furious. I only do it to motivate him. I hit his soft spot."

Her lover's drug addiction persisted, and Ms. West continued to support him financially whenever he needed help. She said she received many indications that this relationship could not make her happy. The man had gone out with other women while dating Ms. West, served a brief jail sentence for selling drugs, and never wanted to engage in mutually entertaining activities, except sex, which was enjoyable. Ms. West had gone to a university, but her lover had never completed high school. She felt that he was like a little child who needed mothering. He would tell her to get lost when she insisted that he stop using drugs, but she continued to call him regularly in spite of his ungrateful behavior. She felt resentful and embittered because of all she had done for him, yet she always helped him when he came back to her, typically late at night, asking for money or assistance. As a result, she said she felt "more like a Mother Teresa than a girlfriend."

Ms. West is now seeing another "exciting" man, also a substance abuser. Although she considers herself "left-wing," her new friend is a collector of Nazi memorabilia. She knew that he treated his previous girlfriend cruelly by being unfaithful and abusive, but she did not think about whether this might happen to her. She has seen this man on and off for a year. He had insisted that he wanted a close relationship but did not tell her he was seeing one of her acquaintances on the side. When she found out about this, she was very upset, but she continues to have an intense interest in him. A number of nicer men who had monogamous intentions have frequently tried to date her, but she has avoided them because they all seemed "boring."

In her other relationships, Ms. West always gives help but never asks for it, even when she is in real need. Most of her friends and ex-boyfriends have been drug addicts or ex-addicts. She herself has never abused drugs. She often visits these people in jail and offers to help them, but when they are released, they hardly ever visit her.

At her job, Ms. West is hardworking and good at solving disputes, but she has sometimes gotten into trouble with her boss for arranging to use the magazine's resources to raise money for needy groups. She feels that her female colleagues "gang up on her" because of envy of her abilities and capacity for hard work, in spite of all the benefits that she has helped them obtain.

Ms. West is the oldest of four children and often had to grudgingly care for her young siblings. She became a "goody two-shoes," while her younger brothers were permitted to "act up." In church and school, she did well and won many awards, until in her teens she rebelled and left home. Her parents predicted that she would "go to hell." She went through a period of "sexual liberation" during which she had about 50 lovers, often in one-night stands, which she rarely enjoyed "because I didn't love those guys." As a young adult, she was always involved in some worthy cause for the underprivileged, the poor, or the politically disadvantaged.

Discussion of "Goody Two-Shoes"

Ms. West seems to have gone through life playing the role of martyr. She has repeatedly been attracted to and chosen boyfriends who are inappropriate and mistreat her. She does not like to take help from others, and this has delayed her seeking treatment, even though she has realized for a long time that her relationships with people are harmful to her. She incites angry responses from others and then feels hurt when she is rejected (telling her boyfriend his failings). She is not interested in boyfriends who treat her well because they are "boring," and she engages in excessive self-sacrifice that is unsolicited by the recipients (visiting people in jail).

Behavior that appears to an outside observer as self-defeating may be observed when a person is in a situation in which they are afraid of being psychologically or physically abused, or when a person is depressed. In Ms. West's case, however, it seems to be a pervasive personality pattern that expresses itself in many situations and relationships of her own choosing. This personality pattern has been called Masochistic Personality Disorder and Self-Defeating Personality Disorder. Many clinicians, particularly those who practice psychodynamically oriented treatment of Personality Disorders, believe that this personality pattern represents a common and important disorder, and occurs nearly as often in men as in women. On the other hand, many clinicians, particularly those concerned with the potential for misuse of psychiatric diagnoses, have argued that the underlying construct of the disorder has no validity and that the diagnosis perpetuates the blaming of victims (primarily women) who have been abused. After much controversy, Self-Defeating Personality Disorder was included in Appendix A ("Proposed Diagnostic Categories Needing Further Study") of DSM-III-R but was eliminated entirely from DSM-IV. Such a case can still be diagnosed according to DSM-5-TR (p. 778) as Other Specified Personality Disorder, because the clinical picture represents a type of personality disorder not included in the DSM classification.

CHAPTER 19

Paraphilic Disorders

A *paraphilia, also* known as a *sexual perversion* or *sexual deviation*, involves intense sexual arousal to atypical or inappropriate objects (e.g., underwear), situations (e.g., inflicting pain, exposing oneself), or individuals (e.g., children). The term comes from the Greek for *para*, meaning "other" or "outside of," and for *philia*, meaning "loving." Central to the concept of "paraphilia" is the value judgment that certain foci of sexual arousal are inherently deviant and therefore pathological. Drawing a clear boundary between sexual interest that is unusual but still "normal" and sexual interest that is considered so atypical as to be pathological is quite challenging and subject to wide variation from one culture to another. Moreover, it appears that the range of possible objects that can be a focus of sexual arousal in an individual is virtually limitless. For example, *forniphilia* involves sexual arousal derived from turning or incorporating a human being into a piece of furniture.

DSM-5-TR makes the important distinction between a paraphilia (i.e., an atypical focus of sexual arousal that does not cause distress or impairment) and a Paraphilic Disorder, which is present when the paraphilic focus of arousal leads to significant negative consequences to the person or to others. DSM-5-TR makes the following distinction:

> A *paraphilic disorder* is a paraphilia that is currently causing distress or impairment to the individual or a paraphilia whose satisfaction has entailed personal harm, or risk of harm, to others. A paraphilia is a necessary but not a sufficient condition for having a paraphilic disorder, and a paraphilia by itself does not necessarily justify or require clinical intervention. (DSM-5-TR, p. 780)

For example, paraphilic imagery may be acted out with a nonconsenting partner in a way that may be injurious to the partner (as in Sexual Sadism Disorder) and may lead to the individual's being subject to arrest and incarceration. In other cases, as in Sexual Masochism Disorder, acting out the paraphilic imagery may lead to self-injury. Social and sexual relationships may suffer if others find the unusual sexual behavior to be shameful or repugnant or if the individual's sexual partner refuses to cooperate in the unusual sexual preferences.

DSM-5-TR includes eight specific Paraphilic Disorders, which have been selected from among the large number of identified paraphilias because they are relatively common in relation to other possible Paraphilic Disorders or involve nonconsenting

471

victims and therefore are relevant to the treatment of sex offenders. These eight disorders include the following, with the related paraphilic focus of sexual arousal noted in parentheses: Voyeuristic Disorder (sexual arousal from observing an unsuspecting person who is naked, disrobing, or engaging in sexual activity), Exhibitionistic Disorder (sexual arousal from the exposure of one's genitals to an unsuspecting person), Frotteuristic Disorder (sexual arousal from touching or rubbing against a nonconsenting person), Sexual Masochism Disorder (sexual arousal from the act of being humiliated, beaten, bound, or otherwise made to suffer), Sexual Sadism Disorder (sexual arousal from the physical or psychological suffering of another person), Pedophilic Disorder (sexual arousal from prepubescent children), Fetishistic Disorder (sexual arousal from the use of nonliving objects or a highly specific focus on nongenital body parts, such as feet), and Transvestic Disorder (sexual arousal from cross-dressing). Table 19–1 lists characteristic features of the Paraphilic Disorders.

Some individuals report that their paraphilic fantasies or stimuli are obligatory for erotic arousal and are always included in sexual activity. Other individuals state that their paraphilic tendencies occur only during periods of stress, and that at other times they are able to function sexually without paraphilic fantasies or stimuli. An individual's pattern of paraphilic interests is often reflected in their choice of pornography.

Paraphilic Disorders are almost exclusively diagnosed in men, except approximately 1 in 20 individuals diagnosed with Sexual Masochism Disorder are women. Most people who develop a paraphilia begin having fantasies about the atypical focus of sexual arousal before they are 13 years old.

19.1
Voyeuristic Disorder

Voyeurism involves sexual arousal from observing an unsuspecting and nonconsenting person who is naked, in the process of disrobing, or engaging in sexual activity. Many people have voyeuristic impulses, but no clinician would consider diagnosing Voyeuristic Disorder in someone who is occasionally sexually aroused by accidentally observing an unsuspecting neighbor disrobe or by watching pornography, in which the actors pretend to be unaware that they are being observed. The DSM-5-TR diagnosis of Voyeuristic Disorder should be made only if the individual experiences an extended period (lasting 6 months or more) of recurrent and intense sexual arousal from voyeurism and only if the individual has acted on these urges with a nonconsenting person or if the urges and fantasies cause clinically significant distress or impairment in functioning.

Because voyeuristic behavior is normal when it occurs in the context of sexual curiosity during adolescence and puberty, the DSM-5-TR diagnosis of Voyeuristic Disorder cannot be made unless the individual is at least 18 years old. Voyeuristic acts are the most common of potentially law-breaking sexual behaviors.

TABLE 19–1. **Characteristic features of specific Paraphilic Disorders**

Disorder	Key characteristics
Voyeuristic Disorder	Sexual arousal from observing an unsuspecting person who is naked, in the process of disrobing, or engaging in sexual activity
	The individual has acted on these urges with a nonconsenting person, or the urges and fantasies cause distress or impairment
Exhibitionistic Disorder	Sexual arousal from the exposure of one's genitals to an unsuspecting person
	The individual has acted on these urges with a nonconsenting person, or the urges and fantasies cause distress or impairment
Frotteuristic Disorder	Sexual arousal from touching or rubbing against a nonconsenting person
	The individual has acted on these urges with a nonconsenting person, or the urges and fantasies cause distress or impairment
Sexual Masochism Disorder	Sexual arousal from the act of being humiliated, beaten, bound, or otherwise made to suffer
	The urges and fantasies cause distress or impairment
Sexual Sadism Disorder	Sexual arousal from the physical or psychological suffering of another person
	The individual has acted on these urges with a nonconsenting person, or the urges and fantasies cause distress or impairment
Pedophilic Disorder	Sexually arousing fantasies, sexual urges, or behaviors involving sexual activity with prepubescent children
	The individual has acted on these urges with a prepubescent child, or the urges and fantasies cause distress or impairment
Fetishistic Disorder	Sexual arousal either from the use of nonliving objects or from a highly specific focus on nongenital body part(s)
	The urges, fantasies, or behaviors cause distress or impairment
Transvestic Disorder	Sexual arousal from cross-dressing
	The urges, fantasies, or behaviors cause distress or impairment

Binoculars

Mark Weber, a 35-year-old business executive, requests psychiatric consultation because of his repeated need to spy on women undressing or engaging in sexual activity. Mr. Weber is an articulate, handsome man who has no difficulty attracting sexual partners. He dates frequently and has sexual intercourse once or twice a week with a variety of women. In addition, however, he is frequently drawn to certain types of situations he finds uniquely arousing. He owns a pair of high-powered binoculars and uses these to peep into neighboring apartments. Sometimes he is rewarded for his efforts, but more frequently he is not, in which case he leaves his apartment and goes to rooftops of large apartment buildings, where he searches with his binoculars until he finds a woman undressing or engaging in sexual activity. He has no desire to enter the apartments he peeps into, and he denies experiencing impulses to rape. If he finds a scene in which he can watch a woman undressing or engaging in sexual activity, he masturbates to orgasm while watching, or immediately afterward, and then returns home. He experiences the voyeuristic situation, in its entirety, as pleasurable, despite the fact that he sometimes encounters potentially hazardous situations. On more than one occasion, he has been nearly apprehended by building staff or police, who took him to be a potential burglar or assailant; once he was chased from a "lovers' lane" by an irate man wielding a tire iron, and another time he barely escaped being shot after he was discovered peeping into a bedroom window in a rural area.

Mr. Weber was reared in a family that included three older sisters. He reports that his family was sexually puritanical. Family members did not disrobe in front of each other, for example, and the parents avoided open displays of activity that could be interpreted as erotic. Still, he recalls that between ages 7 and 10, he watched his mother and sisters undress "as much as possible."

At age 10, Mr. Weber began "peeping," along with many other boys, while at summer camp. He is unable to explain why this particular stimulus subsequently had a continuing appeal for him, whereas other boys seemed to become less interested in peeping as they became more interested in sexual intercourse. He has used binoculars to search for erotically stimulating scenes since he was age 11, but he did not leave his home to do so until age 17.

Mr. Weber notices some relationship between presumed psychological stress and his voyeuristic activity. For example, at times of major life change, such as moving out of his parents' home or finishing a college semester, the activity increased. He is not, however, aware of any relationship between anxiety about having sexual intercourse and the desire to engage in voyeuristic activity. He feels that anxiety is often present in the voyeuristic situation, but it is only a fear of being apprehended. He feels no guilt or shame about his voyeurism and considers it harmless. He is concerned, however, that he might one day go to jail unless he alters his sexual behavior, and for that reason he seeks help.

Discussion of "Binoculars"

Mr. Weber has repeatedly acted on his recurrent and intense voyeuristic urges with individuals who are unaware that they are being spied on and thus are considered "nonconsenting." Moreover, although Mr. Weber experiences no guilt or shame about his voyeurism, considering it "harmless," his fear of ending up in jail because of his behavior eventually has led him to seek treatment.

He thus qualifies for the DSM-5-TR diagnosis of Voyeuristic Disorder (DSM-5-TR, p. 780).

As noted in the introduction to this section, voyeuristic behavior occurring in the context of sexual curiosity during puberty is common and is illustrated in this case by the fact that Mr. Weber began engaging in voyeuristic behavior along with other boys at summer camp when he was age 10. Although the other boys' interest in voyeurism was a temporary phase, Mr. Weber's interest persisted and became a central focus of sexual interest.

As this case also illustrates, although some individuals with a paraphilia can only become sexually aroused when engaged in sexual activities involving their paraphilic focus (e.g., masturbating while surreptitiously watching women undressing or engaging in sexual activity), some people with paraphilias may also get pleasure from nonparaphilic intercourse.

19.2
Exhibitionistic Disorder

Exhibitionism involves sexual arousal from the fantasy or act of exposing one's genitals to an unsuspecting person. The prevalence of presentations that meet the full criteria for Exhibitionistic Disorder (i.e., exhibitionistic sexual urges over a period of at least 6 months that were acted on with an unsuspecting person or that caused distress or impairment) is unknown, although the disorder is thought to be highly unusual in women. Exhibitionistic acts, however, are likely not uncommon. In an internet and telephone survey sample, the lifetime prevalence of exhibitionistic behaviors was reported to be 33% in men and 29% in women. Because this same study found that an "intense desire" and "persistent behavior" occur with much less frequency (prevalence of 5% in men and 0.8% in women) than do exhibitionistic behaviors, the actual prevalence of Exhibitionistic Disorder is likely much lower. The vast majority of people who participate in exhibitionism are men, whereas nearly all of the targets of exhibitionists are women, underage girls, or underage boys. Although the stereotype of an exhibitionist is a "dirty old man in a raincoat," most males arrested for exhibitionism are in their late teens or early 20s. Roughly one-third of all men arrested for sexual offenses in the United States are exhibitionists.

Ashamed

Martin Klein, a 27-year-old engineer, requested consultation because of irresistible urges to exhibit his penis to female strangers. An only child, Mr. Klein had been reared in an orthodox Jewish environment. Sexuality was strongly condemned by both parents as being "dirty." His father, a schoolteacher, was authoritarian and punitive but relatively uninvolved in the home. His mother, a homemaker, was domineering, controlling, and intrusive. She was preoccupied with cleanliness and bathed the patient until he was 10 years old. Mr. Klein remembers that he feared he might have an erection in his mother's presence during one of his baths; however, this did not occur. His mother was opposed to his meeting and dating girls during his adolescence. He was not allowed to bring girls home; according to her, the proper time to bring a woman home was "when she is your wife, and not before." Despite his mother's puritanical values, she frequently walked about the house partially disrobed in his presence. To his shame, he found himself sexually aroused by this stimulation, which occurred frequently throughout his development.

As an adolescent, Mr. Klein was quiet, withdrawn, and studious; teachers described him as a "model child." He was friendly, but not intimate, with a few male classmates. Puberty occurred at age 13, and his first ejaculation occurred at that age during sleep. Because of feelings of guilt, he resisted the temptation to masturbate, and between ages 13 and 18, orgasms occurred only with nocturnal emissions. He did not begin to date women until he moved out of his parents' home, at age 25. During the next 2 years he dated from time to time but was too inhibited to initiate sexual activity.

At age 18, for reasons unknown to himself, during the week before final exams, he first experienced an overwhelming desire to engage in the sexual activity for which he now requested consultation. He sought situations in which he was alone with a woman he did not know. As he would approach her, he became sexually excited. He would then walk up to her and display his erect penis. He found that her shock and fear further stimulated him, and usually he would ejaculate. At other times he fantasized about past encounters while masturbating.

He felt guilty and ashamed after exhibiting himself and vowed never to do so again. Nevertheless, the desire often overwhelmed him, and the behavior recurred frequently, usually at periods of tension. He felt desperate but was too ashamed to seek professional help. Once, when he was age 24, he had almost been apprehended by a policeman, but managed to run away.

For the last 3 years, Mr. Klein managed to resist his exhibitionistic urges. Recently, however, he met a young woman who has fallen in love with him and is willing to have intercourse with him. Never having had intercourse before, he felt panic lest he fail in the attempt. He likes and respects his potential sexual partner, but he also condemns her for being willing to engage in premarital relations. He has once again started to exhibit himself and fears that, unless he stops, he will eventually be arrested.

Discussion of "Ashamed"

One could discuss at great length the childhood experiences that may have contributed to the development of this disorder in this patient. Regarding the diagnosis, however, there can be little speculation. The presence of recurrent and intense sexual arousal from the exposure of the individual's genitals to an unsuspecting person, as manifested by fantasies, urges, or behaviors that are acted on with a nonconsenting person or that cause clinically significant distress or impairment in social, occupational, or other important areas of functioning, establishes the diagnosis of Exhibitionistic Disorder (DSM-5-TR, p. 783). Many clinicians would assume that Mr. Klein has another coexisting Personality Disorder, but without more information about the patient's personality functioning, such a diagnosis cannot be made.

19.3
Frotteuristic Disorder

Frotteuristic Disorder involves the recurrent touching and rubbing up against a nonconsenting person for the purpose of sexual arousal and gratification, a behavior known as frottage. No cases of the disorder have ever been reported in females. The most commonly practiced form of frotteurism is rubbing of the genitals against the victim's thighs or buttocks. A common alternative is to run the hands over the victim's genitals or breasts. Typically, the individual selects a crowded place (e.g., subway, sports event, elevator, shopping mall, busy sidewalk) that has a wide selection of victims. In such settings, the initial rubbing against the woman may not be immediately noticed; the victim usually does not protest because she is not absolutely sure what has happened. Individuals who engage in frottage usually fantasize during the moment of contact that they have an exclusive and caring relationship with their victims. However, once contact is made and broken, the person engaging in frotteurism realizes that escape is important to avoid apprehension. Usually, the paraphilia begins by adolescence. Most acts of frottage occur when the person is ages 15–25 years, after which there is a gradual decline in frequency. Although the prevalence of presentations that meet the full criteria for Frotteuristic Disorder (i.e., frotteuristic sexual urges over a period of at least 6 months that were acted on with an unsuspecting person or that caused distress or impairment) is unknown, frotteuristic acts, including uninvited sexual touching of or rubbing against another individual, may be engaged in by up to 30% of adult men.

Underground Sex

Chad Hughes, a 45-year-old doorman for an apartment building, was referred for psychiatric consultation by his New York City parole officer following his second arrest for rubbing up against a woman in the subway. According to Mr. Hughes, he had a "good" sexual relationship with his wife of 15 years when he began, 10 years ago, to touch women in the subway. A typical episode would begin with his decision to go into the subway to rub up against a woman, usually in her 20s. He would select the woman as he walked into the subway station, move in behind her on the subway platform, and wait for the train to arrive at the station. He would be wearing plastic wrap around his penis so as not to stain his pants after ejaculating while rubbing up against his victim. As riders moved onto the train, he would follow the woman he had selected. When the doors closed, he would begin to push his penis up against her buttocks, fantasizing that they were having intercourse in a normal noncoercive manner. In about half of the episodes, he would ejaculate and then go on to work. If he failed to ejaculate, he would either give up for that day or change trains and select another victim. According to Mr. Hughes, he felt guilty immediately after each episode but would soon find himself ruminating about and anticipating the next encounter. He estimated that he has engaged in this behavior about twice a week for the last 10 years, which would mean that he has rubbed up against approximately 1,000 women.

During the interview, Mr. Hughes expressed extreme guilt about his behavior and often cried when talking about fears that his wife or employer would find out about his second arrest. However, he had apparently never thought about how his victims felt about what he did to them.

His personal history did not indicate any obvious mental problems other than being rather inept and unassertive socially, especially with women.

Discussion of "Underground Sex"

Mr. Hughes has both engaged in frotteuristic behavior with unsuspecting victims and is markedly distressed by his behavior, thus qualifying for the DSM-5-TR diagnosis of Frotteuristic Disorder (DSM-5-TR, p. 785). Mr. Hughes's behavior is typical in that he chooses a crowded place (the subway) that offers a wide variety of victims who likely were not even aware of what was happening to them. This probably explains why Mr. Hughes has only been arrested twice.

19.4
Sexual Masochism Disorder

Sexual fantasies and urges of being humiliated, beaten, bound, or otherwise made to suffer may increase sexual excitement for some people whose sexual life is in all other respects unremarkable. However, when sexually arousing fantasies of this kind are markedly distressing to the person (e.g., causing anxiety, obsessions, guilt, shame) or cause impairment in social or occupational functioning, the diagnosis of Sexual Masochism Disorder is made.

The term *bondage-domination-sadism-masochism* (BDSM) is broadly used to refer to a wide range of behaviors engaged in by individuals with sexual masochism and/or sexual sadism (as well as other individuals with similar sexual interests). Such behaviors include use of restraints or restriction, discipline, spanking, slapping, sensory deprivation (e.g., using blindfolds), and/or dominance-submission role-play involving themes such as master/enslaved person, owner/pet, or kidnapper/victim. Behaviors associated with sexual masochism can be acted out alone (e.g., binding, self-sticking pins, self-administration of electric shock, self-mutilation) or with a partner (e.g., beating, being subjected to verbal abuse).

Sadomasochism involving consenting partners is not considered rare or unusual in the United States, and it often occurs in the absence of a mental disorder. Moreover, such behaviors among consenting partners, occurring in the absence of distress or impairment in important areas of functioning, would not warrant a diagnosis of either Sexual Sadism Disorder or Sexual Masochism Disorder. Sadomasochistic sexual interactions tend to be well planned, with partners deciding on a special "safe word" the masochistic (submissive) person will use to indicate that the sadistic (dominant) partner should stop. Such interactions are often referred to as dominant-submissive relationships. More people consider themselves masochistic than sadistic.

Although masochistic sexual fantasies often begin in childhood, the onset of sexual masochism typically occurs during early adulthood. Sexual masochism is slightly more prevalent in males than in females. In Australia, it has been estimated that 2.2% of men and 1.3% of women had been involved in BDSM behavior in the past 12 months. Although the true association of Sexual Masochism Disorder with suicidal thoughts or behavior is unknown, a study of 321 adults who endorsed BDSM involvement found an association between stigma-related shame and guilt and suicidal ideation. Disorders that commonly co-occur with Sexual Masochism Disorder include other Paraphilic Disorders, such as transvestic fetishism.

A potentially dangerous (and sometimes fatal) masochistic activity is autoerotic partial asphyxiation, in which a person uses ropes, nooses, or plastic bags to induce a state of asphyxia (inadequate oxygenation of the blood from an interruption of breathing) at the point of orgasm. The behavior is meant to enhance orgasm, but accidental deaths sometimes occur.

Bruised

Kathy Romano, a 25-year-old graduate student, asked for a consultation because of depression and marital discord. Ms. Romano had been married for 5 years, during which time both she and her husband were in school. During the past 3 years, her academic performance had been consistently better than his, and she attributed their frequent, intense arguments to this fact. She noted that she experienced a feeling of sexual excitement when her husband screamed at her or hit her in a rage. Sometimes she would taunt him until he had sexual intercourse with her in a brutal fashion, as if she were being raped. She experienced the brutality and sense of being punished as sexually exciting.

One year before the consultation, Ms. Romano had found herself often ending arguments by storming out of the house. On one such occasion she went to a singles bar, picked up a man, and got him to slap her as part of their sexual activity. She found the "punishment" sexually exciting and subsequently fantasized about being beaten while masturbating to orgasm. Ms. Romano then discovered that she enjoyed receiving physical punishment at the hands of strange men more than any other type of sexual stimulus. In a setting in which she could be whipped or beaten, all aspects of sexual activity, including the quality of orgasms, were far in excess of anything she had previously experienced.

This sexual preference was not the primary reason for the consultation, however. She complained that she could not live without her husband yet could not live with him. She had suicidal fantasies stemming from the fear that he would leave her.

Moreover, Ms. Romano recognized that her sexual behavior put her in potentially dangerous situations, and she was very distressed about the potential impact on her marriage if her husband were to find out about her masochistic extramarital activities. She was unaware of any possible reasons for its emergence and was ambivalent about getting treatment to stop the behavior because it gave her so much pleasure.

Discussion of "Bruised"

Ms. Romano experiences recurrent and persistent sexual arousal from being physically beaten, whipped, or punished, especially at the hands of strangers. Although she enjoyed the intensity of these sexual experiences, she is very distressed about the potential negative impact on her marriage. Ms. Romano's ambivalence about being treated for her paraphilia is not uncommon, as individuals with paraphilias are often reluctant to forgo engaging in sexual behaviors that provide such intense pleasure. Given that she has a masochistic pattern of sexual arousal and that she is distressed by its potential negative consequences, the diagnosis of Sexual Masochism Disorder (DSM-5-TR, p. 788) applies in this case.

19.5
Sexual Sadism Disorder

The flip side of sexual masochism is sexual sadism, in which a person is sexually aroused by the physical or psychological suffering of another person. The term *sadism* is derived from the proper name of the Marquis de Sade (1740–1814), a French aristocrat who became notorious for writing novels around the theme of inflicting pain as a source of sexual pleasure. With regard to actual sadistic behavior, the person receiving the pain, suffering, or humiliation may or may not be a willing partner. If the person with a sadistic focus of sexual arousal acts on sadistic urges with an unwilling person (i.e., a victim), then a DSM-5-TR diagnosis of Sexual Sadism Disorder applies. Otherwise, recurrent sadistic fantasies that are not acted on or sadistic behavior with a consenting partner would be considered a disorder only if the sadistic fantasies, urges, or behaviors are markedly distressing to the individual or have a negative impact on relationships (e.g., causing severe strain in a marriage).

The sadistic fantasies or acts typically reflect a desire for sexual or psychological domination of another person. These acts range from behavior that is not physically harmful—although it may be humiliating to the other person (e.g., being urinated on)—to criminal and potentially deadly behavior. Acts of domination may include restraining or imprisoning the other person through the use of handcuffs, cages, chains, or ropes. Other acts and fantasies related to sexual sadism include paddling, spanking, whipping, burning, administering electrical shocks, biting, cutting, rape, murder, and mutilation. In extreme cases, sexual sadism can lead to serious injury or death for the other person.

The extensive use of pornography involving the infliction of pain and suffering is sometimes an associated feature of Sexual Sadism Disorder. Estimates of the population prevalence of Sexual Sadism Disorder are largely based on individuals in forensic settings. Among civilly committed sexual offenders in the United States, fewer than 10% have Sexual Sadism Disorder. Among individuals who have committed sexually motivated homicides, the proportion of homicides involving sexually sadistic behavior is about one-third. In forensic samples, individuals with Sexual Sadism Disorder are almost exclusively men, but in a representative sample of the population in Australia, 2.2% of men and 1.3% of women reported having been involved in BDSM behavior in the previous year. In a population-based sample in Finland, the lifetime prevalence of sexually sadistic behavior was 2.7% among men and 2.3% among women.

Leather

Jason Stavros, a 35-year-old married writer, sought consultation because he feared he might kill someone by acting on sexually sadistic impulses.

Mr. Stavros has been married for 15 years. During the past year, he has had sexual intercourse with his wife approximately every other week. His fantasy life is predominantly homosexual, however, and has been since age 9. He has felt sexually attracted to males since childhood but resisted acting on these impulses until mid-adulthood, when he had his first same-sex encounter long after he married. He reported feeling sexually aroused by homosexual pornography to which he was exposed from mid-adolescence, particularly by pornography with sadistic content. Although he is somewhat responsive to heterosexual pornography, his interest in it has been much lower than his interest in homosexual pornography, and he has never been excited by heterosexual pornography with sadistic content.

Mr. Stavros had married for reasons of social propriety, as well as because he consciously hoped that initiation into regular heterosexual activity would lead to diminution of his sadistic homosexual impulses. Marriage did not stop his impulses, however. These impulses continued periodically to form the basis of his masturbation fantasies. His typical masturbation fantasies were of a man bound, tortured, and killed. Sometimes, the men in his fantasies were people he knew, such as colleagues or teachers, and sometimes movie stars or strangers. These fantasies were more intense at certain times than at others. Mr. Stavros recalls, for example, that he was "wildly" aroused when he read about the activities of a homosexual lust murder as described in a detective magazine. Immediately following this, he masturbated many times a day, always with sadistic homosexual fantasies. After a few weeks, this period of intense arousal subsided, but Mr. Stavros used the scenario of the events described in this magazine in subsequent masturbation fantasies.

About 8 years ago, Mr. Stavros went to a gay bar with an associate from his office. At the time, he was under much pressure at work, and his work was being closely supervised by an aggressive, demanding male superior. Mr. Stavros's associate was openly homosexual, and Mr. Stavros claimed to have gone to the bar with him "as a lark." En route to the particular bar they visited, they passed other bars that, the patient's friend told him, were for "the leather crowd who like S and M." Mr. Stavros had a brief homosexual encounter with someone he picked up in the bar they visited, following which he "put sex out of [his] mind."

Some months later, however, following a week of intense work at his office, Mr. Stavros impulsively sought out one of the "S and M" bars he had previously walked past. There he met a man who was sexually aroused by being beaten, and Mr. Stavros engaged in pleasurable sadistic activity with the understanding that the severity of the beating, administered with a belt, was under the control of his masochistic partner. That incident, occurring when he was 28 years old, was the first episode in a series of sexually sadistic activities, ultimately leading to his consultation. About once a month the patient would frequent a homosexual sadomasochistic bar. He would dress in a leather jacket and wear a leather cap. Once in the bar, he would seek out a masochistic partner and engage in a variety of activities, all of which he experienced as sexually exciting. The activities included binding the partner with ropes, whipping him, threatening to burn him with cigarettes, forcing him to drink urine, and forcing him to "beg for mercy." Mr. Stavros would experience orgasm during these activities, usually by "forcing" his partner to perform fellatio.

During the year before the consultation, Mr. Stavros's wife had become progressively dissatisfied with their marriage. She was unaware of her husband's homosexual interest and sadistic tendencies. She felt, however, that his sexual involvement with her was desultory, and she wondered whether he had a mistress. She also became more hostile and demanding toward him. Mr. Stavros realized that he "needed" his wife, and he did not wish the relationship to end, yet he felt unable to deal with her dissatisfactions directly. He avoided her as much as possible and argued with her when she insisted on talking to him. Mr. Stavros's work pressures increased, and he found, to his dismay, that the intensity of his sadistic impulses had also increased.

On one occasion, Mr. Stavros convinced a partner to agree to being burned. Afterward, he felt guilty and ashamed. Just before the consultation, he bound a partner and cut the man's arm. At the sight of the blood, he experienced a powerful desire to kill his partner. He restrained himself and, alarmed that his sadistic impulses were out of control, sought psychiatric consultation.

Discussion of "Leather"

As recounted in this case, Mr. Stavros had first been aroused by sadistic homosexual fantasies in mid-adolescence. These intense, sexually arousing fantasies persisted, and eventually he began to act on them with consenting partners. He married, hoping that marriage would be an antidote to his sadistic homosexual impulses, but found that this did not occur. He now enters treatment distressed and fearful that the sadistic impulses may become so strong that he will lose control and kill a sexual partner. His marked distress, along with the years of recurrent sadistic sexual arousal, would thus qualify for the DSM-5-TR diagnosis of Sexual Sadism Disorder (DSM-5-TR, p. 790).

19.6
Pedophilic Disorder

When an adult or older adolescent experiences recurrent and intense sexually arousing fantasies, urges, or behaviors involving sexual activity with prepubescent children, they are considered to have a pedophilic pattern of sexual arousal. For such individuals to receive a DSM-5-TR diagnosis of Pedophilic Disorder, one of the following would need to be true: 1) their attraction toward children causes them marked distress (e.g., guilt, anxiety, alienation) or interpersonal difficulty or 2) their urges have caused them to approach children for sexual gratification in real life. Individuals with Pedophilic Disorder may experience an emotional and cognitive affinity with children, sometimes referred to as *emotional congruence* with children. Emotional congruence with children can manifest in different ways, including preferring social interactions with children over such interactions with adults, feeling like the individual has more in common with children than with adults, and choosing occupations or volunteer roles in order to be around children more often.

Adult males with Pedophilic Disorder often indicate that they first became aware of their strong or preferential sexual interest in children around the time of puberty—the same time frame in which males who later prefer physically mature partners become aware of their sexual interest in women or men. The population prevalence of individuals whose presentations meet the full criteria for Pedophilic Disorder is un-known, but is likely lower than 3% among men in international studies. Even less is known about the population prevalence of Pedophilic Disorder in women, but it is likely a small fraction of the prevalence in men. Pedophilia per se (i.e., sexual attrac-tion to children) appears to be lifelong. Pedophilic Disorder, however, includes other elements that may change over time, with or without treatment: subjective distress (e.g., guilt, shame, intense sexual frustration, feelings of isolation), psychosocial im-pairment, the propensity to act out sexually with children, or all three. Therefore, the course of Pedophilic Disorder may fluctuate, or the disorder's intensity may increase or decrease with age. No cure for pedophilia has been developed, but there are ther-apies that can reduce the incidence of an individual committing child sexual abuse.

Child Psychiatrist

Bennett Conrad is a single 36-year-old child psychiatrist. He has been ar-rested and convicted of fondling several neighborhood boys, ages 6–12. Friends and colleagues were shocked and dismayed, because he had been considered by all to be particularly caring and supportive of children. Not only had he chosen a profession involving their care, but he had been a Cub Scout leader for many years and also a member of the local Big Brothers.

His father had also been a physician and was described as a workaholic, spending little time with his three children. When interviewed by a psychiatrist as part of his presentence investigation, Dr. Conrad admitted that he experi-enced little, if any, sexual attraction toward females, either adults or children. Dr. Conrad had never married, and he also denied sexual attraction toward adult men. In presenting the history of his psychosexual development, Dr. Con-rad reported that he had become somewhat dismayed as a child when his male friends began expressing rudimentary awareness of an attraction toward girls. His "secret" at the time was that he was attracted more to other boys and, in fact, during childhood, often played "doctor" with other boys, eventually pro-gressing to mutual masturbation with some of his male friends.

His first sexual experience was at age 6, when a 15-year-old male camp counselor performed fellatio on him several times over the course of the sum-mer, an experience that he had always kept to himself. As he reached his teenage years, he began to suspect that he was homosexual. As he grew older, he was surprised to notice that the age range of males that attracted him sexually did not change, and he continued to have recurrent erotic urges and fantasies about boys between ages 6 and 12. He would fantasize about a boy in that age range whenever he masturbated, would take advantage of situa-tions to fondle them, and on a couple of occasions over the years had felt him-self to be in love with such a youngster.

Intellectually, Dr. Conrad knew that others would disapprove of his many sexual involvements with young boys. He never believed, however, that he had caused any of these youngsters harm, feeling instead that they were simply sharing pleasurable feelings together. He yearned to be able to experience the same sort of feelings toward women, but he never was able to do so. He frequently prayed for help and that his actions would go undetected. He kept promising himself that he would stop, but the temptations were such that he could not. He was so fearful of destroying his reputation, his friendships, and his career that he had never been able to bring himself to tell anyone else about his problem.

Discussion of "Child Psychiatrist"

Dr. Conrad experiences recurrent intense sexual urges and sexually arousing fantasies involving sexual activity with prepubescent boys. He has acted on these fantasies and urges on many occasions, thus justifying the diagnosis of Pedophilic Disorder (DSM-5-TR, p. 792). The diagnosis would also be made if Dr. Conrad had never acted on these fantasies and urges but was markedly distressed by them.

Dr. Conrad, like many other men with Pedophilic Disorder who do not also have Sexual Sadism Disorder, has a genuine interest in children and justified his behavior with the rationalization that he was not harming them in any way.

19.7
Fetishistic Disorder

A *fetish* is an atypical sexual focus on nonliving objects, such as women's undergarments, men's or women's footwear, rubber articles, leather clothing, diapers, or other wearing apparel. Highly eroticized body parts associated with Fetishistic Disorder include feet, toes, and hair. It is not uncommon for sexualized fetishes to include both inanimate objects and body parts (e.g., dirty socks and feet). A sexual fetish may be a nonpathological aid to sexual excitement, but fetish-associated fantasies, sexual urges, or behaviors that cause significant psychosocial distress for the individual or have detrimental effects on important areas of their life are diagnosed as Fetishistic Disorder.

Fetishistic Disorder can involve holding, tasting, rubbing, inserting, or smelling the fetish object while masturbating, or preferring that a sexual partner wear or utilize a fetish object during sexual encounters. It should be noted that many individuals with fetishistic sexual interests also enjoy sexual experiences with their partner without using their fetish object. However, individuals with a fetishistic sexual interest often find that sexual experiences that involve their fetish object are more sexually satisfying than sexual experiences without it. For a minority of people with a fetishistic sexual interest, their fetish object is necessary for becoming sexually aroused or satisfied. Some individuals may acquire extensive collections of highly desired fetish objects. While some paraphilias typically have an onset during puberty, fetishistic sexual interests can develop before adolescence. Fetishistic behaviors have been reported more often in men, but they also occur in women.

Panties

Kurt O'Brien, a single 32-year-old freelance photographer, presented with the chief complaint of an "abnormal sex drive." Mr. O'Brien related that although he was somewhat sexually aroused by women, he was far more aroused by "their panties."

To the best of Mr. O'Brien's memory, sexual excitement began when he was about age 7, when he came upon a pornographic magazine and felt stimulated by pictures of partially nude women wearing panties. His first ejaculation occurred at age 13 via masturbation to fantasies of women wearing panties. He masturbated into his older sister's panties, which he had stolen without her knowledge. Subsequently, he stole panties from her friends and from other women he met socially. He found pretexts to wander into the bedrooms of women during social occasions, and would quickly rummage through their possessions until he found a pair of panties to his satisfaction. He later used these to masturbate into, and then saved them in a "private cache." The pattern of masturbating into women's underwear had been his preferred method of achieving sexual excitement and orgasm from adolescence until the present consultation.

Mr. O'Brien first had sexual intercourse at age 18. Since then, he has had intercourse on many occasions, and his preferred partners were prostitutes who had been paid to wear crotchless panties during the act. On less common occasions, when he attempted sexual activity with a partner who did not wear panties, his sexual excitement was sometimes weak.

Mr. O'Brien felt uncomfortable dating "nice women," because he felt that any friendliness might lead to sexual intimacy and that they would not understand his sexual needs. He avoided socializing with friends who might introduce him to such women. He recognized that his appearance, social style, and profession all resulted in his being perceived as a highly desirable bachelor. He felt anxious and depressed because his social life was limited by his sexual preference.

Mr. O'Brien sought consultation shortly after his mother's sudden and unexpected death. Although he complained of loneliness, he admitted that the pleasure he experienced from his unusual sexual activity made him unsure about whether he wished to give it up.

Discussion of "Panties"

Mr. O'Brien's first remembered sexual arousal was in response to pictures of women wearing panties. Ever since that time, he has had recurrent, intense, sexual urges and sexually arousing fantasies involving the use of nonliving objects (panties, alone or worn by a woman), which indicate fetishism. Whether this arousal pattern should be considered evidence of Fetishistic Disorder (DSM-5-TR, p. 796) depends on whether the fantasies, sexual urges, or behaviors cause clinically significant distress or impairment in the individual's "social, occupational, or other important areas of functioning." In Mr. O'Brien's case, his fetishistic arousal pattern is interfering with his ability to develop an intimate romantic relationship with a woman. Although the case does not specifically explain why, the clinician can assume the interference is caused by Mr. O'Brien's belief that "nice" women would reject him once he revealed his sexual proclivities. Notably, unlike the DSM-5-TR Paraphilic Disorders that involve an unwilling participant or victim and that can be diagnosed simply on the basis of the person's having acted on the paraphilic urges, acting on a fetishistic urge is not enough for the diagnosis of Fetishistic Disorder—there must also be either distress or impairment. Mr. O'Brien's Fetishistic Disorder could therefore be "cured" by his finding a partner who is accepting of his fetishistic desire and who would be willing to incorporate the panties into their sexual interactions. In such a case, Mr. O'Brien would no longer be considered to have Fetishistic Disorder but would instead be considered to have a fetishistic arousal pattern, which is not considered to be a disorder in DSM-5-TR.

Although Mr. O'Brien's chief complaint when he presented for treatment was his "abnormal sex drive," his problem in fact has nothing to do with his sex drive per se (which appears to be normal). His problem is not the intensity of his sex drive but rather the fact that the focus of his sexual arousal is atypical (i.e., involving a focus on women's panties).

19.8
Transvestic Disorder

Transvestism involves being sexually aroused by dressing up in the clothes of the opposite sex (i.e., cross-dressing). The cross-dressing may involve only one or two articles of clothing (e.g., for men, it may involve only women's undergarments), or it may involve dressing completely in the inner and outer garments of the other sex and (in men) may even include the use of women's wigs and makeup. To qualify for a DSM-5-TR diagnosis of Transvestic Disorder, however, the sexual urges to cross-dress or the cross-dressing behavior must cause "clinically significant distress or impairment in social, occupational, or other important areas of functioning"

(p. 798). The presence of distress in individuals with Transvestic Disorder is often indicated by the presence of a "purging and acquisition" pattern of behavior, during which an individual (usually a man) who has spent a great deal of money on women's clothes and other apparel (e.g., shoes, wigs) discards the items (i.e., purges them) in an effort to overcome urges to cross-dress, and then begins acquiring a woman's wardrobe all over again (DSM-5-TR, p. 799).

A diagnosis of Transvestic Disorder does not apply to all individuals who dress as the opposite sex, even those who do so habitually. It applies only to individuals whose cross-dressing or thoughts of cross-dressing are often or always accompanied by sexual excitement and who are emotionally distressed by the fantasies, urges, or behaviors or feel that they impair their social or interpersonal functioning. Individuals with Gender Dysphoria (see "Living as a Man" in Section 14.2), who feel that the gender assigned to them at birth is incongruent with their experienced gender, also typically cross-dress, but prefer to dress in the attire stereotypically characteristic of their experienced gender.

For some individuals with Transvestic Disorder, fantasies or stimuli associated with cross-dressing may always be necessary for erotic arousal and are always included in sexual activity. Other individuals with the disorder might cross-dress only episodically, such as during periods of stress, and be able to function sexually at other times without cross-dressing.

For some individuals diagnosed with Transvestic Disorder, the motivation for cross-dressing may change over time, from a search for sexual excitement to simple relief from stress, depression, or anxiety. In some cases, individuals with Transvestic Disorder may over time develop Gender Dysphoria if they discover that they are unhappy with their biological sex. They may elect to have hormonal and surgical procedures to change their bodies, with some choosing to undergo gender-affirming surgery. Such individuals could be given the additional diagnosis of Gender Dysphoria (see Section 14.2).

In some cases, the course of Transvestic Disorder is continuous, and in others it is episodic. It is not rare for men with Transvestic Disorder to lose interest in cross-dressing when they first fall in love with a woman and begin a relationship, but such abatement usually proves temporary. When the desire to cross-dress returns, so does the associated distress. The prevalence of Transvestic Disorder is unknown; however, the disorder appears to be much more prevalent in men than in women. Fewer than 3% of Swedish men reported having ever been sexually aroused by dressing in women's attire.

X-Dressing

Didier Arnaud, a 65-year-old security guard and formerly a fishing-boat captain from New Brunswick, is distressed about his wife's objections to his wearing a nightgown at home in the evening, now that his youngest child has left home. His appearance and demeanor, except when he is dressing in women's clothes, are always stereotypically masculine, and he is exclusively heterosexual. Occasionally, over the past 5 years, he has worn an inconspic-uous item of female clothing even when dressed as a man, sometimes a pair of panties, sometimes an ambiguous pinkie ring. He always carries a photo-graph of himself dressed as a woman.

Mr. Arnaud's first recollection of an interest in female clothing was putting on his sister's underpants at age 12, an act accompanied by sexual excite-ment. He continued periodically to put on women's underpants, an activity that invariably resulted in an erection, sometimes a spontaneous emission, and sometimes masturbation. Although he occasionally wished to be a girl, he never fantasized himself as one. He was competitive and aggressive with other boys growing up and always acted "masculine." During his single years he was always attracted to girls but was shy about sex. Following his marriage at age 22, he had his first sexual intercourse.

Mr. Arnaud's involvement with female clothes was of the same intensity af-ter his marriage as well. Then, beginning at age 30, after a chance exposure to a magazine called *Transvestia*, he began to increase his cross-dressing ac-tivity. He learned there were other men like himself, and he became more and more preoccupied with female clothing in fantasy and progressed to periodi-cally dressing completely as a woman. More recently, he has become in-volved in a transvestite chat room on the Internet and occasionally attends transvestite parties. Cross-dressing at these parties has been the only time that he has cross-dressed outside his home.

Although Mr. Arnaud is still committed to his marriage, sex with his wife has dwindled over the past 20 years, as his waking thoughts and activities have become increasingly centered on cross-dressing. Over time, this activity has become less eroticized and more an end in itself, but it still is a source of some sexual excitement. He always has an increased urge to dress as a woman when under stress; it has a calming effect. If particular circumstances prevent him from cross-dressing, he feels extremely frustrated.

Mr. Arnaud's parents belonged to different faiths, a fact of some impor-tance to him. He was the eldest of three children, extremely close to his mother, whom he idolized, and angry at his "whoremaster," "alcoholic" father. The parents fought constantly. He is tearful, even now at age 65, when he de-scribes his mother's death when he was age 10. He was the one who found her dead of a massive heart attack, and he says he has been "not the same from that day…always [having] the feeling something's not right." The siblings were reared by three separate branches of the family until the father remar-ried. When the patient was 20, his father died. His brother also died traumati-cally, by drowning in his teens.

Because of the disruptions in his early life, Mr. Arnaud has always treasured the steadfastness of his wife and the order of his home. He told his wife about his cross-dressing practice when they were married, and she was accepting as long as he kept it to himself. Nevertheless, he felt guilty, particularly after he be-gan complete cross-dressing, and periodically he attempted to renounce the practice, throwing out all his female clothes and makeup. His children served as a barrier to his giving free rein to his impulses. Following his retirement from fishing, and in the absence of his children, he finds himself more drawn to cross-dressing, more in conflict with his wife, and more depressed.

Discussion of "X-Dressing"

Mr. Arnaud's case demonstrates the characteristic development and course of the atypical sexual arousal pattern known as transvestism. In the earlier phases of his transvestism, Mr. Arnaud would periodically renounce the practice and throw out the female clothes and makeup that he had acquired. More recently, now that he is retired and his children are no longer in the house, he has found that cross-dressing has taken an even more prominent position in his life, resulting in more conflicts with his wife and depression in himself. Thus, Mr. Arnaud's symptoms qualify for the DSM-5-TR diagnosis of Transvestic Disorder (DSM-5-TR, p. 798), given that the cross-dressing is causing him distress.

CHAPTER 20

Cutting-Edge Conditions

This chapter presents four cutting-edge conditions that were considered for inclusion in DSM-5 but were ultimately omitted as official categories pending future developments. Two of the conditions with proposed diagnostic criteria (Attenuated Psychosis Syndrome and Internet Gaming Disorder) are included in the DSM-5-TR chapter "Conditions for Further Study," for which future research is encouraged. Another condition, Olfactory Reference Disorder, is listed as one of the seven examples in Other Specified Obsessive-Compulsive and Related Disorder. The remaining condition, Compulsive Sexual Behavior Disorder was not included in DSM-5 because there was insufficient evidence to establish the diagnostic criteria and course descriptions needed to identify these behaviors as mental disorders; however, the disorder is included as an official category in the Mental, Behavioral or Neurodevelopmental Disorders chapter in the World Health Organization's International Classification of Diseases, 11th revision (ICD-11), as is Internet Gaming Disorder and Olfactory Reference Disorder. Although ICD-11 was officially endorsed for use by WHO member nations during the 72nd World Health Assembly in May 2019 and officially came into effect on January 1, 2022, each country chooses when to adopt ICD-11. There is currently no proposed timeline for implementation of ICD-11 in the United States. Consequently, for the foreseeable future the official coding system in the United States continues to be the International Classification of Diseases, Tenth Revision, Clinical Modification (ICD-10-CM).

We have included cases for these cutting-edge conditions to increase clinical understanding and awareness and because of clinical and educational interest in them. Table 20-1 lists these conditions in their order of appearance in this chapter, which mirrors their prospective inclusion.

TABLE 20–1.   **Characteristic features of selected cutting-edge conditions (not official diagnoses in DSM-5-TR)**

Condition	Key proposed characteristics
Attenuated Psychosis Syndrome	Attenuated delusions, attenuated hallucinations or attenuated disorganized speech that began or worsened in the past year in an individual whose symptoms have never met criteria for a Psychotic Disorder
	Listed as an example in Other Specified Schizophrenia Spectrum and Other Psychotic Disorder in DSM-5-TR
	Proposed diagnostic criteria included in DSM-5-TR Section III, "Conditions for Further Study"
Olfactory Reference Disorder	Preoccupation with the belief that one is emitting a perceived foul or offensive body odor or breath.
	Listed as an example in Other Specified Obsessive-Compulsive and Related Disorder in DSM-5-TR
	Not an official diagnosis or a proposed condition for further study in DSM-5-TR
	Included as an official diagnosis in ICD-11
Compulsive Sexual Behavior Disorder	Failure to control intense, repetitive sexual impulses or urges resulting in repetitive sexual behavior
	Not an official diagnosis or a proposed condition for further study in DSM-5-TR
	Included as an official diagnosis in ICD-11
Internet Gaming Disorder	Persistent or recurrent use of the internet to engage in games, leading to clinically significant impairment or distress
	Included in DSM-5-TR Section III, "Conditions for Further Study"
	Included as an official diagnosis in ICD-11

20.1
Attenuated Psychosis Syndrome

Attenuated Psychosis Syndrome (APS) is included in DSM-5-TR Section III, in the chapter "Conditions for Further Study." The proposed criteria sets included in this chapter are intended to provide a common language for researchers and clinicians who are interested in studying these disorders. APS was proposed for possible inclusion in DSM-5 but after a careful review, the DSM-5 Task Force determined that there was insufficient evidence to warrant its inclusion as an official mental disorder diagnoses in the main section of DSM-5 (Section II). The rationale for including APS in DSM-5 Section III (and listing as an example in Other Specified Schizophrenia Spectrum and Other Psychotic Disorder) was grounded in two decades of research evidence examining the early phases of illness preceding the onset of psychosis (a period called the "prodrome"). These early phases (also termed "clinical high-risk state for psychosis") characterize a vulnerability stage that may precede the onset of Schizophrenia and other psychotic disorders. It has been the hope that if clinicians could identify individuals who were at high risk for developing Schizophrenia or other psychotic disorders before their onset, perhaps an intervention could be developed to prevent that from happening.

APS is characterized by some of the same types of symptoms that define Schizophrenia (delusions, hallucinations, and disorganized speech)—but these symptoms are not present at the required severity threshold to meet the definition of the delusions, hallucinations, or disorganized speech required for a diagnosis of a psychotic disorder (hence the term *"attenuated* psychosis"). For example, attenuated symptoms are more likely to come and go, and the person harbors doubt and skepticism about the reality of their symptomatic beliefs and perceptions. In the case of attenuated delusions, one way of determining the degree to which a person firmly holds their delusional beliefs is with persistent questioning ("I see that this is how you experience the world—could there be a different explanation?"). The DSM-5-TR proposed definition of APS requires that the attenuated psychotic symptoms must have been present at least once per week for the past month, that the symptoms must have begun or worsened in the past year, and that they are sufficiently distressing and disabling to the individual to warrant clinical attention.

The onset of attenuated psychosis syndrome is usually in mid-to-late adolescence or early adulthood. The experience of attenuated psychotic symptoms is not uncommon. Up to 7% of the general population across a broad range of countries may acknowledge experiencing attenuated delusions or hallucinations. The prevalence of attenuated psychotic symptoms meeting the stricter definitional requirements for the syndrome as defined in DSM-5-TR is much lower. For example, in a study conducted in Switzerland, the prevalence of attenuated psychosis syndrome in non-help-seeking individuals ages 16–40 years was found to be only 0.3%.

High Risk

Martin Albertson, a 17-year-old freshman at an art college, was referred by a general practitioner to a clinic that specializes in the evaluation of individuals who may be at high-risk for developing psychosis. The general practitioner noted a substantial drop in functioning and social withdrawal during the previous 6 months. Martin was 6 months into his freshman year when he reported the workload to be increasingly "tricky," and that he had ended the first semester having failed most of his courses. The general practitioner noted that there was nothing in Martin's developmental history suggesting a problem—Martin appropriately reached developmental milestones and had no family history of a mental disorder, did not report any current or past use of drugs, had never seen a mental health professional for any kind of treatment, and had no significant medical history.

During his assessment, Martin presented as well-kempt. He made appropriate eye contact and answered questions thoroughly and directly; overall, he was engaging and cooperative throughout the interview, showing a good rapport with the clinician doing the assessment. His presenting complaint was that he no longer enjoyed doing things that used to give him pleasure, like playing soccer with his peers. He also reported feeling that he was unable relate to his college classmates or friends. Because of his social withdrawal, his girlfriend recently broke up with him. However, his mood remained euthymic and reactive, and his affect was appropriate; there were no somatic signs of depression-like changes in sleep or appetite. During the assessment, no formal thought disorder was observed.

He disclosed a vague albeit intense feeling of perplexity and derealization described as being in the *Truman Show* (a 2008 film about a man who grew up living an ordinary life that—unbeknownst to him—takes place on a large studio set populated by actors for a television show about him), in that he experienced the surrounding world as somewhat faked and "fabricated." He also had the impression that something uncanny was going on and acknowledged being convinced that random people looked at and talked about him when he was out in public. This feeling was worse with people he did not know well; as a result, he actively avoided people and social situations. He did not think people were trying to harm him, just judging him physically, and he could not pinpoint a particular reason for thinking this. He knew there was no specific reason to be mistrustful of other people. These experiences began around the time he graduated from high school and continued through the start of his freshman year. They were occurring every day, lasting for up to an hour at a time, causing him significant distress. With respect to how strongly he believed that people were looking and talking about him and that his surroundings were in fact not real, he reported that on a scale from 0 to 100 where 0 was "not convinced at all" and 100 was "completely convinced," his level of conviction was about 80% during those times he was actively having these experiences and 40% when he retrospectively looked back at his experiences. He was able to question his beliefs and stated that people were probably commenting on the way he looked, but he did not believe they meant him harm.

Discussion of "High Risk"

Martin presents to the clinic with a number of upsetting thoughts that people are looking at him and talking about him when he is out in public (referential thinking), as well as having feelings of derealization (experiencing the surrounding world as faked and "fabricated"). Despite this, his reality testing (i.e., his ability to evaluate the external environment and differentiate it from his internal world) remained at least partially intact. These symptoms began in the past year and were distressing, leading him to isolate himself socially, which led to the breakdown of significant relationships. Taken together, Martin's presentation meets the proposed research criteria for Attenuated Psychosis Syndrome (DSM-5-TR, p. 903). Although he would not be considered to have a full-blown psychotic disorder at the time he presented to the evaluator, he is at an increased risk of eventually developing a psychotic disorder in the future. In a study of help-seeking individuals, those whose presentations met DSM-5-TR proposed criteria for APS had a 22% risk of developing a psychotic disorder over the next 3 years versus a 1.5% risk in those who presentations did not meet the proposed criteria.

20.2
Olfactory Reference Disorder

DSM-5-TR has a category for disorders that have many of the same characteristics of an Obsessive-Compulsive and Related Disorder, but that do not meet the full criteria for any of the specific disorders in this diagnostic class. Olfactory Reference Disorder (or Syndrome) is listed in DSM-5-TR as an example of a DSM-5-TR Other Specified Obsessive-Compulsive and Related Disorder (DSM-5-TR, p. 294). It is also included as an official ICD-11 disorder in the Mental, Behavioral, and Neurodevelopmental Disorders section.

Olfactory Reference Disorder is characterized by the persistent belief that the affected individual is emitting a foul or offensive body odor or bad breath. In reality, the foul odor or breath is unnoticeable or only slightly noticeable to others. The person with olfactory reference disorder is excessively self-conscious about the perceived odor, often experiences "ideas of reference," believing that others are noticing, judging, or talking about the odor. Because they are preoccupied with these beliefs, the person will engage in repetitive and excessive behaviors, such as constantly checking for body odor or the perceived source of the smell (e.g., smelling themselves or their clothing), seeking reassurance from others that the smell is not too bad, trying to camouflage or otherwise alter the smell (e.g., with perfume, aftershave, or deodorant or excessive showering or use of mouthwash), and avoiding social situations that might trigger distress about the smell (e.g., public transportation or other crowded venues). The preoccupation with body odor results in significant distress or impairment in psychosocial functioning due to extreme embarrassment, self-consciousness, and shame. Individuals with Olfactory Reference Disorder vary in the degree of insight they have about the reality of their beliefs, from being able to consider the possibility that their beliefs may not be true to being totally convinced that they are true.

The prevalence of Olfactory Reference Disorder is not well established but has been estimated to be from 0.5% to 2% in the general population.[1] The disorder usually has an onset in the mid-twenties, but onset during puberty or adolescence is also common. The course of the disorder is chronic and may worsen over time. Individu-

[1]Feusner JD, Phillips KA, Stein DJ: Olfactory reference disorder: issues for DSM-V. *Depression and Anxiety* 27(6):592-599, 2010 20533369.

als with the disorder may often consult non-mental health specialists, such as medical, surgical, or dental practitioners, before their diagnosis is made.

I Stink

Justin Samuels, a 28-year-old man, made an appointment for outpatient psychiatric treatment, because "I stink, and everyone can smell it. My girlfriend and my family say I smell fine, but I don't believe them." Mr. Samuels was convinced that he had trimethylaminuria, a rare condition that causes the body to produce a fishy odor, and he had recently made an appointment to be evaluated for this condition. But he reluctantly agreed to see a psychiatrist because his girlfriend had threatened to end their relationship if he did not do so.

Since age 16, Mr. Samuels had been convinced that he had "foul breath, putrid-smelling sweat especially from my armpits, and a terrible anal odor that people can smell a football field away." These beliefs developed after a school mate called him "stinky" and his uncle told him that he should shower more often.

Mr. Samuels was certain that he smelled bad "because I can smell it myself." He stated that the behavior of other people also convinced him that his belief was correct. When he saw people touching or covering their nose, moving away from him, opening a window, frowning, or sniffing, he was certain that they were reacting to his bad body odor. He also believed that comments such as "It's stuffy in here," or "What's that smell?" referred to his body odor.

Mr. Samuels thought about his supposed body odor for about 8 hours a day. He performed many repetitive and excessive behaviors to check or try to minimize his perceived body odor. He repeatedly sniffed his armpits, blew into his cupped hand to check his breath, washed his clothes three times before wearing them, showered twice a day for an hour each time, and brushed his teeth about ten times a day. He also repeatedly entreated his girlfriend: "I stink, don't I? Can't you smell it??!" When she replied that he didn't stink and that she smelled nothing, her response invariably triggered arguments about his perceived body odor.

Mr. Samuels also attempted to camouflage his perceived body odor by using "gallons of mouthwash" and chewing several packs of mint gum a day. He also used special deodorant soaps, excessive amounts of cologne, and five different deodorants each day. To minimize perceived flatulence and anal odor, he had tried many different diets and had bought Shreddies, underwear that purports to minimize odor caused by flatulence. However, he felt that none of these attempts to mask his perceived body odor were successful.

As Mr. Samuels's preoccupation with body odor intensified during his 20s, he increasingly found it very difficult to be around other people, because he was certain that they perceived and reacted negatively to his body odor. He avoided public transportation and preferred to avoid social activities. Over time, he lost most of his friends because he turned down most social invitations. His relationship with his girlfriend became very strained because of their arguments over whether he smelled and his reluctance to go out and do things with her. He also found it difficult to focus on his job, because he believed that his office co-workers could smell his body odor and that they talked about it and laughed at him behind his back. Eventually, his work performance suffered to the point that he was fired. Mr. Samuels said that his body odor made him feel depressed, anxious, embarrassed, ashamed, and sometimes even suicidal. He said, "When everyone is rejecting you and making fun of you because you stink, what's the point of living?"

Mr. Samuels had sought treatment from many dentists, otolaryngologists, dermatologists, and gastroenterologists. He had tried multiple prescription mouthwashes and deodorants, and gastroenterologists had prescribed probiotics, charcoal, and other treatments. None of these treatments alleviated his body odor preoccupations. Mr. Samuels eventually requested a tonsillectomy, because he thought that his tonsils might be the source of his perceived halitosis (bad breath), but the surgeon was not willing to do a tonsillectomy because he did not agree that Mr. Samuels had halitosis, although he could smell Mr. Samuels's cologne.

At his girlfriend's insistence, Mr. Samuels reluctantly agreed to see a psychiatrist, even though he was skeptical that a psychiatrist could get rid of his body odor. He was treated with fluoxetine (an antidepressant medication that also treats obsessions, compulsive behaviors, anxiety, and other symptoms), gradually reaching a dose of 80 mg a day. He also received cognitive-behavioral therapy (CBT) that focused specifically on his body odor concerns. The CBT and medication significantly decreased Mr. Samuels's body odor preoccupations, excessive repetitive behaviors, and attempts to mask the perceived odors. He was no longer certain that he smelled bad, saying "maybe I don't have bad body odor," and he no longer thought that other people were negatively reacting to his body odor or making fun of him. Mr. Samuels started participating in social activities again and saw friends he had not seen in years. He also went out to do things with his girlfriend again, and they no longer argued about whether he smelled bad. His girlfriend was thrilled with his improvement, which she described as "miraculous."

Discussion of "I Stink"

Mr. Samuels has a long-standing (12 years) belief that he emits foul odors from his breath, his armpits, and his gastrointestinal tract including his anus. These beliefs persist despite reassurance by others, including his girlfriend and family members, that he does not smell. Mr. Samuels, to the contrary, is convinced that everyone anywhere near him—friends, co-workers, strangers on the street—can smell his foul odors. He has the self-referential ideas that when anyone near him talks about "stuffiness" in a room or an unusual smell or covers their nose or opens a window that they are reacting to his bad body odors. Mr. Samuels is preoccupied with his perceived body odors and his behaviors aimed at minimizing his body odors for 8 hours a day (e.g., showering twice a day for an hour each time, brushing his teeth about ten times each day, using "gallons of mouthwash," applying excessive amounts of cologne). He has modified his diet and taken to wearing underwear that minimizes the smell from flatulence.

Some degree of self-consciousness about how one smells is within the range of normality. As is the case with most mental disorders, the diagnosis of Olfactory Reference Disorder should only be given if the preoccupation with having an odor is sufficiently severe to cause significant distress or impairment in the person's functioning. In Mr. Samuels case, he experienced extreme emotional distress, feeling depressed, anxious, embarrassed, ashamed and sometimes even suicidal. Moreover, he had dramatically curtailed his social interactions because he was convinced that others saw him negatively and was fired from work because of poor work performance related to his inability to concentrate on his job.

The persistent preoccupation with emitting offensive body odors, excessive self-consciousness about the perceived odors, repetitive behaviors checking for body odors, excessive attempts to camouflage the odors, and avoidance of social and occupational situations that increased distress about the odors all strongly support the diagnosis of Other Specified Obsessive-Compulsive and Related Disorder, Olfactory Reference Disorder, as noted in DSM-5-TR (p. 294).

20.3
Compulsive Sexual Behavior Disorder

Compulsive sexual behavior was first described by Richard von Krafft-Ebing in his 1886 classic treatise *Psychopathia Sexualis* and has since been included in one form or another, in prior editions of DSM, up to and including DSM-IV-TR. Many terms have been used to refer to such behavior, including some that are dated and pejorative (e.g., nymphomania, satyriasis) and others that are more neutral (e.g., hyperphilia, sexual addiction, hypersexuality, paraphilia-related disorder, impulsive-compulsive sexual disorder, out-of-control sexual behavior). Previous DSM editions included hypersexuality as one of the examples of the Not Otherwise Specified or Not Elsewhere Classified categories of sexual disorders, which were residual categories for sexual disturbances that did not meet criteria for any specific sexual disorder.

A "hypersexual disorder" category—characterized by an increased frequency and intensity of sexual fantasies, urges, and enacted behaviors associated with impulsivity—had been proposed for inclusion in DSM-5. However, there was substantial criticism of the proposal, the main arguments against it being that it represented a pathologizing of a normal variation (i.e., high sex drive), that there was insufficient evidence to establish the diagnostic criteria and course descriptions needed to identify these behaviors as a mental disorder, and fears that the diagnosis could be misused in forensic settings by individuals seeking to evade responsibility for sexual misconduct. Because of concerns of it being misused, "hypersexual disorder" was not included anywhere in DSM-5, not even as an example of an Other Specified Disruptive, Impulse-Control, and Conduct Disorder.

However, ICD-11 includes the category Compulsive Sexual Behavior Disorder (CSBD) in its section on Impulse Control Disorders. CSBD is characterized by a persistent pattern of failure to control intense, repetitive sexual impulses or urges, resulting in a pattern of repetitive sexual behavior. The repetitive sexual activities may become a central focus of the person's life; the person may make numerous unsuccessful attempts to control or reduce these behaviors; and the person may continue these behaviors despite adverse consequences or even despite deriving little or no satisfaction from them.[2] Men are more often affected than women, but both sexes can exhibit CSBD.

Don Juan

J.D. Strong, a 38-year-old married real estate broker, was referred by a therapist who specialized in treating individuals with "compulsive sexual behavior" for evaluation and possible treatment with medication. Mr. Strong was living with his wife but sleeping in a separate bedroom, and had two children in elementary school. His chief complaint was "I need to stop acting out!"

When asked to describe his acting-out behavior, Mr. Strong stated that he was out of control sexually, having intercourse with prostitutes, engaging in multiple affairs, and going to massage parlors where women would manually bring him to orgasm or perform oral sex on him. He reported that on a scale of 0 to 100%, he was only in 10% control of his sexual urges and behavior. He estimated that he had had sexual relations with more than 400 women. He reported that he was constantly thinking about sex, and he masturbated an average of 20 times a week. He also reported that his orgasms had become less pleasurable over time. He denied any history of alcohol or substance abuse or history of bipolar disorder.

Mr. Strong, an only child, was raised by his mother and father. He stated that he was loved as a child but that his mother was beaten by his father, who was an alcoholic. He completed college and had developed a successful real estate business. He was never sexually abused.

Asked about his earliest memories of sex, Mr. Strong stated that as a small boy he was fixated on adult women, looking under their skirts as they sat at tables. He reported that early on he had fantasies of protecting women. When he reached puberty, at the age of 13, these fantasies of protecting women be-

---

[2]World Health Organization: Compulsive sexual behaviour disorder, in Clinical descriptions and diagnostic requirements for ICD-11 mental, behavioural and neurodevelopmental disorders. Geneva, World Health Organization, 2024, pp. 526–527. Available at: https://www.who.int/publications/i/item/9789240077263. Accessed September 10, 2024.

came sexual, and he began masturbating frequently to thoughts of women and their vulnerability. He also began looking at pornography involving adult women engaging in intercourse that he found in his father's night table. He would look at pornography in the evening in his bedroom and would masturbate for hours, often staying up until early in the morning. He was shy and did not date girls in middle school or high school. He had gone to an all-boys high school and had experimented sexually with boys; however, he stated that he was heterosexual in his sexual interests.

After graduating from high school, Mr. Strong went to college in a large city away from home, where he found a way to make money buying and selling airline miles. He used this money initially to engage in phone sex, which he said became "very addictive," leading him to spend many hours a day on the phone. While in college, he began to be more social, going to clubs, meeting young women, and engaging in "one-night stands" with women whom he met at parties or in bars. He stopped using pornography because he preferred engaging in sexual activity with actual women. He also began going to prostitutes and massage parlors.

At the age of 30, Mr. Strong fell in love, married, and stopped sexually acting out. He said that at that time, his sexual life with his wife was "good." However, following the birth of their first child, his wife developed pain on intercourse, and the frequency of their sexual relations decreased dramatically. He again started acting out sexually, stopping at massage parlors on the way home from work and arranging to meet prostitutes in hotel rooms. He also said that while walking around the city, he would constantly be on the lookout for sexy women whom he would sometimes approach and successfully pick up.

Mr. Strong's wife, suspicious of the frequency of his late-night "work meetings," checked his cell phone and found various text exchanges with call girls. Shocked by this revelation, with thoughts of divorce, she insisted on couples therapy, and he promised to stop acting out sexually. He was initially successful in keeping his promise for several months, but his resolve to stop his acting-out behavior weakened, and he surreptitiously resumed having sex with prostitutes and frequenting massage parlors.

Mr. Strong reported that he desperately wanted to stop his behavior and had made many promises to himself to stop, but he could not control his behavior. It was only after his wife contracted a sexually transmitted disease from him and confronted him in couples therapy that he finally admitted that he had resumed his excessive extramarital sexual behavior. She threatened divorce again and insisted that he see a sexual addiction therapist, which he did. The therapist suggested a number of exercises, such as not looking at women on the street for more than 1 second, which decreased his arousal and impulses to approach them. He also began going to 12-step meetings for "sex addicts." He said that initially these meetings were helpful, in that he saw others who were struggling with the same issues that he was. He put into practice some of the suggestions, such as avoiding routes that would bring him in the vicinity of the massage parlors that he used to frequent.

After several months during which he was able to successfully resist the urge to go to massage parlors, Mr. Strong again resumed his previous behavior with a vengeance and started visiting massage parlors multiple times a week. Feeling like a complete failure, he became depressed and hopeless. He began seeing a psychiatrist, who prescribed sertraline, a selective serotonin reuptake inhibitor medication used to treat depression, anxiety, and obsessive-compulsive disorder, with the hope that it might be helpful for both his depression and his sexual acting-out. Although his depression improved, his ability to control his sexual behavior did not. Moreover, he reported that the sertraline made it difficult for him to ejaculate, but said that he continued to have a strong sexual drive.

At the advice of his addiction treatment therapist, he entered an inpatient sex addiction treatment program for 6 weeks in order to receive intensive therapy in a controlled environment. He initially found this therapy to be very helpful, but while in the aftercare outpatient program, he started sexually acting out yet again, saying that he "just could not control himself."

At this point, Mr. Strong was offered androgen deprivation therapy (ADT), which would decrease his testosterone to extremely low levels and also reduce his sexual interest and behavior. Following a thorough medical workup that included a baseline bone-density evaluation (because lowering testosterone levels can result in reductions in bone density), he was started on injections of triptorelin, a gonadotropin-releasing hormone agonist (GnRH) used to treat prostate cancer. After an initial flare-up of sexual arousal (related to the brief surge in testosterone that accompanies initiation of therapy with a GnRH agonist), he reported that his sexual drive and interest decreased dramatically, in parallel with a reduction in his plasma testosterone. He continued in individual therapy with his sex addiction specialist and was seen monthly for medication follow-up. He continued on this medication for a year and was delighted with its effect. "I never felt in so much control of my sexual urges!" He also reported that his continual scanning of his surroundings for attractive women and constant attempts at flirting had stopped after 2 months on the ADT.

Discussion of "Don Juan"

Mr. Strong has clearly experienced intense, repetitive sexual impulses from an early age and has equally clearly been unable to control his impulses to engage in extramarital sexual relations with a large number (estimated to be 400) of women, including many whom he barely knew. Much of his time was spent pursuing sex with attractive women he met on the street, engaging prostitutes, and frequenting massage parlors. Despite wanting to stop these behaviors, he repeatedly fell back into his familiar patterns. His behavior resulted in severe problems in his relationship with his wife that brought his marriage to the brink of divorce. Given that Mr. Strong's behavior persisted far beyond the 6 months required by ICD-11, caused significant distress, and was associated with impairment in family functioning, it would warrant the ICD-11 diagnosis of CSBD.[3] Because this diagnosis does not appear in DSM-5-TR, the corresponding DSM diagnosis (which would be needed for coding purposes) would be Other Specified Disruptive, Impulse-Control, and Conduct Disorder (DSM-5-TR, p. 541), reflecting the failure of such individuals to control their sexual impulses. Although Mr. Strong was treated with antidepressant medication in part for symptoms of depression, there is not enough information to make a Depressive Disorder diagnosis.

20.4
Internet Gaming Disorder

Video gaming has become one of the most popular and accessible leisure activities worldwide, based on which a global multibillion-dollar industry has been built up. In recent years, the gaming landscape has evolved significantly with the rise of multiplayer video games played competitively for spectators and streaming platforms fueled by constant advancements in internet-enabled portable and dedicated home gaming hardware. For the vast majority of players, recreational gaming can confer personal and social benefits, even with relatively high levels of engagement (e.g., daily use for several hours or longer). However, excessive video gaming, characterized by loss of control over gaming behavior, can have negative consequences on physical health, and can impair functioning in social, educational, and occupational domains.

The essential feature of Internet Gaming Disorder is a pattern of excessive and prolonged participation in internet gaming that results in a cluster of cognitive and behavioral symptoms, including progressive loss of control over gaming, with tolerance and withdrawal symptoms analogous to the symptoms of Substance Use Disorders. Internet-based games typically involve competition between groups of players who are often in different global regions, so that extended durations of play are facilitated by time zone independence. Internet gaming often includes a significant amount of social interaction during play, and the "team" aspects of play appear to be a key motivation. Attempts to direct the individual toward schoolwork or interpersonal activities are strongly resisted. Individuals with Internet Gaming Disorder continue to sit at a computer and engage in gaming activities despite neglect of other activities. They typically devote 8–10 hours or more per day to this activity and at least 30 hours per week. If they are prevented from using a computer and returning to the game, they

---

[3]World Health Organization: Compulsive sexual behaviour disorder, in Clinical descriptions and diagnostic requirements for ICD-11 mental, behavioural and neurodevelopmental disorders. Geneva, World Health Organization, 2024, pp. 526–527. Available at: https://www.who.int/publications/i/item/9789240077263. Accessed September 10, 2024.

become agitated and angry. They often go for long periods without food or sleep. Normal obligations (e.g., school, work) and family responsibilities are neglected.

The estimated mean 12-month prevalence of Internet Gaming Disorder is 4.7% across multiple countries, with a range of 0.7%–15.6% across studies. An international meta-analysis of 16 studies found a pooled prevalence of Internet Gaming Disorder among adolescents of 4.6%, with adolescent boys/adult men generally reporting a higher prevalence (6.8%) than adolescent girls/adult women (1.3%).

Health may be neglected because of compulsive gaming. Other diagnoses that may be associated with Internet Gaming Disorder include Major Depressive Disorder, Attention-Deficit/Hyperactivity Disorder, and Obsessive-Compulsive Disorder.

Globally Connected

Patrick Delaney, a 19-year-old college freshman, was referred for an evaluation after failing several classes during his second semester. During his first semester, he had struggled with completing assignments but ultimately passed his final examinations. During the second semester, however, Patrick's performance dramatically worsened because he stopped attending classes or completing any of the coursework. Evaluation revealed that he was spending excessive amounts of time each day playing Fortnite Battle Royale and Minecraft, which were being played among several people around the world. Because of the time zone differences, Patrick tended to play from late at night (beginning at 11 P.M. or so) until morning, averaging about 6–8 hours each day, 7 days a week. Whereas in high school he had tended to play these games for just a few hours each week, the amount of time and emotional investment in these games had increased exponentially during his first year at college. During the time he was not engaged in these games, he either slept or thought about strategies he could employ when he returned to the game.

Patrick recognized that he should be studying and attending classes, but he enjoyed these games and felt "connected" to the global friends he played with. Ironically, Patrick stopped spending time with the friends he had initially made in college, so they no longer asked him to join them in playing basketball at the college gym as he had frequently done a few months earlier. When he failed his midterms, the college counselor had suggested that Patrick stop playing the games for a while so that he could get his schoolwork back on track. He attempted to stop for a few days but reported feeling so anxious that he returned to playing the games.

Patrick's parents were also concerned about him, as they had noticed that he seemed withdrawn and preoccupied when he talked with them on the phone. He lied to them, telling them that he had so much schoolwork that he was feeling overwhelmed by the hours he had to spend on it, and that was why he seemed distracted during telephone calls. He admitted during the evaluation that he was often engaged in a game when his parents called, and he simply was not able to pay attention to them.

When asked why he played the games, Patrick reported that he really enjoyed them, that the games and the people provided a "rush" for him. He also recognized that for whatever reason, he felt really anxious if he did not play each day, which in turn made it difficult to abstain from playing. He also described getting "lost" in the world of the games and losing track of time. He would frequently tell himself that he should only play for an hour or two, and then he would realize that 8 or 10 hours had elapsed, and he had not gone to bed. Patrick reported wanting to study history and get his college degree, but he admitted being ambivalent about stopping—and unable to control—his gaming behavior.

Discussion of "Globally Connected"

Patrick's pattern of game playing on the internet shows all of the hallmarks of a behavioral addiction. The amount of time he spent playing internet games had increased from a few hours each week in high school to 6–8 hours per day, 7 days a week by the time he was a freshman in college. He was so preoccupied with his game playing that when he was not engaged in it, he either slept or would think about strategies he could employ when he returned to the game. He developed intense anxiety when he attempted to stop for a few days, akin to what happens when a person with drug dependence stops using the drug. He had difficulty controlling the amount of time he spent playing games, frequently telling himself that he would play only for 1 or 2 hours, and then emerging from a game to discover that 8 or 10 hours had elapsed and he had still not gone to bed. His school performance dramatically worsened because he simply stopped attending classes or completing any of the coursework. Thus, Patrick's diagnosis is Internet Gaming Disorder (DSM-5-TR, p. 913). Because DSM-5-TR does not offer an "other specified" category for behavioral addictions, for coding purposes one would need to employ the "Other Specified Mental Disorder" diagnosis, which applies to "presentations in which symptoms characteristic of a mental disorder that cause clinically significant distress or impairment in social, occupational, or other important areas of functioning predominate but do not meet the full criteria for any specific mental disorder" (DSM-5-TR, p. 804).

Alphabetical Index
of Case Names

*Case names are listed alphabetically along with the corresponding page number
on which each case begins.*

Alphabetical Index of Diagnoses and Related Cases

This book contains a case for each disorder in DSM-5-TR, as well as disorders in ICD-11. For many disorders, multiple illustrative cases are included. This alphabetical index of diagnoses lists those cases included in the book according to the DSM-5-TR diagnosis given, along with the corresponding page number on which each case begins. Each case name is followed by the age and sex of the patient. Additional distinguishing information about the case (e.g., applicable subtypes and specifiers, comorbid disorders, key features) is also included to help the reader differentiate among the cases included for a particular disorder. Cases are listed in the order that they appear for the corresponding diagnosis.

Index

*Page numbers printed in **boldface type** refer to tables and figures.*